# Vascular Disorders of the Liver

Dominique Valla
Juan Carlos Garcia-Pagan
Andrea De Gottardi • Pierre-Emmanuel Rautou
Editors

# Vascular Disorders of the Liver

## VALDIG's Guide to Management and Causes

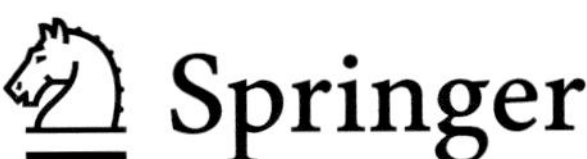

Springer

*Editors*
Dominique Valla
CRI, UMR 1149
Université de Paris and Inserm
75018 Paris, France

Service d'hépatologie
Hôpital Beaujon, APHP
92100 Clichy-la-Garenne, France

Andrea De Gottardi
Gastroenterology and Hepatology
Ente Ospedaliero Cantonale
Lugano, Switzerland

Juan Carlos Garcia-Pagan
Hospital Clinic
Hepatic Hemodynamic Lab Hospital Clinic
Barcelona, Spain

Pierre-Emmanuel Rautou
Université de Paris
Paris, France

Service d'Hépatologie
Centre de Référence des
Maladies Vasculaires du Foie
AP-HP, Hôpital Beaujon
Clichy-la-Garenne, France

Centre de recherche sur
l'inflammation Inserm
UMR 1149
Paris, France

ISBN 978-3-030-82990-2        ISBN 978-3-030-82988-9   (eBook)
https://doi.org/10.1007/978-3-030-82988-9



This Springer imprint is published by the registered company Springer Nature Switzerland AG
The registered company address is: Gewerbestrasse 11, 6330 Cham, Switzerland

# Contents

# Part I
# Vascular Disorders of the Liver and Their Management

# Chapter 1
# Role of Liver Biopsy in the Study of Vascular Disorders of the Liver

Valerie Paradis and Pierre-Emmanuel Rautou

## Introduction

Vascular liver disorders (VLD) encompass a wide spectrum of clinico-pathological entities resulting from damage to the hepatic vascular system, that includes hepatic arteries, portal and hepatic veins, sinusoids, and lymphatics. Among them, the vascular structures most often damaged at liver biopsy examination include portal and hepatic veins, as well as sinusoids.

According to the type of vascular structure involved, specific morphological criteria are recognized, and histological analysis may thus be contributive in the management of patients [1]. In addition to identifying elementary morphological features suggestive of vascular disorders, the analysis of liver biopsy will also assess the extent of changes and their chronicity through the evaluation of fibrosis and architectural distortion. Nevertheless, as for other liver diseases, interpretation of liver histology (i.e. liver biopsy) should be integrated into a multidisciplinary approach including pathologists, clinicians and radiologists.

Recent advances have been made in the description of liver pathological changes associated with portal hypertension in the absence of portal vein thrombosis and cirrhosis, the entity previously recognized as "idiopathic non-cirrhotic portal

V. Paradis
Pathology Department, Beaujon Hospital, Clichy, France

Université de Paris, INSERM UMR 1149, Paris, France

DHU Unity, Clichy, France
e-mail: valerie.paradis@aphp.fr

P.-E. Rautou (✉)
Université de Paris, INSERM UMR 1149, Paris, France

DHU Unity, Clichy, France

Hepatology Department, Beaujon Hospital, Clichy, France
e-mail: pierre-emmanuel.rautou@inserm.fr

© Springer Nature Switzerland AG 2022
D. Valla et al. (eds.), *Vascular Disorders of the Liver*,
https://doi.org/10.1007/978-3-030-82988-9_1

hypertension", for which the denomination "porto-sinusoidal vascular disease" has been recently proposed [2, 3].

This chapter describes the main morphological features observed in VLD, as well as the different patterns associated with each VLD. Indications of liver biopsy will be also recapitulated.

## Pathological Analysis of Liver Biopsy

The histological assessment of liver biopsy for the study of vascular disorders is based on the analysis of serial sections to ensure adequate examination, taking into account potential sampling variability. In addition to standard hematoxylin and eosin staining, which can elucidate most histological features, red Sirius or trichrome for connective tissue staining, and Perls for iron identification are performed. Reticulin staining provides a more accurate evaluation of hepatic architecture than the former, which is most helpful to highlight regenerative processes in a context of vascular disorders.

The interpretation of liver biopsy is based, as in other liver diseases, on a systematic analysis of the different morphological structures of the liver, with a specific attention to centrilobular and portal veins, and sinusoids. As for other chronic liver diseases, morphological lesions in VLD may not be evenly distributed and may vary in their severity, thus challenging the reliability of biopsy. Accordingly, while no specific study has been carried out in the specific context of VLD, a 25-mm biopsy is considered an optimal size for accurate pathological evaluation [4]. Nevertheless, a 15-mm length with at least 10 portal tracts is commonly sufficient [4, 5].

Liver biopsy may be obtained through various routes (transvenous, percutaneous or laparoscopic). Each of them has advantages and limitations. However, in addition to providing access to liver tissue, the transjugular route provides additional information with the measurement of hepatic venous pressure gradient and the identification of hepatic vein to vein communication potentially helpful for diagnosis in patients with VLD [6].

## Elementary Morphological Features of Vascular Liver Disorders

Elementary features associated with VLD are various and may affect portal tracts, centrilobular veins, and sinusoidal spaces. Of note, several terms have been used to describe a same feature, contributing to significant confusion in the literature. Accordingly, in the setting of idiopathic non-cirrhotic portal hypertension (INCPH), an effort has been recently made to propose a standardized nomenclature to homogenize the different terms related to the portal/periportal vascular changes [2].

Although it is reasonable to consider that some of the elementary features are involved in the clinical manifestations (e.g. portal vein loss) it has to be stressed that almost each of them may be observed in patients with chronic liver diseases of different origins, outside the VLD setting. For instance, sinusoidal dilatation may appear as nonspecific, resulting from impaired portal venous blood inflow or severe systemic inflammation syndrome [7].

The terminology and morphological description of the main elementary features described in VLD are detailed in Table 1.1. Of note, in normal liver, most portal tracts contain the classical triad composed of a portal vein, a hepatic artery and a bile duct, the two latter of similar caliber while portal vein being around three times greater in diameter [8].

## Pathological Diagnosis of Vascular Liver Diseases

### *Budd-Chiari Syndrome*

Budd-Chiari syndrome (BCS), or hepatic venous outflow obstruction, is defined as hepatic venous outflow obstruction at any level between small intrahepatic veins and right atrium, excluding sinusoidal obstruction syndrome. BCS is usually diagnosed using imaging procedures. Liver biopsy is restricted to diagnostic uncertainties. When liver biopsy is performed, it shows centrilobular sinusoidal dilatation and congestion (Fig.1.1a, c). Centrilobular thrombi may be seen associated with centrilobular perisinusoidal fibrosis during chronic evolution that may progress towards the development of fibrous septa between adjacent centrilobular areas leading to a

**Table 1.1** Nomenclature and description of morphological features of vascular structures

| Vascular structures | Elementary features | Description |
| --- | --- | --- |
| Portal tracts | • Portal vein stenosis<br>• Herniated portal vein<br>• Hypervascularized PT<br>• Periportal abnormal vessels | Incomplete or complete obliteration of portal vein ± wall thickening<br>A portal vein abutting periportal parenchyma<br>Multiple thin-walled vascular spaces in PT<br>Single or multiple thin-walled vessels at the interface of PT and liver parenchyma |
| Centrilobular veins | • Intimal fibrosis<br>• Obstruction<br>• Thickening of vascular wall | Presence of extracellular matrix within the inner part of the wall<br>Fibrous obliteration of centrilobular vein<br>Fibrous enlargement of the wall |
| Sinusoids | • Dilatation<br>• Congestion<br>• Fibrosis<br>• Peliosis | Sinusoidal lumen >1 liver cell plate wide<br>Presence of red blood cells within sinusoids<br>Sinusoidal walls enlarged by extracellular matrix<br>Cystically dilated spaces lined by hepatocytes and filled with blood cells |

PT (Portal tract)

"reverse nodularity" with hepatocellular nodules centered by portal tracts (Fig. 1.1b). Secondarily, in some cases, portal tracts may be affected and fibrotic. However, all these features are not specific for BCS, being encountered in heart failure, constrictive pericarditis, and to a lesser extent in sinusoidal obstruction syndrome [9].

## *Sinusoidal Obstruction Syndrome*

Sinusoidal obstruction syndrome, also known as veno-occlusive disease (VOD), associates prominent sinusoidal dilatation, congestion and haemorrhage that potentially lead to atrophy or necrosis of hepatocellular plates, with subintimal oedema affecting the sinusoids and the centrilobular vein. Over time, sinusoidal fibrosis in zone 3 and fibrous obliteration of small hepatic venules may be seen (Fig. 1.1d). While SOS is described in well-known settings, including exposure to toxic agents of liver sinusoidal endothelial cells (typically pyrrolizidine alkaloids or oxaliplatin) and conditioning for hematopoietic stem cell transplantation, the lesions are not specific. In the context of chemotherapy-associated liver injury (CALI), a

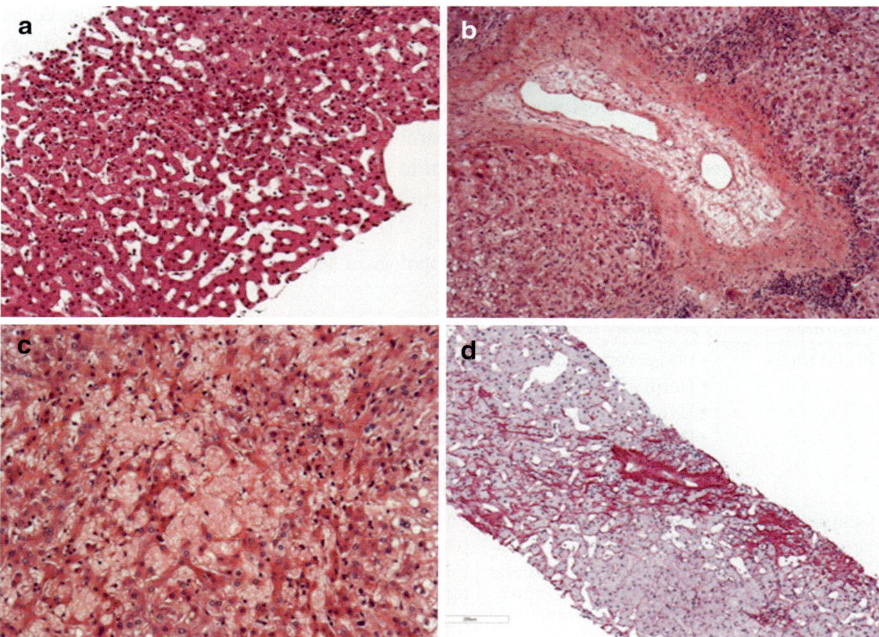

**Fig. 1.1** Centrilobular morphological elementary features. (**a**) Sinusoidal dilatation (Haematoxylin and eosin); (**b**) Fibrous obliteration of a large centrilobular vein (Haematoxylin and eosin); (**c**) Sinusoidal dilatation and congestion leading to cell plate atrophy (Haematoxylin and eosin); (**d**) Fibrous thickening of centrilobular vein associated with perisinusoidal fibrosis (red Sirius). VCL (centrilobular vein)

semi-quantitative scoring system to grade the intensity of lesions has been proposed according to the extent in lobular area according to a 4-grade scale [10].


## *Sinusoidal Dilatation and Peliosis Hepatitis*

Sinusoidal dilatation is defined by a sinusoidal lumen more than one liver cell plate wide, observed in several lobules. It is recognized as a nonspecific feature of impaired portal venous blood inflow, whatever its origin, or can be described in the context of severe systemic inflammatory reaction syndrome [7, 11]. Except in the presence of a "mosaic enhancement pattern" observed at CT or MR imaging after vascular enhancement, a diagnosis of sinusoidal dilatation may only be reached by liver biopsy [12]. The changes are usually observed in centrilobular areas.

By contrast to sinusoidal dilatation where the sinusoidal walls are intact, in peliosis, sinusoidal walls are focally ruptured leading to the random development within the lobule of cystically dilated spaces lined by hepatocytes and filled with blood cells [11]. Conditions associated with peliosis are various, ranging from infectious diseases (e.g. tuberculosis, HIV infection), hematological disorders (e.g. hairy cell leukemia, Hodgkin disease), and toxic injuries related to various agents (e.g. immunosuppressive agents, anabolic steroids, oestrogens).


## *Porto-sinusoidal Vascular Disease*

The entity denominated "porto-sinusoidal vascular disease" (PSVD) has been recently introduced to include various pathologic entities called hepatoportal sclerosis, incomplete septal cirrhosis, non-cirrhotic portal fibrosis obliterative venopathy, and nodular regenerative hyperplasia, and also clinical entities named idiopathic non-cirrhotic portal hypertension (INCPH) [3, 13–15]. Importantly, PSVD can be present in the absence of portal hypertension [16].

The definition of PVSD includes the absence of cirrhosis, the presence of histological lesions suggestive of this disease with or without portal hypertension [3]. Histological diagnosis is based on morphological features initially described as obliterative portal venopathy, nodular regenerative hyperplasia, and incomplete septal cirrhosis [17–19]. Morphologically, the most characteristic elementary features affect the portal and periportal areas. Definition and new nomenclature of these specific changes have been recently proposed in order to improve recognition and allow a better understanding on the pathophysiology of the disease [2]. Accordingly, they include portal stenosis (term recommended instead of phlebosclerosis), herniated portal vein (term recommended instead of aberrant vessel), hypervascularised portal tract (term recommended instead of angiomatosis transformation), and periportal abnormal vessels (term recommended instead of paraportal shunting) (Fig. 1.2). Table 1.1 recapitulates the main elementary morphological features with their recommended terminology. These features may be associated with fibrous changes, characterized by the presence of incomplete, thin, perforated, and poorly cellular septa surrounding hepatocellular nodules without complete nodulation, recapitulating the morphological picture of incomplete septal cirrhosis.

Nodular regenerative hyperplasia (NRH) also belongs to the spectrum of the pathological changes of PSVD, resulting from a diffuse hyperplastic response of the liver parenchyma to vascular injury. It corresponds to a micronodular transformation of the liver with minimal or no parenchymal fibrosis [20, 21]. Macroscopically, NRH may be restricted to a part of the liver or affect the whole organ. Microscopically, numerous small nodules are observed, occasionally centered by portal tracts, throughout the liver without any associated fibrosis. On liver biopsy, the nodules are characterized by thickened cell plates in the center and thinned compressed cell plates, usually associated with sinusoidal dilatation at the periphery (Fig. 1.3). Although such features are much better highlighted on reticulin staining, the histological diagnosis of NRH remains challenging, especially for pathologists with limited experience in liver diseases [15].

The cardinal morphologic feature of PSVD is the absence of cirrhosis. Accordingly, the adequacy of the liver biopsy is a main issue. Although no specific studies have been designed to address such issue, a biopsy specimen at least a 20-mm in length with a minimum of 10 portal tracts is recommended [3]. As for other liver diseases, such cut-offs may appear arbitrary. Indeed, it is conceivable that the minimal prerequisites (length and number of portal tracts) should differ according to the extent and severity of the disease. Thus, the biopsy can be considered adequate for interpretation and accurate for diagnosis by the pathologist even though the length

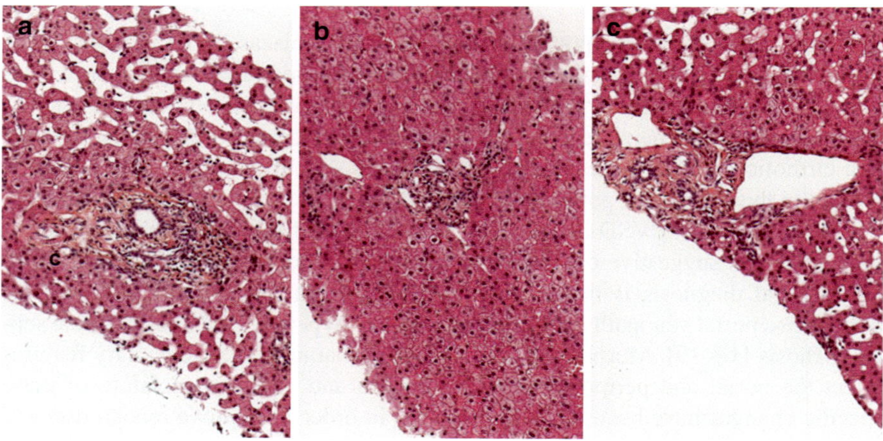

**Fig. 1.2** Portal morphological elementary features. (**a**) Portal vein narrowing (diameter smaller than interlobular bile duct), note the presence of sinusoidal dilatation (Haematoxylin and eosin); (**b**) Abnormal periportal vessels of small caliber with thin walls in a portal tract without patent portal vein (Haematoxylin and eosin); (**c**) Abnormal herniated portal vessels with increased number of arteries (haematoxylin and eosin)

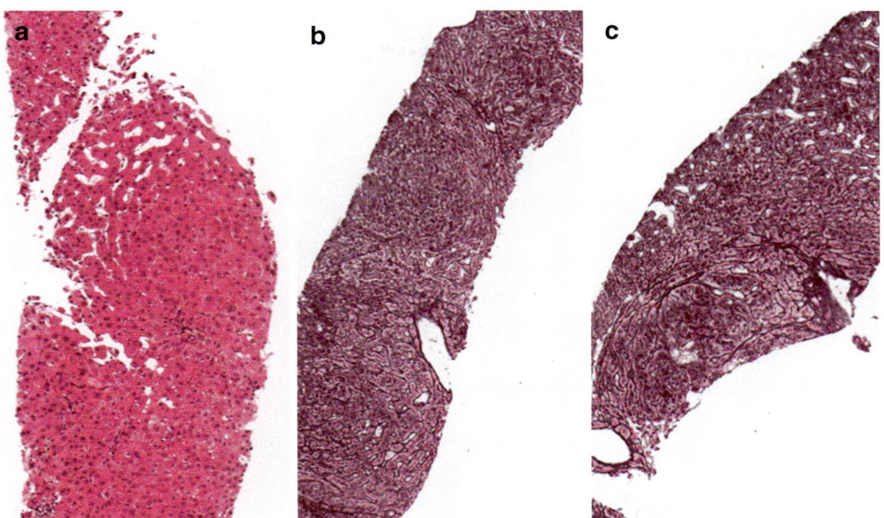

**Fig. 1.3** Regenerative nodular hyperplasia. (**a**, **b**) Low magnification showing several hepatocellular nodules limited by thinned compressed cell plates without extensive fibrosis (**a**, Haematoxylin and eosin; **b**, reticulin); (**c**) At higher magnification hepatocellular nodule surrounded by thin plates and sinusoidal dilatation (reticulin)

biopsy is less than 20 mm and less than 10 portal tracts are included. This is of particular importance since the diagnosis of PSVD can be diagnosed in the absence of portal hypertension, and then relies mostly on liver biopsy [22]. Such a situation may account for around 20% of patients with "cryptogenic" liver disease [22, 16].

In addition to focusing on the morphological lesions suggestive of PVSD, the examination of the biopsy must pay attention to changes possibly related to other chronic liver diseases as they can co-exist with patients with PVSD. Importantly, PVSD changes have been increasingly recognized in patients with HIV and hematological disorders [23, 24].

## Hepatocellular Nodules in VLD

Hepatocellular nodules may develop in the context of VLD, mostly resulting from the imbalance of portal and arterial blood blow. By contrast to other chronic liver diseases, hepatocellular nodules in VLD are usually benign proliferations, corresponding most commonly to focal nodular hyperplasia, but also to hepatocellular adenomas [25, 26] (Fig. 1.4). The incidence of hepatocellular carcinoma varies among vascular liver diseases: in patients with BCS, the incidence of hepatocellular carcinoma is similar to cirrhosis, while it is rare in patients with PSVD or portal vein thrombosis. Chapter 15 is dedicated to the description of hepatocellular

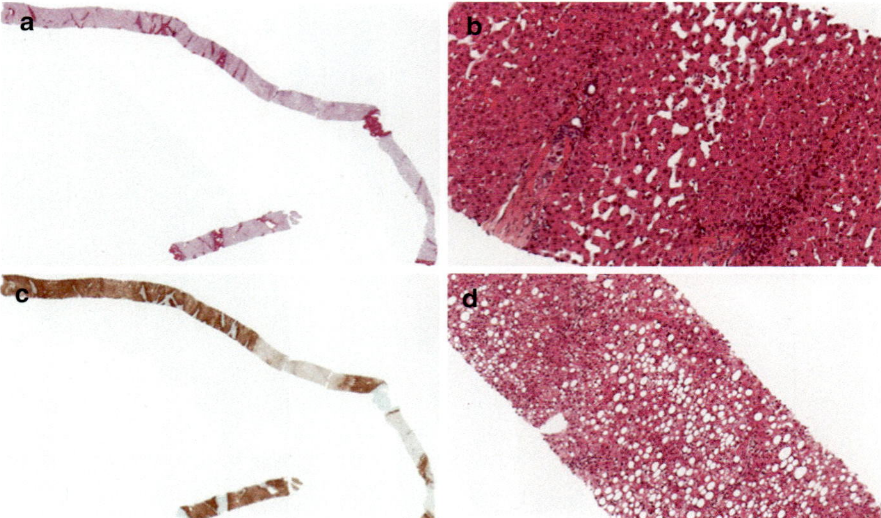

**Fig. 1.4** Hepatocellular adenoma (HCA) developed in porto-sinusoidal vascular disease. (**a–b**) Low magnification of liver biopsy of non tumoral liver (NTL) and nodule: (**a**) NTL showing several portal fibrous septa irregularly distributed and hepatocellular adenomas in two areas (encircled) (red sirius); (**b**) Higher magnification of NTL showing incomplete portal tract without patent portal vein and sinusoidal dilatation (Haematoxylin and eosin); (**c**) LFABP immunostaining showing the normal positivity in NTL contrasting with loss of expression in the nodule; (**d**) Higher magnification of the nodule showing well-differentiated proliferation of steatotic hepatocytes (Haematoxylin and eosin)

nodules. As a definitive diagnosis by imaging alone is difficult, biopsy of both the nodule and the non tumoral liver is frequently required.

# Indications of Liver Biopsy in Vascular Liver Diseases

Liver biopsy is still considered the "gold standard" for accurate diagnosis of liver diseases related to various origins as it provides "at a glance" a complete picture of the morphological lesions allowing to grade (based on activity) and stage (based on fibrosis) the disease. In the context of VLD, in addition to exclude advanced fibrosis or cirrhosis and any possible cause of chronic liver disease, liver biopsy is helpful for (1) the recognition of VLD, (2) the evaluation of the extent of lesions, and (3) the characterization of liver nodules if present. Nevertheless, given the random distribution of pathological features in most of types of VLD, a liver biopsy of sufficient length may show normal liver or subtle changes.

Indications of liver biopsy in VLD are listed in Table 1.2. Generally, in BCS liver biopsy is not indicated if evidence for hepatic venous outflow has been obtained by noninvasive imaging [27]. In portal vein thrombosis, liver biopsy is useful to

**Table 1.2** Indications of liver biopsy in vascular disorders of the liver

| Clinical presentation | Portal and hepatic veins |
| --- | --- |
| Any unexplained liver blood tests abnormalities | Patent |
| Contrast between signs of portal hypertension and absence of liver insufficiency (normal or slightly impaired serum bilirubin or prothrombin time) | |
| Contrast between signs of portal hypertension and low liver stiffness | |
| Elevated liver stiffness or unexplained liver blood test abnormalities or dysmorphic liver | Recent portal vein thrombosis |
| Liver nodule | Patent or portal vein thrombosis or hepatic vein thrombosis |
| Jaundice and/or ascites and/or liver blood test abnormalities following hematopoietic stem cell transplantation | Patent |

identify an underlying liver disease including cirrhosis or PSVD, when liver blood tests, liver stiffness or liver morphology are abnormal. Liver biopsy is required for the diagnosis of SOS even though some diagnostic features, such as fibrous obliteration of small hepatic venules, may be missed. Similarly, liver biopsy is an essential tool for the diagnosis of PSVD as no definite noninvasive tests are currently available. In addition of confirming the absence of cirrhosis, the liver biopsy may show at least one histological feature considered specific or not specific of PSVD depending on the presence of signs or portal hypertension [3]. While biopsy is mandatory for this diagnosis, it should be emphasized that PSVD may be difficult to establish as the morphological changes may be missed given the sampling variability and the uneven distribution of lesions.

# References


1. European Association for the Study of the Liver. Electronic address: easloffice@easloffice.eu. EASL Clinical Practice Guidelines: Vascular diseases of the liver. J Hepatol 2016;64:179–202. doi:https://doi.org/10.1016/j.jhep.2015.07.040.
2. Guido M, Alves VAF, Balabaud C, Bathal PS, Bioulac-Sage P, Colombari R, et al. Histology of portal vascular changes associated with idiopathic non-cirrhotic portal hypertension: nomenclature and definition. Histopathology. 2019;74:219–26. https://doi.org/10.1111/his.13738.
3. De Gottardi A, Rautou P-E, Schouten J, Rubbia-Brandt L, Leebeek F, Trebicka J, et al. Porto-sinusoidal vascular disease: proposal and description of a novel entity. Lancet Gastroenterol Hepatol. 2019;4:399–411. https://doi.org/10.1016/S2468-1253(19)30047-0.
4. Bedossa P, Dargère D, Paradis V. Sampling variability of liver fibrosis in chronic hepatitis C. Hepatol Baltim Md. 2003;38:1449–57. https://doi.org/10.1016/j.hep.2003.09.022.
5. Guido M, Rugge M. Liver fibrosis: natural history may be affected by the biopsy sample. Gut. 2004;53:1878. author reply 1878
6. Seijo S, Reverter E, Miquel R, Berzigotti A, Abraldes JG, Bosch J, et al. Role of hepatic vein catheterisation and transient elastography in the diagnosis of idiopathic portal hypertension.

Dig Liver Dis Off J Ital Soc Gastroenterol Ital Assoc Study Liver. 2012;44:855–60. https://doi.org/10.1016/j.dld.2012.05.005.

7. Saadoun D, Cazals-Hatem D, Denninger M-H, Boudaoud L, Pham B-N, Mallet V, et al. Association of idiopathic hepatic sinusoidal dilatation with the immunological features of the antiphospholipid syndrome. Gut. 2004;53:1516–9. https://doi.org/10.1136/gut.2003.037135.

8. Crawford AR, Lin XZ, Crawford JM. The normal adult human liver biopsy: a quantitative reference standard. Hepatol Baltim Md. 1998;28:323–31. https://doi.org/10.1002/hep.510280206.

9. Cazals-Hatem D, Vilgrain V, Genin P, Denninger M-H, Durand F, Belghiti J, et al. Arterial and portal circulation and parenchymal changes in Budd-Chiari syndrome: a study in 17 explanted livers. Hepatol Baltim Md. 2003;37:510–9. https://doi.org/10.1053/jhep.2003.50076.

10. Rubbia-Brandt L, Audard V, Sartoretti P, Roth AD, Brezault C, Le Charpentier M, et al. Severe hepatic sinusoidal obstruction associated with oxaliplatin-based chemotherapy in patients with metastatic colorectal cancer. Ann Oncol Off J Eur Soc Med Oncol. 2004;15:460–6.

11. Marzano C, Cazals-Hatem D, Rautou P-E, Valla D-C. The significance of nonobstructive sinusoidal dilatation of the liver: impaired portal perfusion or inflammatory reaction syndrome. Hepatol Baltim Md. 2015;62:956–63. https://doi.org/10.1002/hep.27747.

12. Ronot M, Kerbaol A, Rautou P-E, Brancatelli G, Bedossa P, Cazals-Hatem D, et al. Acute extrahepatic infectious or inflammatory diseases are a cause of transient mosaic pattern on CT and MR imaging related to sinusoidal dilatation of the liver. Eur Radiol. 2016;26:3094–101. https://doi.org/10.1007/s00330-015-4124-2.

13. Plessier A, Rautou P-E, Valla D-C. Management of hepatic vascular diseases. J Hepatol. 2012;56(Suppl 1):S25–38. https://doi.org/10.1016/S0168-8278(12)60004-X.

14. Nayak NC, Jain D, Saigal S, Soin AS. Non-cirrhotic portal fibrosis: one disease with many names? An analysis from morphological study of native explant livers with end stage chronic liver disease. J Clin Pathol. 2011;64:592–8. https://doi.org/10.1136/jcp.2010.087395.

15. Schouten JNL, Garcia-Pagan JC, Valla DC, Janssen HLA. Idiopathic noncirrhotic portal hypertension. Hepatol Baltim Md. 2011;54:1071–81. https://doi.org/10.1002/hep.24422.

16. Guido M, Sarcognato S, Sonzogni A, Lucà MG, Senzolo M, Fagiuoli S, et al. Obliterative portal venopathy without portal hypertension: an underestimated condition. Liver Int Off J Int Assoc Study Liver. 2016;36:454–60. https://doi.org/10.1111/liv.12936.

17. Nayak NC, Ramalingaswami V. Obliterative portal venopathy of the liver. Associated with so-called idiopathic portal hypertension or tropical splenomegaly. Arch Pathol. 1969;87:359–69.

18. Mikkelsen WP, Edmondson HA, Peters RL, Redeker AG, Reynolds TB. Extra- and intrahepatic portal hypertension without cirrhosis (hepatoportal sclerosis). Ann Surg. 1965;162:602–20.

19. Hillaire S, Bonte E, Denninger M-H, Casadevall N, Cadranel J-F, Lebrec D, et al. Idiopathic non-cirrhotic intrahepatic portal hypertension in the West: a re-evaluation in 28 patients. Gut. 2002;51:275–80. https://doi.org/10.1136/gut.51.2.275.

20. Steiner PE. Nodular regenerative hyperplasia of the liver. Am J Pathol. 1959;35:943–53.

21. Wanless IR. Micronodular transformation (nodular regenerative hyperplasia) of the liver: a report of 64 cases among 2,500 autopsies and a new classification of benign hepatocellular nodules. Hepatol Baltim Md. 1990;11:787–97.

22. Cazals-Hatem D, Hillaire S, Rudler M, Plessier A, Paradis V, Condat B, et al. Obliterative portal venopathy: portal hypertension is not always present at diagnosis. J Hepatol. 2011;54:455–61. https://doi.org/10.1016/j.jhep.2010.07.038.

23. Chang P-E, Miquel R, Blanco J-L, Laguno M, Bruguera M, Abraldes J-G, et al. Idiopathic portal hypertension in patients with HIV infection treated with highly active antiretroviral therapy. Am J Gastroenterol. 2009;104:1707–14. https://doi.org/10.1038/ajg.2009.165.

24. Krasinskas AM, Eghtesad B, Kamath PS, Demetris AJ, Abraham SC. Liver transplantation for severe intrahepatic noncirrhotic portal hypertension. Liver Transplant Off Publ Am Assoc Study Liver Dis Int Liver Transplant Soc. 2005;11:627–34.; discussion 610-611. https://doi.org/10.1002/lt.20431.

25. Sempoux C, Paradis V, Komuta M, Wee A, Calderaro J, Balabaud C, et al. Hepatocellular nodules expressing markers of hepatocellular adenomas in Budd-Chiari syndrome and

other rare hepatic vascular disorders. J Hepatol. 2015;63:1173–80. https://doi.org/10.1016/j.jhep.2015.06.017.
26. Sempoux C, Balabaud C, Paradis V, Bioulac-Sage P. Hepatocellular nodules in vascular liver diseases. Virchows Arch Int J Pathol. 2018;473:33–44. https://doi.org/10.1007/s00428-018-2373-6.
27. Valla D-C, Cazals-Hatem D. Vascular liver diseases on the clinical side: definitions and diagnosis, new concepts. Virchows Arch Int J Pathol. 2018;473:3–13. https://doi.org/10.1007/s00428-018-2331-3.

# Chapter 2
# Role of Imaging in the Study of Vascular Disorders of the Liver

Valérie Vilgrain, Pierre-Emmanuel Rautou, Maxime Ronot,
and Dominique Valla

## Introduction

It is quite a challenge to explain the role of imaging in vascular disorders of the liver in one chapter as these diseases are multiple, with various causes and consequences. Attention has been paid to define the role of imaging for diagnosing, staging, and evaluating complications as well as explaining the role of Doppler ultrasound often used as first-line examination and CT or MRI.

## Anatomy and Microcirculation

The liver has a rich blood supply that is quite unique. Approximately 20%–25% of the cardiac output goes through the liver. It has a dual blood supply and receives roughly 25% of its blood from the hepatic artery (oxygen-rich blood at high pressure) and the remaining 75% from the portal vein (nutrient-rich blood at low pressure). There is no hepatic capillary network per se and both arterial and portal blood mix in fenestrated sinusoids. These two afferent vascular systems interconnect through trans-sinusoidal and transvasal communications as well as the peribiliary plexuses. From the sinusoids, blood flows into the central veins that drain in the hepatic veins and then in the inferior vena cava. The blood volume in the sinusoids is larger than that in the main vessels [1].

V. Vilgrain (✉) · M. Ronot
Departement of Radiology, Hôpital Beaujon, APHP, Paris, France
e-mail: valerie.vilgrain@aphp.fr; maxime.ronot@aphp.fr

P.-E. Rautou · D. Valla
Departement of Hepatology, Hôpital Beaujon, APHP, Paris, France
e-mail: pierre-emmanuel.rautou@aphp.fr; dominique.valla@aphp.fr

© Springer Nature Switzerland AG 2022
D. Valla et al. (eds.), *Vascular Disorders of the Liver*,
https://doi.org/10.1007/978-3-030-82988-9_2

Liver vasculature is characterized by changes and adaptive mechanisms. The most common are the following ones:

- there is an arterioportal balance called the 'hepatic buffer response' characterized by a compensatory increase in arterial blood flow when portal supply decreases [2].
- An arterial supply decrease is not associated with a compensatory increase in portal blood flow, but induces development of arterial collaterals either from other hepatic branches or extrahepatic arteries.
- The development and progression of liver fibrosis to cirrhosis is associated with micro-architectural vascular changes and modified perfusion: sinusoids gradually convert into continuous non-fenestrated capillaries with an organized basal membrane containing laminin, an increase in vascular resistance and a decrease in portal perfusion, partly compensated by an increase in arterial perfusion and later by an overall decrease in global hepatic perfusion.
- The dual blood inflow explains why liver infarction is very uncommon requiring impairment in both hepatic and portal venous flow.

Besides the hepatic arterial and the portal venous supply, small areas of the liver may be supplied by another venous system (called "third inflow") that is composed of aberrant veins or normal veins that enter directly in the liver independently from the portal venous system. Most of these veins are the right gastric vein, the posterior duodenopancreatic arcade, the veins of Sappey, and or the vein of Burow. These veins can communicate with intrahepatic portal branches focally decreasing portal venous perfusion and therefore can be responsible for pseudolesions. These pseudolesions are usually seen around the gallbladder fossa, around the falciform ligament, close to the hilum mostly in segment 4, segment 1, and the left liver lobe [3]. Some of these lesions are fatty (focal fatty steatosis) or present with focal fatty sparing related to differences in the portal venous inflow [4].

## Imaging Modalities

Three imaging modalities are essential to diagnose vascular liver diseases: ultrasound (US), multiphasic CT and MRI.

Doppler US is usually the first-line modality for evaluating flow in liver vessels. It allows vessel exploration using B mode image to detect any abnormal hyperechogenicity that would be associated to clotting or tumoral obstruction and flow analysis. Interestingly, each major vessel's waveform is characteristic of the vascular system, sometimes referred to as its "signature" appearance. The normal hepatic arterial waveform is pulsatile, antegrade throughout the entire cardiac cycle with low resistive index. The hepatic venous waveform is triphasic alternating antegrade-retrograde flow, which is related to the cardiac cycle. While the majority of hepatic venous blood flow is antegrade to get back to the heart, retrograde reflux is seen during the atrial contraction. This flow pulsatility is reduced or absent with significant liver fibrosis or cirrhosis since the fibrotic parenchyma compresses the veins. The portal venous flow is antegrade (also called hepatopetal), gently undulated with low mean velocity [5].

In advanced chronic liver diseases, portal venous flow can be retrograde (hepatofugal). Doppler US has many advantages. It is part of the routine liver US examinations. It allows assessing flow direction easily. Yet, exploration of the extrahepatic portal venous system can be difficult and parenchymal liver consequences cannot be seen. The latter can be partially overcome by contrast-enhanced US.

Multiphasic CT is a highly suitable technique for vascular liver diseases. CT protocol should include at least two-phase (arterial and portal venous phase) evaluation of liver parenchyma. On hepatic arterial phase, (20–30 s after the initiation of IV contrast material administration), aorta and hepatic arteries are enhanced while the liver shows minimal enhancement. On portal venous phase (60–80 s after the initiation of IV contrast material administration), the portal vein is strongly enhanced as well as the liver. Contrast material reaches hepatic veins. This multiphasic evaluation allows detecting transient hepatic parenchymal enhancement, which helps identifying vascular anomalies. Hence, multiphasic CT is crucial in vascular liver diseases because it does not only show vessel patency but can also demonstrate alterations in the dynamics of hepatic blood flow [6].

MRI is a multiparametric imaging modality and there are several techniques that are useful to analyse liver vasculature [7]. The classical one is multiphasic contrast-enhanced MRI that acts as multiphasic CT analyzing both vessels and liver enhancement. By using serial, high temporal resolution acquisition MRI can go beyond qualitative evaluation of contrast behaviour and quantify liver perfusion. Another technique is phase-contrast MRI sequences, which is routinely used in cardiovascular and brain. It can assess hepatic flow velocity with high spatial resolution. While these techniques can be implemented easily for portal venous hemodynamics, they are more challenging in smaller vessels such as hepatic arteries. Compared to CT, MRI has advantages because it can show vessel patency on unenhanced sequences (white-blood sequences or black-blood sequences) but the spatial resolution is inferior to CT. Except for flow quantification, MRI is mostly performed in patients with impaired renal function.

## Focal Vascular Anomalies of the Liver

Focal liver lesions or pseudolesions related to anomalies of liver vasculature can be divided in two patterns: those that exhibit transient hepatic parenchymal enhancement and those that do not.

## *Transient Hepatic Parenchymal Enhancement*

Hyperenhancing pseudotumors on hepatic arterial phase may be misdiagnosed as true tumors and therefore should be recognized.

### Hepatic Arterioportal Shunts

Hepatic arterioportal shunts are communications between the hepatic artery and the portal venous system at different levels: transinusoidal, transvasal, or transtumoral and may be due to various causes, most commonly cirrhosis, tumors, inflammation, and trauma including liver biopsy [8]. Occlusion of the small hepatic venules and retrograde filling of portal flow by arterioportal anastomosis is the suggested mechanism of hepatic arterioportal shunts in cirrhosis. Arterioportal shunts are seen as a transient increase in enhancement of the parenchyma during the arterial phase on contrast-enhanced CT or MR images with early enhancement of the corresponding portal vein branch (Fig. 2.1). Certain imaging features are highly suggestive of hepatic arterioportal shunts. First, increased hepatic parenchymal enhancement predominates on the periphery of the liver and is usually small and wedge-shaped with a straight margin corresponding to lobar, segmental, or subsegmental landmarks. Second, the altered parenchyma returns to normal or nearly normal during the portal venous and delayed phases, which is different from liver tumors and hepatocellular carcinoma in particular. Third, there is usually no focal abnormal signal intensity in the region of hyperenhancement on unenhanced T1- and T2-weighted MR images. Recognition of wedge-shaped enhancement is not always easy on axial CT or MR images and multiplanar reconstruction images are helpful. However, hepatic arterioportal shunts may also be atypical with nodular enhancement and slightly hyperintense T2-weighted images [9, 10]. In difficult cases, gadoxetic acid–enhanced hepatocyte-phase MR imaging can help confirm the diagnosis of hepatic arterioportal shunts. Very few (5%–15%) are hypointense during the hepatocyte phase, and in these cases, the level of signal intensity is not as low as hepatocellular carcinoma [11, 12].

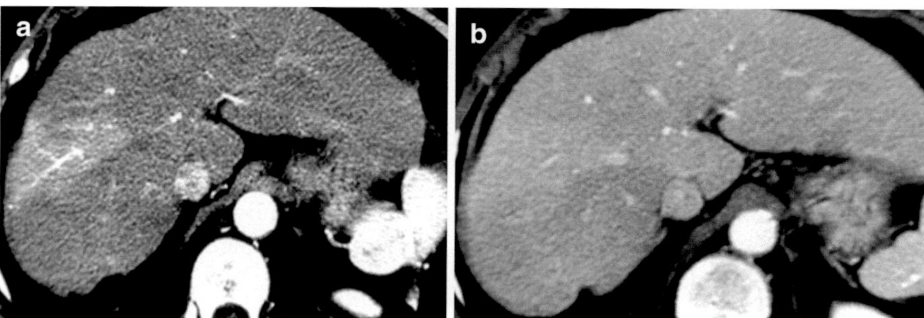

**Fig. 2.1** Arterioportal shunt. On contrast-enhanced CT the shunt appears as a transient increase in enhancement of the parenchyma during the arterial phase (**a**) and enhances as the adjacent liver on portal venous phase (**b**). Note the early enhancement of the corresponding portal vein branch on (**a**)

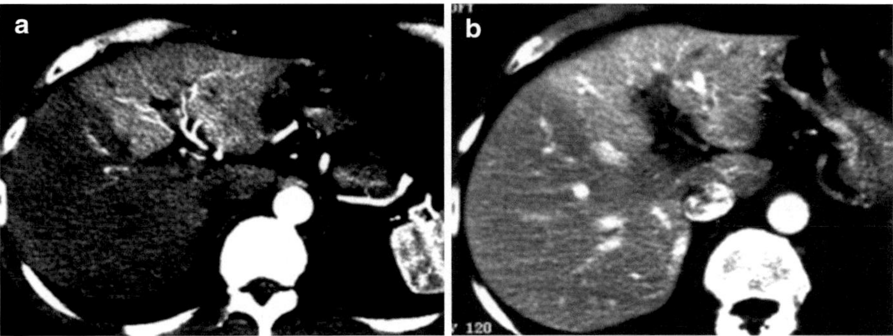

**Fig. 2.2** Obstruction of the left portal branch. On contrast-enhanced CT there is a hyperenhancement of the corresponding territory of hepatic parenchyma during the arterial phase (**a**). Conversely to hepatic arterioportal shunts, the portal vein branch does not enhance on portal venous phase (**b**)

## Subsegmental, Segmental or Lobar Portal Venous Thrombosis

Intrahepatic portal venous thrombosis is also associated with a transient increase in enhancement of the corresponding territory of hepatic parenchyma during the arterial phase on contrast-enhanced CT or MR images. Conversely to hepatic arterioportal shunts, the portal vein branch within the hyperenhancement does not enhance and appears a linear hypoattenuation on portal venous phase (Fig. 2.2). On acute phase (up to 1 month after venous obstruction), clotting can be hyperattenuating on unenhanced CT. Features suggesting intraluminal venous invasion (mostly seen in hepatocellular carcinoma) are marked enlargement of the obstructed vein, enhancement of the obstructed vein on hepatic arterial phase, and hypersignal on diffusion-weighted MRI [13].

Any cause of portal venous compression may cause transient increase in enhancement of the liver. For instance, marked dilatation of intrahepatic bile ducts can compress intrahepatic portal branches and be responsible for perfusion disorders.

## Obstruction of the Superior Vena Cava

During chronic obstruction of the superior vena cava, collateral pathways develop to maintain venous drainage. In particular, the cavoportal collateral pathway diverts the flow from the superior vena cava to the portal vein on two different tracks: caval-superficial-umbilical-portal and caval-mammary-phrenic–hepatic capsular–portal [14]. These collaterals are clearly visualized on contrast-enhanced CT and MR images and may be associated with increased enhancement in the liver (a so-called "hot spot" on nuclear medicine images) mimicking hypervascular tumors. This increased enhancement of the liver can be seen in up to 29% of the patients with obstruction of the superior vena cava [15]. Besides visualization of the venous collaterals, the location of increased enhancement helps identify it as a vascular abnormality because it is mainly found in the anterior part of segment 4 but can also be seen in the subdiaphragmatic portion of the liver [16].

## Increased Hepatic Enhancement Around Liver Tumors

Hypervascular liver tumors may increase the hepatic arterial blood supply of the surrounding liver. On hepatic arterial phase, the hepatic parenchyma adjacent to the tumor shows transient increased enhancement compared to other liver segments. It may be seen in malignant tumors such as hepatocellular carcinoma, hypervascular liver metastases but also in benign hypervascular tumors such as focal nodular hyperplasia or rapidly-filling hemangioma (Fig. 2.3).

## Increased Hepatic Enhancement Related to Inflammation

Local inflammation can cause hyperemia with increase in hepatic artery inflow and decrease in portal venous inflow as in acute cholecystitis, cholangitis, and liver abscess. On CT or MR imaging, the liver next to the inflammation shows hyperenhancement on hepatic arterial phase and returns to normal on portal venous phase [6].

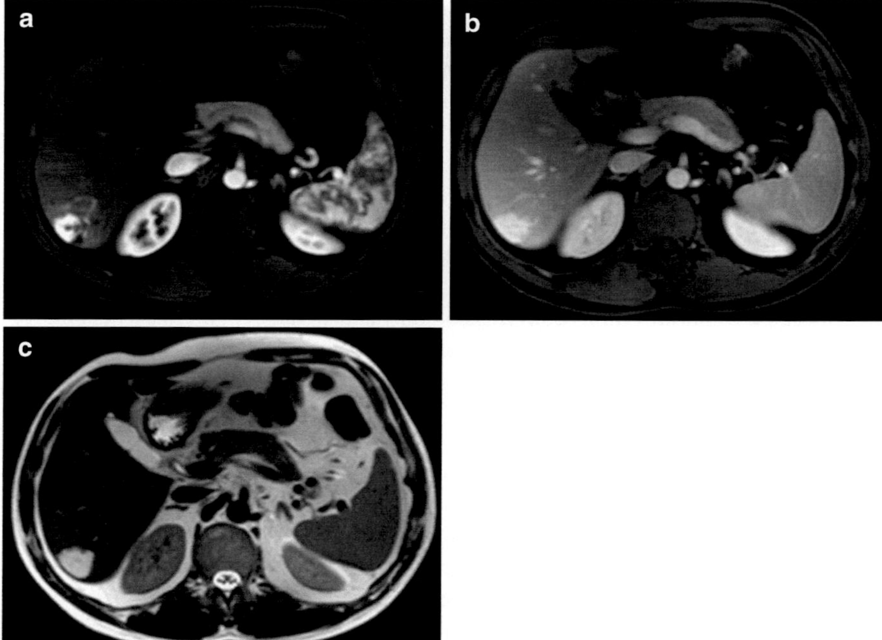

**Fig. 2.3** Increased hepatic enhancement around rapid-filling hemangioma. On contrast-enhanced MRI during the arterial phase, there is an early enhancement of the lesion with increased hepatic enhancement around the hemangioma (**a**). On portal venous phase, the hemangioma is homogeneously hyperintense and the perfusion disorder is no longer seen (**b**). Typical strong hyperintensity of the hemangioma on T2-weighted MR sequence (**c**)

**Other Transient Hepatic Parenchymal Enhancement**

Portal blood flow is reduced when there is increased pressure on hepatic parenchyma due to the low portal pressure. Ribs or diaphragm may compress the liver especially during deep inspiration. It is seen as a hypoattenuation area in the subcapsular region and has been reported in 14% of patients [17].

## *Pseudolesions*

Pseudolesion is defined as a focal mass-like finding seen only on imaging studies without real parenchymal change [18]. Pseudolesions related to vascular anomalies are usually seen in specific locations.

**Pseudolesions Around the Falciform Ligament**

They have been described at CT, CT arterial portography, and MR imaging for years. They are seen in up to 20% at CT or MR imaging liver examinations [19, 20]. Visualization is best on portal venous phase images. They appear as a focal low attenuation or signal intensity on CT or MR images and can also be identified at the arterial phase. Initially thought to be due to focal fat, these pseudolesions are probably related to anomalous venous drainage [20]. Moreover, an inferior vein of Sappey (which drains venous blood flow from the anterior part of the abdominal wall into the liver) is often encountered in these pseudolesions [19].

**Pseudolesion Adjacent to the Hilum**

A focal liver lesion located in the posterior part of segment 4 or the left liver lobe suggests focal fatty sparing or focal steatosis. They are explained by abnormal venous supply coming not from the portal vein itself, but portal venous tributaries [4, 21–24]. When aberrant right gastric vein (with low insulin concentration) drains directly into a liver segment it may result in focal fatty sparing in an otherwise fatty liver (Fig. 2.4). Conversely, when aberrant duodenopancreatic arcade (with high insulin concentration) drains directly into the liver, it may result in focal fatty steatosis.

**Pseudolesions Around the Gallbladder**

In patients with steatosis, focal fatty sparing may be seen around the gallbladder fossa in segments 4 and 5. Interestingly, these pseudolesions are much more frequent in patients with an intact gallbladder than in those who have undergone cholecystectomy (78% vs. 33%) [25]. Focal fatty sparing around the gallbladder is also

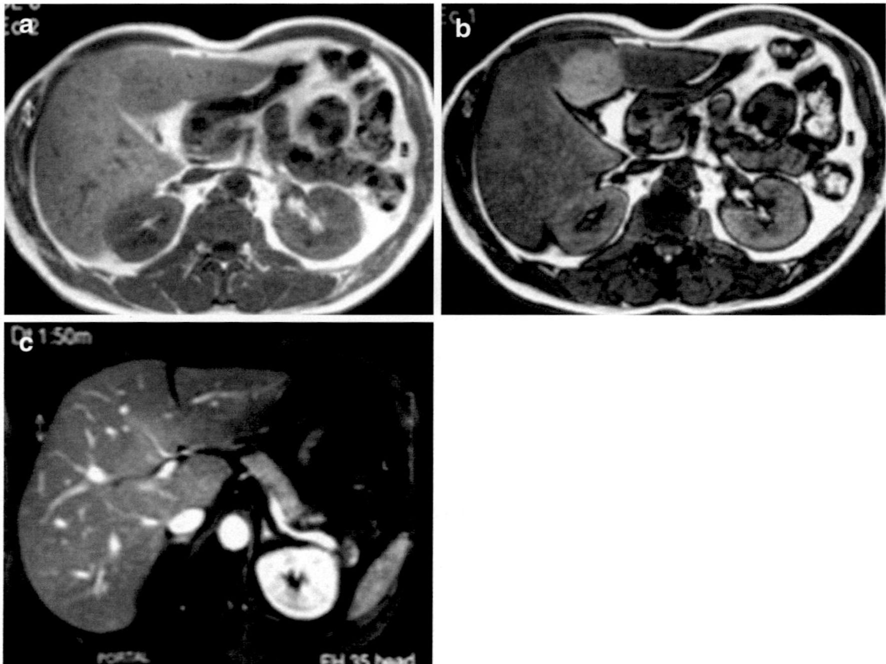

**Fig. 2.4** Focal fatty sparing in an otherwise fatty liver. In—(**a**) and opposed (**b**) phase T1-weighted MR sequence showing drop in signal intensity of the liver indicating steatosis. The posterior part of segment 4 does not contain fat due to its abnormal venous supply coming not from the portal vein itself but from aberrant right gastric vein seen on portal venous phase (**c**)

probably related to venous drainage because there are almost always small cystic veins (with low insulin concentration) that drain directly into the liver and are interrupted by cholecystectomy.

## Diffuse Vascular Liver Diseases

Most diffuse vascular liver diseases are due to venous impairment—either portal vein or hepatic veins—rather than anomalous hepatic arteries.

## *Extrahepatic Portal Vein Thrombosis*

Although local inflammatory diseases may induce portal vein thrombosis, most cases are related to coagulation disorders, myeloproliferative diseases, or cirrhosis. Imaging is important because clinical symptoms are not specific. Ultrasound typically demonstrates absence of flow within the vessel. CT or MRI shows lack of enhancement within the vessel. As above discussed for intrahepatic portal venous obstruction, recent clotting may appear as hyperattenuating on unenhanced CT (Fig. 2.5). Imaging is also important to grade the venous obstruction (complete vs. incomplete), and to assess its length (portal vein only or extensive with obstruction of branches and/or tributaries). In patients with complete obstrution of the superior mesenteric vein and/or splenic vein, radiologists should carefully analyze the small bowel enhancement as well as look for splenic infarcts.

If acute complete extrahepatic portal vein obstruction does not resolve (with or without anticoagulation), small collateral veins rapidly develop in the porta hepatis to maintain portal blood to the liver. These veins are known as cavernous transformation of the portal vein or portal cavernoma. They appear in the first days after

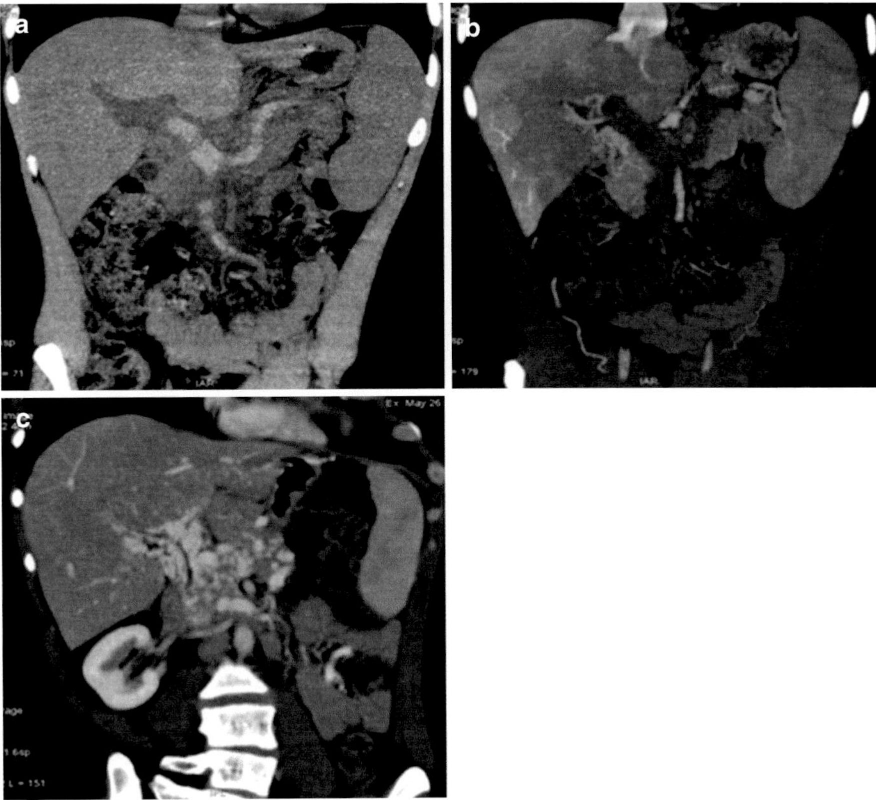

**Fig. 2.5** Extrahepatic portal vein thrombosis. Acute onset (**a** and **b**). Unenhanced CT (**a**) showing spontaneous hyperattenuation indicating recent clotting. On portal venous phase, (**b**) no enhancement is seen within the portal vein. Differences in liver enhancement are seen on multiphasic CT corresponding to the portal deprivation in liver segments remote from the hilum and consequent increased arterial inflow. Several months later, the portal cavernoma has developed and is mainly observed around the common bile duct (**c**)

vessel occlusion, and grow over time. They are well depicted on ultrasound showing multiple vessels in the hepatoduodenal ligament. On Doppler US, they show portal venous flow patterns. On contrast-enhanced CT or MRI, portal cavernoma is best seen on portal venous phase. It typically develops around the common bile duct and the gallbladder. Sometimes, portal cavernoma is more difficult to diagnose due to pseudotumorous appearance.

Besides the direct signs of venous obstruction and venous collaterals, differences in liver enhancement are seen on multiphasic CT or MRI. On hepatic arterial phase, the liver segments close to the hilum normally enhance because the portal blood flow is maintained while the liver segments remote from the hilum (right liver segments and left liver lobe) have reduced portal venous flow and show hyperenhancement that disappears on portal and delayed phases.

In chronic complete extrahepatic portal vein thrombosis, morphologic changes of the liver may mimic cirrhosis: atrophy of the right liver, hypertrophy of segment 1, and signs or portal hypertension. However, the atrophy-hypertrophy complex is peculiar because the hypertrophy is central (segment 1 and 4) and is explained by the different inflows [26]. As portal cavernoma is mostly developed around the common bile duct, intrahepatic bile duct dilatation along with cholestasis may be seen with downstream strictures caused by portal cavernoma. This frequent complication is called portal cavernoma cholangiopathy or portal biliopathy. Biliary symptoms such as pruritus, and rarely jaundice are seen in patients with biliary stenosis and dilation on MRCP [27]. It seems that portal cavernoma cholangiopathy develops and stabilises early after portal vein thrombosis [28].

## *Budd-Chiari Syndrome*

Budd-Chiari Syndrome (BCS) is defined by clinical and laboratory signs associated with partial or complete impairment of hepatic venous drainage. Primary BCS is the most common type and is a complication of hypercoagulable states, in particular myeloproliferative neoplasms. BCS may have several clinical presentations: acute, chronic, the latter being the most common. Imaging is key for the diagnosis combining direct signs of venous obstruction and indirect ones such as morphologic changes or portal hypertension. Ultrasound is particularly hepful for direct signs of venous involvement while contrast-enhanced CT or MRI is very accurate for hepatic consequences and nodule characterization. Angiography is no longer performed for diagnostic purposes but is indeed the first step before endovascular treatment.

In acute BCS, obstructed hepatic veins or IVC are enlarged. At the site of the obstruction, the veins appear hyperechoic and do not enhance on CT or MRI or appear stenotic. Although rare, acute hepatic venous thrombosis may be seen as hyperattenuation on unenhanced CT. Upstream to the obstruction, hepatic venous flow patterns are variable either stagnant or inverted on Doppler US. Venous collaterals that drain flow from obstructed veins to patent veins may not be seen at that stage. The liver is enlarged and heterogeneous on multiphasic CT or MRI. Enhancement of the obstructed liver parenchyma is reduced and delayed due to congestion contrasting with the non obstructed segments such as the segment 1, whose hepatic venous flow is usually preserved [29] (Fig. 2.6). Perfusion anomalies often predominate at the periphery of the liver, defining the zonal enhancement. MRI is useful because it allows sequence acquisition in various planes such as coronal ones that best show IVC and non-contrast sequences that can easily depict vessel obstruction as already referred as black-blood and white-blood sequences.

In chronic BCS, imaging findings are different. Obstructed hepatic veins are no longer visible or are seen as fibrous cords. The major vascular feature and the most sensitive one is the development of collateral network that can be seen both intra- and extrahepatically [30]. They can drain the hepatic venous flow into another hepatic vein, directly into the IVC, in other veins such as right adrenal vein or pass directly through the diaphragm to reach the right atrium. These venous collaterals are easily recognized because they are tortuous, have irregular shape and are more horizontal-oriented than the normal hepatic veins. On Doppler US, their flow is variable: continuous pseudoportal or triphasic. Although they are very specific of BCS, they have been described in other conditions such as portosinusoidal disease [31]. Hepatic changes associated with chronic BCS are prominent. First, morphologic changes, which show marked atrophy-hypertrophy consistent with obstructed/non

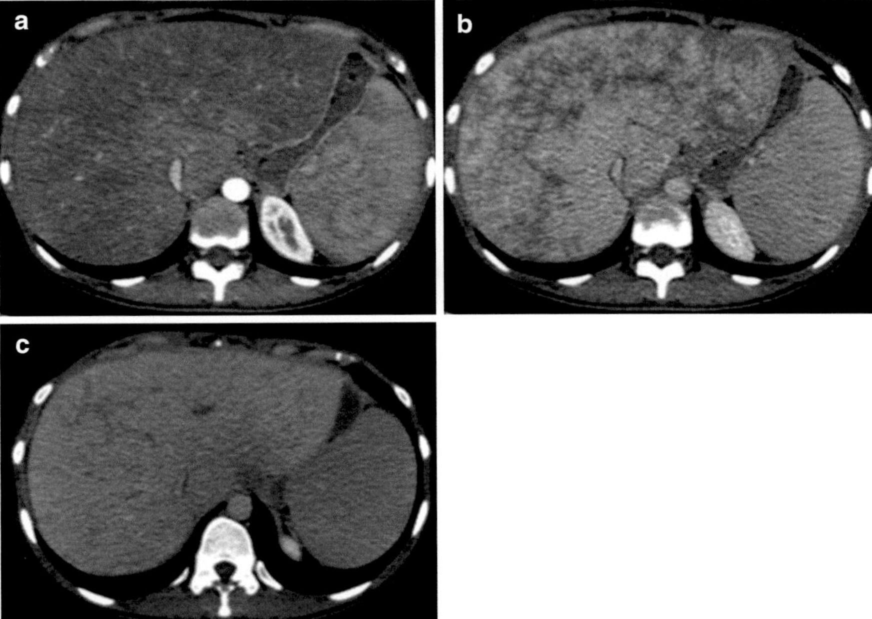

**Fig. 2.6** Subacute Budd-Chiari syndrome. On multiphasic contrast-enhanced CT differences in liver enhancement are minimal on arterial—(**a**) and delayed phases (**c**) while they are prominent on portal venous phase (**b**) with reduced enhancement of the obstructed liver parenchyma due to congestion contrasting with the non obstructed segments such as the segment 1, whose hepatic venous flow is usually preserved

obstructed liver segments. Indeed, segment 1 is enlarged in most cases and hepatic veins draining the segment 1 are often dilated (>3 mm) but these features are not specific. Second, liver enhancement often has a "mosaic" enhancement pattern that is a reticulated enhancement on arterial/portal venous enhancement followed by homogeneous liver enhancement on delayed phase.

Other imaging findings may be seen, some related to portal hypertension: porto-caval varices, splenomegaly, the latter being also related to myeloproliferative disorders, and ascites; liver nodules that will be described later; and portal vein thrombosis (reported in about 15% of BCS) [32].

Secondary BCS is another entity usually caused by vascular compression (cyst, benign solid tumor…) or invasion by intrahepatic tumor (hepatocellular carcinoma in particular) or extrahepatic ones mostly originating from the kidney, adrenal, and IVC. Visualization of a tumor helps make the proper diagnosis.

Imaging is also extremely important to plan and monitor transjugular intrahepatic portosystemic shunt.

## Other Causes of Sinusoidal Dilatation

One important imaging finding of BCS is the "mosaic pattern" that is related to sinusoidal dilatation. It presents with a reticular enhancement of the liver seen on late arterial phase or portal venous phase. On hepatobiliary phase, sinusoidal dilatation is characterized by a reticular hypointense appearance of the liver.

Yet, this finding is not specific of BCS as any obstruction of venous outflow obstruction between the heart and the sinusoids causes congestion of the vessels such as pericardial diseases, epicardial adipose tissue hypertrophy, heart failure, and patients who received Fontan procedure [33]. Conversely to BCS, hepatic veins are patent and often dilated, as well as the IVC.

Non obstructive sinusoidal dilatation can be also seen in non-hepatic acute inflammatory disease such as pyelonephritis, cholecystitis, pneumonia, pancreatitis, and inflammatory bowel disease as well as in chronic conditions. On imaging, the mosaic appearance seen on contrast-enhanced CT or MRI disappears when inflammation resolves.

Oral contraceptives are also associated with hepatic sinusoidal dilatation.

## Sinusoidal Obstruction Syndrome

Sinusoidal obstruction syndrome (SOS) is an endothelial sinusoidal damage often related to cytoreductive therapy prior to hematopoietic stem cell transplantation, several drugs including platin-based chemotherapy. On contrast-enhanced CT or MRI, liver enhancement is heterogeneous with or without mosaic appearance. SOS is more evident on hepatobiliary phase with a reticular hypointense pattern that correlates well with pathologic grades. Yet, nodular regenerative hyperplasia that is associated with the most severe grade of SOS is usually not seen on imaging. Elastography-based ultrasound has been reported useful in this indication [34].

Peliosis hepatis is characterized by multiple blood-filled cystic lesions at the level of the sinusoids, randomly distributed throughout the lobule, with loss of endothelium. Many conditions may lead to peliosis: hematological diseases, infectious disorders. Imaging features show tumor-like lesions with variable enhancement on multiphasic CT or MRI [35]. Most lesions are strongly hyperintense on T2-weighted MR sequences.

## *Portosinusoidal Disease*

Portosinusoidal disease is a recently described entity based on the absence of cirrhosis together with signs of portal hypertension and/or histological lesions characteristic for this disease. It comprises the diseases previously known as obliterative venopathy, nodular regenerative hyperplasia or incomplete septal cirrhosis [36]. This disease involves the portal venules and/or the sinusoids.

Imaging findings may include common features of portal hypertension, namely splenomegaly and porto-systemic collaterals and no classical morphologic changes of the liver seen in cirrhosis, although the disease is not necessarily associated with portal hypertension. Liver surface is ususally smooth. The striking imaging features are intrahepatic portal vein abnormalities consisting of a reduced caliber, occlusive thrombosis, or and lack of visibility (Fig. 2.7) [37]. Interestingly, liver stiffness values are much lower than the cut-offs for clinically significant portal hypertension in cirrhosis, and spleen to liver stiffness ratio is higher than in other chronic liver diseases.

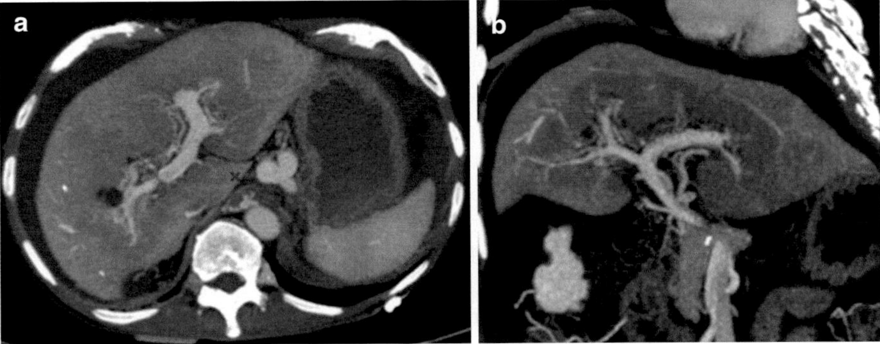

**Fig. 2.7** Portosinusoidal disease. Contrast-enhanced CT during portal venous phase shows intrahepatic portal vein abnormalities consisting of a reduced caliber and signs of portal hypertension (**a**). On coronal view (**b**), differences in liver enhancement are explained by reduced portal venous flow in the periphery of the liver

## *Congenital Portosystemic Shunts*

Congenital portosystemic shunts are rare vascular malformations that create an abnormal connection between portal and systemic veins. They can be located intra- or extrahepatically. Then portal vein flow is completely or partially diverted into the systemic venous system. According to the type and the amount of portal flow diversion, it can be diagnosed prenatal, in childhood or in adult patients [38]. Several classifications exist, regarding extrahepatic shunts, the Abernethy classification is a well-known one: type I (end-to-side), and type II (side-to-side). The presence of remnant hepatopetal portal venous flow is essential to assess.

Imaging is important to diagnose congenital portosystemic shunts and to stage the shunt as surgical closure or interventional radiology play an important role to restore portal venous flow. Ultrasound is often the first imaging modality that shows communication between the two venous systems. Precise mapping is obtained on contrast-enhanced CT or MRI showing the type of communication, the afferent vein, the efferent vein. Major portal deprivation often causes the development of liver nodules that could disappear after shunt occlusion. When treatment is indicated, angiography with occlusion test is the first step especially when intrahepatic portal branches are not visible before the procedure as they can appear during occlusion test.

## *Hereditary Hemorrhagic Telangiectasia*

Hereditary hemorrhagic telangiectasia (HHT) or Rendu–Osler–Weber disease is an autosomal dominant disorder characterized by widespread cutaneous, mucosal, and visceral telangiectasias. The primary lesion of HHT is the telangiectasia, arising from the dilation of a postcapillary venule that fuses directly with an arteriole, bypassing the capillary vessels [39]. The diagnosis is based on the Curacao criteria. Liver vascular malformations are found in 41–74% of HHT. Liver involvement is more frequent in the HHT2 genotype than in the HHT1 genotype and is seen more commonly in women than men. Liver vascular malformations are variable from small telangiectasias to large shunting and any type of shunting can be seen (hepatic artery to portal vein, hepatic artery to hepatic vein and/or portal vein to hepatic vein). The most important clinical findings are highoutput cardiac failure, portal hypertension, encephalopathy, biliary ischemia, and mesenteric ischemia. Liver regeneration can induce nodular regenerative hyperplasia and/or focal nodular hyperplasia. On Doppler US, the diagnoses relies on the combination of dilated hepatic arteries (common hepatic artery >7 mm and intrahepatic arterial hypervascularization) and anomalous flow patterns in hepatic artery, portal vein (pulsatility), and or hepatic veins (biphasic or continuous patterns) [40, 41].

On contrast-enhanced CT or MRI, one key imaging finding is the prominent hepatic artery possibly associated with dilated hepatic and/or portal veins (Fig. 2.8).

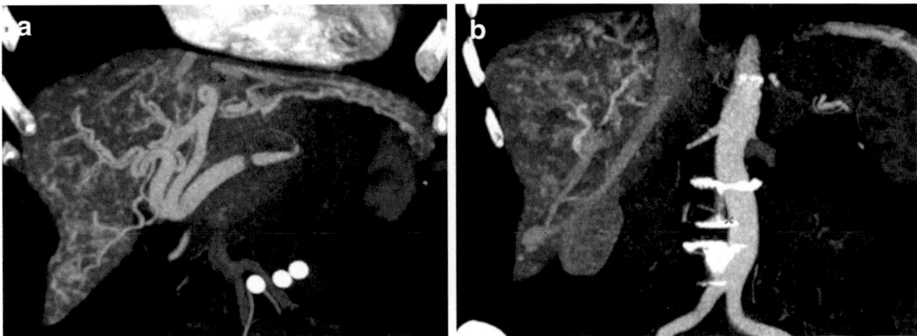

**Fig. 2.8** Hereditary hemorrhagic telangiectasia. Contrast-enhanced CT during arterial phase shows dilated hepatic arteries and arteriovenous shunts (with early enhancement of hepatic veins) (**a**). Telangiectasias are well seen on coronal image (**b**)

The multiphasic analysis allows recognition of liver shunting. They also both analyze the signs of portal hypertension and look for the biliary complications (ischemic cholangitis and bilomas) induced by the blood flow steal through arteriovenous shunting. Angiography is no longer a diagnostic tool and should be performed only if embolization of vascular malformations is scheduled. As this procedure is complex and risky in those patients, decision has to be taken by expert multidisciplinary team.

## Liver Cirrhosis

Liver cirrhosis is known to alter normal hepatic blood flow dynamics, resulting in increased arterial flow and decreased portal venous flow to the liver as well as distortion of hepatic veins. On imaging, the hepatic artery is frequently enlarged and tortuous, and Doppler US can easily demonstrate increased flow. Arterioportal shunts (described earlier) are also quite common. Hepatic veins decrease in size with the severity of fibrosis and their flow is less modulated by the cardiac cycle.

## Thrombosis, Stenosis, Dissection of the Hepatic Artery

Acute thrombosis of hepatic artery is generally induced by surgical or radiologic interventions. In most cases, there are no consequences owing to the rich and extensive collateral arterial supply from other hepatic branches, celiac artery, or extrahepatic arteries. It is completely different in transplanted livers as the arterial supply cannot develop immediately after liver transplantation. This is why serial Doppler US is systematically performed after liver transplantation. On Doppler US, this complication is suspected when no flow can be recorded within the hepatic artery or when reduced resistive index (<0.50) is associated with long systolic acceleration time (>80 ms). Specificity is improved when the tardus parvus pattern is combined with a peak systolic velocity less than or equal to 48 cm/s [42].

Hepatic artery dissection is rare and favored by surgical or radiologic interventions. On contrast enhanced CT or MRI, the hepatic artery is enlarged with a linear low-attenuated filling defect within the lumen [43].

## *Hepatic artery Aneurysm*

The hepatic artery is the second most common visceral artery for the development of aneurysms, after the splenic artery [44]. Hepatic aneurysm formation is rarely due to atherosclerosis and other diseases such segmental arterial mediolysis, and vasculitis should be searched. It can also be iatrogenic (intervention radiology, liver transplantation) or inflammatory. On Doppler US, the hepatic artery appears focally enlarged. Contrast-enhanced CT or MRI is useful to define the extent of the aneurysm.

## *Portal Vein Aneurysm*

Portal vein aneurysms are uncommon and account for only 3% of all venous aneurysms [43]. They may be congenital or acquired, cirrhosis, trauma, portal hypertension, surgery, and pancreatitis being the most common causes. On imaging, they appear as a focal dilatation of the portal vein containing turbulent flow.

## *Nodules Associated with Liver Diseases*

Many vascular liver disorders can induce hepatocellular tumors. They may be related to portal venous deprivation, venous outflow obstruction or arterial diseases. Their common feature is an imbalance between hepatic arterial and portal venous blood flow leading to an increased hepatic arterial inflow. The vascular liver disorders that commonly develop hepatocellular nodules are BCS, congenital portosystemic shunt, and hereditary hemorrhagic telangiectasia [45]. Liver lesions can also be seen in cavernous transformation of the portal vein, portosinusoidal disease, congenital hepatic fibrosis, and sinusoidal obstruction syndrome [46]. Focal nodular hyperplasia-like lesions are the most common (Fig. 2.9) but other benign tumors may also be found including focal nodular regenerative hyperplasia and hepatocellular adenomas. Imaging and especially MRI plays a major role in the diagnosis, which diagnosis can still be more difficult than in normal livers. A histopathological examination may be required. The size and number of these benign lesions may

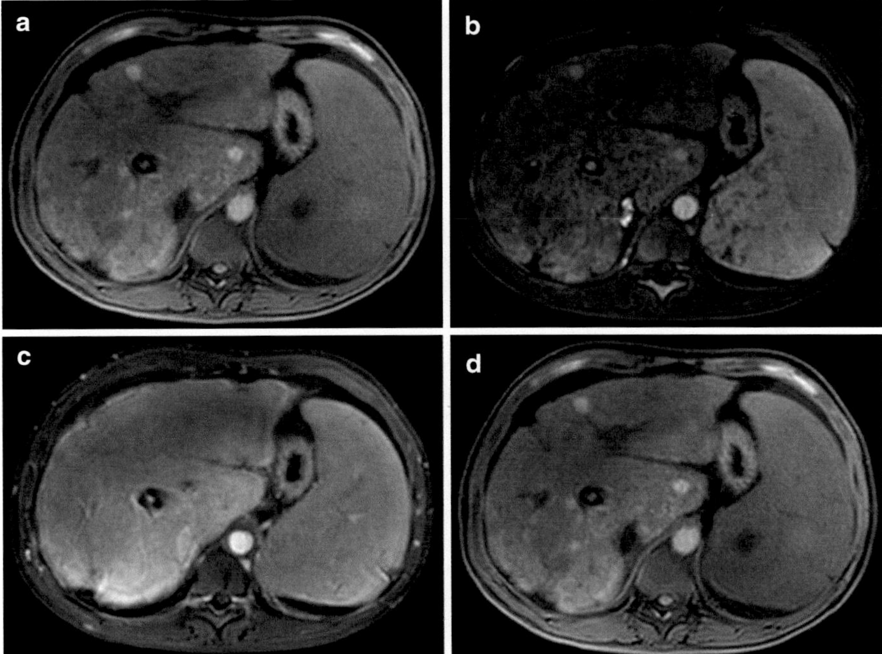

**Fig. 2.9** Focal nodular hyperplasia-like in Budd-Chiari syndrome. Multiple small-sized liver nodules that are hyperintense on T1-weighted MR sequence (**a**), hyperenhancing on arterial phase (**b**), iso-intense on portal venous phase (**c**), and hyperintense on hepatobiliary phase T1-weighted MR sequence (**d**)

increase over time making the diagnosis often difficult. Hepatocellular carcinoma is rare except in patients with BCS or following a Fontan procedure [45].

In conclusion, Doppler US, CT and MRI are essential to diagnose vascular disorders of the liver. They allow proper diagnosis, which is often difficult clinically as clinical symptoms are non specific. They are also helpful to define the extent of the disease, evaluate the complications and choose the optimal treatment. Image interpretation may be difficult and often requires expertise. As in oncology, expert multidisciplinary board provides the best patient management.

# References


1. Kan Z, Madoff DC. Liver anatomy: microcirculation of the liver. Semin Intervent Radiol. 2008;25(2):77–85.
2. Itai Y, Matsui O. Blood flow and liver imaging. Radiology, 1997. 202(2):306–14.
3. Yoshimitsu K, Honda H, Kuroiwa T, Irie H, Aibe H, Shinozaki K, et al. Unusual hemodynamics and pseudolesions of the noncirrhotic liver at CT. Radiographics. 2001;21:S81–96.
4. Vilgrain V, Lagadec M, Ronot M. Pitfalls in liver imaging. Radiology. 2015;278(1):34–51.

5. McNaughton DA, Abu-Yousef MM. Doppler US of the liver made simple. Radiographics. 2011;31(1):161–88.
6. Quiroga S, Sebastia C, Pallisa E, Castella E, Perez-Lafuente M, Alvarez-Castells A. Improved diagnosis of hepatic perfusion disorders: value of hepatic arterial phase imaging during helical CT. Radiographics. 2001;21(1):65–81. questionnaire 288–94
7. Chouhan MD, Lythgoe MF, Mookerjee RP, Taylor SA. Vascular assessment of liver disease-towards a new frontier in MRI. Br J Radiol. 2016;16:20150675.
8. Choi BI, Lee KH, Han JK, Lee JM. Hepatic arterioportal shunts: dynamic CT and MR features. Korean J Radiol. 2002;3(1):1–15.
9. Yu JS, Kim KW, Jeong MG, Lee JT, Yoo HS. Nontumorous hepatic arterial-portal venous shunts: MR imaging findings. Radiology. 2000;217(3):750–6.
10. Matsuo M, Kanematsu M, Kondo H, Maeda S, Goshima S, Suenaga I, et al. Arterioportal shunts mimicking hepatic tumors with hyperintensity on T2-weighted MR images. J Magn Reson Imaging. 2002;15(3):330–3.
11. Sun HY, Lee JM, Shin CI, Lee DH, Moon SK, Kim KW, et al. Gadoxetic acid-enhanced magnetic resonance imaging for differentiating small hepatocellular carcinomas (< or =2 cm in diameter) from arterial enhancing pseudolesions: special emphasis on hepatobiliary phase imaging. Invest Radiol. 2010;45(2):96–103.
12. Motosugi U, Ichikawa T, Sou H, Sano K, Tominaga L, Muhi A, et al. Distinguishing hypervascular pseudolesions of the liver from hypervascular hepatocellular carcinomas with gadoxetic acid-enhanced MR imaging. Radiology. 2010;256(1):151–8.
13. Catalano OA, Choy G, Zhu A, Hahn PF, Sahani DV. Differentiation of malignant thrombus from bland thrombus of the portal vein in patients with hepatocellular carcinoma: application of diffusion-weighted MR imaging. Radiology. 2009;254(1):154–62.
14. Kapur S, Paik E, Rezaei A, Vu DN. Where there is blood, there is a way: unusual collateral vessels in superior and inferior vena cava obstruction. Radiographics. 2010;30(1):67–78.
15. Siegel Y, Schallert E. Prevalence and etiology of focal liver opacification in patients with superior vena cava obstruction. J Comput Assist Tomogr. 2013;37(5):805–8.
16. Sheth S, Ebert MD, Fishman EK. Superior vena cava obstruction evaluation with MDCT. Am J Roentgenol. 2010;194(4):W336–46.
17. Yoshimitsu K, Honda H, Kuroiwa T, Irie H, Tajima T, Jimi M, et al. Pseudolesions of the liver possibly caused by focal rib compression: analysis based on hemodynamic change. Am J Roentgenol. 1999;172(3):645–9.
18. Kobayashi S, Gabata T, Matsui C. Radiologic manifestation of hepatic pseudolesions and pseudotumors in the third inflow area. Imaging. 2010;2(5):519–28.
19. Genchellac H, Yilmaz S, Ucar A, Dursun M, Demir MK, Yekeler E. Hepatic pseudolesion around the falciform ligament: prevalence, aberrant venous supply, and fatty infiltration evaluated by multidetector computed tomography and magnetic resonance imaging. J Comput Assist Tomogr. 2007;31(4):526–33.
20. Macari M, Yeretsian R, Babb J. Assessment of low signal adjacent to the falciform ligament on contrast-enhanced MRI. Am J Roentgenol. 2007;189(6):1443–8.
21. Hashimoto M, Heianna J, Tate E, Nishii T, Iwama T, Ishiyama K. Small veins entering the liver. Eur Radiol. 2002;12(8):2000–5.
22. Matsui O, Kadoya M, Yoshikawa J, Gabata T, Takahashi S, Ueda K, et al. Aberrant gastric venous drainage in cirrhotic livers: imaging findings in focal areas of liver parenchyma. Radiology. 1995;197(2):345–9.
23. Gabata T, Matsui O, Kadoya M, Ueda K, Kawamori Y, Yoshikawa J, et al. Aberrant gastric venous drainage in a focal spared area of segment IV in fatty liver: demonstration with color Doppler sonography. Radiology. 1997;203(2):461–3.
24. Nevalainen PI, Kallio T, Lahtela JT, Mustonen J, Pasternack AI. High peritoneal permeability predisposes to hepatic steatosis in diabetic continuous ambulatory peritoneal dialysis patients receiving intraperitoneal insulin. Perit Dial Int. 2000;20(6):637–42.
25. Aubin B, Denys A, Lafortune M, Dery R, Breton G. Focal sparing of liver parenchyma in steatosis: role of the gallbladder and its vessels. J Ultrasound Med. 1995;14(2):77–80.

26. Vilgrain V, Condat B, Bureau C, Hakime A, Plessier A, Cazals-Hatem D, et al. Atrophy-hypertrophy complex in patients with cavernous transformation of the portal vein: CT evaluation. Radiology. 2006;241(1):149–55.
27. Condat B, Vilgrain V, Asselah T, O'Toole D, Rufat P, Zappa M, et al. Portal cavernoma-associated cholangiopathy: a clinical and MR cholangiography coupled with MR portography imaging study. Hepatology. 2003;37(6):1302–8.
28. Llop E, de Juan C, Seijo S, García-Criado A, Abraldes JG, Bosch J, et al. Portal cholangiopathy: radiological classification and natural history. Gut. 2011;60(6):853–60.
29. Van Wettere M, Bruno O, Rautou PE, Vilgrain V, Ronot M. Diagnosis of Budd-Chiari syndrome. Abdom Radiol (NY). 2018;43(8):1896–907.
30. Valla DC. The diagnosis and management of the Budd-Chiari syndrome: consensus and controversies. Hepatology. 2003;38(4):793–803.
31. Seijo S, Reverter E, Miquel R, Berzigotti A, Abraldes JG, Bosch J, et al. Role of hepatic vein catheterisation and transient elastography in the diagnosis of idiopathic portal hypertension. Dig Liver Dis. 2012;44(10):855–60.
32. Darwish Murad S, Valla DC, de Groen PC, Zeitoun G, Haagsma EB, Kuipers EJ, et al. Pathogenesis and treatment of Budd-Chiari syndrome combined with portal vein thrombosis. Am J Gastroenterol. 2006;101(1):83–90.
33. Brancatelli G, Furlan A, Calandra A, Dioguardi BM. Hepatic sinusoidal dilatation. Abdom Radiol (NY). 2018;43(8):2011–22.
34. Dietrich CF, Trenker C, Fontanilla T, Gorg C, Hausmann A, Klein S, et al. New ultrasound techniques challenge the diagnosis of sinusoidal obstruction syndrome. Ultrasound Med Biol. 2018;44(11):2171–82.
35. Iannaccone R, Federle MP, Brancatelli G, Matsui O, Fishman EK, Narra VR, et al. Peliosis hepatis: spectrum of imaging findings. Am J Roentgenol. 2006;187(1):W43–52.
36. De Gottardi A, Rautou PE, Schouten J, Rubbia-Brandt L, Leebeek F, Trebicka J, et al. Vascular portosinusoidal disease: a position paper from the vascular liver disease interest group (Valdig). Lancet Gastroenterol. 2019 (in press).
37. Glatard AS, Hillaire S, d'Assignies G, Cazals-Hatem D, Plessier A, Valla DC, et al. Obliterative portal venopathy: findings at CT imaging. Radiology. 2012;263(3):741–50.
38. Franchi-Abella S, Gonzales E, Ackermann O, Branchereau S, Pariente D, Guerin F. Congenital portosystemic shunts: diagnosis and treatment. Abdom Radiol (NY). 2018;43(8):2023–36.
39. Buscarini E, Gandolfi S, Alicante S, Londoni C, Manfredi G. Liver involvement in hereditary hemorrhagic telangiectasia. Abdom Radiol (NY).
40. Caselitz M, Bahr MJ, Bleck JS, Chavan A, Manns MP, Wagner S, et al. Sonographic criteria for the diagnosis of hepatic involvement in hereditary hemorrhagic telangiectasia (HHT). Hepatology. 2003;37(5):1139–46.
41. Buscarini E, Danesino C, Olivieri C, Lupinacci G, De Grazia F, Reduzzi L, et al. Doppler ultrasonographic grading of hepatic vascular malformations in hereditary hemorrhagic telangiectasia—results of extensive screening. Ultraschall Med. 2004;25(5):348–55.
42. Park YS, Kim KW, Lee SJ, Lee J, Jung DH, Song GW, et al. Hepatic arterial stenosis assessed with doppler US after liver transplantation: frequent false-positive diagnoses with tardus parvus waveform and value of adding optimal peak systolic velocity cutoff. Radiology. 2011;260(3):884–91.
43. Onur MR, Karaosmanoglu AD, Akca O, Ocal O, Akpinar E, Karcaaltincaba M. Imaging features of non-traumatic vascular liver emergencies. Jpn J Radiol. 2017;35(5):215–24.
44. Virmani V, Ramanathan S, Virmani VS, Kielar A, Sheikh A, Ryan J. Non-neoplastic hepatic vascular diseases: spectrum of CT and MRI appearances. Clin Radiol. 2014;69(5):538–48.
45. Vilgrain V, Paradis V, Van Wettere M, Valla D, Ronot M, Rautou PE. Benign and malignant hepatocellular lesions in patients with vascular liver diseases. Abdom Radiol (NY). 2018;43(8):1968–77.
46. Furlan A, Brancatelli G, Dioguardi Burgio M, Grazioli L, Lee JM, Murmura E, et al. Focal nodular hyperplasia after treatment with oxaliplatin: a multiinstitutional series of cases diagnosed at MRI. Am J Roentgenol. 2018;210(4):775–9.

# Chapter 3
# Hepatic Artery Occlusion and Ischemic Cholangiopathy

Pierre Deltenre

## Pathophysiology

The anatomy of the blood vessel systems that serve the liver and bile ducts provides clues to understanding the pathophysiology of ischemic cholangiopathy. About half of the blood carried by the hepatic artery is destined to the biliary tree. The other half is distributed to the liver capsule, the vasa vasora, and to hepatic venous tracts [1, 2]. The intrahepatic arteries run close to the bile ducts. The arterial supply to the bile ducts also comes from retroduodenal and retroportal arteries [2, 3]. The terminal small branches of these arteries resolve into a rich microvascular network surrounding the bile ducts, the peribiliary plexus, which drains into venules joining the intrahepatic portal system.

The exclusive arterial supply of the biliary system contrasts with the dual blood supply of the hepatic parenchyma coming from hepatic arteries and portal vein [1, 2, 4]. This anatomical particularity explains why hepatic artery occlusion mainly affects the bile ducts. In theory, any kind of injury to the hepatic artery may cause ischemic damage to the bile ducts. However, outside the transplant setting, occlusion of the main hepatic artery rarely causes ischemic damage to the biliary tree [2]. This is due to the fact that, in normal conditions, a number of compensatory mechanisms exist or develop in cases of proximal blockade of the hepatic artery. First, numerous small arterial branches coming from splanchnic and non-splanchnic arteries enter the liver through its surface. These may serve as a compensatory mechanism in case of main hepatic artery occlusion [2]. Second, blood may be supplied in a retrograde manner from the portal venous system. This is supported by the observation that retrograde bleeding from the donor hepatic artery occurs after

P. Deltenre (✉)
Department of Gastroenterology, Hepatopancreatology and Digestive Oncology, CUB Hôpital Erasme, Université Libre de Bruxelles, Brussels, Belgium

Department of Gastroenterology and Hepatology, Clinique Saint-Luc, Bouge, Belgium

© Springer Nature Switzerland AG 2022
D. Valla et al. (eds.), *Vascular Disorders of the Liver*,
https://doi.org/10.1007/978-3-030-82988-9_3

portal reperfusion during liver transplantation [5]. Third, rapid development of arterial collaterals can be observed as early as 10–15 h after hepatic artery ligation [6–9]. By contrast, distal blockade of hepatic arteries is usually followed by bile duct injury. Numerous animal and human data indicate that embolization of small particles (<200 μm) may be responsible for ischemic damage to the bile ducts [2]. In addition to the blockade of small hepatic arteries that feed the peribiliary plexus, these particles may also suppress arterioportal shunts which constitute another compensatory mechanism for bile duct oxygenation [10].

## Conditions Associated with Injury of the Arterial Blood Supply of the Bile Ducts Susceptible to Induce Ischemic Cholangiopathy

Conditions associated with injury of the arterial blood supply of bile ducts susceptible to induced ischemic damage have been extensively reviewed elsewhere [2]. They can be divided into two groups according to the degree of evidence that ischemia is the pathophysiological mechanism leading to bile duct injury (Table 3.1).

### *Conditions Associated with Definite Ischemic Cholangiopathy*

Conditions associated with definite ischemic cholangiopathy include diseases in which primary lesions of the blood vessels supplying the bile ducts have been demonstrated. This group includes liver transplantation [11–15], hepatic arterial

**Table 3.1** Conditions associated with injury of the arterial blood supply susceptible to induced ischemic cholangiopathy

| Conditions associated with definite ischemic cholangiopathy | Conditions associated with possible ischemic cholangiopathy |
| --- | --- |
| Liver transplantation | Post-cholecystectomy biliary strictures |
| Hepatic arterial chemotherapy infusion, embolization or chemoembolization of toxic agents | Systemic diseases with microvascular involvement (sickle cell disease, Kawasaki disease, Schönlein-Henoch purpura, systemic lupus, antiphospholipid syndrome, paroxysmal nocturnal hemoglobinuria, hypereosinophilic syndrome) |
| Acquired immune deficiency syndrome | Cholangiopathy occurring after prolonged intensive care |
| Hereditary hemorrhagic telangiectasia | |
| Radiotherapy on main bile duct area | |
| Polyarteritis nodosa | |
| Atherosclerosis associated with cholesterol-crystal embolism | |

chemotherapy infusion, embolization or chemoembolization of toxic agents [16–20], acquired immune deficiency syndrome (AIDS) [21–26], hereditary hemorrhagic telangiectasia [27–29], radiotherapy on the main bile duct area [30, 31], polyarteritis nodosa [32–34], and arteriosclerosis associated with cholesterol-crystal embolism [35–37]. The ischemic process of AIDS-related cholangiopathy is supported by the observation of CMV inclusions in arterioles close to bile ducts, which may induce vasculitis. All these conditions are characterized by the presence of focal or diffuse abnormalities of the bile ducts that cannot be explained by other causes, as well as by the presence of primary lesions of the blood vessels supplying the bile ducts.

Liver transplantation is the condition in which ischemic cholangiopathy has been most extensively described. It occurs in 2% to 30% of transplanted patients [11–13, 38–40]. The incidence of ischemic biliary lesion following liver transplantation is higher in cases where donation followed circulatory death than in cases where donation followed brain death [41–46]. In the former, the length of time during which bile ducts are exposed to ischemia is higher, and incidence rates of biliary complications up to 50% have been reported in the transplanted liver. The most severe forms of ischemic cholangiopathy have been observed in cases of early and acute thrombosis of the hepatic artery because the interruption of the arterial blood flow coming from the hepatic artery occurs too quickly to allow the development of arterial collaterals before the development of bile duct lesions. This condition is often associated with severe bile duct damage including bile duct necrosis and biliary casts [14, 15]. On the other hand, when hepatic artery thrombosis occurs progressively, hepatic collaterals may develop and protect patients against re-transplantation [47, 48]. A number of additional features explain why bile ducts are susceptible to ischemic injury after liver transplantation. First, the donor biliary tree may be injured during the preservation and reperfusion process, which may induce ischemic and thrombotic lesions [5]. Lesions occurring during preservation and reperfusion can be mediated by immune reactions as well since the frequency of these lesions is increased when an ABO incompatible graft is transplanted [5, 49–51]. Both IgM and C1q have been observed in the endothelium of the hepatic artery of ABO incompatible grafts suggesting that ABH antigens could be expressed on the endothelia of the transplanted liver [52]. Thus, the immunological process related to ABO incompatibility may induce vascular injury resulting in ischemic lesions of the biliary tree. Second, the biliary tree is even more susceptible to ischemia in transplanted patients than in non-transplanted patients because the transplanted liver has been devascularized from all hepatic arteries entering the liver through capsule, which interrupts possible pathways for collateralization [2]. Third, CMV infection is likely responsible for ischemic damage to bile duct epithelia as CMV DNA has been found to be expressed in endothelial cells of small arteries near bile duct lesions [53]. Furthermore, CMV infection has been associated with late hepatic artery thrombosis [54]. Thus, different processes for arterial injury can combine, resulting in bile duct damage following liver transplantation, strongly suggesting that ischemia is the main pathophysiological mechanism responsible for bile duct lesions after liver transplantation.

The mechanisms implicated in other conditions associated with definite ischemic cholangiopathy have been reviewed in detail elsewhere [2].

## Conditions Associated with Possible Ischemic Cholangiopathy

Conditions associated with possible ischemic cholangiopathy comprise diseases in which biliary involvement due to microvascular injury is plausible but not proven. This group includes post-cholecystectomy strictures [55–58], systemic diseases with microvascular involvement such as sickle cell disease [59], Kawasaki disease [60], Schönlein-Henoch purpura [61], systemic lupus [62–65], antiphospholipid syndrome [66], paroxysmal nocturnal hemoglobinuria [67], hypereosinophilic syndrome [68], and cholangiopathy occurring after a prolonged stay in intensive care [69–73]. In these conditions, lesions of the vessels providing blood to the bile ducts have not been reported. However, most of these conditions are characterized by several patho-physiological mechanisms that may induce ischemia or damage to small hepatic arteries and, thus, blood deprivation to the bile ducts leading to ischemic lesions.

Cholangiopathy occurring after a prolonged stay in intensive care has been identified only in recent years. One reason why cholangiopathy occurring after a prolonged stay in intensive care is increasingly recognized is probably related to the more frequent use of aggressive reanimation techniques in more compromised patients that survive long enough to develop ischemic bile duct lesions. Although other mechanisms may explain bile duct damage, several lines of evidence indicate that ischemia plays an important role in bile duct lesions. First, severe hemodynamic instability that compromises the blood supply to many organs has been observed in most of the patients with this condition [73]. Second, all patients received high doses of vasopressors which reduces splanchnic blood flow [73, 74]. Third, most of the patients experienced a long duration of mechanical ventilation, often with the need for an inspired oxygen fraction greater than 80% and with lung protective mechanical ventilation (low tidal volume, prone positioning, high positive end-expiratory pressure), which may further decrease splanchnic blood flow [70, 74].

Cholangiopathy occurring after a prolonged stay in intensive care usually has a poor prognosis (see below). Most patients have rapid progression to cirrhosis overs weeks or months and a significant proportion of them die during the intensive care stay [75]. However, patients surviving beyond the intensive care period may have few or no symptoms. In a recent series of 16 critically ill patients surviving beyond the intensive care period, most patients had jaundice but other had only cholestasis without jaundice or even normal liver tests, which suggests that this type of cholangiopathy may still be underrecognized [76].

When a liver biopsy is performed, morphological changes are usually nonspecific and include peribiliary inflammatory infiltrates and cholestatic features with or without fibrosis or cirrhosis. Overall, these findings are suggestive of biliary obstruction but they are not indicative of an ischemic injury as occlusion of small hepatic arteries has usually not been observed. In a single case, the arteries supplying damaged bile ducts showed sclerosing arteriopathy with intimal fibrous thickening and narrowing of the lumina [70]. This observation brings additional evidence that a conjunction of features susceptible to compromise arterial blood supply to the bile ducts may induce bile duct ischemic damage during a prolonged stay in intensive care.

The mechanisms implicated in other conditions associated with possible ischemic cholangiopathy have been reviewed in detail elsewhere [2].

## Clinical, Laboratory, Radiological, and Histological Findings Associated with Ischemic Cholangiopathy

Manifestations of ischemic cholangiopathy are closely related to the speed and the extent of hepatic arterial involvement and to the stage of the disease [38]. In the acute stage, bile duct necrosis and biliary casts are frequently observed. Clinical manifestations include pain, fever, and jaundice, with or without signs of bacterial cholangitis or multi-organ failure. At this stage, laboratory examinations show features of cholestasis and/or sepsis, and radiological findings show intra-hepatic defects due to biliary casts, dilated bile ducts, and/or biloma corresponding to collections of necrotic bile-stained material (Fig. 3.1).

Latter stages are characterized by biliary strictures responsible for jaundice, itching, or bacterial cholangitis. Some patients may be pauci-symptomatic or even asymptomatic. If biliary obstruction persists, secondary biliary cirrhosis may occur. Laboratory findings are consistent with bile duct obstruction and radiological findings include diffuse and/or multiple stenosis of the bile duct, often localized to the middle third of the common bile duct or to the biliary confluence, the parts of the biliary tree most vulnerable to ischemic damage (Fig. 3.2) [77–79].

When a histological examination is performed, desquamation of the necrotic epithelium may be observed at the acute stage, as well as biliary casts, biloma and, in case of abrupt interruption of the arterial blood flow, necrosis of the bile duct wall. At latter stages, features associated with bile duct obstruction, ductopenia, and/or biliary fibrosis or cirrhosis can be seen. Due to the heterogeneous distribution of the lesions, a liver biopsy often fails to sample tissues where lesions of arterial blood vessels supplying the bile ducts are located [38]. On some occasions, damage of small arteries located near bile duct lesions provide evidence to support the ischemic pathophysiological mechanism of the bile duct injury.

## Differential Diagnosis

Ischemic cholangiopathy should be differentiated from cholestasis occurring during ischemic conditions [80–83]. In this circumstance, expression of hepatocellular transporters for biliary compounds is reduced in the absence of bile duct lesions. The differential diagnosis between impaired bile formation during ischemic

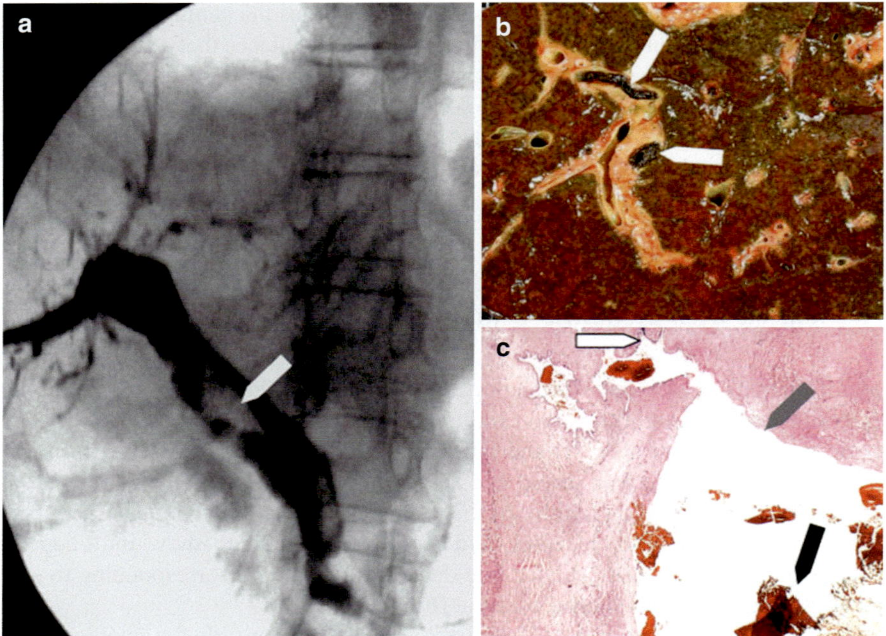

**Fig. 3.1** Biliary casts. (**a**) Typical appearance on endoscopic retrograde cholangiopancreatography in a patient with ischemic cholangiopathy following liver transplantation. Filling defects (white arrow) can be seen in dilated bile ducts, with mildly irregular margins. (**b**) Gross appearance at sectioning in an excised liver. Solid brown material can be seen within large bile ducts (white arrows). (**c**) Microscopic appearance of a large bile duct. Biliary epithelium is lacking in some areas (gray arrow) and is preserved in other areas (white arrow). Solid, bile-stained material is observed within the lumen (black arrow). (Courtesy of Dr. Annie Sibert, Service de Radiologie, and Dr. Valérie Paradis, Service d'Anatomie et de Cytologie pathologiques, Hôpital Beaujon, Clichy, France)

conditions and ischemic cholangiopathy is usually not a matter of concern with the exception of unstable circulatory states that require high doses of catecholamines in patients with prolonged stays in intensive care in which both diseases may be encountered. In this situation, imaging of the bile ducts using magnetic resonance cholangiopancreatography can lead to the right diagnosis.

For patients presenting with bile duct stenosis, differential diagnosis should be made for primary sclerosing cholangitis, IgG4 cholangiopathy, and cholangiocarcinoma [38]. If the diagnosis is quite easy in the context of a disease that is known to cause injury to bile duct vessels, it may be much more difficult in the absence of such a context. Of note, biliary casts have not been reported in cases of primary biliary sclerosis and in IgG4 cholangiopathy [71, 72]. When biliary lesions only consist of strictures, the localization of bile duct lesions to the middle third of the common bile duct or on the biliary confluence is an argument suggesting the ischemic nature of the bile duct injury. Aside from bile duct lesions, imaging techniques allow for the identification of thrombosis of the main hepatic arteries, which should always be looked at in liver-transplant recipients, although a patent artery does not rule out the

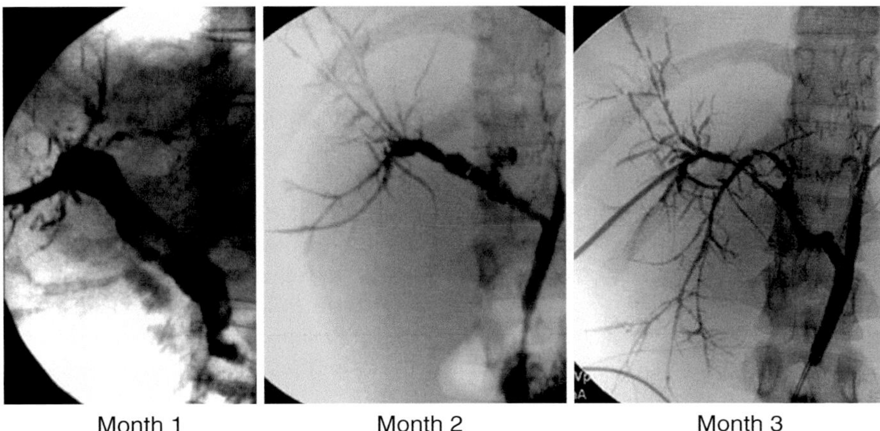



**Fig. 3.2** Course of cholangiographic appearance in a patient with hepatic artery thrombosis following liver transplantation. Treatment consisted of thrombolytic therapy and stenting of the hepatic artery. Month 1: Biliary casts. Months 2 and 3: Progressive development of diffuse stenoses, mimicking primary sclerosing cholangitis. (Courtesy Dr. Annie Sibert, Service de Radiologie, Hôpital Beaujon, Clichy, France)

---

Clinical context of pain, fever, and jaundice, with or without signs of bacterial cholangitis and presence of a condition that may compromise bile duct blood supply

↓

Exclusion of cholestasis occurring during ischemic conditions

↓

Laboratory findings consistent with biliary obstruction and/or bacterial cholangitis

↓

Imaging techniques showing bile duct necrosis, biliary casts, bilomas in casesof acute stage disease, or diffuse and/or multiple stenosis of the bile duct in chronic stages, preferentially localized in the middle third of the common bile duct or on the biliary confluence

↓

Liver biopsy in cases of uncertain diagnosis

↓

Established or probable ischemic cholangiopathy according to the condition suspected to be involved in the damage of the bile duct blood supply

---

**Fig. 3.3** Proposed algorithm for diagnosing ischemic cholangiopathy

diagnosis ischemic cholangiopathy. A liver biopsy may be required in cases of uncertain diagnosis, such as for ruling out cholangiocarcinoma, for example. An algorithm for diagnosing ischemic cholangiopathy is proposed in Fig. 3.3.

## Prognosis and Available Therapeutic Options

The outcomes of patients with ischemic cholangiopathy depends on the rapidity and the extent of the injury to the bile duct blood supply and on the underlying disease [38]. Prognostic data are very limited for many conditions associated with ischemic cholangiopathy. Within the particular context of ischemic cholangiopathy following liver transplantation, mortality rates vary between 23% and 55% [13, 38–40]. Up to 30% of these patients require re-transplantation. Donations that were made after cardiac death carry higher rates of graft failure due to ischemic biliary lesions compared to donations that were made after brain death [42, 45]. The prognosis for patients with ischemic cholangiopathy occurring after septic shock has been recently reviewed [71]. This condition is associated with rapid progression to cirrhosis and poor survival rates without liver transplantation [75]. Mortality rates higher than 50% have been reported in some series and only a few patients were eligible for liver transplantation. When transplanted, the survival rate at 1 year is 85%, comparable with that of patients transplanted for other reasons.

Outside the very rare situation in which a therapeutic option is available for the causal condition, therapeutic modalities aim to deal with biliary complications of the disease [38]. In rare instances, therapies aiming at restoring the arterial supply to the bile ducts may be attempted. This is especially indicated in cases of main hepatic artery thrombosis in a liver-transplant recipient. In this situation, thrombolysis, anticoagulation therapy, and/or angioplasty may be considered [38]. Antiplatelet or anticoagulant therapy may also be indicated. When small arteries are involved in the injury process, available options are much more limited. Antibiotics are needed in bacterial cholangitis and endoscopic and/or percutaneous procedures are often required to remove biliary casts and to treat strictures that are accessible. Surgical procedures may be needed for bile duct reconstruction. These procedures consist of various surgical anastomoses on the larger bile ducts, often at the hepatic confluence, a site that is frequently involved in cases of ischemic damage. Ideally, these procedures should not compromise liver transplantation which remains the last therapeutic option for patients with the most severe forms of bile duct injury that make surgical reconstruction impossible, or with decompensated secondary biliary cirrhosis.

Attention should also be given to strategies reducing the incidence of ischemic biliary lesions in circumstances at risk for ischemic damage of the bile ducts. This is the case for patients who require intraarterial infusion of toxic agents to treat liver metastases. As the risk of ischemic damage to the bile ducts seems to be particularly high after intra-arterial chemotherapy in combination with embolization, this association should be avoided [2]. Preventive strategies can also be useful to prevent ischemic cholangiopathy following liver transplantation, especially after circulatory death donation. Recent data indicate that, in cases of donation after circulatory death, the use of machine preservation systems could reduce the risk of ischemic cholangiopathy [84–86]. In the same line, the use of a protocol that includes thrombolytic therapy administered into the donor hepatic artery at the time of portal vein reperfusion also reduces the incidence of ischemic biliary lesions and allows more frequent effective endoscopic management than that without thrombolysis [43]. Although these results need to be confirmed in further studies, these approaches may constitute an attractive way to prevent ischemic bile duct injury following liver transplantation.

For asymptomatic or pauci-symptomatic patients, no therapeutic intervention may be required and observation seems a reasonable option [38].

An algorithm for the management of ischemic cholangiopathy is proposed in Fig. 3.4.

## Conclusion

Hepatic artery occlusion mainly affects the bile ducts. Ischemic cholangiopathy may be observed in various conditions in which an injury to the bile duct blood supply may occur. Circumstances in which vascular lesions could contribute to bile duct injury should be ruled out when primary sclerosing cholangitis, IgG4 cholangiopathy, or cholangiocarcinoma are suspected. Prognosis depends on the rapidity and the extent of the injury to bile duct blood supply. Endoscopic, percutaneous, and surgical procedures are the main therapeutic options for treating bile duct complications. Liver transplantation is the only therapeutic option in cases of diffuse involvement or decompensated biliary cirrhosis.

| Preventive therapies in conditions in which such an approach is feasible (Avoidance of the use of intra-arterial chemotherapy in combination with embolization for the treatment of liver metastases, strategies aiming at improving liver function in case of donation after circulatory death for liver transplantation) |
| --- |

↓

| Therapies aimed at restoring blood supply to the bile ducts (thrombolytic therapy in acute thrombosis of the main hepatic artery, angioplasty, antiplatelet, and/or anticoagulant therapy) |
| --- |

↓

| Antibiotics for septic complications |
| --- |

↓

| Endoscopic, percutaneous, and/or surgical procedures aimed at correcting bile duct lesions (percutaneous drainage of obstructed bile ducts, endoscopic removal of biliary casts or stones, dilatation or stenting of main biliary strictures, hepaticojejunostomy, various surgical bilioenteric anastomoses) |
| --- |

↓

| Liver transplantationin cases of recurrent complications due to impossible bile duct reconstruction or in cases of decompensated secondary biliary cirrhosis |
| --- |

**Fig. 3.4** Proposed algorithm for managing ischemic cholangiopathy

**Competing Interests** The author declares he has no competing interests.

**Writing Assistance** The author acknowledges the contribution of Sandy Field, Ph.D., for her assistance concerning English-language editing.

# References

1. Takasaki S, Hano H. Three-dimensional observations of the human hepatic artery (Arterial system in the liver). J Hepatol. 2001;34(3):455–66.
2. Deltenre P, Valla DC. Ischemic cholangiopathy. J Hepatol. 2006;44(4):806–17.
3. Terblanche J, Allison HF, Northover JM. An ischemic basis for biliary strictures. Surgery. 1983;94(1):52–7.
4. Northover JM, Terblanche J. A new look at the arterial supply of the bile duct in man and its surgical implications. Br J Surg. 1979;66(6):379–84.
5. Fisher A, Miller CH. Ischemic-type biliary strictures in liver allografts: the Achilles heel revisited? Hepatology. 1995;21(2):589–91.
6. Bengmark S, Rosengren K. Angiographic study of the collateral circulation to the liver after ligation of the hepatic artery in man. Am J Surg. 1970;119(6):620–4.
7. Koehler RE, Korobkin M, Lewis F. Arteriographic demonstration of collateral arterial supply to the liver after hepatic artery ligation. Radiology. 1975;117(1):49–54.
8. Mays ET, Wheeler CS. Demonstration of collateral arterial flow after interruption of hepatic arteries in man. N Engl J Med. 1974;290(18):993–6.
9. Redman HC, Reuter SR. Arterial collaterals in the liver hilus. Radiology. 1970;94(3):575–9.
10. Demachi H, Matsui O, Kawamori Y, Ueda K, Takashima T. The protective effect of portoarterial shunts after experimental hepatic artery embolization in rats with liver cirrhosis. Cardiovasc Intervent Radiol. 1995;18(2):97–101.
11. Cameron AM, Busuttil RW. Ischemic cholangiopathy after liver transplantation. Hepatobiliary Pancreat Dis Int. 2005;4(4):495–501.
12. Pascher A, Neuhaus P. Bile duct complications after liver transplantation. Transpl Int. 2005;18(6):627–42.
13. Roos FJM, Poley JW, Polak WG, Metselaar HJ. Biliary complications after liver transplantation; recent developments in etiology, diagnosis and endoscopic treatment. Best Pract Res Clin Gastroenterol. 2017;31(2):227–35.
14. Abbasoglu O, Levy MF, Vodapally MS, Goldstein RM, Husberg BS, Gonwa TA, et al. Hepatic artery stenosis after liver transplantation—incidence, presentation, treatment, and long term outcome. Transplantation. 1997;63(2):250–5.
15. Valente JF, Alonso MH, Weber FL, Hanto DW. Late hepatic artery thrombosis in liver allograft recipients is associated with intrahepatic biliary necrosis. Transplantation. 1996;61(1):61–5.
16. Hohn DC, Stagg RJ, Friedman MA, Hannigan JF Jr, Rayner A, Ignoffo RJ, et al. A randomized trial of continuous intravenous versus hepatic intraarterial floxuridine in patients with colorectal cancer metastatic to the liver: the northern California oncology group trial. J Clin Oncol. 1989;7(11):1646–54.
17. Iwata M, Sasaki M, Harada K, Kaneko S, Kobayashi K, Adachi K, et al. Intrahepatic cholangitis and arteritis after transcatheter arterial embolization in a patient with tumor-like lesion-associated autoimmune hepatitis. Pathol Res Pract. 2001;197(1):59–63.
18. Kemeny N, Daly J, Reichman B, Geller N, Botet J, Oderman P. Intrahepatic or systemic infusion of fluorodeoxyuridine in patients with liver metastases from colorectal carcinoma. A randomized trial. Ann Intern Med. 1987;107(4):459–65.
19. Kemeny N, Huang Y, Cohen AM, Shi W, Conti JA, Brennan MF, et al. Hepatic arterial infusion of chemotherapy after resection of hepatic metastases from colorectal cancer. N Engl J Med. 1999;341(27):2039–48.

20. Kemeny N, Seiter K, Niedzwiecki D, Chapman D, Sigurdson E, Cohen A, et al. A randomized trial of intrahepatic infusion of fluorodeoxyuridine with dexamethasone versus fluorodeoxyuridine alone in the treatment of metastatic colorectal cancer. Cancer. 1992;69(2):327–34.
21. Cello JP. Acquired immunodeficiency syndrome cholangiopathy: spectrum of disease. Am J Med. 1989;86(5):539–46.
22. Golden MP, Hammer SM, Wanke CA, Albrecht MA. Cytomegalovirus vasculitis. Case reports and review of the literature. Medicine (Baltimore). 1994;73(5):246–55.
23. Margulis SJ, Honig CL, Soave R, Govoni AF, Mouradian JA, Jacobson IM. Biliary tract obstruction in the acquired immunodeficiency syndrome. Ann Intern Med. 1986;105(2):207–10.
24. Morgello S, Cho ES, Nielsen S, Devinsky O, Petito CK. Cytomegalovirus encephalitis in patients with acquired immunodeficiency syndrome: an autopsy study of 30 cases and a review of the literature. Hum Pathol. 1987;18(3):289–97.
25. Schneiderman DJ, Arenson DM, Cello JP, Margaretten W, Weber TE. Hepatic disease in patients with the acquired immune deficiency syndrome (AIDS). Hepatology. 1987;7(5):925–30.
26. Viteri AL, Greene JF Jr. Bile duct abnormalities in the acquired immune deficiency syndrome. Gastroenterology. 1987;92(6):2014–8.
27. Bauer T, Britton P, Lomas D, Wight DG, Friend PJ, Alexander GJ. Liver transplantation for hepatic arteriovenous malformation in hereditary haemorrhagic telangiectasia. J Hepatol. 1995;22(5):586–90.
28. Blewitt RW, Brown CM, Wyatt JI. The pathology of acute hepatic disintegration in hereditary haemorrhagic telangiectasia. Histopathology. 2003;42(3):265–9.
29. Garcia-Tsao G, Korzenik JR, Young L, Henderson KJ, Jain D, Byrd B, et al. Liver disease in patients with hereditary hemorrhagic telangiectasia. N Engl J Med. 2000;343(13):931–6.
30. Chandrasekhara KL, Iyer SK. Obstructive jaundice due to radiation-induced hepatic duct stricture. Am J Med. 1984;77(4):723–4.
31. Cherqui D, Palazzo L, Piedbois P, Charlotte F, Duvoux C, Duron JJ, et al. Common bile duct stricture as a late complication of upper abdominal radiotherapy. J Hepatol. 1994;20(6):693–7.
32. Barquist ES, Goldstein N, Zinner MJ. Polyarteritis nodosa presenting as a biliary stricture. Surgery. 1991;109(1):16–9.
33. Griffith GC, Vural IL. A correlation of clinical and postmortem findings in seventeen cases. Circulation. 1951;3(4):481–91.
34. Reidbord HE, McCormack LJ, O'Duffy JD. Necrotizing angiitis. II. Findings at autopsy in twenty-seven cases. Cleve Clin Q. 1965;32(4):191–204.
35. Char D, Mohan E, George R, Gambarin S. Common bile duct necrosis after cardiac catheterization. Am J Gastroenterol. 1998;93(12):2597–8.
36. Hashikura Y, Makuuchi M, Kawasaki S, Miwa S, Kobayashi A, Imai Y, et al. Benign stricture of the intrahepatic bile duct with arterial involvement. Hepato-Gastroenterology. 1994;41(1):79–81.
37. Saiura A, Umekita N, Inoue S, Maeshiro T, Miyamoto S, Matsui Y, et al. Benign biliary stricture associated with atherosclerosis. Hepato-Gastroenterology. 2001;48(37):81–2.
38. Deltenre P, Valla DC. Ischemic cholangiopathy. Semin Liver Dis. 2008;28(3):235–46.
39. Fujiki M, Hashimoto K, Palaios E, Quintini C, Aucejo FN, Uso TD, et al. Probability, management, and long-term outcomes of biliary complications after hepatic artery thrombosis in liver transplant recipients. Surgery. 2017;162(5):1101–11.
40. Dominguez Bastante M, Molina Raya A, Vilchez Rabelo A, Villar Del Moral J, Exposito Ruiz M, Fundora SY. Analysis of ischemic cholangiopathy after treatment of arterial thrombosis in liver transplantation in our series. Transplant Proc. 2018;50(2):628–30.
41. Chan EY, Olson LC, Kisthard JA, Perkins JD, Bakthavatsalam R, Halldorson JB, et al. Ischemic cholangiopathy following liver transplantation from donation after cardiac death donors. Liver Transpl. 2008;14(5):604–10.
42. O'Neill S, Roebuck A, Khoo E, Wigmore SJ, Harrison EM. A meta-analysis and meta-regression of outcomes including biliary complications in donation after cardiac death liver transplantation. Transpl Int. 2014;27(11):1159–74.
43. Bohorquez H, Seal JB, Cohen AJ, Kressel A, Bugeaud E, Bruce DS, et al. Safety and outcomes in 100 consecutive donation after circulatory death liver transplants using a protocol that includes thrombolytic therapy. Am J Transplant. 2017;17(8):2155–64.

44. DeOliveira ML, Jassem W, Valente R, Khorsandi SE, Santori G, Prachalias A, et al. Biliary complications after liver transplantation using grafts from donors after cardiac death: results from a matched control study in a single large volume center. Ann Surg. 2011;254(5):716–22. discussion 22-3

45. Jay CL, Lyuksemburg V, Ladner DP, Wang E, Caicedo JC, Holl JL, et al. Ischemic cholangiopathy after controlled donation after cardiac death liver transplantation: a meta-analysis. Ann Surg. 2011;253(2):259–64.

46. Detry O, Donckier V, Lucidi V, Ysebaert D, Chapelle T, Lerut J, et al. Liver transplantation from donation after cardiac death donors: initial Belgian experience 2003-2007. Transpl Int. 2010;23(6):611–8.

47. Hesselink EJ, Klompmaker IJ, Pruim J, van Schilfgaarde R, Slooff MJ. Hepatic artery thrombosis after orthotopic liver transplantation—a fatal complication or an asymptomatic event. Transplant Proc. 1989;21(1 Pt 2):2462.

48. Wozney P, Zajko AB, Bron KM, Point S, Starzl TE. Vascular complications after liver transplantation: a 5-year experience. AJR Am J Roentgenol. 1986;147(4):657–63.

49. Sebagh M, Farges O, Kalil A, Samuel D, Bismuth H, Reynes M. Sclerosing cholangitis following human orthotopic liver transplantation. Am J Surg Pathol. 1995;19(1):81–90.

50. Sanchez-Urdazpal L, Batts KP, Gores GJ, Moore SB, Sterioff S, Wiesner RH, et al. Increased bile duct complications in liver transplantation across the ABO barrier. Ann Surg. 1993;218(2):152–8.

51. Sanchez-Urdazpal L, Sterioff S, Janes C, Schwerman L, Rosen C, Krom RA. Increased bile duct complications in ABO incompatible liver transplant recipients. Transplant Proc. 1991;23(1 Pt 2):1440–1.

52. Demetris AJ, Jaffe R, Tzakis A, Ramsey G, Todo S, Belle S, et al. Antibody mediated rejection of human liver allografts: transplantation across ABO blood group barriers. Transplant Proc. 1989;21(1 Pt 2):2217–20.

53. Lautenschlager I, Hockerstedt K, Jalanko H, Loginov R, Salmela K, Taskinen E, et al. Persistent cytomegalovirus in liver allografts with chronic rejection. Hepatology. 1997;25(1):190–4.

54. Gunsar F, Rolando N, Pastacaldi S, Patch D, Raimondo ML, Davidson B, et al. Late hepatic artery thrombosis after orthotopic liver transplantation. Liver Transpl. 2003;9(6):605–11.

55. Alves A, Farges O, Nicolet J, Watrin T, Sauvanet A, Belghiti J. Incidence and consequence of an hepatic artery injury in patients with postcholecystectomy bile duct strictures. Ann Surg. 2003;238(1):93–6.

56. Bismuth H, Lazorthes F. 83rd congress of the French surgical society (Paris, 21-24 September 1981). Second report. Operative injuries of the common biliary duct. J Chir (Paris). 1981;118(10):601–9.

57. Chen WJ, Ying DJ, Liu ZJ, He ZP. Analysis of the arterial supply of the extrahepatic bile ducts and its clinical significance. Clin Anat. 1999;12(4):245–9.

58. Northover J, Terblanche J. Bile duct blood supply. Its importance in human liver transplantation. Transplantation. 1978;26(1):67–9.

59. Hillaire S, Gardin C, Attar A, Attassi M, Terris B, Belghiti J, et al. Cholangiopathy and intrahepatic stones in sickle cell disease: coincidence or ischemic cholangiopathy? Am J Gastroenterol. 2000;95(1):300–1.

60. Gear JH, Meyers KE, Steele M. Kawasaki disease manifesting with acute cholangitis. A case report. S Afr Med J. 1992;81(1):31–3.

61. Viola S, Meyer M, Fabre M, Tounian P, Goddon R, Dechelotte P, et al. Ischemic necrosis of bile ducts complicating Schonlein-Henoch purpura. Gastroenterology. 1999;117(1):211–4.

62. Alberti-Flor JJ, Jeffers L, Schiff ER. Primary sclerosing cholangitis occurring in a patient with systemic lupus erythematosus and diabetes mellitus. Am J Gastroenterol. 1984;79(11):889–91.

63. Lamy P, Valla D, Bourgeois P, Rueff B, Benhamou JP. Primary sclerosing cholangitis and systemic lupus erythematosus. Gastroenterol Clin Biol. 1988;12(12):962–4.

64. Audan A, Bruley Des Varannes S, Georgelin T, Sagan C, Cloarec D, Serraz H, et al. Primary sclerosing cholangitis and systemic lupus erythematosus. Gastroenterol Clin Biol. 1995;19(1):123–6.

65. Heyman SN, Spectre G, Aamar S, Rubinger D, Pappo O, Ackerman Z. Autoimmune cholangiopathy associated with systemic lupus erythematosus. Liver. 2002;22(2):102–6.

66. Kirby DF, Blei AT, Rosen ST, Vogelzang RL, Neiman HL. Primary sclerosing cholangitis in the presence of a lupus anticoagulant. Am J Med. 1986;81(6):1077–80.

67. Le Thi HD, Valla D, Franco D, Wechsler B, De Gramont A, Auperin A, et al. Cholangitis associated with paroxysmal nocturnal hemoglobinuria: another instance of ischemic cholangiopathy? Gastroenterology. 1995;109(4):1338–43.

68. Scheurlen M, Mork H, Weber P. Hypereosinophilic syndrome resembling chronic inflammatory bowel disease with primary sclerosing cholangitis. J Clin Gastroenterol. 1992;14(1):59–63.

69. Engler S, Elsing C, Flechtenmacher C, Theilmann L, Stremmel W, Stiehl A. Progressive sclerosing cholangitis after septic shock: a new variant of vanishing bile duct disorders. Gut. 2003;52(5):688–93.

70. Gelbmann CM, Rummele P, Wimmer M, Hofstadter F, Gohlmann B, Endlicher E, et al. Ischemic-like cholangiopathy with secondary sclerosing cholangitis in critically ill patients. Am J Gastroenterol. 2007;102(6):1221–9.

71. Gudnason HO, Bjornsson ES. Secondary sclerosing cholangitis in critically ill patients: current perspectives. Clin Exp Gastroenterol. 2017;10:105–11.

72. Leonhardt S, Veltzke-Schlieker W, Adler A, Schott E, Eurich D, Faber W, et al. Secondary sclerosing cholangitis in critically ill patients: clinical presentation, cholangiographic features, natural history, and outcome: a series of 16 cases. Medicine (Baltimore). 2015;94(49):e2188.

73. Leonhardt S, Veltzke-Schlieker W, Adler A, Schott E, Hetzer R, Schaffartzik W, et al. Trigger mechanisms of secondary sclerosing cholangitis in critically ill patients. Crit Care. 2015;19:131.

74. Lin T, Qu K, Xu X, Tian M, Gao J, Zhang C, et al. Sclerosing cholangitis in critically ill patients: an important and easily ignored problem based on a German experience. Front Med. 2014;8(1):118–26.

75. Martins P, Verdelho MM. Secondary sclerosing cholangitis in critically ill patients: an underdiagnosed entity. GE Port J Gastroenterol. 2020;27(2):103–14.

76. Laurent L, Lemaitre C, Minello A, Plessier A, Lamblin G, Poujol-Robert A, et al. Cholangiopathy in critically ill patients surviving beyond the intensive care period: a multicentre survey in liver units. Aliment Pharmacol Ther. 2017;46(11–12):1070–6.

77. Aldrighetti L, Arru M, Ronzoni M, Salvioni M, Villa E, Ferla G. Extrahepatic biliary stenoses after hepatic arterial infusion (HAI) of floxuridine (FUdR) for liver metastases from colorectal cancer. Hepato-Gastroenterology. 2001;48(41):1302–7.

78. Hohn D, Melnick J, Stagg R, Altman D, Friedman M, Ignoffo R, et al. Biliary sclerosis in patients receiving hepatic arterial infusions of floxuridine. J Clin Oncol. 1985;3(1):98–102.

79. Shea WJ Jr, Demas BE, Goldberg HI, Hohn DC, Ferrell LD, Kerlan RK. Sclerosing cholangitis associated with hepatic arterial FUDR chemotherapy: radiographic-histologic correlation. AJR Am J Roentgenol. 1986;146(4):717–21.

80. Geier A, Fickert P, Trauner M. Mechanisms of disease: mechanisms and clinical implications of cholestasis in sepsis. Nat Clin Pract Gastroenterol Hepatol. 2006;3(10):574–85.

81. Trauner M, Fickert P, Stauber RE. Inflammation-induced cholestasis. J Gastroenterol Hepatol. 1999;14(10):946–59.

82. Fouassier L, Beaussier M, Schiffer E, Rey C, Barbu V, Mergey M, et al. Hypoxia-induced changes in the expression of rat hepatobiliary transporter genes. Am J Physiol Gastrointest Liver Physiol. 2007;293(1):G25–35.

83. Wagner M, Zollner G, Trauner M. Ischemia and cholestasis: more than (just) the bile ducts! Transplantation. 2008;85(8):1083–5.

84. De Carlis R, Di Sandro S, Lauterio A, Ferla F, Dell'Acqua A, Zanierato M, et al. Successful donation after cardiac death liver transplants with prolonged warm ischemia time using normothermic regional perfusion. Liver Transpl. 2017;23(2):166–73.

85. Dutkowski P, Polak WG, Muiesan P, Schlegel A, Verhoeven CJ, Scalera I, et al. First comparison of hypothermic oxygenated perfusion versus static cold storage of human donation after cardiac death liver transplants: an international-matched case analysis. Ann Surg. 2015;262(5):764–70. discussion 70-1

86. Patrono D, Lavezzo B, Molinaro L, Rizza G, Catalano G, Gonella F, et al. Hypothermic oxygenated machine perfusion for liver transplantation: an initial experience. Exp Clin Transplant. 2018;16(2):172–6.

# Chapter 4
# Hepatic Vascular Malformations in Hereditary Hemorrhagic Telangiectasia

Elisabetta Buscarini, Guido Manfredi, and Saverio Alicante

**Hereditary hemorrhagic telangiectasia** (HHT) or Rendu-Osler-Weber disease is an autosomal dominant disorder characterized by widespread cutaneous, mucosal and visceral telangiectasias, with an estimated frequency of 1/5000. The pathophysiological mechanism appear to be the inability of a blood vessel to mature appropriately [1].

The primary lesion of HHT is the telangiectasia, arising from the dilation of a postcapillary venule that fuses directly with an arteriole, bypassing the capillary vessels.

Clinical presentation and prognosis varies greatly depending on the number, type and location of telangiectasias or vascular malformations (VMs) with their inherent potential morbidities and mortalities [2].

The clinical criteria for diagnosing HHT, the Curaçao criteria, were established by a panel of experts [3] (Table 4.1). Currently, five types of HHT are recognized.

Most HHT patients have mutations in one of two known disease-related genes, endoglin (ENG, HHT1) or activin A receptor type II-like 1 (ACVRL1, HHT2), which are both involved in the TGFβ pathway. One to two percent of cases have mutations in SMAD4; these mutations also cause the gastrointestinal epithelial precancerous state of juvenile polyposis [4]. There are at least two further unidentified genes [5–7].

All classical features of HHT can be seen in both HHT1 and HHT2, but the prevalence of specific vascular abnormalities varies according to genotype. Pulmonary AVMs are more common in HHT1 than in HHT2 [8, 9]. HHT1 patients are also more commonly affected by cerebral AVMs [10, 11], but have a lesser prevalence of hepatic AVMs [9–14].

E. Buscarini (✉) · G. Manfredi · S. Alicante
Gastroenterology Department, VASCERN HHT Reference Center, Maggiore Hospital, ASST Crema, Crema, Italy
e-mail: elisabetta.buscarini@asst-crema.it; guido.manfredi@asst-crema.it; saverio.alicante@asst-crema.it

© Springer Nature Switzerland AG 2022
D. Valla et al. (eds.), *Vascular Disorders of the Liver*,
https://doi.org/10.1007/978-3-030-82988-9_4

**Table 4.1** The Curaçao criteria [3][a]

| Criteria | |
| --- | --- |
| Epistaxis | Spontaneous, recurrent nosebleeds |
| Telangiectases | Multiple at characteristic sites (lips, oral cavity, fingers, nose) |
| Visceral lesions | Pulmonary VMs, liver VMs, cerebral VMs, spinal VMs, gastrointestinal telangiectases (with or without bleeding) |
| Family history | A first degree relative with HHT with these criteria |
| HHT diagnosis is | |
| Definite | if 3 criteria |
| Possible/ suspected | if 2 criteria |
| Unlikely | if fewer than 2 criteria |

[a]All offspring of an individual with HHT are at risk of having the disease since HHT may not manifest until late in life. If there is any concern regarding the presence of physical signs, an experienced physician should be consulted

## Liver VMs in HHT

Hepatic VMs are found in 41–74% of HHT patients [15, 16]. Hepatic VMs and severe disease due to hepatic VMs are significantly more frequent in the HHT2 genotype than in the HHT1 genotype [12–14]. The penetrance of HHT is age-related and the mean age of patients with hepatic VMs was 48 years [13, 15], and symptoms of hepatic VMs generally occur around age 50 [12, 15]. Data reported in the literature show a strong predominance of hepatic VMs in females with HHT, with a male/female ratio of 1/4.5.

## Pathogenesis

Hepatic VMs unique to HHT involve the liver diffusely and can evolve from small telangiectasias to large arteriovenous malformations. Three different and often concomitant types of intrahepatic shunting (hepatic artery to portal vein, hepatic artery to hepatic vein and/or portal vein to hepatic vein) can lead to different and potentially concomitant clinical features, including high-output cardiac failure (HOCF), portal hypertension (PH), encephalopathy, biliary ischemia and mesenteric ischemia; the latter two are due to a blood flow steal through arteriovenous shunting [17, 18].

Livers with HHT may show either diffuse or partial hepatocellular regenerative activity [19], leading to nodular regenerative hyperplasia or focal nodular hyperplasia, respectively.

It has recently been reported that the prevalence of focal nodular hyperplasia in patients with HHT is 100-fold greater than in general population [20]. The combination of fibrosis (around abnormal vessels), nodular regenerative hyperplasia and portal hypertension may lead to a misdiagnosis of cirrhosis. However, the liver involvement unique to HHT, is not cirrhosis and is not associated with liver insufficiency [17, 18, 20].

## Clinical Manifestations

Only 8% of patients with liver VMs are symptomatic at baseline, as shown by cross-sectional surveys [15, 16]. However, in a longitudinal cohort study regarding the disease course in 154 patients with a long follow-up (median 44 months, range 12–181), median survival was 175 months (24–181, 95% CI 66–283); along follow up 1% underwent OLT, 5% died, 21% had liver vascular malformations worsening, 25% had complications of liver VMs and 48% unchanged liver VMs; incidence of fatal outcome and of morbidity were 1.1 and 3.6% person/years respectively with a median event-free survival of 90 months (10–181, 95% CI 44–135). HOCF represents the predominant complication associated with HHT, but complicated PH occurs at a rate comparable to that of HOCF (1.4 and 1.2, per 100 person-years, respectively); HOCF and complicated PH each account for about half of hepatic VM–associated fatalities [13, 18]; none of those complications were observed in the control group represented by patients without liver VMs. In patients with chronic cardiac overload due to liver VMs atrial fibrillation had a 1.6 incidence rate per 100 person-years, suggesting that this arrhythmia in patients with liver VMs is not purely coincidental and should be approached with special caution [13]. Much rarer presentations of liver VMs in HHT are encephalopathy, mesenteric angina and ischemic cholangitis that can cause bilomas or more ominously lead to a catastrophic complication termed "hepatic disintegration" [18, 21–24].

Portal hypertension due to arterioportal shunts can manifest itself with severe recurrent variceal bleeding; however both a case series and a cohort study have shown that GI bleedings in patients with liver VMs were due rather to bleeding from GI telangiectasias than to variceal bleeding [13, 17].

Anicteric cholestasis is observed in one third of patients with liver VMs; its entity shows linear correlation with the severity of vascular malformations and their complications [13, 25, 26].

## Diagnosis of Liver VMs in HHT

Diffuse liver VMs are unique to HHT and their presence should always lead to the search of HHT diagnostic criteria.

Investigations for liver VMs are to be completed in HHT patients with symptoms/signs suggestive of complicated liver VMs.

Screening for hepatic AVMs in asymptomatic individuals with suspected or certain HHT has been recommended as there is a totally non-invasive and effective screening tool (Doppler US), and because a correct diagnosis can help to clarify the diagnosis of HHT and improve subsequent patient management [18, 24].

The diagnosis of liver involvement in HHT requires laboratory assessment and liver imaging. Echocardiographic evaluation is also recommended to estimate of hemodynamic impact of liver VMs. Further testing (either one or a combination of the following: GI endoscopy, CT, magnetic resonance, angiography, cardiac catheterization, portal pressure measurement with hepatic venous pressure gradient) may be required depending either on the presence of focal liver lesions or on the severity of liver VMs and their hemodynamic impact [18] (Fig. 4.1).

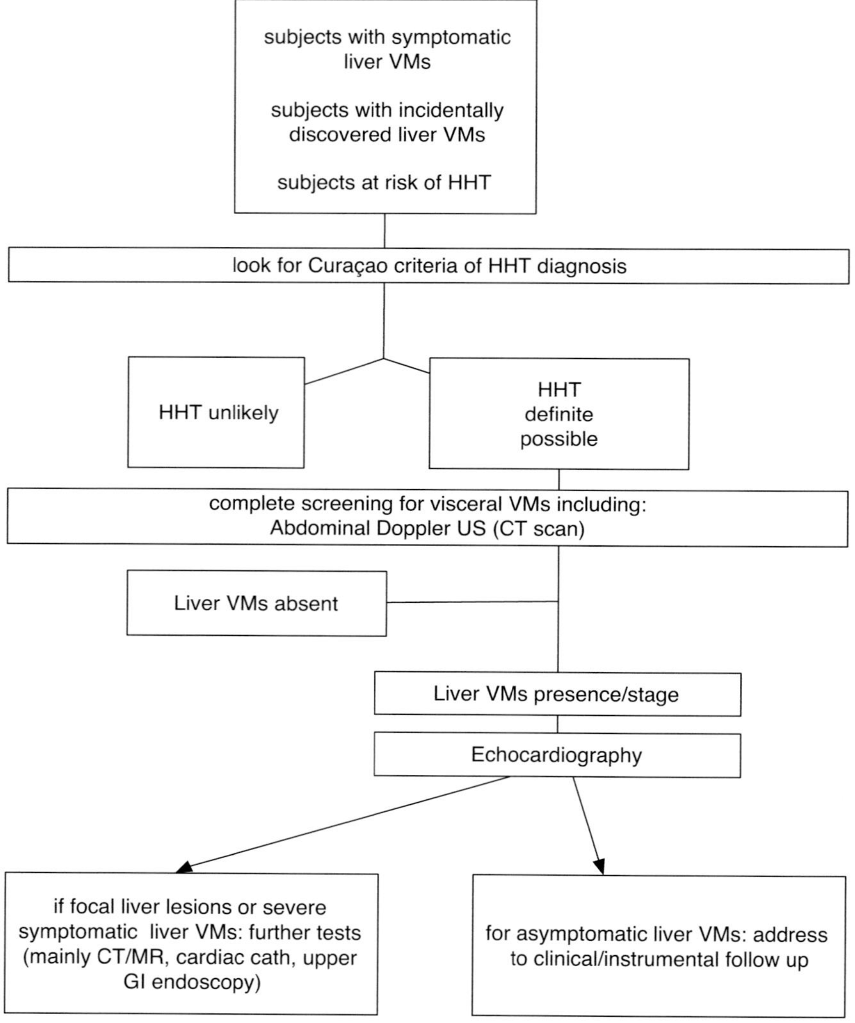


**Fig. 4.1** Diagnostic approach to liver VMs in HHT

## Doppler US Evaluation of Liver VMs in HHT

Doppler ultrasound (US) has been proposed as the ideal first-line investigation for the assessment of liver VMs due to its safety, tolerability, low costs and accuracy for the detection of liver VMs [18].

Doppler US findings of liver VMs in HHT have been reported since the 1990s [25, 27].

A combination of various features of liver VMs have been proposed as US criteria for the hepatic involvement in HHT. Anomalies of liver vessels have been classified with Doppler US according to the criteria proposed by Buscarini [15]; the combination of hepatic vessel abnormalities and anomalous flow patterns leads to a severity grading from 0.5 to 4 (Table 4.2) of liver VMs. Caselitz et al. [28] defined

**Table 4.2**  Doppler US grading of severity of hepatic VMs in HHT (modified, 15)

| VMs grade | scheme | Doppler US criteria |
|---|---|---|
| 0+ | ha | • HA diameter > 5 < 6 mm, and/or<br>• PFV > 80 cm/sec, and/or<br>• RI < 0.55, and/or<br>• Peripheral hepatic hypervascularization |
| 1 | ha | • HA dilatation, only extrahepatic >6 mm, and<br>• PFV > 80 cm/s, and/or<br>• RI < 0.55 |
| 2 | ha | • HA dilatation, extra- and intrahepatic ("double channel" aspect) and<br>• PFV > 80 cm/s<br>• Possibly associated with moderate flow abnormality of hepatic and/or portal veins |
| 3 | ha | • Complex changes in hepatic artery and its branches (tortuous and tangled) with marked flow abnormalities<br>• Abnormality of hepatic and/or portal vein flow |
| 4 | hv / pv | Decompensation of arteriovenous shunt associated with:<br>• Dilatation of hepatic and/or portal vein<br>• Marked flow abnormalities in both arteries and vein/s |

Veno-venous shunts may be found and do not imply a VM up-grading. Nodular transformation of hepatic parenchyma progresses along with liver VMs severity, and it is generally found in grade 4
*HA* hepatic artery, *PV* portal vein, *HV* hepatic vein

two major criteria for the dilated common hepatic artery >7 mm and intrahepatic arterial hypervascularization. The minor criteria are either Vmax in hepatic artery >110 cm/s, RI of the proper hepatic artery <0.60, Vmax of the portal vein >25 cm/s, or tortuous course of the extrahepatic hepatic artery. Two major criteria or one major and two minor criteria are required for the diagnosis of liver VMs in HHT.

Hepatic artery diameter >4 mm is accurate for differentiation of HHT patients with VMs from HHT patients without VMs, cirrhotic patients and normal subjects; this represents a very sensitive diagnostic parameter for hepatic VMs in HHT. The unique advantage of pulsed and color Doppler US over other imaging modalities is that it allows rapid analysis of the flow pattern of hepatic VMs, including: (1) qualitative parameters, such as flow direction and turbulence, (2) quantitative parameters, such as the angle-corrected flow velocities, and, (3) semiquantitative measures, such as the resistivity and pulsatility index [15, 28, 29] (Fig. 4.2).

Either hepatic artery to portal vein shunts or to hepatic veins cause changes in the Doppler waveform of the veins; the portal and/or hepatic veins are dilated in severe and decompensated liver arteriovenous shunt. Ascites can be associated with severe decompensated liver VMs (Figs. 4.3 and 4.4). Portosystemic shunts can also be found.

Liver size can be enlarged in liver VMs in HHT, whereas spleen is usually normal. US evaluation of liver parenchyma can show either focal isoechoic lesions compatible with FNH (Figs. 4.5 and 4.6) or, in more severe VMs, diffuse margin nodularity with a coarse heterogeneous echo pattern (Figs. 4.7 and 4.8).

The sensitivity of different Doppler US criteria [15, 28, 29] has been recently compared using CT or MR as the reference standard in a series of 18 patients; the Caselitz and Buonamico criteria missed 16% and 27% of liver VMs, respectively, whereas the Buscarini criteria [15] did not miss any liver VMs [30].

A controlled interobserver study showed very good interobserver agreement for Doppler US diagnosis of the presence/absence of liver VMs, with a K value of 0.85–0.93 [31].

The Doppler US classification of liver VMs [15, 32, 33] providing severity grading of hepatic VMs has been shown to be a predictor of clinical outcome [13], and it can be useful for tailoring patient management and follow-up [32, 33].


## Non invasive and Invasive Assessment of Cardiac Hemodynamics

Echocardiographic evaluation of cardiac function and morphology, particularly cardiac index and pulmonary arterial pressures, is crucial to estimate the haemodynamic impact of liver VMs, also allowing repeated evaluations during follow-up, in contrast with invasive measurement of cardiac hemodynamics by cardiac catheterization [25, 34]. Moreover, a close correlation has been demonstrated between echocardiography and cardiac catheterization in assessing cardiac output in a series of HHT patients with liver VMs [28].

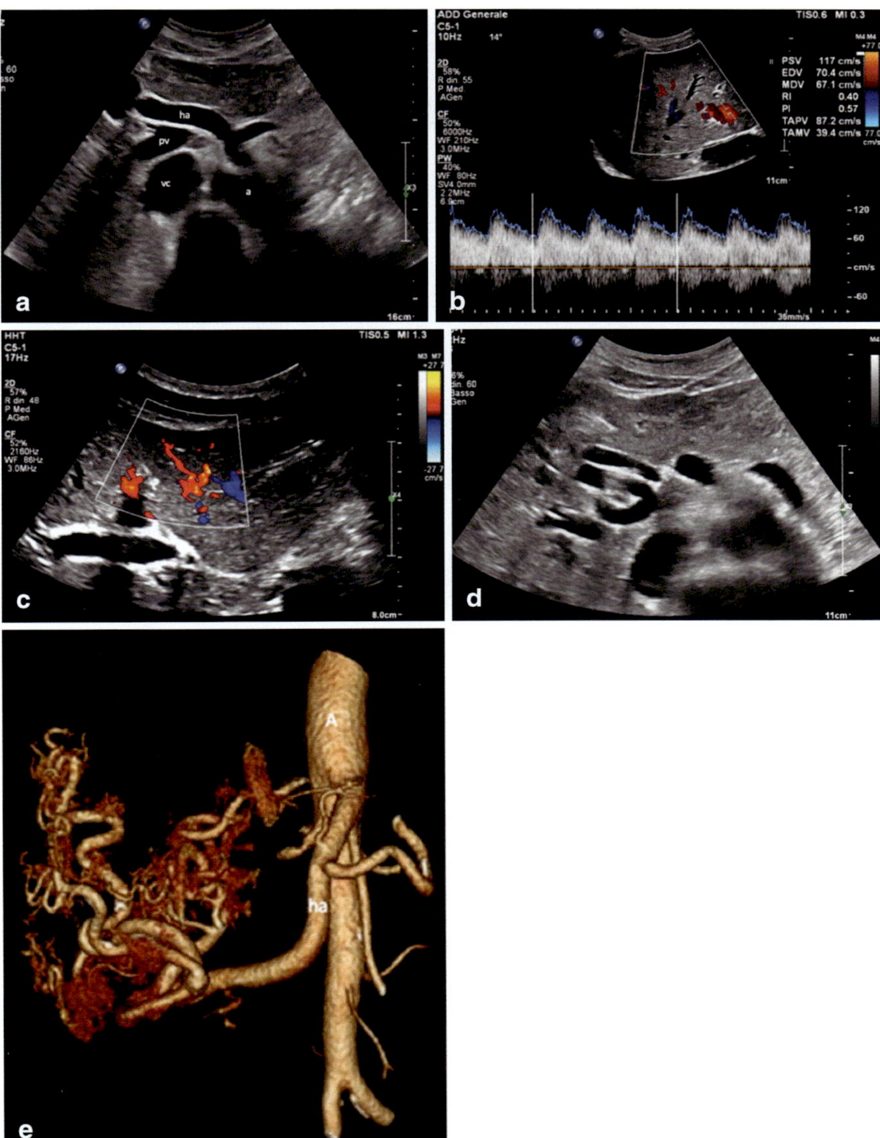

**Fig. 4.2** (**a**) Hepatic artery (ha) dilation is a typical hallmark of liver VMs in HHT; (**b**) Doppler US analysis of hepatic artery flow, in the hepatic artery, a very high Vmax with high diastolic phase and low RI is demonstrated; (**c**) Intrahepatic hypervascularization is demonstrated by color Doppler, with prominent peripheral arteries; (**d**) prominent intrahepatic branches of the hepatic artery; (**e**) Celiac angiogram obtained during CT, early arterial phase, shows dilated common hepatic artery with tangled and prominent intrahepatic branches. *Ha* hepatic artery, *vc* vena cava, *pv* portal vein, *a* aorta

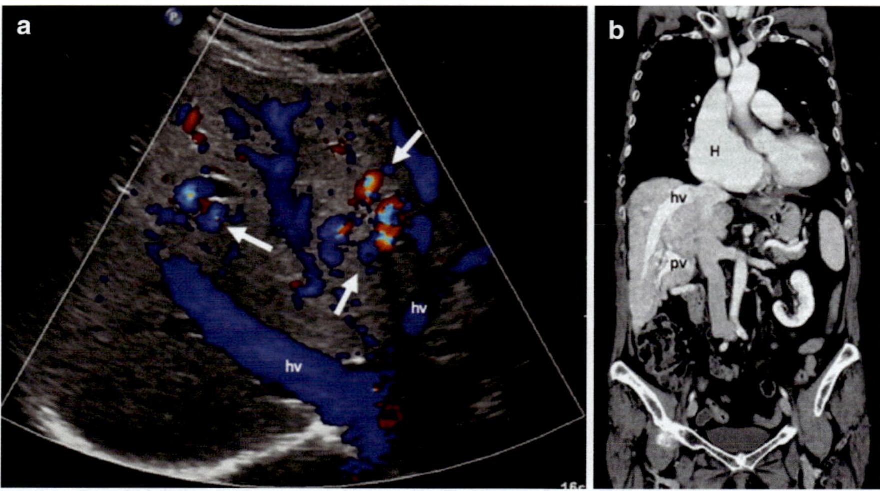



**Fig. 4.3** (**a**) Color Doppler US analysis in grade 4 liver VMs with predominant arteriohepatic shunt: tangled arterial branches (arrows) surrounding dilated hepatic vein (hv); (**b**) Triple-phase CT: markedly dilated hepatic veins (hv) in a patient with grade 4 liver VMs, predominantly arteriohepatic: note the substantially enlarged heart (H), marked liver enlargement, with nodular margins, and diffuse VMs throughout the liver. pv, portal vein

Echocardiography in HHT patients may suggest pulmonary hypertension (i.e., right ventricular enlargement and increased tricuspid regurgitant peak velocity) [35, 36].

Increased pulmonary artery pressures invariably accompany and likely predispose to high output cardiac failure, entail a severe condition that significantly reduces survival on HHT patients, and should be screened in all HHT patients with liver VMs [18].

Right heart catheterization is always to be done in HHT patients with complicated liver VMs who are evaluated for OLT: specific pulmonary hemodynamic patterns with normal or reduced pulmonary vascular resistances are consistent with secondary pulmonary hypertension which accompanies liver VMs in HHT, that is a post-capillary pulmonary hypertension with pulmonary artery systolic pressure >40 mmHg; OLT is allowed with pulmonary vascular resistance <240 dynes s cm$^{-5}$ [18].

Right heart catheterization is also essential in differentiating a form of primary pre-capillary pulmonary artery hypertension characterized by very high pulmonary vascular resistances which can be associated to HHT [35, 37].

## CT

X-ray exposure and potential adverse reactions to contrast make multiphase CT recommended wherever expertise in Doppler US is lacking for investigation of symptomatic liver VMs in HHT. CT may also be required, depending on either the

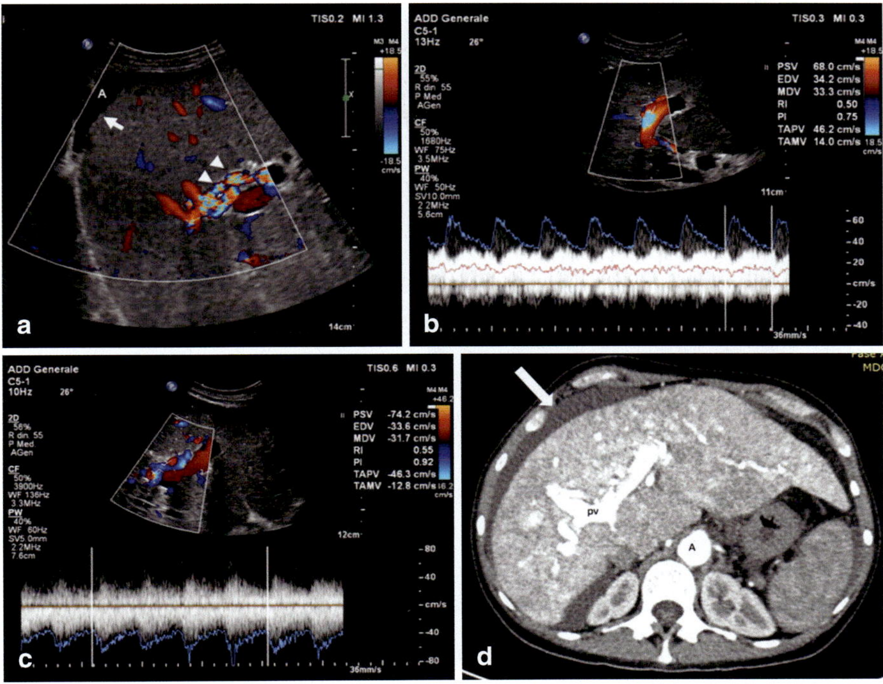

**Fig. 4.4** (**a**), grade 4 liver VMs with predominant arterioportal shunt, portal vein is surrounded by prominent and tortuous arterial branches (arrowheads); liver margins are nodular (arrow). (**a**) ascites. (**b**) spectral analysis shows a pulsatile and phasically reverted flow in the portal vein, with high mean velocity. (**c**) high velocity and low RI in arterial branches surrounding portal vein; (**d**) CT scan shows early filling of portal vein (pv) in arterial phase; diffuse VMs throughout the liver, liver nodular margins, ascites (arrow)

**Fig. 4.5** In a HHT patient with grade 3 liver VMs, US shows slightly hypoechoic round lesions (arrows) of right liver lobe

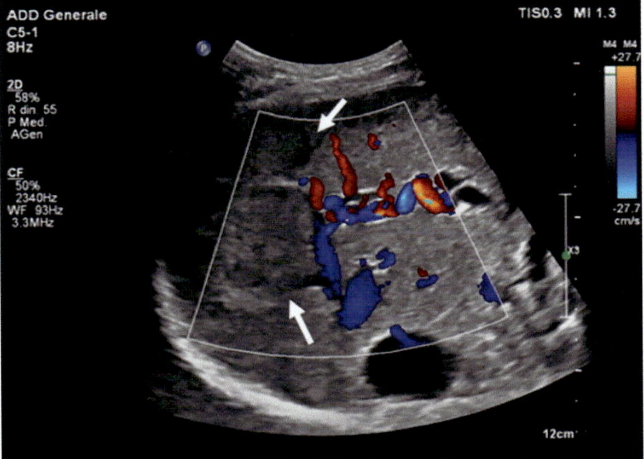

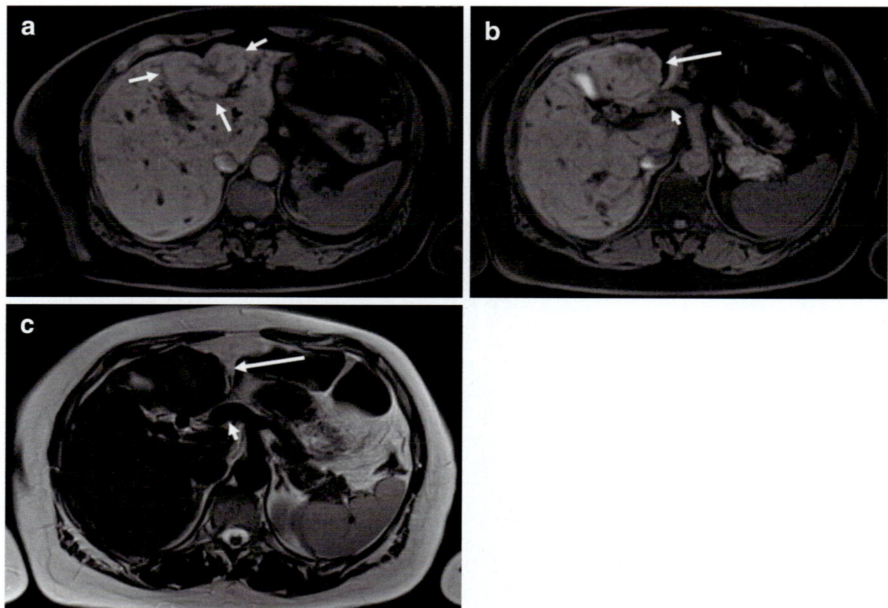

**Fig. 4.6** MR findings consistent with FNH in a HHT patient with liver VMs: (**a**) T1 weighed MR, axial image, shows a hyperintense liver lesion (arrows), with central scar; (**b**) T2 MR and (**c**) T2 blade MR, show the lesion (long arrow) and prominent hepatic artery (short arrow)

**Fig. 4.7** In a patient with grade 4 liver VMs, with prominent and tortuous peripheral arteries, liver margin is nodular (arrows), and the liver echotexture is coarse

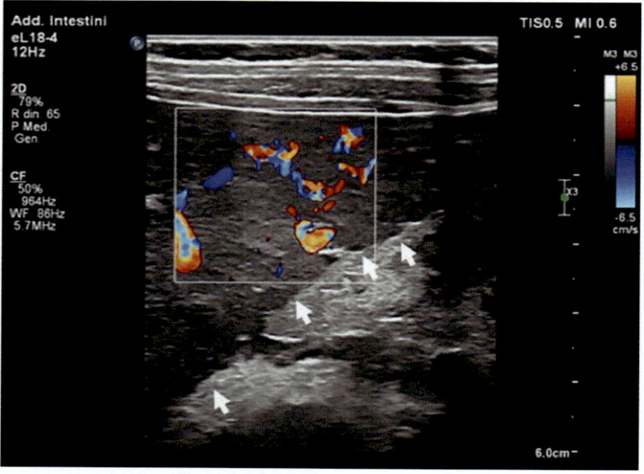


presence of focal liver lesions or on the severity of liver VMs and their hemodynamic impact; it is always used in complicated liver VMs considered for OLT (Figs. 4.3 and 4.4) [18]. Contrast-enhanced multiphase multirow CT angiography can show a prominent hepatic artery possibly associated with dilated hepatic and/or

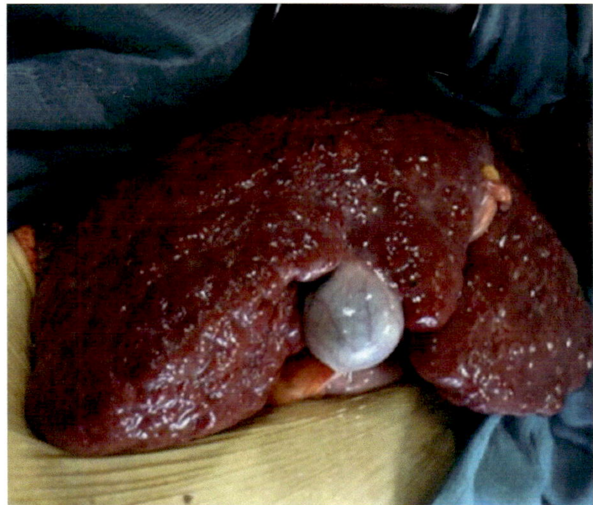

**Fig. 4.8** In a HHT patient submitted to OLT for complicated and refractory liver VMs note the liver enlargement with nodular surface, during liver transplantation

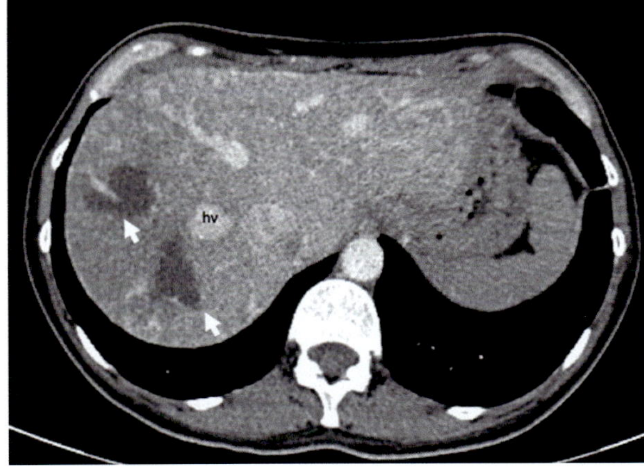



**Fig. 4.9** Triple-phase CT angiography, venous phase in a severely ill patient with grade 4 liver VMs: bilomas (arrows) are demonstrated; note the dilated hepatic veins (hv), liver enlargement, with nodular margins, and diffuse VMs throughout the liver

portal veins. Multirow CT and reconstructions depict the complex hepatic vascular alterations typical of HHT, different types of shunts and parenchymal perfusion disorders, together with evaluation of the spleen, gastroesophageal varices and other venous collaterals [16, 25, 38]. CT can also accurately display the most ominous complication of liver VMs in HHT, i.e., necrotizing cholangitis with formation of bilomas, shown on CT as single or multiple low-density lesions with ill-defined boundaries and no enhancement (Fig. 4.9).

Interpretation of focal liver lesions typical of liver involvement in HHT requires a combination of morphologic features (size, shape, liver margins deformation) and careful evaluation of dynamic data because the filling kinetics can be perturbed due to abnormalities of hepatic flow unique to liver involvement in HHT. The combination of various imaging techniques, particularly Doppler US and CT/MR, can greatly assist the characterization of focal hepatic lesions in HHT [32].

Liver VMs unique to HHT do not predispose a patient to hepatocellular carcinoma; however, HHT patients may need multiple transfusions because of chronic bleeding, and in the past decades, they were at risk for viral hepatitis. Therefore, the presence of chronic liver disease predisposing to hepatocellular carcinoma should be investigated to properly interpret imaging findings [39].

A diagnosis of hepatic focal nodular hyperplasia in the context of liver VMs is made if lesions are isodense or slightly hypodense with a hypodense central scar in unenhanced CT, becoming hyperdense in the arterial phase of contrast-enhanced CT [40]; regenerative nodules are usually diffuse with deformation of the liver surface and show specific dynamic characteristics [41].

## MR

MR imaging can also show hepatic VMs. The abnormalities are better depicted on MR angiograms and dynamic MR images, providing a map of anomalous vessels and analysis of filling kinetics; MR has been proven to be as accurate as multirow CT over which it has the advantage of the absence of ionizing radiation [25, 42].

MR diagnostic criteria for focal nodular hyperplasia and regenerative nodules are appreciated according to phase-specific and dynamic characteristics (Fig. 4.6) [40, 41].

## Celiac Angiography

Angiography, which can easily depict liver and mesenteric VMs, was once considered the gold standard for diagnosis of liver VMs, but has been replaced by less invasive CT or MR angiograms (Fig. 4.2) [18, 25].

## Endoscopy and Invasive Evaluation of Portal Hypertension

GI bleeding in HHT patients with portal hypertension due liver VMs is generally caused by GI telangiectases rather than to gastroesophageal varices [13], which are seldom found in these patients probably because of spontaneous liver portosystemic shunts.

Portal pressure measurement with hepatic venous pressure gradient is reserved to selected patients with complicated liver VMs when evaluated for OLT [18].

## Liver Biopsy

Liver biopsy is not necessary for the diagnosis of hepatic VMs related to HHT; if it is necessary for other reasons in a patient with known or suspected HHT, the risk of increased bleeding with the percutaneous transcapsular route has to be considered in view of the high prevalence of liver VMs in HHT [18].

A liver mass in the context of HHT can be characterized noninvasively by weighing epidemiological (high prevalence of FNH in HHT), clinical and laboratory data (including serum tumor markers, hepatitis B and C markers) as well as imaging (at least two examinations—whether Doppler US, MR or CT—showing suggestive findings) [18].

## Differential Diagnosis

Rare syndromes as Klippel-Trénaunay-Weber syndrome, can be associated to liver VMs.

Enlarged hepatic artery is not totally specific for the diagnosis of HHT. Other hypervascular lesions of the liver (large FNH or hemangiomas, some liver malignancies) can be associated with enlarged hepatic artery. The combination of either arterial and venous hepatic vascular abnormalities and the diffusion of liver VMs to the entire liver facilitate differential diagnosis [43, 44].

Congenital or acquired arterioportal shunts (more commonly iatrogenic), unlike liver VMs unique to HHT, are typically focal and can be associated with portal hypertension [33].

Three HHT patients evaluated 10, 8 and 8 years respectively after OLT, asymptomatic, showed hepatic vascular malformations at imaging in the transplanted livers, and the hypothesis of a relapse of VMs was made, with hepatic peliosis as alternative diagnosis [45, 46]. Peliosis is an uncommon benign vascular disease that is usually asymptomatic, even if it may be associated with high mortality, especially in major and diffuse forms; it is characterized by blood-filled cavities distributed randomly throughout the liver, with "swiss cheese" features. The lesions can be focal, segmental, or diffusely disseminated in hepatic sinusoids [44]; the imaging features of peliosis are nonspecific and differ from one another and it is hard to properly assess them by imaging only [47]. The size of lesions ranges from a few millimeters to several centimeters and may even occupy most of the liver. In a few cases, the number or size of peliotic lesions could increase in a short period and disseminate throughout the liver, resembling the progress of liver carcinoma or metastases [48]. It has been suggested that prolonged use of various kinds of drugs may cause peliosis (mainly steroids, immunosuppressants, and oral contraceptives) [49]. Peliosis should be considered, instead of recurrence of VMs, in the rare HHT patients who show multiple liver vascular dilatations after OLT, similarly to what described in other transplant recipients [50, 51].

## Treatment

Presently, no treatment is recommended for asymptomatic liver VMs.

An intensive therapeutic approach is recommended for symptomatic liver involvement in HHT [18]. The specific approach depends on the type of complication present. HOCF is first treated medically by administration of diuretics and beta blockers. If indicated, measures are taken to correct anemia and manage any arrhythmia, such as atrial fibrillation. Management of portal hypertension is analogous to that recommended for the same complication in patients with cirrhosis. Biliary necrosis, which is associated with a poor prognosis, is an indication for antibiotics. The treatment outcome in 55 complications observed in 39 patients with symptomatic liver VMs in HHT has been complete response in 35 (63.7%), partial response in 12 (21.8%) and no response (with progression to death) in 8 (14.5%)[6]. These data support the recommendation to consider invasive therapies for liver involvement by HHT only for otherwise intractable complications, after the judgment of response to first line treatment has been made, generally within 6–12 months [18].

Amongst invasive therapies which are considered in patients failing to respond to first-line intensive treatment, staged embolization of arteriovenous hepatic fistulas [52] is not currently recommended because it is palliative and can entail ominous complications, such as hepatic or biliary necrosis; it can be considered for patients who are not candidates for OLT [18].

Nowadays OLT remains the only definitive curative option for patients with HHT who have intractable cardiac failure, complicated portal hypertension, and/or biliary ischemia due to liver VMs. Outcomes of OLT for liver VMs in HHT are excellent (Table 4.3) [53–61]. Liver VMs in HHT are not associated to liver insufficiency, and are included in MELD (Model for End Stage Liver Disease) exceptions [18]; a MELD score for liver involvement in HHT has been proposed [62] with a score of 22 for intractable HOCF/PH, and 40 for ischemic biliary necrosis. Insofar priority for patients with liver VMs requiring OLT should be assessed with experts of HHT [18, 24]. Right heart catheterization is always to be done in patients with HHT evaluated for OLT to exclude severe pre-capillary pulmonary hypertension: OLT is allowed with pulmonary vascular resistance <240 dynes s cm$^{-5}$ [18, 24].

Potential morbidity and mortality rates associated with OLT are a cause for concern and the optimal timing for OLT in HHT with symptomatic liver involvement is a matter of debate. Actually, the puzzling decision of enlisting a patient for OLT could be supported by predictors. In a prospective longitudinal cohort of 154 HHT patients with liver involvement with a mean follow-up of 44 months (range 12–181) the outcome predictors were: stage 4 liver VMs at baseline and genotype HHT2 (ALK1). In a retrospective cohort [63] of 41 HHT patients with HOCF due to liver VMs, with a mean follow-up of 6 years (range 4–8), 27 (66%) died, with a mean age at death of 69 (range 34–86). The median survival time was 7 years (95% CI: 5.15–9.67) and the suggested outcome predictors were age at presentation, pulmonary artery systolic pressure, total bilirubin, weight loss, GI bleeding and any biliary ischemia. In a prospective cohort of 171 patients [26], with a mean follow up of 18 months (range 2–48), criteria of clinically significant liver involvement were: age

**Table 4.3** Outcomes of OLT for symptomatic liver involvement in HHT

| Author | Date of inclusion | Number of cases | Sex F/M | Age Mean (min-max) | Indication | Graft survival rate (%) | Cause of death |
|---|---|---|---|---|---|---|---|
| Lerut, 2006 | 1985–2003 | 40 (14 centers) | 35/5 | 48 (27–71) | HOCF 14 Biliary necrosis: 12 HOCF and biliary necrosis: 6 Portal hypertension: 5 HOCF and PH: 2 HOCF and PH and biliary necrosis: 1 | 82.5 | Intraoperative bleeding (1) Acute rejection (1) Heart failure (1) Cerebral hemorrhage (1) Gastric AVM rupture (1) Others (2) |
| Dupuis-Girod, 2010 | 1993–2007 | 13[a] (1 center) | 12/1 | 51.8 (33.1–64.5) | HOCF: 9 Biliary necrosis: 2 Hemobilia: 1 HOCF and biliary necrosis: 1 | 92 | Cardiac failure (1) |
| Nunez Viejo MA, 2010 | 2004 | 1 | 1/0 | 48 | HOCF: 1 | 100 | – |
| Lee M, 2010 | 2010 | 1 | | | | | |
| Cag M, 2011 | 2002–2008 | 4 | 1/3 | 57 (40–65) | HOCF: 3 Associated viral Hepatitis B: 1 | 100 | – |
| Maggi U, 2013 | 2008–2011 | 2 | 2/0 | 44–62 | HOCF: 2 | 100 | – |
| Elwir S, 2015 | | 1 | 1/0 | 54 | HOCF | 100 | – |
| Maestraggi Q, 2015 | | 1 | 1/0 | 63 | Biliary necrosis | 100 | – |
| Felli E, HPB 2017 | 2015 | 1 | 1/0 | 66 | HOCF | 100 | – |
| Total | | 61 | F 54 | | HOCF 50%/ biliary necrosis 24%/PH 8%/ mixed 18% | 5-year survival rate 82–100% | |

[a]3 pts reported in Lerut

at presentation >47, female gender, hemoglobin level at presentation <8 g/dL and alkaline phosphatase level at presentation >300 UI/L. Clearly, whereas prospective assessment of a cohort over a long follow up allows to extrapolate predictors, clinical features resulting from either retrospective analysis or short follow up can be valuable for diagnosis but not for prognosis. Therefore OLT enlisting of HHT patients with otherwise intractable complicated liver VMs requires careful weighing of reported predictors of bad outcome, including further clinical worrisome features: atrial fibrillation, high blood transfusion requirement, weight loss, right upper quadrant pain, high bilirubin levels, and sepsis [13, 63].

Looking for a potential alternative to invasive therapies for cure of symptomatic liver VMs in HHT, recently bevacizumab (an antivascular endothelial growth factor monoclonal antibody) was evaluated in HHT patients with severe liver involvement [64–66].

These preliminary studies suggested that bevacizumab may be a therapeutic option in the treatment of complicated liver VMs in HHT; however, potential adverse events related to bevacizumab need careful consideration: a multicenter European survey has evaluated adverse events in 69 HHT patients treated with bevacizumab, 37 for HOCF in hepatic AVMs, and 32 for HHT-related bleeding; the 69 patients received bevacizumab for a mean of 11 months for a total of 63.8 person/years treatment; an average incidence rate of 50 adverse events grade 1–3 and a 1.5 fatal adverse events per 100 person-years were captured [67].

Furthermore, also rates of no or partial response to bevacizumab, and the symptoms/signs recurrence after drug withdrawal make this drug unsuitable to replace OLT to cure complicated liver VMs in HHT. On the other hand bevacizumab may show a potential "bridging" role where severe liver VMs critically worsen clinical condition of the patient: if bevacizumab obtains a complete response with resolution of the liver VM complication OLT would be scheduled within the following few months [68, 69]. The timing of this decision is critical as bevacizumab is known to impair wound healing and anastomoses repair and insofar every elective surgery is delayed of at least 2 months after the treatment end; on the other hand recurrence of VMs symptoms/signs is the rule after treatment end (within 6–12 months in reported cases). The right "OLT window" after bevacizumab in severe complicated liver VMs in HHT should therefore be between 2 and 6 months after the last drug administration (Fig. 4.10).

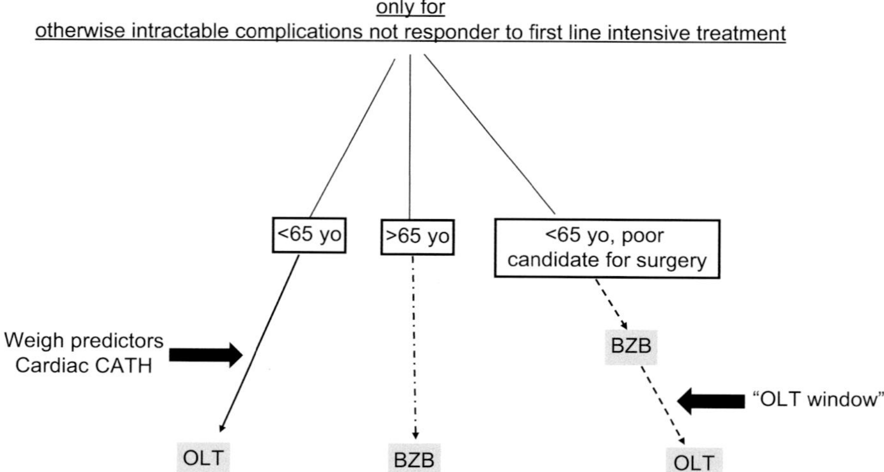


**Fig. 4.10** Therapeutic algorithm for complicated and refractory liver VMs in HHT

In conclusion, it has to be underscored that considering the condition complexity and the scant available literature data, any major treatment decision regarding liver VMs, and notably liver transplant, has to be done only after conferring with a medical team with expertise in HHT.

# References


1. Park S, Wankhede M, Lee Y, et al. Real-time imaging of de novo arteriovenous malformation in a mouse model of hereditary hemorrhagic telangiectasia. J Clin Invest. 2009;119:3487–96.
2. Mahmoud M, Allinson K, Zhai Z, et al. Pathogenesis of arteriovenous malformations in the absence of endoglin. Circ Res. 2010;106:1425–33.
3. Shovlin CL, Guttmacher AE, Buscarini E, et al. Diagnostic criteria for hereditary hemorrhagic telangiectasia (Rendu-Osler-Weber syndrome). Am J Med Genet. 2000;91:66–7.
4. Gallione C, Repetto GM, Legius E, et al. A combined syndrome of juvenile polyposis and hereditary haemorrhagic telangiectasia is associated with mutations in MADH4 (SMAD4). Lancet. 2004;363:852–9.
5. Cole SG, Begbie ME, Wallace GMF, et al. A new locus for hereditary haemorrhagic telangiectasia (HHT3) maps to chromosome 5. J Med Genet. 2005;42:577–82.
6. Govani F, Shovlin C. Fine mapping of the hereditary haemorrhagic telangiectasia (HHT)3 locus on chromosome 5 excludes Sprouty 4, VE-cadherin 2 and other interval genes. J Angiogenes Res. 2010;2:15.
7. Bayrak-Toydemir P, McDonald J, Akarsu N, et al. A fourth locus for hereditary hemorrhagic telangiectasia maps to chromosome 7. Am J Med Genet. 2006;140:2155–62.
8. Kjeldsen AD, Møller TR, Brusgaard K, et al. Clinical symptoms according to genotype amongst patients with hereditary haemorrhagic telangiectasia. J Int Med. 2005;258:349–55.
9. Letteboer TGW, Mager JJ, Snijder RJ, et al. Genotype–phenotype relationship in hereditary haemorrhagic telangiectasia. J Med Genet. 2006;43:371–7.
10. Bayrak Toydemir P, McDonald J, Markewitz B, et al. Genotype–phenotype correlation in hereditary hemorrhagic telangiectasia. Am J Med Genet. 2006;140:463–70.
11. Sabbà C, Pasculli G, Lenato GM, et al. Hereditary hemorrhagic telangiectasia: clinical features in ENG and ALK1 mutation carriers. J Thromb Haemost. 2007;5:1149–57.
12. Lesca G, Olivieri C, Burnichon N, et al. Genotype-phenotype correlations in hereditary hemorrhagic telangiectasia: data from the French-Italian HHT network. Genet Med. 2007;9:14–22.
13. Buscarini E, Leandro G, Conte D, et al. Natural history and outcome of hepatic vascular malformations in a large cohort of patients with hereditary hemorrhagic teleangiectasia. Dig Dis Sci. 2011;56:2166–78.
14. Gincul R, Lesca G, Gelas-Dore B, et al. Evaluation of previously nonscreened hereditary hemorrhagic telangiectasia patients shows frequent liver involvement and early cardiac consequences. Hepatology. 2008;48:1377–9.
15. Buscarini E, Danesino C, Olivieri C, et al. Doppler ultrasonographic grading of hepatic vascular malformations in hereditary hemorrhagic telangiectasia—results of extensive screening. Ultraschall Med. 2004;25:348–55.
16. Memeo M, Stabile Ianora AA, Scardapane A, et al. Hepatic involvement in hereditary hemorrhagic telangiectasia: CT findings. Abdom Imaging. 2004;29:211–20.
17. Garcia-Tsao G, Korzenik JR, Young L, et al. Liver disease in patients with hereditary hemorrhagic telangiectasia. N Engl J Med. 2000;343:931–6.
18. European Association for the Study of the Liver, Garcia-Pagàn JC, Buscarini E, Janssen HL, et al. Vascular diseases of the liver. J Hepatol. 2016;64:179–202.
19. Wanless IR, Gryfe A. Nodular transformation of the liver in hereditary hemorrhagic telangiectasia. Arch Pathol Lab Med. 1986;110:331–5.

20. Buscarini E, Danesino C, Plauchu H, et al. High prevalence of hepatic focal nodular hyperplasia in subjects with hereditary hemorrhagic telangiectasia. Ultrasound Med Biol. 2004;30:1089–97.
21. Blewitt RW, Brown CM, Wyatt JI. The pathology of acute hepatic disintegration in hereditary hemorrhagic telangiectasia. Histopathology. 2003;42:265–9.
22. Bueres Dominguez I, Annet L, et al. Extensive ischemic liver necrosis complicating hereditary hemorrhagic telangiectasia: a rare indication for liver transplantation. Liver Int. 2005;25:677–9.
23. Lerut J, Orlando G, Adam R, et al. Liver transplantation for hereditary hemorrhagic telangiectasia: report of the European liver transplant registry. Ann Surg. 2006;244:854–62.
24. Faughnan ME, Palda VA, Garcia-Tsao G, et al. International guidelines for the diagnosis and management of hereditary haemorrhagic telangiectasia. J Med Genet. 2011;48:73–87.
25. Buscarini E, Buscarini L, Danesino C, et al. Hepatic vascular malformations in hereditary hemorrhagic telangiectasia: Doppler sonographic screening in a large family. J Hepatol. 1997;26:111–8.
26. Singh S, Swanson KL, Hathcock MA, et al. Identifying the presence of clinically significant hepatic involvement in hereditary haemorrhagic telangiectasia using a simple clinical scoring index. J Hepatol. 2014;61:124–31.
27. Buscarini E, Buscarini L, Civardi G, et al. Hepatic vascular malformations in hereditary hemorrhagic telangiectasia: imaging findings. AJR Am J Roentgenol. 1994;163:1105–10.
28. Caselitz M, Bahr MJ, Bleck JS, et al. Sonographic criteria for the diagnosis of hepatic involvement in hereditary hemorrhagic telangiectasia (HHT). Hepatology. 2003;37:1139–46.
29. Buonamico P, Suppressa P, Lenato GM, et al. Liver involvement in a large cohort of patients with hereditary hemorrhagic telangiectasia: echo-color-Doppler vs multislice computed tomography study. J Hepatol. 2008;48:811–20.
30. Schelker RC, Barreiros AP, Hart C, et al. Macro- and microcirculation patterns of intrahepatic blood flow changes in patients with hereditary hemorrhagic telangiectasia. World J Gastroenterol. 2017;23:486–95.
31. Buscarini E, Gebel M, Ocran K, et al. Interobserver agreement in diagnosing liver involvement in hereditary hemorrhagic telangiectasia by Doppler ultrasound. Ultrasound Med Biol. 2008;34:718–25.
32. Buscarini E, Gandolfi S, Alicante S, et al. Liver involvement in hereditary hemorrhagic telangiectasia. Abdom Radiol. 2018;10:1671–4.
33. De Gottardi A, Berzigotti A, Buscarini E, et al. Ultrasonography in liver vascular disease. Ultraschall Med. 2018;39:382–405.
34. Gincul R, Lesca G, Gelas-Dore B, et al. Evaluation of previously non screened hereditary hemorrhagic telangiectasia patients shows frequent liver involvement and early cardiac consequences. Hepatology. 2008;48:1570–6.
35. Olivieri C, Lanzarini L, Pagella F, et al. Echocardiographic screening discloses increased values of pulmonary artery systolic pressure in 9 of 68 unselected patients affected with hereditary hemorrhagic telangiectasia. Genet Med. 2006;8:183–90.
36. Sopeña B, Pérez-Rodríguez MT, Portela D, et al. High prevalence of pulmonary hypertension in patients with hereditary hemorrhagic telangiectasia. Eur J Intern Med. 2013;24:30–4.
37. Trembath RC, Thomson JR, Machado RD, et al. Clinical and molecular genetic features of pulmonary hypertension in patients with hereditary hemorrhagic telangiectasia. N Engl J Med. 2001;345:325–34.
38. Siddiki H, Doherty MG, Fletcher JG, et al. Abdominal findings in hereditary hemorrhagic telangiectasia: pictorial essay on 2D and 3D findings with isotropic multiphase CT. Radiographics. 2008;28:171–84.
39. Vilgrain V, Paradis V, Van Wettere M, et al. Benign and malignant hepatocellular lesions in patients with vascular liver diseases. Abdom Radiol. 2018; 19.
40. Dioguardi Burgio M, Ronot M, Salvaggio G, et al. Imaging of hepatic focal nodular hyperplasia: pictorial review and diagnostic strategy. Semin Ultrasound CT MR. 2016;37:511–24.

41. Brancatelli G, Federle MP, Grazioli L, et al. Large regenerative nodules in Budd-Chiari syndrome and other vascular disorders of the liver: CT and MR imaging findings with clinicopathologic correlation. AJR Am J Roentgenol. 2002;178:877–83.
42. Scardapane A, Stabile Ianora A, Sabbà C, et al. Dynamic 4D MR angiography versus multislice CT angiography in the evaluation of vascular hepatic involvement in hereditary haemorrhagic telangiectasia. Radiol Med. 2012;117:29–45.
43. Tian JL, Zhang JS. Hepatic perfusion disorders: etiopathogenesis and related diseases. World J Gastroenterol. 2006;12:3265–70.
44. Kamaya A, Maturen KE, Tye GA, et al. Hypervascular liver lesions. Semin Ultrasound CT MR. 2009;30:387–407.
45. Ulus S, Arslan A, Karaarslan E, et al. De novo vascular lesions after liver transplant in a case with hereditary hemorrhagic telangiectasia and fibropolycystic liver disease: long-term follow-up with magnetic resonance imaging and magnetic resonance angiography. Exp Clin Transplant. 2016; https://doi.org/10.6002/ect.2016.0024.
46. Sabbà C, Gallitelli M, Longo A, et al. Orthotopic livertransplantation and hereditary hemorrhagic telangiectasia: do hepatic vascular malformations relapse? A long term follow up study on two patients. J Hepatol. 2004;41:687–9.
47. Dai YN, Ren ZZ, Song WY, et al. Peliosis hepatis: 2 case reports of a rare liver disorderand its differential diagnosis. Medicine (Baltimore). 2017;96:e6471.
48. Kootte AM, Siegel AM, Koorenhof M. Generalised peliosis hepatis mimicking metastases after long-term use of oral contraceptives. Neth J Med. 2015;73:41–3.
49. Crocetti D, Palmieri A, Pedullà G, et al. Peliosis hepatis: personal experience and literature review. World J Gastroenterol. 2015;21:13188–94.
50. Cavalcanti R, Pol S, Carnot F, et al. Impact and evolution of peliosis hepatis in renal transplant recipients. Transplantation. 1994;58:315–6.
51. Yu CY, Chang LC, Chen LW, et al. Peliosis hepatis complicated by portal hypertension following renal transplantation. World J Gastroenterol. 2014;20:2420–5.
52. Chavan A, Luthe L, Gebel M, et al. Complications and clinical outcome of hepatic artery embolisation in patients with hereditary haemorrhagic telangiectasia. Eur Radiol. 2013;23:951–7.
53. Lerut J, Orlando G, Adam R, et al. Liver transplantation for hereditary hemorrhagic telangiectasia: report of the European liver transplant registry. Ann Surg. 2006;244:854–62.
54. Dupuis-Girod S, Chesnais AL, Ginon I, et al. Long-term outcome of patients with hereditary hemorrhagic telangiectasia and severe hepatic involvement after orthotopic liver transplantation: a single-center study. Liver Transpl. 2010;16:340–7.
55. Núñez Viejo MA, Fernández Montes A, Hernández Hernández JL, et al. Rendu-Osler disease with hepatic involvement: first transplant in Spain. Med Clin. 2010;135:552–5.
56. Lee M, Sze DY, Bonham CA, et al. Hepatic arteriovenous malformations from hereditary hemorrhagic telangiectasia: treatment with liver transplantation. Dig Dis Sci. 2010;55:3059–62.
57. Cag M, Audet M, Saouli AC, et al. Successful liver transplantation for Rendu-Weber-Osler disease, a single Centre experience. Hepatol Int. 2011;5:834–40.
58. Maggi U, Conte G, Nita G, et al. Arterial anastomosis in liver transplantation for Rendu-Osler-Weber disease: two case reports. Transplant Proc. 2013;45:2689–91.
59. Elwir S, Martin C, Chinnakotla S, et al. Liver transplantation for high output heart failure secondary to HHT: a case report and review of the literature. J Gastrointest Dig Syst. 2015;5:331.
60. Maestraggi Q, Bouattour M, Toquet S, et al. Bevacizumab to treat cholangiopathy in hereditary hemorrhagic telangiectasia: be cautious: a case report. Medicine (Baltimore). 2015;94:e1966.
61. Felli E, Addeo P, Faitot F, et al. Liver transplantation for hereditary hemorrhagic telangiectasia: a systematic review. HPB (Oxford). 2017;19:567–72.
62. Garcia-Tsao G, Gish RG, Punch J. Model for end-stage liver disease (MELD) exception for hereditary hemorrhagic telangiectasia. Liver Transpl. 2006;12:S108–9.
63. Young LH, Henderson K, Pollak JS, et al. Predictors of death in patients with HHT, liver vascular malformations and symptomatic heart failure. Abstr: 10th International hereditary hem-

orrhagic telangiectasia scientific conference 2013; Cork, Ireland Hematology Reports 2013; 5(s1):6.
64. Dupuis-Girod S, Ginon I, Saurin JC, et al. Bevacizumab in patients with hereditary hemorrhagic telangiectasia and severe hepatic vascular malformations and high cardiac output. JAMA. 2012;307:948–55.
65. Mitchell A, Adams LA, MacQuillan G, et al. Bevacizumab reverses need for liver transplantation in hereditary hemorrhagic telangiectasia. Liver Transpl. 2008;14:210–3.
66. Vlachou PA, Colak E, Koculym A, et al. Improvement of ischemic cholangiopathy in three patients with hereditary hemorrhagic telangiectasia following treatment with bevacizumab. J Hepatol. 2013;59:186–9.
67. Buscarini E, Botella LM, Geisthoff U, et al. Safety of thalidomide and bevacizumab in patients with hereditary hemorrhagic telangiectasia. Orphanet J Rare Dis. 2019 (in press).
68. Muller YD, Oppliger R, Breguet R, et al. Hereditary haemorrhagic telangiectasia: to transplant or not to transplant – is there a right time for liver transplantation? Liver Int. 2016;36:1735–40.
69. Dupuis-Girod S, Buscarini E. Hereditary hemorrhagic telangiectasia: to transplant or not to transplant? Liver Int. 2016;36:1741–4.

# Chapter 5
# Congenital Extrahepatic Portosystemic Shunts: Abernethy Malformation


Anna Baiges, Fanny Turon, Virginia Hernández-Gea, and Juan Carlos Garcia-Pagan


## Introduction

Congenital extrahepatic portosystemic shunts (CEPS), also known as Abernethy malformation, are a rare condition in which most of the intestinal and splenic venous blood bypasses the portal vein and the liver, draining directly into systemic veins through abnormal communications. CEPS were first described by John Abernethy in 1793 as a post-mortem finding in a 10 month-old girl that presented several malformations, including the termination of the portal vein in an end-to-side shunt to the inferior vena cava [1]. Since then, less than 300 cases of congenital extrahepatic portosystemic shunts have been reported in the literature, most of them published in the last decades, probably in relation to the improvement and wide use of imaging studies in clinical practice leading to an increased detection of shunts. The vast majority of published cases are single case reports providing only a transversal description without follow-up and, despite some series have been reported [2–5], most of them are small and mix patients with both extrahepatic and intrahepatic congenital shunts. It is important to underline that extrahepatic and intrahepatic portosystemic shunts (IPSS) should be considered different entities because they might have a different natural history. While CEPS can have a wide range of manifestations (from completely asymptomatic patients to severe shunt-related complications including hepatocellular carcinoma), IPSS are more frequently asymptomatic and can undergo spontaneous closure during infancy (<2 years old). Moreover, there are no reports of malignant liver tumours in IPSS [6, 7]. Trying to address this issue, an international retrospective study still published in abstract form [8] collected 66 patients with CEPS and evaluated their natural history since diagnosis until adulthood.


A. Baiges (✉) · F. Turon · V. Hernández-Gea · J. C. Garcia-Pagan
Barcelona Hepatic Hemodynamic Laboratory, Liver Unit, Hospital Clínic de Barcelona, IDIBAPS, CIBERehd, Universitat de Barcelona, Barcelona, Spain
e-mail: abaigesa@clinic.cat; fturon@clinic.cat; vihernandez@clinic.cat; jcgarcia@clinic.cat



© Springer Nature Switzerland AG 2022
D. Valla et al. (eds.), *Vascular Disorders of the Liver*,
https://doi.org/10.1007/978-3-030-82988-9_5

The real prevalence of CEPS is not known as it is not routinely screened for. In countries regularly performing neonatal screening for hereditary galactosemia it has been estimated that the incidence of congenital portosystemic shunts is around 1 in 30,000 births [9, 10] (high levels of galactose can be found in newborns with congenital portosystemic shunts because galactose bypasses the liver), but these data cannot differentiate intra and extrahepatic shunts and may underestimate its real prevalence since not all patients with CEPS harbour hypergalactosemia.

## Etiology

The development of the portal vein and the inferior vena cava is a complex process that takes place simultaneously during the fourth and tenth weeks of embryonic life, the portal venous system arising from the extraembryonic and umbilical veins and the systemic veins developing from intraembryonic structures [11]. The embryonic veins (umbilical, vitelline and cardinal veins) form complex networks creating intra and extrahepatic connections that later selectively involute and evolve to the fully developed portal vein [12]. The complicated process, multiple interactions and the close relationship between these two systems may explain the occurrence of abnormal communications [13] that are probably a result from incomplete involution of these embryonic vessels. An abnormal involution may result in a duplicated portal vein while, on the contrary, excessive involution may result in a complete absence or attenuation of the portal vein [14, 15]. As a result, congenital portosystemic shunts can involve different veins and can have different anatomies, can be single or multiple and can induce partial or complete diversion of the portal blood to the systemic circulation.

CEPS frequently can appear in the setting of multiple congenital malformative processes or in patients with associated genetic disorders such as Down or Turner syndrome. The most frequently reported associations are cardiac malformations, polysplenia syndrome, renal malformations, and musculoskeletal defects [8, 13, 16–21]. Cardiac anomalies are present in approximately one third of patients and include ventricular and atrial septal defects, patent ductus arteriosus and foramen ovale [22]. The presence of other vascular anomalies and chromosomal anomalies have also been reported [23].

## Diagnosis

The diagnosis of Abernethy malformation is often missed on initial presentation due to low level of suspicion and wide variability in clinical presentation. Some patients (around 20%) are diagnosed after presenting symptoms potentially attributable to CEPS (hepatic encephalopathy, dyspnea) [8] but diagnosis is usually reached through imaging tests performed because of different unrelated reasons that casually demonstrate the presence of the portosystemic shunt. The initial diagnosis is usually suspected through Doppler ultrasonography (US) finding absence or non-visibility of intrahepatic portal branches, as well as slow or absent portal flow and a compensatory dilatation of the hepatic artery. The imaging evaluation must be completed to further assess the exact anatomy and location of the shunt with a computed tomography (CT) or a magnetic resonance imaging (MRI). Angiography with temporary balloon occlusion of the shunt is an invasive imaging technique that better depicts the presence and pattern of the shunt [3, 5, 24].

CEPS is usually diagnosed during childhood [2–5]. However, patients with CEPS may be undiagnosed until adulthood or even until an advanced age because they can remain asymptomatic until late in the disease. Indeed, in a recent cohort [8] 45% of patients with CEPS with more than 50 years of age remained asymptomatic. CEPS can also be diagnosed at prenatal ultrasound [4, 25, 26]. Prenatal US can assess the anatomical origin and drainage of the fetal umbilical vein, portal vein, ductus venosus and hepatic venous systems, as well as the integrity of the intrahepatic portal venous system.

Liver function is usually preserved although blood tests can be slightly altered, most frequently with hyperbilirubinemia or mild elevation of liver enzymes. Hyperammonemia is present in almost all patients with CEPS as a consequence of shunting [8, 27].

## Anatomical Classification

Morgan and Superina [28], and afterwards Howard and Davenport [13], classified CEPS into two types according to its anatomical morphology (Fig. 5.1). Type I CEPS is characterized by the absence of intrahepatic portal vein branches and an end-to-side portocaval shunt, while in type II CEPS the intrahepatic veins are hypoplastic but patent and a side-to side shunt diverts blood from the portal vein to the inferior vena cava. Type I CEPS can be further classified into type Ia, when the superior mesenteric and splenic vein drain separately into inferior cava veins (IVC), and type Ib, when these veins form a common trunk before draining into the IVC. The first published case reports stated that type I CEPS was most frequent in females while type II CEPS was most frequent in males [13, 16]. This association

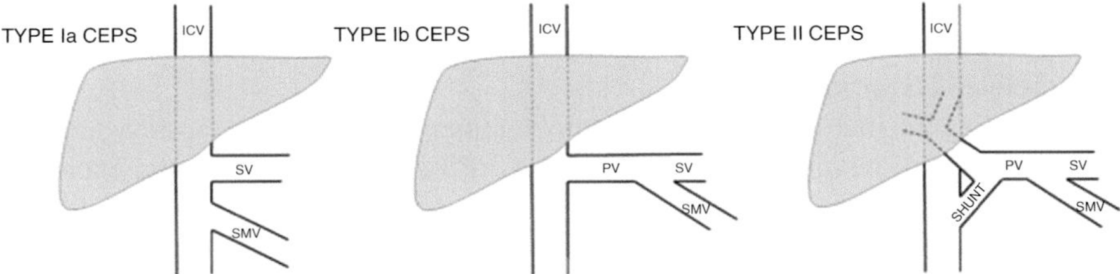


**Fig. 5.1** Classical CEPS classification

has not been reproduced in more extensive and recent series that show a more balanced gender ratio [8].

Lately, other more detailed anatomical subclassifications by Lautz [3] and Blanc (the Bicêtre surgical classification) [5] have been described correlating the anatomy of the shunt to the surgical approach required for its closure. The Bicêtre classification initially focuses on whether the shunt is a porto-caval shunt or whether it is originated from a different vein of the splanchnic system. Shunts are further subclassified into end-to-side shunt, side-to-side shunt or an H type shunt. However, it has also been recognized that to accurately assess the patency of intrahepatic veins, an angiography with temporary balloon occlusion of the shunt needs to be performed, to distinguish if the assumed absence of intrahepatic veins in type I CEPS could in fact be concealing remnant hypoplastic hepatic branches not visible on CT or MRI [3, 5, 24]. Establishing confidently the presence or absence of intrahepatic veins is highly relevant when evaluating possible therapeutic options, as classically was considered that type I patients could only be treated with liver transplantation. Performing an angiography could allow a reclassification of CEPS type and thus enable the consideration of other treatment options for these patients.

## Liver Pathology

In patients with CEPS the liver is usually small and with a certain degree of atrophy, which could be in the context of systemic shunting of splanchnic venous blood leading to an impaired development and function of the liver. Moreover, lack of hepatotrophic factors supplied by portal venous blood could also have a role in liver atrophy [18, 29].

Liver histology can be normal but structural changes as fibrosis and steatosis have also been reported [30]. The most typical findings in liver biopsies are absent or hypoplastic portal vein branches combined with congestive sinusoids and large arterial branches [31–33].

## CEPS Complications

CEPS can present with a wide range of clinical manifestations, from completely asymptomatic patients or only mild hepatic dysfunction to severe portosystemic shunt related complications.

Regarding the incidence of CEPS complications, a recent study shows a cumulative incidence of having at least one major CEPS complication (hepatic encephalopathy, pulmonary arterial hypertension, hepatopulmonary syndrome, hepatocellular carcinoma or hepatocellular adenoma) is 35%, 45% and 58%, at 20, 30 and 40 years respectively [8]. However, it is also certain that, as data from a systematic population screening is not available, the prevalence of CEPS complications cannot be confidently inferred and asymptomatic patients with CEPS might remain under diagnosed.

CEPS complications can be explained, at least in part, due to the fact that toxic compounds generated in the gastrointestinal tract that would be normally metabolized in the liver, in CEPS are diverted into systemic circulation with accumulative deleterious effects.

## *Hepatic Encephalopathy*

Hepatic encephalopathy (HE) is one of the most frequent CEPS complications [30, 34] affecting nearly 30% of patients with CEPS [8]. It can present as an acute or chronic event, but it usually presents as persistent HE. HE is probably due to venous shunting of circulating ammonia not metabolized by the liver [30, 35, 36], resulting in abnormal neurologic symptoms, behaviour alterations (irritability, agitation, disorientation) or learning impairment, among others. The risk of encephalopathy is probably related to the degree of portosystemic shunting [6], but no differences between type I and type II CEPS in the prevalence of HE have been found. It is important to take into account that in patients also presenting genetic or malformative disorders with intellectual disability, HE (and especially minimal HE) may be challenging to diagnose if not specifically looked for. In this context, it has been explored if serum ammonia levels could relate to the development of HE but, until now, it has not been possible to identify any clinical or biochemical parameter able to predict HE development [8]. In brain MRI, high globus pallidum intensity on T1-weighted images has been associated to the presence of HE [2, 33]. Furthermore, it has been suggested that the finding of high globus pallidum intensity in brain MRI could identify those patients at a higher risk of developing HE or that may have minimal subclinical HE, but this finding still has to be confirmed [8].

## *Pulmonary Arterial Hypertension (PaHT) and Hepatopulmonary Syndrome (HPS)*

Effects of circulating endotoxins [37] might contribute to the development of either hepatopulmonary syndrome (HPS) with chronic hypoxemia or pulmonary arterial hypertension (PaHT). The development of HPS and PaHT, although not fully understood, could be in relation to intestinal vasoactive mediators [37–39] that, having bypassed the liver and not being properly metabolized, reached the pulmonary vascular bed. These vasoactive mediators would induce a long-standing pulmonary vasoconstriction in the case of PAHT [39, 40] or, on the contrary, pulmonary vasodilation in the case of HPS. Development of pulmonary complications in CEPS has not been associated to neither the presence of other congenital cardiac malformations nor to the type of CEPS. PaHT has been estimated to be present in around 20% of patients with CEPS [8, 34], but it is important to underline that it may be underestimated if not specifically looked for because most patients are asymptomatic in the early stages of the disease. Severe PaHT leading to death has been reported [33].

## *Liver Nodules*

Liver nodules are a frequent CEPS complication, affecting around 50–70% of patients. Nodules can be unique or multiple and can present at all ages. Liver nodules are probably a reaction to uneven perfusion due to the misbalanced excessive increase of arterial blood flow trying to compensate the diminished portal blood flow. The misbalanced flow would result in atrophy of ischemic areas and nodule formation in well perfused areas [41]. The diagnosis and characterization of liver nodules in patients with CEPS is reached as usual using current radiographic imaging techniques as well as histochemical and immunohistochemical analysis of the nodules. Most of the reported nodules (although not always supported by histological proof), have been described as focal nodular hyperplasia and regenerative nodular hyperplasia (70%). Hepatocellular carcinoma (HCC, 10%) and adenomas (20%) are also found, although in a lower proportion [2, 40, 42–45]. Less frequently, hepatoblastoma and sarcomas have also been reported [27]. However, in the context of better imaging accuracy in the recent years, the incidence of reported neoplastic nodules is increasing, especially in patients reaching adulthood.

Previous observations suggested that the development of liver nodules was more frequent in type I CEPS than in type II CEPS [42, 45, 43]. Interestingly however, recent data suggest that this is the case only for HCC: HCC appears almost exclusively in type I CEPS, probably in the abovementioned setting of more severe alterations in liver perfusion in type I CEPS [46, 47]. It has also been proposed that HCCs are more frequent in men while adenomas usually present in women [8].

It is well known that adenomas have a risk of malignant transformation to HCC and it is important to take into account this possibility when monitoring patients with CEPS [42, 43]. In this regard, adenomas with β-catenin mutations are considered to be at a higher risk of malignant transformation when compared to other subtypes, and this has also been proved in nodules arising on a background of CEPS independently of their size and histological appearance [42]. Overall, these data support the need of performing a careful and periodic screening for liver nodules in patients with CEPS. Nodule biopsy should be considered if imaging characterization is inconclusive.

## Management and Treatment

There are no clinical guidelines addressing CEPS management and therefore its treatment is highly variable among different centres. CEPS complications such as hepatic encephalopathy, HPS, PaHT or neoplastic nodules can be approached with their usual standard medical treatment. However, what remains controversial is whether shunt closure is necessary in all cases (including asymptomatic patients), in which patients it can be performed and in which patients it would be preferable to perform a liver transplantation.

Shunt closure can be performed either radiologically or surgically, although usually radiological endovascular closure is the first-line option because it is considered to be less invasive and safer [5].

Published data suggest that shunt closure and the restoration of portal blood flow to the liver have a huge efficacy managing most CEPS complications (regression of HE and hepatopulmonary syndrome, disappearance of benign nodules). However, shunt closure should be considered early in the evolution of the disease because it is not clear whether chronic long-established complications could fully reverse in spite of shunt closure. Indeed, divergent results have been reported in the field of pulmonary arterial hypertension as in some patients regression of PaHT can be difficult to achieve, and this has been related to the severity and duration of the disease [8]. As expected, no changes in established neoplastic nodules have been reported after shunt closure.

Although further data is needed to confirm these findings, some reports also suggest that pre-emptive shunt closure could prevent the development of CEPS complications [12, 40], thus supporting the recommendation of closing the shunt even in asymptomatic patients.

Formerly, it was considered that the only curative treatment for patients with type I CEPS was liver transplantation. However, the incorporation of recent imaging techniques such as angiography and the possibility to perform a radiological shunt occlusion test, have shown that, even in previously misdiagnosed type I CEPS, there are sometimes hypoplastic remnant intrahepatic portal branches [3, 5, 24]. Intrahepatic portal flow could be restored in patients with hypoplastic veins with a low incidence of complications if a trial occlusion test with pressure measurements and assessment of the physiologic consequences of sudden cessation of flow through the shunt was performed [3]. In this regard, a recently published pediatric report including 42 patients has helped to reinforce the concept that preoperative venography delineates shunt morphology and balloon occlusion simulates closure hemodynamics. This data is necessary to determine whether definitive closure should be performed through endovascular or surgical methods an whether closure should be performed in a single or staged setting [48].

Concerning shunt closure complications, some authors have suggested that prophylactic anticoagulation could also be useful to prevent thrombosis after shunt closure [2, 4].

Liver transplantation has also been reported to be a successful treatment for CEPS but its indication is currently being reduced to patients with neoplastic nodules (especially hepatocelular carcinoma) or with technical difficulties for shunt closure.

# References


1. Abernethy J. Account of two instances of uncommon formation in the viscera of the human body. Phil Trans R Soc. 1793;83:59–66.
2. Franchi-Abella S, Branchereau S, Lambert V, Fabre M, Steimberg C, Losay J, et al. Complications of congenital portosystemic shunts in children: therapeutic options and outcomes. J Pediatr Gastroenterol Nutr. 2010;51(3):322–30.
3. Lautz TB, Tantemsapya N, Rowell E, Superina RA. Management and classification of type II congenital portosystemic shunts. J Pediatr Surg [Internet]. 2011;46(2):308–14. https://doi.org/10.1016/j.jpedsurg.2010.11.009.
4. Chocarro G, Virginia M, Jose A, Encinas L, Vilanova A, Hernandez F, et al. Congenital portosystemic shunts: clinic heterogeneity requires an individual management of the patient. Eur J Pediatr Surg. 2016;26(1):74–80.
5. Blanc T, Guerin F, Franchi-Abella S, Jacquemin E, Pariente D, Soubrane O, et al. Congenital portosystemic shunts in children: a new anatomical classification correlated with surgical strategy. Ann Surg. 2014;260(1):188–98.
6. Uchino T, Matsuda I, Endo F. The long-term prognosis of congenital portosystemic venous shunt. J Pediatr. 1999;135(2 Pt 1):254–6.
7. Francois B, Gottrand F, Lachaux A, Boyer C, Benoit B, De Smet S. Outcome of intrahepatic portosystemic shunt diagnosed prenatally. Eur J Pediatr [Internet]. 2017;176(12):1613–8. http://www.ncbi.nlm.nih.gov/pubmed/28913555
8. Baiges A, Turon F, Simón-Talero M, Stephanie T, Javier B, Kamal Z, et al. Congenital extrahepatic portosystemic shunts (Abernethy malformation). An international observational study. Hepatology. 2020;71(2):658–69.
9. Gitzelmann R, Forster I, Willi UV. Hypergalactosaemia in a newborn: self-limiting intrahepatic portosystemic venous shunt. Eur J Pediatr [Internet]. 1997;156(9):719–22. http://www.ncbi.nlm.nih.gov/pubmed/9296538
10. Ono H, Mawatari H, Mizoguchi N, Eguchi T, Sakura N. Clinical features and outcome of eight infants with intrahepatic porto-venous shunts detected in neonatal screening for galactosaemia. Acta Paediatr [Internet]. 1998;87(6):631–4. http://www.ncbi.nlm.nih.gov/pubmed/9686654
11. Joyce AD, Howard ER. Rare congenital anomaly of the portal vein. Br J Surg [Internet]. 1988;75(10):1038–9. http://www.ncbi.nlm.nih.gov/pubmed/2851363.
12. Franchi-Abella S, Gonzales E, Ackermann O, Branchereau S, Pariente D, Guérin F, et al. Congenital portosystemic shunts: diagnosis and treatment. Abdom Radiol (New York) [Internet]. 2018;43(8):2023–36. http://www.ncbi.nlm.nih.gov/pubmed/29730740
13. Howard ER, Davenport M. Congenital extrahepatic portocaval shunts – the Abernethy malformation. J Pediatr Surg. 1997;32(3):494–7.
14. Benedict M, Rodriguez-Davalos M, Emre S, Walther Z, Morotti R. Congenital extrahepatic portosystemic shunt (abernethy malformation type Ib) with associated 2 hepatocellular carcinoma: case report and literature review. Pediatr Dev Pathol [Internet]. 2016. https://doi.org/1 0.2350/16-01-1761-CR.1
15. Bhargava P, Vaidya S, Kolokythas O, Katz DS, Dighe M. Pictorial review. Hepatic vascular shunts: embryology and imaging appearances. Br J Radiol [Internet]. 2011. 84(1008):1142–52. http://www.ncbi.nlm.nih.gov/pubmed/22101582

16. Ikeda S, Sera Y, Ohshiro H, Uchino S, Uchino T, Endo F. Surgical indications for patients with hyperammonemia. J Pediatr Surg. 1999;34(6):1012–5.
17. Witters P, Maleux G, George C, Delcroix M, Hoffman I, Gewillig M, et al. Congenital veno-venous malformations of the liver: widely variable clinical presentations. J Gastroenterol Hepatol. 2008;23(8 PART2).
18. Shinkai M, Ohhama Y, Nishi T, Yamamoto H, Fujita S, Take H, et al. Congenital absence of the portal vein and role of liver transplantation in children. J Pediatr Surg. 2001;36(7):1026–31.
19. Bas S, Guran T, Atay Z, Haliloglu B, Abali S, Turan S, et al. Premature pubarche, hyper-insulinemia and hypothyroxinemia: novel manifestations of congenital portosystemic shunts (Abernethy malformation) in children. Horm Res Paediatr. 2015;83(4):282–7.
20. Konstas AA, Digumarthy SR, Avery LL, Wallace KL, Lisovsky M, Misdraji J, et al. Congenital portosystemic shunts: imaging findings and clinical presentations in 11 patients. Eur J Radiol. 2011;80(2):175–81.
21. Stringer MD. The clinical anatomy of congenital portosystemic venous shunts. Clin Anat. 2008;21(2):147–57.
22. Schaeffer DF, Laiq S, Jang HJ, John R, Adeyi OA. Abernethy malformation type II with nephrotic syndrome and other multisystemic presentation: an illustrative case for understanding pathogenesis of extrahepatic complication of congenital portosystemic shunt. Hum Pathol [Internet]. 2013;44(3):432–7. https://doi.org/10.1016/j.humpath.2012.08.018
23. Hu GH, Shen LG, Yang J, Mei JH, Zhu YF. Insight into congenital absence of the portal vein: is it rare? World J Gastroenterol. 2008;14(39):5969–79.
24. Kanazawa H, Nosaka S, Miyazaki O, Sakamoto S, Fukuda A, Shigeta T, et al. The classification based on intrahepatic portal system for congenital portosystemic shunts. J Pediatr Surg [Internet]. 2015;50(4):688–95. http://www.ncbi.nlm.nih.gov/pubmed/25840084.
25. Athanasiadis A, Karavida A, Chondromatidou S, Tsitouridis J, Tarlatzis B. Prenatal diagnosis of Abernethy malformation by three-dimensional ultrasonography. Ultrasound Obstet Gynecol. 2015;46(5):638–9.
26. Achiron R, Kivilevitch Z. Fetal umbilical-portal-systemic venous shunt: in-utero classification and clinical significance. Ultrasound Obstet Gynecol [Internet]. 2016;47(6):739–47. http://www.ncbi.nlm.nih.gov/pubmed/25988346.
27. Franchi-Abella S, Gonzales E, Ackermann O, Branchereau S, Pariente D, Guérin F. Congenital portosystemic shunts: diagnosis and treatment. Abdom Radiol. 2018;43(8):2023–36.
28. Glyn Morgan RS. Congenital absence of the portal vein: two cases and a proposed classification system for portasystemic vascular anomalies. J Pediatr Surg [Internet]. 1994;29(9):1239–41. https://doi.org/10.1016/0022-3468(94)90812-5.
29. Starzl TE, Francavilla A, Halgrimson CG, Francavilla FR, Porter KA, Brown TH, et al. The origin, hormonal nature, and action of hepatotrophic substances in portal venous blood. Surg Gynecol Obstet [Internet]. 1973;137(2):179–99. http://www.ncbi.nlm.nih.gov/pubmed/4353133
30. Bernard O, Franchi-Abella S, Branchereau S, Pariente D, Gauthier F, Jacquemin E. Congenital portosystemic shunts in children: recognition, evaluation, and management. Semin Liver Dis. 2012;32(4):273–87.
31. Murray CP, Yoo SJ, Babyn PS. Congenital extrahepatic portosystemic shunts. Pediatr Radiol. 2003;33(9):614–20.
32. Sanada Y, Mizuta K, Kawano Y, Egami S, Hayashida M, Wakiya T, et al. Living donor liver transplantation for congenital absence of the portal vein. Transplant Proc [Internet]. 2009;41(10):4214–9. http://linkinghub.elsevier.com/retrieve/pii/S0041134509014237
33. Matsuura T, Takahashi Y, Yanagi Y, Yoshimaru K, Yamamura K, Morihana E, et al. Surgical strategy according to the anatomical types of congenital portosystemic shunts in children. J Pediatr Surg [Internet]. 2016;51(12):2099–104. http://www.ncbi.nlm.nih.gov/pubmed/27697318
34. Guérin F, Blanc T, Gauthier F, Abella SF, Branchereau S. Congenital portosystemic vascular malformations. Semin Pediatr Surg [Internet]. Elsevier Inc.; 2012;21(3):233–44. https://doi.org/10.1053/j.sempedsurg.2012.05.006

35. Akahoshi T, Nishizaki T, Wakasugi K, Mastuzaka T, Kume K, Yamamoto I, et al. Portal-systemic encephalopathy due to a congenital extrahepatic portosystemic shunt: three cases and literature review. Hepatogastroenterology [Internet]. 47(34):1113–6. http://www.ncbi.nlm.nih.gov/pubmed/11020891.

36. Elnekave E, Belenky E, Van der Veer L. Noncirrhotic extrahepatic portosystemic shunt causing adult-onset encephalopathy treated with endovascular closure. Case Rep Radiol. 2015;2015:852853.

37. Morikawa N, Honna T, Kuroda T, Kitano Y, Fuchimoto Y, Kawashima N, et al. Resolution of hepatopulmonary syndrome after ligation of a portosystemic shunt in a pediatric patient with an Abernethy malformation. J Pediatr Surg. 2008;43(2).

38. Fu L, Wang Q, Wu J, Guo Y, Huang M, Liu T, et al. Congenital extrahepatic portosystemic shunt: an underdiagnosed but treatable cause of hepatopulmonary syndrome. Eur J Pediatr. 2016;175(2):195–201.

39. Yi J-E, Jung H-O, Youn H-J, Choi JY, Chun HJ, Lee JY. A case of pulmonary arterial hypertension associated with congenital extrahepatic portocaval shunt. J Korean Med Sci. 2014;29(4):604–8.

40. Sokollik C, Bandsma RHJ, Gana JC, van den Heuvel M, Ling SC. Congenital porto-systemic shunt: characterization of a multisystem disease. J Pediatr Gastroenterol Nutr. 2013;56(6):675–81.

41. Grazioli L, Alberti D, Olivetti L, Rigamonti W, Codazzi F, Matricardi L, et al. Congenital absence of portal vein with nodular regenerative hyperplasia of the liver. Eur Radiol. 2000;10(5):820–5.

42. Sharma R, Suddle A, Quaglia A, Peddu P, Karani J, Satyadas T, et al. Congenital extrahepatic portosystemic shunt complicated by the development of hepatocellular carcinoma. Hepatobiliary Pancreat Dis Int. 2015;14(5):552–7.

43. Sorkin T, Strautnieks S, Foskett P, Peddu P, Thompson RJ, Heaton N, et al. Case report: multiple beta-catenin mutations in hepatocellular lesions arising in Abernethy Malformation. Hum Pathol [Internet]. 2016;53:153–8. http://www.sciencedirect.com/science/article/pii/S0046817716300089

44. Happaerts S, Foucault A, Billiard JS, Nguyen B, Vandenbroucke-Menu F. Combined hepatocellular-cholangiocarcinoma in a patient with Abernethy malformation and tetralogy of Fallot: a case report. Hepatology [Internet]. 2016;2015–7. https://doi.org/10.1002/hep.28656

45. Sinakos E, Hytiroglou P, Chourmouzi D, Akriviadis E. Focal nodular hyperplasia in an individual with Abernethy malformation type 1b. Dig Liver Dis [Internet]. Editrice Gastroenterologica Italiana; 2015;47(12):1089. https://doi.org/10.1016/j.dld.2015.07.046

46. Gülşen Z, Yiğit H, Demir P. Multiple regenerative nodular hyperplasia in the left infrarenal vena cava accompanied by abernethy malformation. Surg Radiol Anat [Internet]. 2016;38(3):373–8. https://doi.org/10.1007/s00276-015-1460-5.

47. Alonso-Gamarra E, Parrón M, Pérez A, Prieto C, Hierro L, López-Santamaría M. Clinical and radiologic manifestations of congenital extrahepatic portosystemic shunts: a comprehensive review. Radiographics [Internet]. 2011;31(3):707–22. http://www.ncbi.nlm.nih.gov/pubmed/21571652.

48. Rajeswaran S, Johnston A, Green J, Riaz A, Thornburg B, Mouli S, Lautz T, Lemoine C, Superina R, Donaldson J. Abernethy malformations: evaluations and management of congenital portosystemic shunts. J Vasc Interv Radiol. 2020;31(5):788–94.

# Chapter 6
# Budd-Chiari Syndrome: Hepatic Venous Outflow Tract Obstruction

Virginia Hernández-Gea, Anna Baiges, Fanny Turon, and Juan Carlos Garcia-Pagan

## Introduction

Hepatic venous outflow tract obstruction (HVOTO) or Bud-Chiari syndrome (BCS) is characterized by the hepatic venous outflow obstruction anywhere from the small hepatic veins (HV) to the junction of the inferior vena cava (IVC) and the right atrium in the absence of cardiac or pericardial obstruction and hepatic veno-occlusive disease [1–3]. Although it can be rarely caused by extrinsic compression or intraluminal mass (tumoral, infectious or parasitic), this review is focused on primary BCS, in which obstruction originates in the vein caused by an endoluminal venous lesion (thrombosis or vascular web).

## Etiology and Risk Factors

BCS is a rare disease affecting mainly young people (median age at diagnosis 35–40 years) [4–6] with an incidence of 1 per million per year and usually associated with a prothrombotic condition [4]. Underlying disorders including hereditary and acquired hypercoagulable states and a miscellanea of other causes can be found in about 75% of patients with BCS [3].

An extensive etiological study of prothrombotic systemic disorder (Table 6.1) is mandatory at the diagnosis of BCS. Moreover in at least 35% of BCS patients more than one prothrombotic condition can be identified [4, 7] justifying that even when one causal factor is identified, additional factors should be investigated.

V. Hernández-Gea · A. Baiges · F. Turon · J. C. Garcia-Pagan (✉)
Barcelona Hepatic Hemodynamic Laboratory, Liver Unit, Hospital Clínic de Barcelona, IDIBAPS, CIBERehd, European Reference Network for Rare Vascular Liver Diseases, Universitat de Barcelona, Barcelona, Spain
e-mail: vihernandez@clinic.cat; abaigesa@clinic.cat; fturon@clinic.cat; jcgarcia@clinic.cat

© Springer Nature Switzerland AG 2022
D. Valla et al. (eds.), *Vascular Disorders of the Liver*,
https://doi.org/10.1007/978-3-030-82988-9_6

**Table 6.1** Prevalence of prothrombotic disorders in two recent European BCS cohort studies with 69 and [5, 58] 99 BCS patients

| | N tested | % Positive |
|---|---|---|
| *Acquired disorders* | | |
| Myeloproliferative neoplasms | 168 | 41 |
| Antiphospholipid syndrome | 165 | 10 |
| Paroxysmal nocturnal hemoglobinuria | 152 | 7 |
| *Inherited disorders* | | |
| Factor V Leiden | 165 | 8 |
| Factor II gene mutation | 168 | 3 |
| Protein C deficiency | 150 | 5 |
| Protein S deficiency | 147 | 4 |
| Antithrombin deficiency | 153 | 1 |
| External factors | | |
| Recent pregnancy | 168 | 1 |
| Oral contraceptive use | 168 | 22 |
| *Systemic disease*[a] | 168 | 6 |
| *Local factor* | | |
| Inflammatory intra-abdominal lesions[b] | 168 | 2 |
| Intra-abdominal surgery | 168 | 1 |
| Abdominal trauma | 168 | 2 |
| *No cause*[c] | 168 | 24 |
| *>1 risk factor* | 168 | 19 |

[a]Connective tissue disease, celiac disease, Behçet's disease, mastocytosis, inflammatory bowel disease, human immunodeficiency virus infection, sarcoidosis, myeloma
[b]Acute pancreatitis, biliary or intestinal infection/inflammation
[c]Including oral contraceptive use and pregnancy

There are also a variable number of patients in whom no risk factor can be identified, although the percentage has significantly decreased in recent studies suggesting an improvement in their detection [1, 8]. Identically, recent data coming from Asia, where the prevalence of prothrombotic disorders was traditionally low, show a higher detection probably due to an improvement in their detection [9, 10].

In more than 40% of European patients with BCS an underlying myeloproliferative neoplasm (MPN) can be detected. Indeed, BCS is 10,000-fold more common in patients with MPN than in the general population [11] both in Western and Eastern countries, with the exception of China where it is less common [9]. Among MPN, polycythemia vera is the most prevalent type associated with BCS, whereas essential thrombocythemia and myelofibrosis are less commonly identified [12].

Due to the very high prevalence of underlying somatic mutation in patients with MPN, identification of JAK2 V617F, JAK2 exon 12 and Calreticulin mutations are the major diagnostic criteria for MPN diagnosis. In BCS patients with typical hematological features of MPN, JAK2 can be found in up to 30–40% and even in the absence of hematological alterations it can be detected in 17% of the cases [13].

Additionally, Next-generation sequencing (NGS) has recently described as a potential useful tool capable of detecting JAK2 exon 12 mutations not previously detected by conventional techniques in this setting [14]. This is of special consideration as $JAK2^{V617F}$ in BCS is associated with poor prognosis and more severe presentation [15].

Other prothrombotic disorders have been associated with BCS, mainly factor V Leiden that is twice as high in patients with BCS than in general population both in Western and Eastern countries (except for China) [16]. Other less common associated disorders are paroxysmal nocturnal hemoglobinuria (HPN) and antiphospholipid syndrome. A study evaluated cytometry of 10 patients with HPN and BCS and showed that in all but one patient more than a half of the circulating granulocytes were affected by PNH (PNH-clone size >50%). Patients with HPN and PBH-clone size >50% are considered those with greater clinical expression of the disease and candidates for prophylactic treatments [17]. Inherited protein C/S or antithrombin deficiencies can also be found although its detection in patients with chronic liver disease is challenging [18, 19]. The ratio of protein C antigen, protein S antigen or antithrombin value to (factor II + factor X)/2 below 0.7 suggested the presence of hereditary deficiencies and it is recommended to investigate it [18].

Another systemic disease associated with BCS is Behcet's disease, a disorder characterized by the presence of recurrent oral and genital ulcerations and eye lesions [20].

Local factors such as abdominal infection or inflammatory diseases and local trauma have been reported in 11–25% of BCS patients, less frequently than in patients with thrombosis of the porto-mesenteric axis [1, 4, 7, 21].

Oral contraceptives, pregnancy and immediate postpartum are well-known prothrombotic factors that may increase the risk of BCS development; however when it develops other underlying thrombophilia has to be exhaustively sought [22, 23].


## Manifestations


Obstruction of the hepatic venous outflow leads to venous stasis and congestion increasing hepatic sinusoidal pressure and causing portal hypertension. Presentation may vary from asymptomatic cases to fulminant liver failure depending on the extent and rapidity of vein obstruction and the development of decompressive venous collaterals. Frequently, the diagnosis is made after portal hypertension related complications arise. Abdominal pain (61%), hepatomegaly (67%) and ascites (83%) is the most frequent clinical triad in European patients [1]. Moreover, esophageal varices can be detected in more than 50% of patients at diagnosis [1]. 15% of the cases can remain asymptomatic due to partial thrombosis accompanied by the formation of decompressive venous collaterals with frequent atrophy of the affected liver and hypertrophy of those segments well drained. These patients are usually incidentally diagnosed when studying mild alteration of liver enzymes [1,

24]. Conversely, if the thrombosis is rapidly formed and extensive, acute liver failure may arise with high mortality if not adequately treated. It is not infrequent, despite severe acute onset, to find signs of chronic liver disease as thrombosis can recur in a patient with previous hepatic vein occlusion that initially achieved enough hepatic outflow to maintain the patient compensated.

Blood test may reveal mild transaminases elevation and decrease prothrombin time in severe cases. Low cellularity and high protein content ascites may also help in the diagnosis of BCS [25, 26].

In eastern countries however, the most frequent presentation are clinical decompensation of portal hypertension, abdominal portosystemic collaterals and lower limb edema or ulcers as the main common site of thrombosis is the inferior vena cava alone or combined with hepatic vein obstruction [27, 28].

Up to 60–80% of patients with BCS have regenerative nodules in imaging exams. Typically they are multiple (more than 10 lesions), small in size (under 4 cm), hypervascularized and disseminated throughout the liver [7]. Malignant transformation may occur during follow up, with a 5-year cumulative incidence of 7% [29]. In a recent systematic review addressing prevalence, rates ranged from 2–46%, probably due to heterogeneity of the studies included [30]. A higher risk of hepatocellular carcinoma (HCC) development has been described in patients with long-term IVC obstruction [31], although predisposing factors remain unknown. Radiological diagnosis of BCS-associated nodules remains challenging. Benign nodules may present the typical radiological features and vascular enhancement pattern of HCC in cirrhosis and may increase in number and size over time [29, 32, 33]. Consequently, HCC diagnosis in a patient with BCS always requires histological confirmation. A level of alpha-fetoprotein above 15 ng/ml has been suggested as biomarker for HCC in BCS patients, although it cannot be recommended in clinical practice until validated in larger studies [2, 29].

# Diagnosis

Clinical manifestations are very heterogeneous, justifying suspicion in any patient with acute or chronic liver disease of unknown origin and/or with an underlying prothrombotic condition (Fig. 6.1). Diagnosis requires demonstration of hepatic venous flow obstruction and non-invasive imagining techniques (Doppler ultrasonography, CT-Scan or MRI) are the mainstay of diagnosis. Doppler ultrasound, performed by an experienced operator, has a sensitivity higher than 75% and should be the first choice option [2]. Typical ultrasound features of venous obstruction are: identification of thrombus, non-visualization of the HV, collateral veins and transformation of the HV into a cord lacking flow signals, caudate lobe hypertrophy and a caudate vein greater than 3 mm [34, 35]. Usually, the role of MRI and CT-Scan is

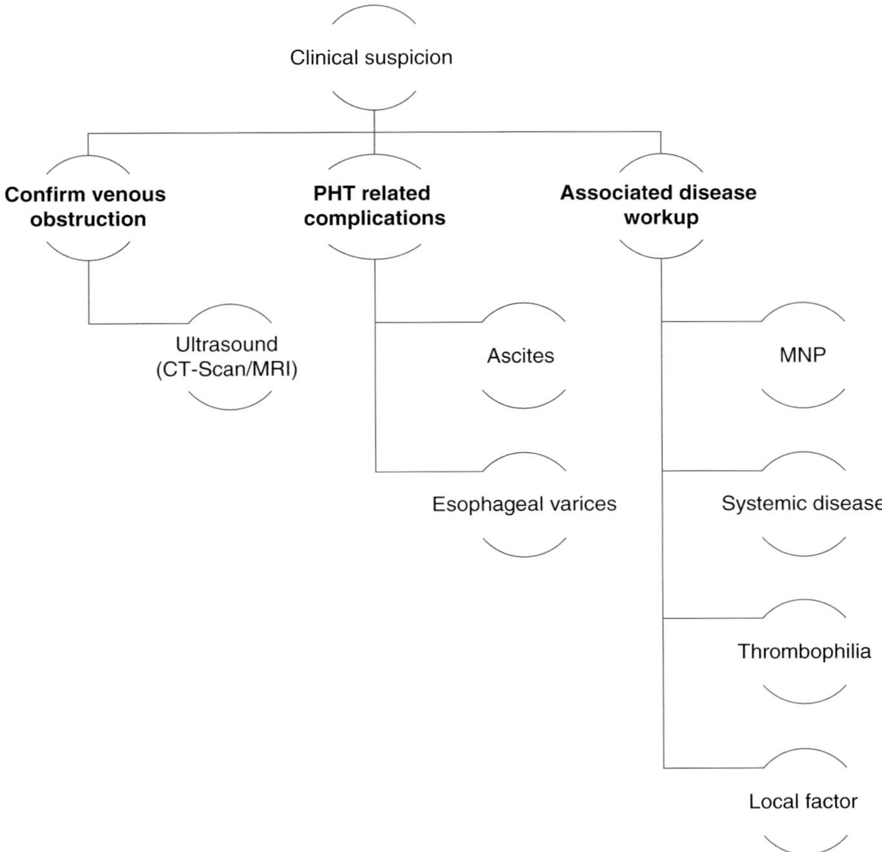


**Fig. 6.1** Proposed diagnostic algorithm for Budd-Chiari syndrome

diagnosis confirmation and should be of choice in the absence of an experience US operator. They can depict a rapid clearance of dye from the caudate lobe and patchy hepatic enhancement due to uneven portal perfusion.

Hepatic venography may be helpful in cases of uncertain diagnosis and the most typical sign is the presence of a spiderweb pattern drawing collateral circulation (Fig. 6.2).

Liver biopsy is not necessary for diagnosis unless BCS due to small intrahepatic veins obstruction is suspected. In these patients, liver histology is the only way to achieve diagnosis. In the other circumstances, histological changes are supportive but not pathognomonic (congestion, coagulative necrosis or simple loss of hepato-cytes without inflammatory infiltrates and/or fibrosis) as they may be found in other

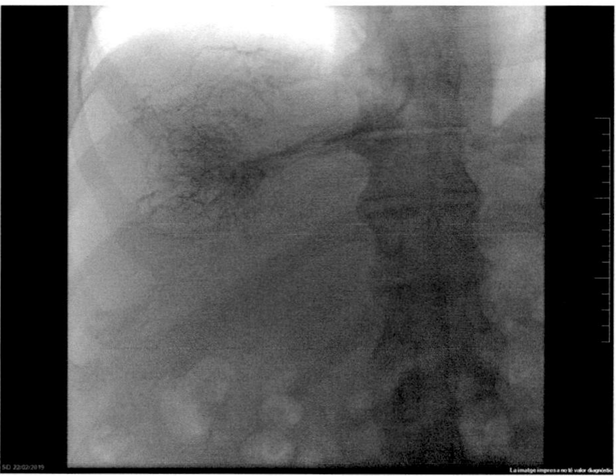

**Fig. 6.2** Presence of a spiderweb pattern drawing collateral circulation in a patients with BCS

congestive etiologies. Histologic findings are also no reflective of disease severity as liver damage maybe patchy and very heterogeneous [2].

## Treatment

Treatment of BCS is based on three mainstays: management of portal hypertension, treatment of the underlying disease and restoring hepatic venous outflow.

5.1. Portal hypertension complications (treatments of ascites, prophylaxis of variceal bleeding…) should be managed as recommended for liver cirrhosis [2, 36].
5.2. Management of the underlying prothrombotic disorder. A prompt diagnosis of the underlying prothrombotic disorders and its specific treatment should be the main goal in BCS as it markedly influences the outcome and/or prevent thrombosis progression.
5.3. Hepatic venous outflow restoration. The most recommended and supported approach is a progressive therapeutic strategy [2, 8, 36] stepping from less to more invasive treatments according to the clinical response of the patient. However, the main challenge is to recognize the good time to step forward in a given patient, representing an important reason why these patients should be managed in referral centers with a dedicated multidisciplinary team of hepatologist, radiologists, hematologist and specialist in systemic disorders.

    5.3.1 Anticoagulation represents the first step, with the aim of achieving vein recanalization but mainly of preventing thrombosis progression. All patients with diagnosis of BCS even in the absence of symptoms or of a recognized prothrombotic disorder should receive anticoagulation. Just with the use of early and long-term anticoagulation a 5-year intervention free survival with control of the disease is achieved in approximately 25% of patients, especially in mild/moderate cases in both Western and Eastern patients. Low molecular weight heparin followed by vitamin k antagonist, once the patient is in stable conditions, is the most frequent anticoagulation approach. Unfractionated heparin should be avoided due to risk of heparin-induced thrombocytopenia [8]. Data with DOACS are very limited, although promising, but BCS is not an approved indication yet [37, 38].

5.3.2 Thrombolysis. In selected cases of recent and incomplete thrombosis, and always at experienced centers, local instillation of recombinant tissue plasminogen activator after catheterization of the thrombosed hepatic vein and in combination with another interventional procedure (e.g. angioplasty, stenting) may help to restore venous outflow [39]. Bleeding complications can occur and can even be fatal. Thus, this strategy is contraindicated in patients with a potentially hemorrhagic condition or who had any invasive procedure in the previous 24 h.

5.3.3 Percutaneous angioplasty. In cases of segmental stenosis, percutaneous transluminal angioplasty with or without stenting may restore hepatic vein outflow relieving symptoms with an adequate safety profile. However, in the European population this therapeutic approach only account for 10% of the cases [6]. In Asia, where IVC obstruction predominates, combination of angioplasty and stenting can achieve patency in more than 80% of the patents at 5 years [40]. A recent RCT suggested that routine stenting with angioplasty is superior to angioplasty alone in patients with Budd-Chiari syndrome with short hepatic vein stenosis and this approach should be the first choice treatment [41]. However, this study has been challenged by the fact that no changes in survival were observed with this approach and in 60% of patients receiving angioplasty alone no reestenosis was observed [42]. Therefore, current evidence shows that there is still room for trying angioplasty first and reserving stenting for failures [42]. Similarly, it has been suggested that retrievable stents may prevent long-term occlusions and stenosis, however data need to be confirmed before their recommendation [43].

5.3.4 Derivative techniques that convert the portal system into an outflow tract aimed to decompress the liver may be necessary when all the above fails. Mesocaval surgical shunts or mesoatrial shunt (by passing the inferior vena cava when the obstruction is localized also at this level) were the only derivative techniques available before the 90s

[44, 45]. These surgical procedures are associated with a high early morbi-mortality. Indeed, patients requiring decompresive surgery are in poor conditions developing frequent surgical complications. Moreover, shunts frequently thrombose. A variable percentage of patients (32%–68%) in whom the shunt remained patent during follow up had excellent outcome [46, 47]. Currently, decompressive surgery has been almost completely replaced by the less invasive transjugular intrahepatic portosystemic shunt (TIPS) which has demonstrated to be more effective in maintaining patency (67% at 2 years using PTFE-covered stents). TIPS however should be placed in centers of expertise due to technical difficulty, as it often requires a transcaval approach for the portal vein puncture. In a European cohort of 157 patients with BCS, 40% required treatment with TIPS. In most patients (73%), TIPS was placed during the first 6 months after diagnosis due to persistence of symptoms despite medical therapy. In this cohort, 5-year survival without need of liver transplant (requiring TIPS and/or angioplasty in association to anticoagulation) was of 72% [6]. In Asian countries, TIPS is less frequently needed as the main site of obstruction is the IVC requiring angioplasty/stenting obtaining similar outcome than in the European cohorts [48, 49].

5.3.5 Liver transplantation (OLT) represents the last therapeutic option in those patients in whom the previous mentioned approach fails. In addition, OLT may be the first step in patients with fulminant hepatic failure. As it happens with TIPS, OLT in BCS may be technically difficult due to retroperitoneal fibrosis, increased size of the caudate lobe and occlusion of the HV ostia. Post OLT survival rate has improved over the years and in European patient. In a large cohort of patients in whom OLT was in most cases used as a first treatment option (previous TIPS was only performed in a few patients) the overall survival was 76%, 71% and 68% at 1 year, 5 years and 10 years respectively [50]. These survival rates were similar to those observed when using a stepwise treatment and accordingly only applying OLT to 7% of patients reinforcing the benefit of the stepwise approach while saving a large number of liver graft for other indications [51]. Interestingly, the previous use of TIPS does not seem to worsen post-OLT prognosis if patients finally require OLT [51].

Management of the underlying prothrombotic disease leading to BCS becomes relevant after OLT. Indeed, it may be cured with the transplant such as in the case of protein C or S deficiency but also may impact the outcome post-OLT if not adequately treated such as in the case of MPN. Thus, patients with MPN may require long-term post-OLT anticoagulation, aspirin or antiproliferative treatment depending of the thrombotic risk and should be closely monitored to prevent/detect recurrent thrombotic complications [52, 53].

## Pregnancy

Good outcome has been demonstrated in patients with BCS during pregnancy, hence it should not be contraindicated although risk of miscarriage and premature birth are increased [22]. Patients should be managed by a multidisciplinary team including obstetricians experienced in high risk pregnancies. Anticoagulation during pregnancy and postpartum should be maintained if patient was already under anticoagulation. Low molecular weight heparins are the preferred agent for anticoagulation during pregnancy while vitamin K antagonists are not recommended since it cross the placental barrier and carry teratogenicity. In patients with no previous anticoagulation, its initiation should be evaluated individually depending in prothrombotic state and obstetrical history.

Assisted vaginal delivery remains the recommended strategy [22]. Patients should be screened for portopulmonary hypertension, as it can be worsen during pregnancy. Screening for esophageal varices is recommended during second trimester if patient is not on beta-blockers to apply proper prophylaxis.

## Prognosis

The outcome of BCS has improved in the last decades due to a higher degree of suspicion leading to early stage diagnosis but also to a better management. 5 years survival in the largest prospective multicenter cohort of European BCS patients was 85% [6]. Although initially suggested, the presence of lesions at liver biopsy does not contribute to predict outcome in BCS [54].

Liver function is an independent predictor of outcome in BCS [54, 55]. ALT $\geq 5 \times$ ULN at presentation has been associated with a poor outcome if there is not a rapid decrease in ASAT levels in the following few days [11, 56]. Specific BCS prognostic scores are useful for predicting transplant-free survival of futility for invasive therapy (Table 6.2). However, none of these prognostic scores can predict individual prognosis and cannot be used to guide individualized management [57].

**Table 6.2** Specific BCS prognostic scores

| Score | Formula | Cut-off | Predicted survival rate | References |
|---|---|---|---|---|
| Clichy prognostic index | Ascites score[a] × 0.75) + (Pugh score×0.28) + (age × 0.037) + (creatinine × 0.0036) | 5.4 (range from 3.4 to 9.1) | At 5y $\leq$5.4: 95% > 5.4: 65% | [59] |
| New Clichy prognostic index | 0.95 × ascites score+0.35 × Pugh score + 0.0 47 × age+0.0045 × serum creatinine+2.2 × type III[b]—2.6 | 5.1 (range from 2.0 to 9.7) | At 5y <5.1: 100% $\geq$ 5.1: 65% | [60] |
| Rotterdam BCS index | 1.27 × encephalopathy+1.04 × ascites + 0.72 × prothrombin time + 0.004 × bilirubin | Class I: 0–1.1 Class II: 1.1–1.5 Class III: $^3$1.5 (range from 0.02 to 4.03) | At 5y Class I 89% Class II 74% Class III 42% | [61] |
| TIPS-BCS prognostic index | Age ((years) × 0.08 + bilirubin (mg/dL) × 0.16 + international normalized ratio (INR) × 0.63 | 7 | 1-year OLT-free survival $\leq$7 95% >7 12% | [51] |
| BCS-intervention-free survival prognostic score | Ascites [yes = 1, no = 0]*1.675 + ln creatinine [umol/L]*0.613 + ln bilirubin [umol/ L]*0.440) | Interval I: £5 Interval 2: 5–6 Interval 3: $\geq$ 6 | Intervention-free survival Interval I 78.3% Interval 2 27.8% Interval 3 6.8% | [6] |
| BCSurvival score | Age/10*0.370 + ln creatinine [umol/L]*0.809 + ln bilirubin [umol/L]*0.496) | Interval I: $\leq$7 Interval 2: 7–8 Interval 3 $\geq$ 8 | Probability survival 87.5% 63.3% 42.9% | [6] |

[a]Ascites score: 1, absent with free sodium intake and no diuretic agents; 2, easy to control with sodium restriction or diuretic agents; and 3, resistant to this treatment because of hyponatremia or functional renal failure

[b]Type III' is a binary variable coded as 1 for patients with clinicopathological findings of acute injury superimposed on chronic lesions, and 0 for the other patients

# References


1. Murad SDSD, Plessier A, Hernandez-Guerra M, Fabris F, Eapen CECEE, Bahr MJMJJ, et al. Etiology, management, and outcome of the Budd-Chiari syndrome. Ann Intern Med [Internet]. 2009;151(3):167–75. http://www.ncbi.nlm.nih.gov/pubmed/19652186.
2. European Association for the Study of the liver. EASL clinical practice guidelines: vascular diseases of the liver. J Hepatol. 2016;64(1):179–202.
3. Menon KVN, Shah V, Kamath PS. The Budd–Chiari syndrome. N Engl J Med. 2004;350:578–85.
4. Ollivier-Hourmand I, Allaire M, Goutte N, Morello R, Chagneau-Derrode C, Goria O, et al. The epidemiology of Budd–Chiari syndrome in France. Dig Liver Dis [Internet]. 2018;50(9):931–7. https://doi.org/10.1016/j.dld.2018.04.004
5. Turon F, Cervantes F, Colomer D, Baiges A, Hernandez-Gea V, Garcia-Pagan JC, et al. Role of calreticulin mutations in the aetiological diagnosis of splanchnic vein thrombosis. J Hepatol [Internet]. 2015;62(1600–0641 (electronic)):72–4. http://www.ncbi.nlm.nih.gov/pubmed/25173966
6. Seijo S, Plessier A, Hoekstra J, Era AD, Mandair D, Rifai K, et al. Good long-term outcome of Budd-Chiari syndrome with a step-wise management. Hepatology [Internet]. 2013;57(5):1962–8. http://www.ncbi.nlm.nih.gov/pubmed/23389867
7. Valla D-C. Budd–Chiari syndrome/hepatic venous outflow tract obstruction. Hepatol Int [Internet]. 2018;12(S1):168–80. http://www.ncbi.nlm.nih.gov/pubmed/28685257
8. Plessier A, Sibert A, Consigny Y, Hakime A, Zappa M, Denninger M-HH, et al. Aiming at minimal invasiveness as a therapeutic strategy for Budd-Chiari syndrome. Hepatology [Internet]. 2006;44(5):1308–16. http://www.ncbi.nlm.nih.gov/pubmed/17058215
9. Qi X, Wu F, Ren W, He C, Yin Z, Niu J, et al. Thrombotic risk factors in Chinese Budd-Chiari syndrome patients. An observational study with a systematic review of the literature. Thromb Haemost. 2013;109(0340–6245 (Print)):878–84.
10. Pati HP, Dayal S, Srivastava A, Pande GK, Acharya SK. Spectrum of hemostatic derangements, in Budd-Chiari syndrome. Indian J Gastroenterol [Internet]. 2003;22(2):59–60. http://www.ncbi.nlm.nih.gov/pubmed/12696825
11. Parekh J, Matei VM, Canas-Coto A, Friedman D, Lee WM, Acute Liver Failure Study Group. Budd-chiari syndrome causing acute liver failure: a multicenter case series. Liver Transpl [Internet]. 2017;23(2):135–42. https://doi.org/10.1002/lt.24643
12. Valla D, Casadevall N, Lacombe C, Varet B, Goldwasser E, Franco D, et al. Primary myeloproliferative disorder and hepatic vein thrombosis. A prospective study of erythroid colony formation in vitro in 20 patients with Budd-Chiari syndrome. AnnInternMed. 1985;103(0003–4819 (Print)):329–34.
13. Smalberg JH, Arends LR, Valla DC, Kiladjian JJ, Janssen HL, Leebeek FW. Myeloproliferative neoplasms in Budd-Chiari syndrome and portal vein thrombosis: a meta-analysis. Blood. 2012;120(1528–0020 (Electronic)):4921–8.
14. Magaz M, Alvarez-Larrán A, Colomer D, López-Guerra M, García-Criado MÁ, Mezzano G, et al. Next-generation sequencing in the diagnosis of non-cirrhotic splanchnic vein thrombosis. J Hepatol [Internet]. 2020;15:S0168-8278. https://doi.org/10.1016/j.jhep.2020.06.045.
15. Kiladjian JJJ-JJ, Cervantes F, Leebeek FWGWFWG, Marzac C, Cassinat B, Chevret S, et al. The impact of JAK2 and MPL mutations on diagnosis and prognosis of splanchnic vein thrombosis: A report on 241 cases. Blood. 2008;111(1528–0020 (Electronic)):4922–9.
16. Deltenre P, Denninger MH, Hillaire S, Guillin MC, Casadevall N, Briere J, et al. Factor V Leiden related Budd-Chiari syndrome. Gut. 2001;48(2):264–8.
17. Ragasol A. Budd-Chiari syndrome and paroxysmal nocturnal hemoglobinuria. MedChir Dig. 1974;3(0047–6412 (Print)):405–7.
18. Janssen HL, Meinardi JR, Vleggaar FP, van Uum SH, Haagsma EB, Der Meer FJ, et al. Factor V Leiden mutation, prothrombin gene mutation, and deficiencies in coagulation inhibitors associated with Budd-Chiari syndrome and portal vein thrombosis: results of a case-control study. Blood. 2000;96(7):2364–8.

19. Qi XHGL. Ulcer in Budd-Chiari syndrome. Am J Gastroenterol. 2016;111:25.
20. Seyahi E, Caglar E, Ugurlu S, Kantarci F, Hamuryudan V, Sonsuz A, et al. An outcome survey of 43 patients with Budd-Chiari syndrome due to Behçet's syndrome followed up at a single, dedicated center. Semin Arthritis Rheum [Internet]. 2015;44(5):602–9. https://linkinghub.elsevier.com/retrieve/pii/S0049017214002558
21. Plompen EPC, Valk PJMPJM, Chu I, Murad SD, Plessier A, Turon F, et al. Somatic calreticulin mutations in patients with Budd-Chiari syndrome and portal vein thrombosis. Haematologica [Internet]. 2015;100(1592–8721 (electronic)). http://www.ncbi.nlm.nih.gov/pubmed/25682604
22. Bissonnette J, Durand F, de Raucourt E, Ceccaldi PF, Plessier A, Valla D, et al. Pregnancy and vascular liver disease. J Clin Exp Hepatol. 2015;5(1):41–50.
23. Valla D, Le MG, Poynard T, Zucman N, Rueff B, Benhamou JP. Risk of hepatic vein thrombosis in relation to recent use of oral contraceptives. A case-control study. Gastroenterology. 1986;90(0016–5085 (Print)):807–11.
24. Hadengue A, Poliquin M, Vilgrain V, Belghiti J, Degott C, Erlinger S, et al. The changing scene of hepatic vein thrombosis: recognition of asymptomatic cases. Gastroenterology [Internet]. 1994;106(4):1042–7. http://www.ncbi.nlm.nih.gov/pubmed/8143970
25. Hernández-Gea V, De Gottardi A, Leebeek FWG, Rautou PE, Salem R, Garcia-Pagan JC. Current knowledge in pathophysiology and management of Budd-Chiari syndrome and non-cirrhotic non-tumoral splanchnic vein thrombosis. J Hepatol [Internet]. 2019;71(1):175–99. https://doi.org/10.1016/j.jhep.2019.02.015.
26. Mitchell MC, Boitnott JK, Kaufman S, Cameron JL, Maddrey WC. Budd-Chiari syndrome: etiology, diagnosis and management. Med. 1982;61(0025–7974 (Print)):199–218.
27. Qi X, Han G, Guo X, De Stefano V, Xu K, Lu Z, et al. Review article: the aetiology of primary Budd-Chiari syndrome – differences between the West and China. Aliment Pharmacol Ther [Internet]. 2016;44(11–12):1152–67. https://doi.org/10.1111/apt.13815
28. Okuda K. Inferior vena cava thrombosis at its hepatic portion (obliterative hepatocavopathy). Semin Liver Dis. 2002;22(0272–8087 (Print)):15–26.
29. Moucari R, Rautou P-EE, Cazals-Hatem D, Geara A, Bureau C, Consigny Y, et al. Hepatocellular carcinoma in Budd-Chiari syndrome: characteristics and risk factors. Gut [Internet]. 2008;(1468–3288 (electronic)):828–35. http://www.ncbi.nlm.nih.gov/pubmed/18218675
30. Ren W, Qi X, Jia J, Yang MHG. Prevalence of hepatocellular carcinoma in Chinese Budd-Chiari syndrome patients: an extended systematic review using Chinese-language databases. Eur J Gastroenterol Hepatol. 2013;25:1241–3.
31. Paul SB, Shalimar, Sreenivas V, Gamanagatti SR, Sharma H, Dhamija E, et al. Incidence and risk factors of hepatocellular carcinoma in patients with hepatic venous outflow tract obstruction. Aliment Pharmacol Ther [Internet]. 2015;41(10):961–71. https://doi.org/10.1111/apt.13173
32. Cazals-Hatem D, Vilgrain V, Genin P, Denninger MH, Durand F, Belghiti J, et al. Arterial and portal circulation and parenchymal changes in Budd-Chiari syndrome: a study in 17 explanted livers. Hepatology. 2003;37(0270–9139 (Print)):510–9.
33. Brancatelli G, Federle MP, Grazioli L, Golfieri R, Lencioni R. Benign regenerative nodules in Budd-Chiari syndrome and other vascular disorders of the liver: radiologic-pathologic and clinical correlation. Radiographics [Internet]. 2002;22(4):847–62. http://www.ncbi.nlm.nih.gov/pubmed/12110714
34. Bargalló X, Gilabert R, Nicolau C, García-Pagán JC, Bosch J, Brú C, et al. Sonography of the caudate vein: value in diagnosing Budd-Chiari syndrome. Am J Roentgenol [Internet]. 2003;181(6):1641–5. file:///f/HEMHEPAT/PDF reference manager/JC2/PDF articles Nostres/Budd-chiari-TP/AJR Am.J.Roentgenol-2003(1641-1645pag).pdf
35. Miller WJ, Federle MP, Straub WH, Davis PL. Budd-Chiari syndrome: imaging with pathologic correlation. Abdom Imaging [Internet]. 1993;18(4):329–35. http://www.ncbi.nlm.nih.gov/pubmed/8220030.
36. De Franchis R, Abraldes JG, Bajaj J, Berzigotti A, Bosch J, Burroughs AK, et al. Expanding consensus in portal hypertension: report of the Baveno VI consensus workshop: stratifying

risk and individualizing care for portal hypertension. J Hepatol [Internet]. 2015;63(3):743–52. http://linkinghub.elsevier.com/retrieve/pii/S0168827815003499

37. Taguchi E, Koyama J, Kajiwara M, Inoue M, Horibata Y, Nishigami K, et al. Successful Vascular Intervention Without Embolic Complications in Budd-Chiari Syndrome. Circ J [Internet]. 2018;82:602–3. https://www.jstage.jst.go.jp/article/circj/82/2/82_CJ-17-0333/_pdf/-char/en

38. De Gottardi A, Trebicka J, Klinger C, Plessier A, Seijo S, Terziroli B, et al. Antithrombotic treatment with direct-acting oral anticoagulants (DOACs) in patients with splanchnic vein thrombosis and cirrhosis. Liver Int [Internet]. 2016;37(5):694–9. https://doi.org/10.1111/liv.13285.

39. Sharma S, Texeira A, Texeira P, Elias E, Wilde J, Olliff SP. Pharmacological thrombolysis in Budd Chiari syndrome: a single centre experience and review of the literature. J Hepatol. 2004;40(1):172–80.

40. Han G, Qi X, Zhang W, He C, Yin Z, Wang J, et al. Percutaneous recanalization for Budd-Chiari syndrome: an 11-year retrospective study on patency and survival in 177 Chinese patients from a single center. Radiology. 2013;266(2):657–67.

41. Wang Q, Li K, He C, Yuan X, Luo B, Qi X, et al. Angioplasty with versus without routine stent placement for Budd-Chiari syndrome: a randomised controlled trial. Lancet Gastroenterol Hepatol [Internet]. 2019;4(9):686–97. https://doi.org/10.1016/S2468-1253(19)30177-3.

42. Ferrusquía-Acosta J, Hernández-Gea V, Turón F, García-Pagán JC. Budd-Chiari syndrome with short-length stenosis: still room for the angioplasty and wait-and-see strategy. Lancet Gastroenterol Hepatol [Internet]. 2019;4(11):823. https://doi.org/10.1016/S2468-1253(19)30296-1

43. Bi Y, Chen H, Ding P, Ren J, Han X. Comparison of retrievable stents and permanent stents for Budd-Chiari syndrome due to obstructive inferior vena cava. J Gastroenterol Hepatol [Internet]. 2018;33(12):2015–21. https://doi.org/10.1111/jgh.14295

44. Klein AS, Molmenti EP. Surgical treatment of Budd-Chiari syndrome. Liver Transpl [Internet]. 2003;9(9):891–6. https://doi.org/10.1053/jlts.2003.50156

45. Bachet J, Condat B, Consigny Y, Belghiti J, Valla D. Long-term portosystemic shunt patency as a determinant of outcome in Budd – Chiari syndrome. J Hepatol. 2007;46:60–8.

46. Panis Y, Belghiti J, Valla D, Benhamou JP, Fekete F. Portosystemic shunt in Budd-Chiari syndrome: long-term survival and factors affecting shunt patency in 25 patients in Western countries. Surgery. 1994;115(3):276–81.

47. Chen H, Zhang F, Ye Y, Cheng Y, Chen Y. Long-term follow-up study and comparison of meso-atrial shunts and meso-cavo-atrial shunts for treatment of combined Budd-Chiari syndrome. J Surg Res [Internet]. 2011;168(1):162–6. http://linkinghub.elsevier.com/retrieve/pii/S002248040900393X

48. Qi X, Guo W, He C, Zhang W, Wu F, Yin Z, et al. Transjugular intrahepatic portosystemic shunt for Budd-Chiari syndrome: techniques, indications and results on 51 Chinese patients from a single centre. Liver Int [Internet]. 2014;34(1478–3231 (Electronic)):1164–75. http://www.ncbi.nlm.nih.gov/pubmed/24256572

49. He F, Zhao H, Dai S, Wu Y, Wang L, Huang H, et al. Transjugular intrahepatic portosystemic shunt for Budd–Chiari syndrome with diffuse occlusion of hepatic veins. Sci Rep [Internet]. 2016;6(1):36380. http://www.ncbi.nlm.nih.gov/pubmed/27805025

50. Mentha G, Giostra E, Majno PE, Bechstein WO, Neuhaus P, Grady JO, et al. Liver transplantation for Budd – Chiari syndrome: a European study on 248 patients from 51 centres *. J Hepatol. 2006;44(2005):520–8.

51. Garcia-Pagan JC, Heydtmann M, Raffa S, Plessier A, Murad S, Fabris F, et al. TIPS for Budd-Chiari syndrome: long-term results and prognostics factors in 124 patients. Gastroenterology [Internet]. 2008;135(3):808–15. http://www.ncbi.nlm.nih.gov/pubmed/18621047.

52. Melear JM, Goldstein RM, Levy MF, Molmenti EP, Cooper B, Netto GJ, et al. Hematologic aspects of liver transplantation for Budd-Chiari syndrome with special reference to myeloproliferative disorders. Transplantation. 2002;74(0041–1337 (Print)):1090–5.

53. Chinnakotla S, Klintmalm GB, Kim P, Tomiyama K, Klintmalm E, Davis GL, et al. Long-term follow-up of liver transplantation for Budd-Chiari syndrome with antithrombotic therapy

based on the etiology. Transplantation [Internet]. 2011;92(3):341–5. http://www.ncbi.nlm.nih.gov/pubmed/21659946.

54. Tang TJ, Batts KP, de Groen PC, van Hoek B, Haagsma EB, Hop WC, et al. The prognostic value of histology in the assessment of patients with Budd-Chiari syndrome. J Hepatol. 2001;35(0168–8278 SB–IM):338–43.

55. Darwish MS, Kim WR, de Groen PC, Kamath PS, Malinchoc M, Valla DC, et al. Can the model for end-stage liver disease be used to predict the prognosis in patients with Budd-Chiari syndrome? Liver Transplant. 2007;13(1527–6465 (Print)):867–74.

56. Denié C, Douarin L, Francoz C, Durand F, Ozenne V, Rautou P, et al. Levels and initial course of serum alnaine aminotransferase can predict outcome of patients with Budd-Chiari syndrome. Clin Gastroenterol Hepatol [Internet]. 2009;7(11):1230–5. http://www.ncbi.nlm.nih.gov/pubmed/19560555.

57. Rautou PE, Moucari R, Escolano S, Cazals-Hatem D, Denie C, Chagneau-Derrode C, et al. Prognostic indices for Budd-Chiari syndrome: valid for clinical studies but insufficient for individual management. Am J Gastroenterol. 2009;104(1572–0241 (Electronic)):1140–6.

58. Poisson J, Plessier A, Kiladjian JJ, Turon F, Cassinat B, Andreoli A, et al. Selective testing for calreticulin gene mutations in patients with splanchnic vein thrombosis: a prospective cohort study. J Hepatol [Internet]. 2017;67(3):501–7. https://doi.org/10.1016/j.jhep.2017.04.021.

59. Zeitoun G, Escolano S, Hadengue A, Azar N, El Younsi M, Mallet A, et al. Outcome of Budd-Chiari syndrome: a multivariate analysis of factors related to survival including surgical portosystemic shunting. Hepatology [Internet]. 1999;30(0270–9139 SB–M):84–9. http://www.ncbi.nlm.nih.gov/pubmed/10385643.

60. Langlet P, Escolano S, Valla D, Coste-zeitoun D, Denie C, Mallet A, et al. Clinicopathological forms and prognostic index in Budd-Chiari syndrome. J Hepatol. 2003;39:496–501.

61. Darwish Murad S, Valla DC, de Groen PC, Zeitoun G, Hopmans JAM, Haagsma EB, et al. Determinants of survival and the effect of portosystemic shunting in patients with Budd-Chiari syndrome. Hepatology [Internet]. 2004;39(2):500–8. http://www.ncbi.nlm.nih.gov/pubmed/14768004.

# Chapter 7
# Extrahepatic Portal Vein Obstruction: Recent Portal Vein Thrombosis and Portal Cavernoma in the Absence of Cirrhosis

Aurélie Plessier

## Abbreviations

| | |
|---|---|
| CT scan | Computerized tomography scan |
| DOACS | Direct oral anticoagulants |
| EHPVO | Extrahepatic portal vein obstruction |
| HCC | Hepatocellular carcinoma |
| HCA | Hepatic cell adenoma |
| MPN | Myeloproliferative neoplasm |
| MRI | Magnetic resonance imaging |
| SIRS | Systemic inflammatory response syndrome |
| TIPS | Transjugular porto systemic shunt |
| PSVD | Porto sinusoidal vascular disease |

## Definition and Epidemiology of Recent (or Acute) and Chronic Extrahepatic Portal Vein Obstruction

Extrahepatic portal vein obstruction (EHPVO) is the obstruction of the extrahepatic portal vein, and/or right or left branches, associated or not to obstruction of other segments of the splanchnic venous axis. It does not include isolated thrombosis of the splenic or superior mesenteric veins. EHPVO secondary to malignant tumor (frequently but improperly referred to as malignant thrombosis) is considered as a

A. Plessier (✉)
Centre de Référence des Maladies Vasculaires du Foie, Inserm U1149, Centre de Recherche sur l'Inflammation (CRI), Université Paris 7-Denis-Diderot, Paris, France

Fil-foie, ERN Rare Liver, Clichy, France
e-mail: aurelie.plessier@aphp.fr

© Springer Nature Switzerland AG 2022
D. Valla et al. (eds.), *Vascular Disorders of the Liver*,
https://doi.org/10.1007/978-3-030-82988-9_7

different entity, related to encasement or invasion of the veins by malignant tumors, including primary hepatobiliary malignancy most often in the presence of cirrhosis.

We will here discuss non-malignant EHPVO in the absence of cirrhosis. In this context, portal venous obstruction is due to thrombosis or fibrous stenosis of these veins. EHPVO is either recognized at a recent stage (so called acute) or at a chronic stage, as a sequel of portal vein obstruction, most often recognized by porto-portal collaterals (so called portal cavernoma). Acute EHPVO refers to recent obstruction while chronic EHPVO refers to a long standing obstruction. We prefer using the term "recent EHPVO" rather than acute EHPVO. Indeed, precise determination of the date of occurrence of acute EHPVO is difficult, the diagnosis being often made during a 1–2 weeks period of time, based on symptoms and imaging. Moreover, acute portal vein thrombosis (rethrombosis) may also occur in patients with preexisting chronic obstruction of the portal venous system (ref *manifestations*).

Nonmalignant EHPVO in the absence of cirrhosis is a rare disease, the incidence of which has been estimated in Europe 0.7 and 3/100,000 inhabitants per year, and the prevalence 3/100,000 inhabitants [1, 2]. Malignant and cirrhotic portal vein obstruction is much more frequent. In a Swedish autopsy series of portal vein obstruction, 28% had cirrhosis, 23% had primary and 44% secondary hepatobiliary malignancy [3]. In both Swedish and Italian registry series, 31–35% had cirrhosis and 21%–40% had primary or secondary hepatobiliary malignancy [2, 3]. Causes of non-malignant EHPVO will only be overviewed in this chapter as they are described in part 2 of this book. In Europe, a general prothrombotic condition and a local factor are identified in approximately 60% and 30% of adult patients, respectively. In adults, several factors can be found simultaneously in the same patient. No cause is identified in 1/3 of patients. Suffice to emphasize here that a local factor is more frequently present than in thrombosis of the hepatic veins and that a general factor is found in one third of patients with a local factor in patients with recent portal vein obstruction [4]. Among local risk factors, inflammatory, malignancy, or surgical trauma to the portal venous system (at portosystemic shunting or splenectomy particularly in patients with portal hypertension) are most commonly incriminated. Appendicitis, diverticulitis, inflammatory bowel disease, acute CMV infection, pancreatitis, cholecystitis, and cholangitis can cause septic or nonseptic, recent EHPVO. Moreover, portal vein obstruction occurs in 10–50% of patients with portosinusoidal vascular disease (PSVD) and PSVD is found in 20% of patients who had a liver biopsy for abnormal liver tests, or dysmorphic liver in the context of acute portal vein obstruction [4]. In Europe, myeloproliferative neoplasm is the most prevalent risk factor for non-cirrhotic, non-malignant EHPVO. In a recent study including 312 patients with vascular liver disease (99 with Budd Chiari syndrome and 213 with EHPVO), Jak2 $^{V617F}$ mutation was present in 19%. Combining enlarged spleen (bipolar diameter >16 cm) and platelet counts >200,000/μL had a positive predictive value of 56% (5/9) and a negative predictive value of 100% (0/233) for the identification of CALR mutations [5]. In children, etiological investigations usually failed to document an underlying condition.

## Manifestations, Outcome and Complications

Manifestations range in severity from the absence of symptom to intestinal infarction, and this diversity is related to the time (recent or long standing) and site of obstruction, the extension of thrombosis to mesenteric vein and radicles, and to the presence of a pre-existing cavernoma [6].

Due to an improved availability and sensitivity of non-invasive imaging, the diagnosis of EHPVO is now more frequently done at an early stage of recent portal EHPVO [7].

### *Recent EHPVO*

In a prospective multicentre European survey, the main clinical features recorded in patients with recent portal vein thrombosis were abdominal pain (present in 90% of patients), and a systemic inflammatory response syndrome (SIRS) (in 85%) [4]. These features contrast with local or systemic infection, being present in only 20% of these patients. Nausea, anorexia, asthenia and ileus, are common. Mild ascites is present in 50% of patients, and usually only visible on imaging. On physical examination, most patients have spleen enlargement. Forty percent of these patients have an MPN [4]. Therefore, finding spleen enlargement may increase the suspicion of a MPN, or the suspicion of previously existing portal hypertension. The abdomen may be distended. The absence of guarding, contrasting with the severity of abdominal pain, has long been considered as a feature suggestive for mesenteric venous thrombosis. Liver tests are usually normal or only mildly elevated. Septic pylephlebitis is associated when there is a superimposed bacterial or fungal infection of the thrombus. In this context, blood cultures most frequently grow *Streptococcus viridans, Escherichia coli, or Bacteroides fragilis*. Polymicrobial infection is present in 25% of the patients with septic pylephlebitis, and a liver abscess can be associated [8].

Intestinal infarction is a severe early complication, with a high risk for intestinal resection (and short bowel syndrome as a sequel) and high mortality rate in the absence of anticoagulation therapy. Intestinal infarction occurs only when EHPVO extends to the superior mesenteric vein [9]. Persisting severe abdominal pain despite adequate anticoagulation therapy, organ failure (shock, renal failure, metabolic acidosis, elevated arterial lactates), guarding or contracture, massive ascites, rectal bleeding, are features suggestive for intestinal infarction. In a recent study, factors independently associated with transmural necrosis were: organ failure, serum lactate levels >2 mmol/l and bowel loop dilation on computerized tomography scan [10]. Transmural necrosis rate increased from 3% to 38%, 89%, and 100% in patients with 0, 1, 2, and 3 of these factors, respectively [10]. In another study, diabetes was the only factor independently associated with intestinal resection [11]. In a Swedish autopsy series of 270 patients with porto-mesenteric thrombosis, infarction was associated with venous thrombo-embolism in other sites [9].

## *Chronic EHPVO (Portal Cavernoma)*

Complications of chronic EHPVO have been assessed in a recently reported retrospective study [12]. Associated portal hypertension features were an enlarged spleen, reduced blood-cell counts, gastroesophageal varices, or portosystemic collaterals at abdominal imaging. Gastrointestinal bleeding were the most frequent complications.

In children, chronic EHPVO is most often diagnosed in the presence of thrombocytopenia, splenomegaly and inaugural hemorrhages. Growth retardation and occult encephalopathy have also been described [13, 14].

In patients without varices, the probability of developing varices was 2%, 22%, and 22% at 1, 3, and 5 years, respectively. In those with small esophageal varices, growth to large oesophageal varices (LEV) was observed in 13%, 40%, and 54% at 1, 3, and 5 years, respectively. In patients with LEVs on primary prophylaxis, the probability of bleeding was 9%, 20%, and 32% at 1, 3, and 5 years, respectively [12]. Ascites is usually triggered by gastrointestinal bleeding or infection, and contrasts with features of otherwise preserved liver function.

A retrospective study analyzed the risk of recurrent thrombosis in patients with EHVPO [15]. Among 119 such patients, incidence rate of recurrent thrombosis (all types of thrombotic events) was 3.4 (95% CI, 0.1–6.7) per 100 patient-years during the first year after portal vein thrombosis, 6.4 (95% CI, 1.3–11.5) per 100 patient-years during the second year, and 7.7 (95% CI, 1.6–13.8) per 100 patient-years during the third year [15]. The incidence of recurrent thrombotic events in the portal venous system was 0.64 and 1.87 per 100 patient-years in patients with and without anticoagulant therapy, respectively (RR, 2.9; 95% CI, 0.6–14).

Portal cavernoma cholangiopathy corresponds to biliary obstruction ascribed to extrinsic compression or to ischemia caused by portal collateral vessels, leading to fixed stricture formation in the setting of chronic EHPVO. The Indian Association for the Study of the Liver consensus statement defines it as abnormalities in the extrahepatic biliary system including the cystic duct and gallbladder with or without abnormalities in the first and second generation biliary ducts [19]. It most commonly occurs in non-cirrhotic patients with obstruction of the portal and mesenteric vein or splenic vein, but it has also been described in cirrhotic portal vein thrombosis [20, 21]. The majority of patients is asymptomatic. Biliary symptoms related to portal cavernoma cholangiopathy such as biliary pain, pancreatitis, cholecystitis, cholangitis are less frequently encountered (in 5–20% of the patients) than portal hypertension related complications [15–18]. Symptoms seem to occur rapidly in patients with severe imaging strictures (grade 3 cholangiopathy) or in patients with long lasting disease [18, 21]. Biliary pain, cholangitis, or detectable jaundice may be secondary to bile duct stones (5–20%) or cholangitis. As compared with asymptomatic patients, patients with symptomatic portal cavernoma cholangiopathy are older, have a longer duration of disease, gallbladder stones, dilated segments of bile ducts, presence of gallstones and common bile duct stones and abnormal liver function tests [19, 22]. Recurrent, progressive disease is frequent in symptomatic patients.

Lastly, cardiovascular complications such as intra-pulmonary shunts and pulmonary hypertension have been reported in EHPVO [23, 24].

# Diagnosis of EHPVO

**1. Imaging Doppler Ultrasound, Contrast-Enhanced Computerized Tomography (CT) Scan and Magnetic Resonance Imaging (MRI)** *How to establish a diagnosis of EHPVO?*

A diagnosis of EHPVO can be stablished.

1. when there is evidence for a thrombus in the portal vein lumen; or,
2. in the absence of visible lumen corresponding to the portal vein, when there are numerous, serpiginous porto-portal collaterals in the porta hepatis or hilus region.

Nonspecific signs of EHPVO inslude extrahepatic porto-systemic collateral circulation, perfusion abnormalities, a dysmorphic liver, a mild irregular dilatation of the bile ducts and signs of portal hypertension [25, 26]. Pancreatic cavernoma may mimic pancreatic cancer at imaging due to heterogeneous enlargement, of the pancreas and irregularities of the main pancreatic duct [27]. Cystic cavernoma may mimic cholecystitis by enlarging its wall which enhances at the portal phase due to portoportal collaterals running in its wall.

Doppler ultrasound has a sensibility and specificity for the diagnosis of EHPVO in adults and children of 80% to 100%. Some limitations have to be kept in mind. Diagnostic sensitivity is lower in patients with incomplete obstruction, as well as with recent thrombosis or isolated mesenteric obstruction; furthermore, visualization is reduced in obese patients, and in patients with abundant bowel gas, but reliability improves with informed and experienced radiologists [25, 28]. At Doppler ultrasound, specific signs for EHPVO include a hypo/isoechogenic thrombus in the lumen, or/and the absence of flow within part or all the lumen of the portal vein, or the absence of visible lumen corresponding to the portal vein; and the presence of numerous, tortuous, hepatofugal neo-veins in porta hepatis. Contrast CT evaluation adds valuable information, to confirm diagnosis and assess extension of thrombosis. Recent EHPVO on unenhanced CT scan is spontaneously a hyperdense clot in the portal vein lumen which persists at least 30 days after symptoms [6, 29, 30]. At the portal phase of contrast-enhanced cross-sectional imaging, acute EHPVO manifests as a filling defect within the obstructed vein. On both CT and MRI, the vein may be dilated with acute non enhancing thrombus and may be associated with edge enhancement of the thrombosed vein. Associated changes in hepatic perfusion may be seen as an increased parenchymal enhancement of the peripheral parts of the liver at the arterial phase with homogeneous decreased enhancement at a later phase. With long-standing thrombosis, non-visible portal vein is the most common finding on contrast-enhanced imaging, associated to the presence of numerous, serpiginous porto-portal neo-veins [25].

*How to exclude malignant obstruction?*

Differential diagnosis of non-tumoral EHPVO is malignant obstruction of the portal vein. Evidence for tumor invasion of the portal vein by hepato-biliary malignancy include arterial neovascularization within the thrombus at color and pulsed Doppler ultrasound and/or internal enhancement within the thrombus, associated to a typical surrounding neoplastic mass at arterial phase CT and MRI [38]. In rare occasions, biopsy of the portal thrombus may be needed to definitively establish the differential diagnosis.

*How to assess complications?*

CT scan provides additional information regarding the extent of the thrombus to the mesenteric veins and arches, the presence of a local factor, or of congestion and ischemia of the bowel. Features more frequently encountered in patients who will have intestinal resection include:

- distal thrombosis (occlusion of second order radicles of superior mesenteric vein),
- intestinal anomalies (homogeneous wall thickening with heterogeneous hypoattenuation or hyperattenuation, dilatation of intestinal loop, abnormal or absent wall enhancement),
- large volume ascites, pneumatosis, and portal venous gas [11].

Many classifications are currently used in clinical trials to characterize the extension of EHPVO, but these classifications, elaborated in, and applying to patients with cirrhosis, are not helpful to assess prognosis in clinical practice [31, 32].

In patients with suspected portal cholangiopathy, a cholangio-MRI helps assessing prognosis. Imaging features of cholangiopathy are present in 80–100% of patients with portal cavernoma, but biliary disease is symptomatic in less than 30% of the patients [18]. A recent study has shown that strictures with dilatation (intrahepatic duct >4 mm or extrahepatic duct >7 mm), is associated with symptomatic cholangiopathy [18]. Portal cholangiopathy can mimic the MRI aspect of primary sclerosing cholangitis. The severity of visible strictures may contrast with the absence of clinical or laboratory features of biliary disease. Similarly, cavernoma can mimic the aspect of a tumor when developed at the hepatic hilum like a solid mass, so called a tumor-like cavernoma that can be confused with carcinoma of the main bile duct [20].

In the setting of portal blood flow deprivation, and arterial buffer compensation, regenerative nodules may occur. They are often multiple, with variable size (but frequently <3 cm), usually homogeneous, hyperintense on T1-weighting on MRI, with homogeneous hyperenhancement on arterial phase on IV contrast-enhanced CT or MRI, without washout during the portal and late phases. On T2-weighted MR images, they may appear to be isointense or have slight hyperintensity. In a series of 58 EHPVO adult patients, screening for regenerative nodules, identified 12 (21%) patients with FNH like lesions and one with hepatic cell adenoma (HCA) [33]. In a pediatric series of 45 children with porto-systemic surgery (15%) liver nodules were identified in 7 patients within a median 80-months follow-up, including 2 with HCA [34]. HCC has been exceptionally described in patients with EHPVO. Differential diagnosis with HCC or adenoma is challenging, central scar is often lacking in HNF nodules due to their small size, although the diagnostic value of iso- or hyperintense lesions on hepatobiliary phase MR is good [35–37].

*How to rule out cirrhosis.*

Hypertrophy of the caudate lobe combined to signs of portal hypertension mimic advanced chronic liver disease, but left lateral segment atrophy, a normal or enlarged segment IV and smooth liver surface are distinctive findings of cavernous transformation [27]. Therefore, when diagnosing primary EHPVO, ruling out cirrhosis is needed but sometimes difficult without the help of liver stiffness, hepatic venous pressure measurement and liver biopsy (refer to Chap. 9) [7].

**2. Noninvasive and Invasive Tools**

Liver stiffness (LS) and spleen stiffness (SS) measurements using FibroScan transient elastography can be used as a noninvasive tool to rule out cirrhosis, and to assess the risk of bleeding. Indeed, in a recent study, mean liver stiffness in non-cirrhotic EHPVO was significantly lower (6.4 ± 2.2 kPa) than in cirrhosis (40.9 ± 20.5 kPa), or PSVD (8.4 ± 3.3 kPa) [38]. In another study, LS and SS in patients with EHPVO (6.7 kPa ± 2.3 and 51.7 kPa ± 21.5, respectively) were low but still higher than in control subjects (4.6 kPa ± 0.7 and 16.0 kPa ± 3.0, respectively). Patients with a history of bleeding had a higher SS than did those without a bleed (60.4 kPa ± 5.4 vs. 30.3 kPa ± 14.2), a value >42.8 kPa predicted variceal bleed with a 88% sensitivity, and a 94% specificity [39]. Nevertheless in another study, still 31% of EHPVO had LS indicative of compensated advanced chronic liver disease (>10 kPa) as defined by Baveno VI. These patients with EHPVO and high LS had a significantly higher free hepatic vein pressure (11 ± 3 vs. 6 ± 4 mm Hg) [40]. Therefore, even though liver stiffness is significantly lower in patients with EHPVO in the absence of cirrhosis, in 1/3 of the patients who still have ambiguous results, liver biopsy may still be needed to rule out cirrhosis or PSVD.

Mean hepatic venous pressure gradient (HVPG) can also be a useful tool to rule out cirrhosis. In a recent study assessing HPVG in PSVD, EHPVO and cirrhosis, HVPG in EHPVO was markedly lower than in cirrhosis (3.5 ± 2 vs. 17 ± 3 mm Hg, $p < 0.001$), and significantly lower than in PSVD (3.5 ± 2 vs. 7 ± 3) [38]. In this study, hepatic vein-to-vein communications were found in 49% PSVD patients precluding adequate hepatic venous pressure gradient measurements in 44% of the patients [38].

# Therapy

Therapeutic strategy varies according to the age of the patient, the age of thrombosis, the severity of complications and response to therapy.

In recent EHPVO, the aims of therapy is to prevent the extension of the thrombus or thrombi and thereby to prevent or limit ischemic damage to the gut and to obtain a rapid and as complete as possible recanalization of the obstructed vessels to prevent or limit the development of portal hypertension.

# *Anticoagulation, Thrombolysis, Surgery: Efficacy and Complications*

## Recent EHPVO

Spontaneous recanalization of the portal vein is rare in adults or children with symptomatic obstruction, whereas it is very frequent in neonates once an umbilical vascular catheter has been removed [15, 41]. There is no randomized study to confirm the efficacy of anticoagulation therapy in recent EHPVO. Nevertheless, available data support immediate initiation of anticoagulation therapy in patients with recent EHPVO. Underlying prothrombotic conditions are common. Furthermore, outcome has improved since the introduction of routine anticoagulation therapy, as recanalization of the portal vein and superior mesenteric vein occurs in 40% and 50% of patients, respectively and the incidence of mesenteric infarction was about 2% [4] vs. 40% in older series [6, 42, 43]. Bleeding complications are rare (9–15%) [4, 6, 42, 43]. Predictive factors for no recanalization were an abundant ascites at diagnosis or extensive thrombosis [4]. Therefore administration of low molecular heparin followed by coumarine derivatives is currently used in most centers, whatever the underlying thrombotic risk factor [6]. Heparin-induced thrombocytopenia (HIT) has been reported to occur in up to 20% of EHPVO patients treated with unfractionated heparin, a much higher rate compared to HIT in patients without EHPVO [6], which justifies close monitoring of platelet counts. Available data on DOACs are retrospective and limited to a small number of patients (refer to Chap. 17). In a retrospective study on 38 patients treated for EHPVO in the absence of cirrhosis, no major bleeding complication of DOACS has been observed [44]. Caution should be made regarding drug interaction, renal failure, and the doses of DOAC to be used in this situation.

Patients with persistent abdominal pain despite anticoagulation, bloody diarrhoea and lactic acidosis have increased risk of intestinal infarction and organ failure, and therefore repermeabilization or resection of the necrotic gut are often needed [45]. Recently, three criteria (organ failure, serum lactate levels >2 mmol/l and bowel loop dilation on computerized tomography) [10] have been described and may also be helpful to decide timing for surgery. Death rate remains high (42–52%), in surgical series, in particular in patients with higher ASA classification, age > 70 years, late presentation, and high serum lactate levels [46, 47]. When septic pylephlebitis is diagnosed, prolonged treatment with antibiotic therapy adapted to isolated bacteria or to anaerobic digestive flora is needed. In a surgical series of 96 patients with recent EHPVO, in whom the diagnosis of septic pylephlebitis was established in 44% of the patients by positive blood cultures, mortality rate was only 11%, 67% of the patients having been treated with a combination of anticoagulation and antibiotic therapy. In the absence of sepsis or septic EHPVO, recent data suggest to associate oral antibiotics to diminish bacterial translocation in acute mesenteric ischemia: [10].

Over half the patients (55%) not achieving recanalization with anticoagulation therapy will develop gastroesophageal varices during their follow-up, with a 2-year actual probability of variceal bleeding and ascites of 12% and 16% respectively [48]. Radiologically severe portal cholangiopathy, developed in 30% of patients with acute PVT within 1 year [18].

To avoid these complications, recanalization attempt of recent EHPVO, to reestablish a physiological venous outflow in so called "uncontrollable severe symptoms" or mesenteric ischemia or patients with extensive EHPVO, has been described (Table 7.1). The procedure consisted of either percutaneous, transjugular, transhepatic, transsplenic, transileocolic, or omental vein access to the portal venous system in order to proceed to portal vein recanalization. Available data are limited to small series of less than 20 patients for the largest. Furthermore, indication for thrombolysis or TIPS was not always clear, as indicated in Table 7.1: progressive extension of the thrombus appears to be the most objective criteria [35–39]. In 3 recently reported series of respectively 12, 17 patients and 11 patients with acute EHPVO, complete recanalization was obtained in respectively 60%, 52%, 20%, partial recanalization in 90–100%. Complication rate varies from 50% severe bleeding [49] to 30% other complications in Klinger's study [50] (including 1 artery pseudoanevrysm, and 2 gut resections), and 30% thrombosis of TIPS idem [50–52]. Interestingly, in these studies, patients with complete recanalization were free of portal hypertension complications and did not have recurrent symptoms over several years.

## Chronic EHPVO

Long term anticoagulation is controversial in chronic EHPVO. Anticoagulation is mainly administered either in patients treated for 6 months after acute EHPVO but with no or incomplete recanalization, or in patients diagnosed at the stage of cavernoma. Three retrospective cohort studies on non-cirrhotic PVT patients, showed that long-term anticoagulation was associated with a reduced risk of recurrent thrombosis [15, 53, 54] and significantly improved survival in one study [55]. Recurrent thrombosis was more frequent in the presence of a prothrombotic state [15, 49, 50]. In only one of these three studies, anticoagulation was associated to an increased bleeding risk [53]. European guidelines recommend to consider permanent anticoagulation in patients with a strong prothrombotic condition (based on personal and familial history of unprovoked deep vein thrombosis, and on findings of isolated or combined prothrombotic conditions), or past history suggesting intestinal ischemia or recurrent thrombosis on follow-up [6]. In all other patients, several factors including a familial or personal history of thrombosis, the identification of a permanent cause for thrombosis, the extension of the thrombus, probably need to be considered and discussed for individual patient's decision in multidisciplinary meeting board discussion. The weight of each of these factors or of pro thrombotic scores such as Padua or Dash

**Table 7.1** Interventional radiology recanalization (thrombolysis through transhepatic or transjugular access) in recent EHPVO (patients with cirrhosis or chronic EHPVO are excluded)

Recent EHPVO in the absence of cirrhosis

| | Hollingshead 2005 [49] | Smalberg 2008 [51] | Wang 2009 [73] | Liu 2009 [74] | Cao 2013 [75] | Rosenquist 2016 [76] | Klinger 2017 [50] | Wolter 2018 [52] |
|---|---|---|---|---|---|---|---|---|
| N | 20 | 4 | 2 | 32 | 12 | 4 | 17 | 11 |
| Indication recanalisation | – Progressive thrombus<br>– Pain (persisting with anticoagulation)<br>– Stable imaging<br>– Extensive thrombus | – Progressive thrombus<br>– Extensive thrombus | – Pain (persisting or worsened with anticoagulation) | – Different degrees of abdominal pain, fullness, and anorexia | Postoperative Thrombosis | – Intestinal ischemia | – Imminent intestinal infarction<br>– Progressive Thrombus<br>– Concomitent BCS | – Failure of adequate response anticoagulation |
| Intestinal ischemia | 20 | NA | 2 | NA | NA | 4 | 10 | 10 |
| Associated TIPS | 0 | 1 | 0 | 26 | 0 | 1 + 2 later | 8 | 7 |
| Recanalisation complete | 3 | 1 | 2 | 26 | 10 | 0 | 9 | 7 |
| Partial | 12 | 1 | 0 | 6 | 1 | 4 | 7 | 2 |
| Failure | 5 | 2 | 0 | 0 | 1 | 0 | 1 | 2 |
| Gut resection | 0 | NA | 0 | NA | NA | 1 | 2 | NA |
| Complications | 12 major (bleeding, death from sepsis) | 2 bleeding | 0 | 1 death sepsis | 1 death respiratory distress | 3 bleeding | 2 HIT | 1 encephalopathy |
| Thrombosis | 0 | NA | 0 | 3 | 5 | 3TIPS occlusion 2 Cavernoma | 1 hepatic artery pseudoaneurysm | 1 MOF |

score, mainly used in patients with deep vein thrombosis in other territories [56, 57] have not yet been assessed in EHPVO and randomised studies are critically needed in this situation.

The course of gastroesophageal varices in chronic noncirrhotic, nontumoral EHPVO appears to be similar to that in cirrhosis (as above described in section "Manifestations") [12]. Therefore, recommendations for treatment of portal hypertension complications are similar to those recommendations for patients with cirrhosis. The use of β-blocker treatment in EHPVO is supported by the following arguments: (1) a clinically significant reduction in the pressure gradient from spleen pulp to the free hepatic vein [58]; (2) the reduction of the bleeding risk [15]; and (3) a significantly improved survival when associated to anticoagulation therapy [55]. In an Indian therapeutic trial in patients with non-cirrhotic portal hypertension, mostly chronic EHPVO, not treated with anticoagulation, after a median follow-up period of 23 months, rates of recurrence of bleeding were similar when comparing beta-blockers and endoscopic variceal ligation (EVL) (EVL, 23.5%; propranolol, 18%; $p = 0.625$) [59].

In patients with persisting complications of portal hypertension, refractory to first line therapy, more invasive procedures such as portal vein recanalization (Table 7.2) have been proposed. One recent study shows promising results: indications for recanalization were portal hypertension bleeding in 6 patients, symptomatic biliopathy in 2 and preoperative portal decompression in 4 patients: 13/15 patients with EHPVO diagnosed since 44 months, had a successful recanalization of the portal vein, with 2 mild complications. More importantly, portal hypertension bleeding resolved in 5/6 patients, bilirubin normalised in one patient with severe jaundice and biliopathy, and 5 patients had no complications of abdominal surgery. In patients with extensive intrahepatic obstruction to segmental and distal branches, recanalization was either not feasible or systematic recurrent obstruction was seen. Preoperative imaging lacked diagnostic accuracy in predicting feasibility. Conversely, portography performed at the beginning of the procedure may be helpful to identify patients with extensive intrahepatic obstruction [60]. Adding TIPS insertion to trans-splenic portal vein recanalization (PVR-TIPS) has been

**Table 7.2** Interventional radiology recanalization (associated or not to TIPS) in chronic EHPVO

| | Qi 2012 [62] | Denys 2018 [60] | Kallini 2016 [61] |
|---|---|---|---|
| N | 20 | 15 | 5 |
| Associated TIPS | 20 | 0 | 5 |
| Recanalization success | 7 + 2 in collaterals | 13 | 5 |
| Complications | 1 bleeding<br>2 TIPS dysfunction | 1 liver haematoma<br>1 hyperamylasemia from wirsungo portal fistula | 0 |
| Late complications | 2 deaths liver related<br>1 death from systemic infection | 4 PV obstructions<br>(only ¼ recurrent PHT symptoms) | 0 |

performed, with a recanalization possible in 50–100% of cases, but once again the number of patients is limited, with series of less than 20 patients, and a total of patients less than 50 reported patients [61, 62]. Age of obstruction and extension of thrombosis does not seem to preclude recanalization feasibility, which mostly relies on distal intrahepatic obstruction.

Management of portal cholangiopathy is based on endoscopic management in symptomatic patients [63–65]. Endoscopic treatment includes endoscopic sphincterotomy, stone extraction, mechanical lithotripsy and biliary stricture dilatation with or without stent [22]. Sphincterotomy and endoscopic stone removal was demonstrated to be a safe procedure, with only few instances of hemobilia [19]. Administration of ursodeoxycholic acid (UDCA) has been reported to be useful in a few (less than 40) symptomatic patients, with an improvement of cholestasis, with no controlled study. In patients with recurring symptoms despite endoscopy therapy, decompressive shunt surgery has also been performed and relieved biliary obstruction 65% of patients [66], although management may currently differ in the era of interventional radiology. Biliary-bypass and supra mesocolic surgery although performed in very experienced surgical teams, with satisfactory results in term of survival, are still at risk of severe portal hypertension and bleeding complications [67, 68]. Hence, INASL recommendations are to perform endoscopy therapy in first line, and to perform decompressive surgery if there is a shuntable vein available, with non-selective shunts and to perform second-stage biliary drainage surgery (hepaticojejunostomy or choledochoduodenostomy) only in patients who continue to have biliary obstruction and remain symptomatic despite shunt procedure. Although not mentioned in these recommendations, interventional radiology should likely be considered before surgery (see above).

In children with chronic EHPVO, arguments for long term anticoagulation are scarce (significant thrombophilia is rare, and a local cause or a congenital malformation frequent); therefore anticoagulation therapy is not indicated. Conversely, surgical restauration of portal blood flow is rapidly considered, as thrombophilia is scarce and portal hypertension long term complications frequent. Portal reperfusion by meso-Rex anastomosis (bypass between the superior mesenteric vein and the recess of Rex with a large autologous venous conduit is currently the procedure of choice), when it is conceivable, is indicated in children for primary and secondary prophylaxis of gastrointestinal haemorrhage, and in case of portal cavernoma cholangiopathy or cardiopulmonary complication. It is highly successful when Rex's recess is permeable and in the absence of extension of thrombosis to the splenic and mesenteric veins [69]. Portal reperfusion by meso-Rex anastomosis showed a 100% efficacy to prevent variceal bleeding, a potential reversal of cavernoma cholangiopathy, resolution of hypersplenism, coagulopathy, and hepato renal syndrome, improvement of minimal hepatic encephalopathy, but uncertain effect on porto pulmonary hypertension. Meso rex bypass has also been performed in adults, and although data is limited, it seems that adult patients may benefit from this experience [70–72].

## Conclusion

Management of EHPVO has dramatically changed in the last 30 years, aiming at minimal invasiveness, in diagnosis and therapeutics. Imaging tools are very sensitive and specific, in the hands of informed, trained radiologists. The prognostic value of liver stiffness measurements is helpful to discard cirrhosis and probably in assessing prognosis. Anticoagulation therapy has largely improved the outcome in patients with recent EHPVO, and might also be beneficial in patients with chronic EHPVO although more data are needed on patients' selection and on the effects of direct anticoagulants. Interventional procedures could prove of interest in patients with refractory manifestations but additional data are needed. Management in children, which has differed from that of adults until now, is centered by the encouraging results of surgical reperfusion of intrahepatic portal venous system that have also to be further evaluated in adult patients. Long term management needs special focus on the management of causal factors, anticoagulation therapy and the management of portal hypertension related complications. A recently presented randomized controlled trial in patients with past portal vein thrombosis or cavernoma, in the absence of major risk factors for thrombosis demonstrated full prevention from recurrent thrombosis using rivaroxaban 15 mg daily for 24 to 48 months, compared to patients not receiving anticoagulation. There was no increase in major bleeding or portal hypertension related bleeding while the incidence of minor bleeding was increased in rivaroxaban treated group compared to the patients receiving no anticoagulation [77]. These data suggest that anticoagulation should be considered in patients with past portal vein thrombosis or cavernoma even in the absence of major risk factors for thrombosis.

## References


1. Rajani R, Björnsson E, Bergquist A, Danielsson A, Gustavsson A, Grip O, et al. The epidemiology and clinical features of portal vein thrombosis: a multicentre study. Aliment Pharmacol Ther. 2010;32(9):1154–62.
2. Ageno W, Dentali F, Pomero F, Fenoglio L, Squizzato A, Pagani G, et al. Incidence rates and case fatality rates of portal vein thrombosis and Budd-Chiari Syndrome. Thromb Haemost. 2017.
3. Ogren M, Bergqvist D, Björck M, Acosta S, Eriksson H, Sternby NH. Portal vein thrombosis: prevalence, patient characteristics and lifetime risk: a population study based on 23,796 consecutive autopsies. World J Gastroenterol. 2006;12(13):2115–9.
4. Plessier A, Darwish-Murad S, Hernandez-Guerra M, Consigny Y, Fabris F, Trebicka J, et al. Acute portal vein thrombosis unrelated to cirrhosis: a prospective multicenter follow-up study. Hepatol Baltim Md. 2010;51(1):210–8.
5. Poisson J, Plessier A, Kiladjian J-J, Turon F, Cassinat B, Andreoli A, et al. Selective testing for calreticulin gene mutations in patients with splanchnic vein thrombosis: a prospective cohort study. J Hepatol. 2017;5
6. European Association for the Study of the Liver. Electronic address: easloffice@easloffice.eu. EASL clinical practice guidelines: vascular diseases of the liver. J Hepatol. 2016;64(1):179–202.

7. Khoury T, Massarwa M, Hazou W, Daher S, Hakimian D, Benson AA, et al. Acute portal vein thrombosis predicts concomitant diagnosis of hepatocellular carcinoma in cirrhotic patients. J Gastrointest Cancer. 2018;25

8. Choudhry AJ, Baghdadi YMK, Amr MA, Alzghari MJ, Jenkins DH, Zielinski MD. Pylephlebitis: a review of 95 cases. J Gastrointest Surg Off J Soc Surg Aliment Tract. 2016;20(3):656–61.

9. Acosta S, Alhadad A, Verbaan H, Ogren M. The clinical importance in differentiating portal from mesenteric venous thrombosis. Int Angiol J Int Union Angiol. 2011;30(1):71–8.

10. Nuzzo A, Maggiori L, Ronot M, Becq A, Plessier A, Gault N, et al. Predictive factors of intestinal necrosis in acute mesenteric ischemia: prospective study from an intestinal stroke center. Am J Gastroenterol. 2017;112(4):597–605.

11. Elkrief L, Corcos O, Bruno O, Larroque B, Rautou P-E, Zekrini K, et al. Type 2 diabetes mellitus as a risk factor for intestinal resection in patients with superior mesenteric vein thrombosis. Liver Int Off J Int Assoc Study Liver. 2014;34(9):1314–21.

12. Noronha Ferreira C, Seijo S, Plessier A, Silva-Junior G, Turon F, Rautou P-E, et al. Natural history and management of esophagogastric varices in chronic noncirrhotic, nontumoral portal vein thrombosis. Hepatol Baltim Md. 2016;63(5):1640–50.

13. Sharma P, Sharma BC, Puri V, Sarin SK. Natural history of minimal hepatic encephalopathy in patients with extrahepatic portal vein obstruction. Am J Gastroenterol. 2009;104(4):885–90.

14. Rangari M, Gupta R, Jain M, Malhotra V, Sarin SK. Hepatic dysfunction in patients with extrahepatic portal venous obstruction. Liver Int. 2003;23(6):434–9.

15. Condat B, Pessione F, Hillaire S, Denninger MH, Guillin MC, Poliquin M, et al. Current outcome of portal vein thrombosis in adults: risk and benefit of anticoagulant therapy. Gastroenterology. 2001;120(2):490–7.

16. Resseguier AS, André M, Orian Lazar EA, Bommelaer G, Tournilhac O, Delèvaux I, et al. Natural history of portal cavernoma without liver disease. A single Centre retrospective study of 32 cases. Rev Med Interne. 2016;37(6):394–8.

17. Condat B, Vilgrain V, Asselah T, O'Toole D, Rufat P, Zappa M, et al. Portal cavernoma-associated cholangiopathy: a clinical and MR cholangiography coupled with MR portography imaging study. Hepatol Baltim Md. 2003;37(6):1302–8.

18. Llop E, de Juan C, Seijo S, García-Criado A, Abraldes JG, Bosch J, et al. Portal cholangiopathy: radiological classification and natural history. Gut. 2011;60(6):853–60.

19. Dhiman RK, Saraswat VA, Valla DC, Chawla Y, Behera A, Varma V, et al. Portal Cavernoma Cholangiopathy: consensus statement of a working Party of the Indian National Association for study of the liver. J Clin Exp Hepatol. 2014;4(Suppl 1):S2–14.

20. Walser EM, Runyan BR, Heckman MG, Bridges MD, Willingham DL, Paz-Fumagalli R, et al. Extrahepatic portal biliopathy: proposed etiology on the basis of anatomic and clinical features. Radiology. 2011;258(1):146–53.

21. Khuroo MS, Rather AA, Khuroo NS, Khuroo MS. Portal biliopathy. World J Gastroenterol. 2016;22(35):7973–82.

22. Dhiman RK, Behera A, Chawla YK, Dilawari JB, Suri S. Portal hypertensive biliopathy. Gut. 2007;56(7):1001–8.

23. Flores-Calderón J. Guidelines for the diagnosis and treatment of extrahepatic portal vein obstruction (EHPVO) in children. Ann Hepatol. 2013;12.

24. Lejealle C, Paradis V, Bruno O, de Raucourt E, Francoz C, Soubrane O, et al. Evidence for an association between intrahepatic vascular changes and the development of hepatopulmonary syndrome. Chest. 2018;

25. Jha RC, Khera SS, Kalaria AD. Portal vein thrombosis: imaging the Spectrum of disease with an emphasis on MRI features. AJR Am J Roentgenol. 2018;211(1):14–24.

26. Vilgrain V, Condat B, Bureau C, Hakimé A, Plessier A, Cazals-Hatem D, et al. Atrophy-hypertrophy complex in patients with cavernous transformation of the portal vein: CT evaluation. Radiology. 2006;241(1):149–55.

27. Vilgrain V, Condat B, O'Toole D, Plessier A, Ruszniewski P, Valla DC. Pancreatic portal cavernoma in patients with cavernous transformation of the portal vein: MR findings. Eur Radiol. 2009;19(11):2608–13.

28. Margini C, Berzigotti A. Portal vein thrombosis: the role of imaging in the clinical setting. Dig Liver Dis Off J Ital Soc Gastroenterol Ital Assoc Study Liver. 2017;49(2):113–20.
29. Plessier A, Rautou P-E, Valla D-C. Management of hepatic vascular diseases. J Hepatol. 2012;56(Suppl 1):S25–38.
30. Senzolo M, Riggio O, Primignani M. Italian Association for the Study of the liver (AISF) ad hoc. Vascular disorders of the liver: recommendations from the Italian Association for the Study of the liver (AISF) ad hoc committee. Dig Liver Dis Off J Ital Soc Gastroenterol Ital Assoc Study Liver. 2011;43(7):503–14.
31. Sarin SK, Philips CA, Kamath PS, Choudhury A, Maruyama H, Nery FG, et al. Toward a comprehensive new classification of portal vein thrombosis in patients with cirrhosis. Gastroenterology. 2016;151(4):574–7.e3.
32. Yerdel MA, Gunson B, Mirza D, Karayalçin K, Olliff S, Buckels J, et al. Portal vein thrombosis in adults undergoing liver transplantation: risk factors, screening, management, and outcome. Transplantation. 2000;69(9):1873–81.
33. Marin D, Galluzzo A, Plessier A, Brancatelli G, Valla D, Vilgrain V. Focal nodular hyperplasia-like lesions in patients with cavernous transformation of the portal vein: prevalence, MR findings and natural history. Eur Radiol. 2011;21(10):2074–82.
34. Guérin F, Porras J, Fabre M, Guettier C, Pariente D, Bernard O, et al. Liver nodules after portal systemic shunt surgery for extrahepatic portal vein obstruction in children. J Pediatr Surg. 2009;44(7):1337–43.
35. Vilgrain V, Paradis V, Van Wettere M, Valla D, Ronot M, Rautou P-E. Benign and malignant hepatocellular lesions in patients with vascular liver diseases. Abdom Radiol. 2018;43(8):1968–77.
36. Sempoux C, Paradis V, Komuta M, Wee A, Calderaro J, Balabaud C, et al. Hepatocellular nodules expressing markers of hepatocellular adenomas in Budd-Chiari syndrome and other rare hepatic vascular disorders. J Hepatol. 2015;63(5):1173–80.
37. Amarapurkar P, Bhatt N, Patel N, Amarapurkar D. Primary extrahepatic portal vein obstruction in adults: a single center experience. Indian J Gastroenterol. 2014;33(1):19–22.
38. Seijo S, Reverter E, Miquel R, Berzigotti A, Abraldes JG, Bosch J, et al. Role of hepatic vein catheterisation and transient elastography in the diagnosis of idiopathic portal hypertension. Dig Liver Dis Off J Ital Soc Gastroenterol Ital Assoc Study Liver. 2012;44(10):855–60.
39. Sharma P, Mishra SR, Kumar M, Sharma BC, Sarin SK. Liver and spleen stiffness in patients with extrahepatic portal vein obstruction. Radiology. 2012;263(3):893–9.
40. Vuppalanchi R, Mathur K, Pyko M, Samala N, Chalasani N. Liver stiffness measurements in patients with non-cirrhotic portal hypertension – the devil is in the details. Hepatol Baltim Md. 2018.
41. Cabannes M, Bouissou A, Favrais G, Sembély-Taveau C, Morales L, Favreau A, et al. Systematic ultrasound examinations in neonates admitted to NICU: evolution of portal vein thrombosis. J Perinatol Off J Calif Perinat Assoc. 2018;6
42. Condat B, Pessione F, Helene Denninger M, Hillaire S, Valla D. Recent portal or mesenteric venous thrombosis: increased recognition and frequent recanalization on anticoagulant therapy. Hepatol Baltim Md. 2000;32(3):466–70.
43. Hall TC, Garcea G, Metcalfe M, Bilk D, Rajesh A, Dennison A. Impact of anticoagulation on outcomes in acute non-cirrhotic and non- malignant portal vein thrombosis: a retrospective observational study. Hepato-Gastroenterology. 2013;60(122):311–7.
44. De Gottardi A, Trebicka J, Klinger C, Plessier A, Seijo S, Terziroli B, et al. Antithrombotic treatment with direct-acting oral anticoagulants in patients with splanchnic vein thrombosis and cirrhosis. Liver Int Off J Int Assoc Study Liver. 2016;25
45. de Franchis R. Expanding consensus in portal hypertension. J Hepatol. 2015;63(3):743–52.
46. Adaba F, Askari A, Dastur J, Patel A, Gabe SM, Vaizey CJ, et al. Mortality after acute primary mesenteric infarction: a systematic review and meta-analysis of observational studies. Color Dis. 2015;17(7):566–77.
47. Kassahun WT, Schulz T, Richter O, Hauss J. Unchanged high mortality rates from acute occlusive intestinal ischemia: six year review. Langenbeck's Arch Surg. 2008;393(2):163–71.
48. Turnes J, García-Pagán JC, González M, Aracil C, Calleja JL, Ripoll C, et al. Portal hypertension-related complications after acute portal vein thrombosis: impact of early anticoagulation. Clin Gastroenterol Hepatol Off Clin Pract J Am Gastroenterol Assoc. 2008;6(12):1412–7.

49. Hollingshead M, Burke CT, Mauro MA, Weeks SM, Dixon RG, Jaques PF. Transcatheter thrombolytic therapy for acute mesenteric and portal vein thrombosis. J Vasc Interv Radiol JVIR. 2005;16(5):651–61.

50. Klinger C, Riecken B, Schmidt A, De Gottardi A, Meier B, Bosch J, et al. Transjugular local thrombolysis with/without TIPS in patients with acute non-cirrhotic, non-malignant portal vein thrombosis. Dig Liver Dis Off J Ital Soc Gastroenterol Ital Assoc Study Liver. 2017;49(12):1345–52.

51. Smalberg JH, Spaander MVMCW, Jie K-SG, Pattynama PMT, van Buuren HR, van den Berg B, et al. Risks and benefits of transcatheter thrombolytic therapy in patients with splanchnic venous thrombosis. Thromb Haemost. 2008;100(6):1084–8.

52. Wolter K, Decker G, Kuetting D, Trebicka J, Manekeller S, Meyer C, et al. Interventional treatment of acute portal vein thrombosis. ROFO Fortschr Geb Rontgenstr Nuklearmed. 2018;190(8):740–6.

53. Spaander MCW, Hoekstra J, Hansen BE, Van Buuren HR, Leebeek FWG, Janssen HLA. Anticoagulant therapy in patients with non-cirrhotic portal vein thrombosis: effect on new thrombotic events and gastrointestinal bleeding. J Thromb Haemost. 2013;11(3):452–9.

54. Amitrano L, Guardascione MA, Scaglione M, Pezzullo L, Sangiuliano N, Armellino MF, et al. Prognostic factors in noncirrhotic patients with splanchnic vein thromboses. Am J Gastroenterol. 2007;102(11):2464–70.

55. Orr DW, Harrison PM, Devlin J, Karani JB, Kane PA, Heaton ND, et al. Chronic mesenteric venous thrombosis: evaluation and determinants of survival during long-term follow-up. Clin Gastroenterol Hepatol Off Clin Pract J Am Gastroenterol Assoc. 2007;5(1):80–6.

56. Barbar S, Noventa F, Rossetto V, Ferrari A, Brandolin B, Perlati M, et al. A risk assessment model for the identification of hospitalized medical patients at risk for venous thromboembolism: the Padua prediction score. J Thromb Haemost. 2010;8(11):2450–7.

57. Tosetto A, Testa S, Martinelli I, Poli D, Cosmi B, Lodigiani C, et al. External validation of the DASH prediction rule: a retrospective cohort study. J Thromb Haemost. 2017;15(10):1963–70.

58. Sørensen M, Larsen LP, Villadsen GE, Aagaard NK, Grønbæk H, Keiding S, et al. β-Blockers Improve Presinusoidal Portal Hypertension. Dig Dis Sci. 2018.

59. Sarin SK, Gupta N, Jha SK, Agrawal A, Mishra SR, Sharma BC, et al. Equal efficacy of endoscopic variceal ligation and propranolol in preventing variceal bleeding in patients with noncirrhotic portal hypertension. Gastroenterology. 2010;139(4):1238–45.e1.

60. Marot A, Barbosa JV, Duran R, Deltenre P, Denys A. Percutaneous portal vein recanalization using self-expandable nitinol stents in patients with non-cirrhotic non-tumoral portal vein occlusion (in press Diagnostic and Interventional Imaging).

61. Kallini JR, Gabr A, Kulik L, Ganger D, Lewandowski R, Thornburg B, et al. Noncirrhotic complete obliterative portal vein thrombosis: novel management using trans-splenic transjugular intrahepatic portosystemic shunt with portal vein recanalization. Hepatol Baltim Md. 2016;63(4):1387–90.

62. Qi X, Han G, Yin Z, He C, Wang J, Guo W, et al. Transjugular intrahepatic portosystemic shunt for portal cavernoma with symptomatic portal hypertension in non-cirrhotic patients. Dig Dis Sci. 2012;57(4):1072–82.

63. Perlemuter G, Béjanin H, Fritsch J, Prat F, Gaudric M, Chaussade S, et al. Biliary obstruction caused by portal cavernoma: a study of 8 cases. J Hepatol. 1996;25(1):58–63.

64. Mutignani M, Shah SK, Bruni A, Perri V, Costamagna G. Endoscopic treatment of extrahepatic bile duct strictures in patients with portal biliopathy carries a high risk of haemobilia: report of 3 cases. Dig Liver Dis. 2002;34(8):587–91.

65. Dumortier J, Vaillant E, Boillot O, Poncet G, Henry L, Scoazec J-Y, et al. Diagnosis and treatment of biliary obstruction caused by portal cavernoma. Endoscopy. 2003;35(5):446–50.

66. Agarwal AK, Sharma D, Singh S, Agarwal S, Girish SP. Portal biliopathy: a study of 39 surgically treated patients. HPB. 2011;13(1):33–9.

67. Vibert E, Azoulay D, Aloia T, Pascal G, Veilhan L-A, Adam R, et al. Therapeutic strategies in symptomatic portal biliopathy. Ann Surg. 2007 Jul;246(1):97–104.

68. Dokmak S, Aussilhou B, Sauvanet A, Lévy P, Plessier A, Ftériche FS, et al. Safety of supra-mesocolic surgery in patients with portal cavernoma without portal vein decompression. Large single Centre experience. HPB. 2016;18(7):623–9.
69. Shneider BL, de Ville de Goyet J, Leung DH, Srivastava A, Ling SC, Duché M, et al. Primary prophylaxis of variceal bleeding in children and the role of MesoRex bypass: summary of the Baveno VI pediatric satellite symposium. Hepatology. 2016;63(4):1368–80.
70. Chaves IJ, Rigsby CK, Schoeneman SE, Kim ST, Superina RA, Ben-Ami T. Pre- and post-operative imaging and interventions for the meso-Rex bypass in children and young adults. Pediatr Radiol. 2012;42(2):220–32. quiz 271–2
71. Ha T-Y, Kim K-M, Ko G-Y, Oh SH, Kwon T-W, Cho Y-P, et al. Variant meso-Rex bypass with transposition of abdominal autogenous vein for the management of idiopathic extrahepatic portal vein obstruction: a retrospective observational study. BMC Surg [Internet]. 2015;15. https://www.ncbi.nlm.nih.gov/pmc/articles/PMC4609139/
72. Han D, Tang R, Wang L, Li A, Huang X, Shen S, et al. Case report of a modified Meso-Rex bypass as a treatment technique for late-onset portal vein cavernous transformation with portal hypertension after adult deceased-donor liver transplantation. Medicine (Baltimore). 2017;96(25):e7208.
73. Wang M-Q, Lin H-Y, Guo L-P, Liu F-Y, Duan F, Wang Z-J. Acute extensive portal and mesen-teric venous thrombosis after splenectomy: treated by interventional thrombolysis with tran-sjugular approach. World J Gastroenterol. 2009;15(24):3038–45.
74. Liu F-Y, Wang M-Q, Fan Q-S, Duan F, Wang Z-J, Song P. Interventional treatment for symp-tomatic acute-subacute portal and superior mesenteric vein thrombosis. World J Gastroenterol WJG. 2009;15(40):5028–34.
75. Cao G, Ko G-Y, Sung K-B, Yoon H-K, Gwon DI, Kim J-H. Treatment of postoperative main portal vein and superior mesenteric vein thrombosis with balloon angioplasty and/or stent placement. Acta Radiol Stockh Swed 1987. 2013;54(5):526–32.
76. Rosenqvist K, Eriksson L-G, Rorsman F, Sangfelt P, Nyman R. Endovascular treatment of acute and chronic portal vein thrombosis in patients with cirrhotic and non-cirrhotic liver. Acta Radiol Stockh Swed 1987. 2016;57(5):572–9.
77. Plessier A, Goria O, et al. Prophylaxis of recurrent thrombosis by rivaroxabanin patients with non-cirrhotic chronic portal vein thrombosis (PVT): a multicentre randomized controlled study testing rivaroxaban vs no anticoagulation (GS-613). J Hepatol. 2021;75(Supplement 2): S197.

# Chapter 8
# Portal Vein Thrombosis in Patients with Cirrhosis

**Filipe Nery**

## Epidemiology, Diagnosis and Classification

PVT has been described to be more frequent in patients with more severe and advanced liver disease. Actually, a bulk of epidemiological data are derived from studies conducted in patients with advanced severe chronic liver disease, e.g. wait-listed for liver transplantation (LT). In the latter context, 1-year incidence of 7.4% [1] has been reported, but prevalence by the time of LT has been estimated between 15.9 and 26% [2, 3]. In a mixed population of patients with cirrhosis stage Child-Pugh A to C, Zocco et al. observed a 1-year incidence of 16.4% [4]. A similar 1-year incidence of 17.9% was found in another cohort of patients with decompensated liver disease [5]. Yet, PVT is also a concern in more stable patients, as it has been found to occur in up to 4.6%, 8.2% and 10.7% at respectively 1-, 3- and 5-years, in a population of mostly compensated liver disease patients [6].

As PVT is more commonly a clinically silent event, it is mostly uncovered at Doppler ultrasound (DUS) performed for hepatocellular carcinoma (HCC) screening. Outside the context of LT, there is currently no recommendation to routinely screen for PVT in patients with cirrhosis [7]. PVT diagnosis is generally made by DUS. DUS sensitivity in detecting PVT increases with the degree of occlusion and extension [8]. It may be difficult to differentiate bland thrombi from malignant

F. Nery (✉)
Centro Hospitalar Universitário do Porto – Hospital de Santo António, Porto, Portugal

Instituto de Ciências Biomédicas de Abel Salazar – Universidade do Porto, Porto, Portugal

EPI Unit, Institute of Public Health, University of Porto, Porto, Portugal

Laboratory for Integrative and Translational Research in Population Health (ITR), Porto, Portugal

© Springer Nature Switzerland AG 2022
D. Valla et al. (eds.), *Vascular Disorders of the Liver*,
https://doi.org/10.1007/978-3-030-82988-9_8

portal vein invasion. Increased diameter of the vessel, evident vessel wall disruption or adjacent malignant liver parenchyma infiltration may contribute to differentiate the two types of portal venous obstruction. Arterial phase enhancement after contrast injection in HCC invasion is the most accurate differential feature. Contrast-enhanced ultrasound is superior to DUS in making this differentiation, allowing a final diagnosis in more than 97% of the patients [9]. CT scan (Fig. 8.1) or MRI (Fig. 8.2) are useful in evaluating extension, allowing the application of different classification scores [10]. The most widely used classification of PVT in patients with cirrhosis was proposed by Yerdel et al., two decades ago [8]. Being simple and reproducible, this anatomical classification takes into account the site, degree of occlusion and extension of the thrombus, which is relevant in choosing the operative management at LT [8]. A recent anatomic and functional classification has been proposed, outside the transplant setting, precising PVT location, grade of occlusion and extension, as well as clinical presentation and functional relevance, also allowing to select patients who would benefit most of anticoagulation therapy [11]. Further validation of the latter classification is needed.

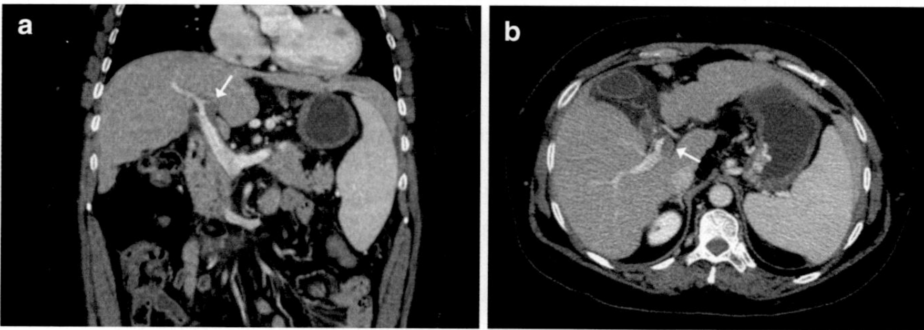

**Fig. 8.1** Partial trunk portal vein thrombosis (arrows) documented in a CT-scan. (**a**) Coronal CT sequence; (**b**) Axial CT sequence

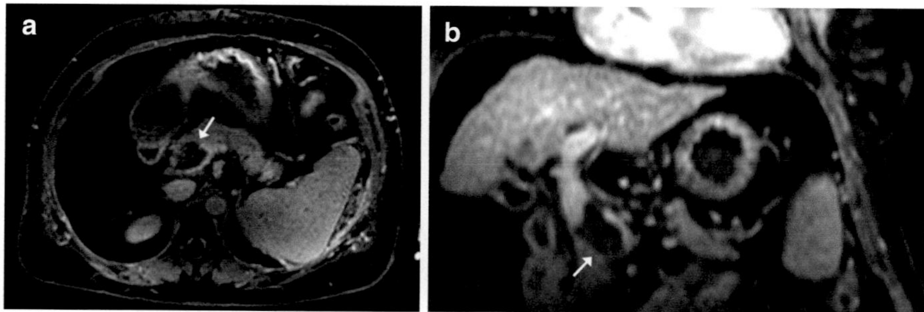

**Fig. 8.2** Portal vein thrombosis with extension to splenoportal venous confluence and superior mesenteric vein (arrows) documented in Magnetic Resonance Imaging. (**a**) Axial T1-weigthed image; (**b**) Coronal view

# Risk Factors

Understanding of venous thrombosis development irrespective of the site of occurrence is based on the work of ancient haematologists, probably the most recognized being the one by Rudolf Virchow, conducted in the mid-nineteenth century [12]. Clot formation occurs in the presence of factors related to blood stasis, a hypercoagulable state and endothelial damage, the pillars of the Virchow's triad [12]. The combination of such factors, rather than one factor acting alone may also be considered for PVT, viewed as a multifactorial entity (Fig. 8.3).

**Blood Stasis** The increased intrahepatic resistance that is characteristic of liver cirrhosis, and responsible for portal hypertension, induces a slowdown of the portal vein blood flow. Portal vein blood flow velocity decreases proportionally to the severity of the liver disease (as assessed by Child-Pugh classification) [13] and higher degrees of fibrosis [14]. A portal vein blood flow velocity of 15 cm/s or less has been found to be predictive for subsequent PVT development [4, 5, 15]. It has been proposed that a decreased blood flow would lead to an increased concentration of thrombin at the level of the portal vein tract, contributing to PVT development [4]. However, a decreasing [6, 16] or low [17] portal vein blood flow velocity was not found to be independently related to subsequent PVT development by other investigators. Well-known limits in assessing portal blood flow velocity with percutaneous DUS may account for these disparate results. An increased flow volume in collateral vessels was independently linked to PVT development in a cohort of patients with cirrhosis related to viral hepatitis [18]. However, the authors do not

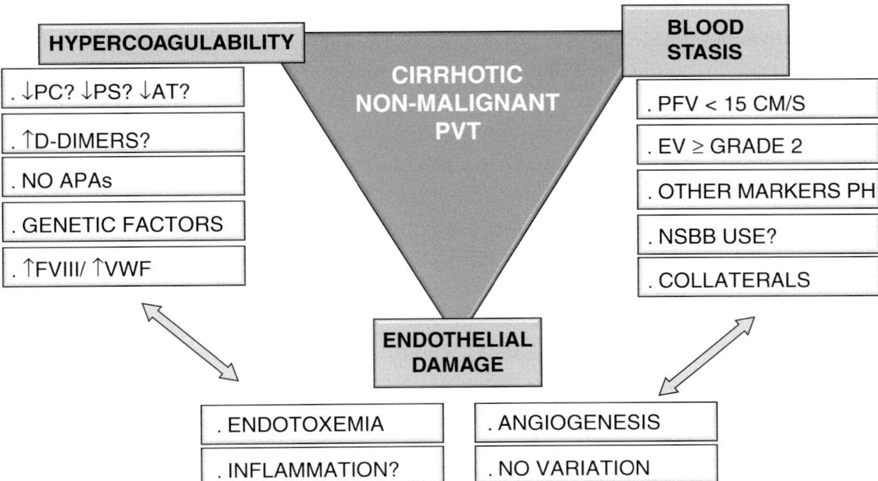


**Fig. 8.3** Virchow's triad applied to portal vein thrombosis genesis. *PVT* portal vein thrombosis, *PC* protein C, *PS* protein S, *AT* Antithrombin, *APAs* Antiphospholipid antibodies, *FVIII* Factor VIII, *VWF* von Willebrand factor, *NO* Nitric oxide, *PFV* portal vein flow, *EV* esophageal varices, *PH* portal hypertension, *NSBB* non-selective beta-blockers

mention the impact of this deviation of blood from the portal tract on a possible decrease in portal vein blood flow [18]. Thus, hemodynamic factors related to portal vein blood flow stasis although an attractive hypothesis to explain PVT, require further assessment.

Other factors related to severe portal hypertension and/or portal blood flow stasis have also been found to be associated to PVT, including low platelet count [1, 5], increased splenic thickness [5] or spleen size [18], previous variceal bleeding [1], presence of medium or large-sized esophageal varices [6] and of ascites [18].

Non-selective beta-blockers (NSBB), generally used for primary or secondary variceal bleeding prophylaxis, have been proposed to decrease portal blood flow via a reduced cardiac output and increased splanchnic vasoconstriction [19]. A recent longitudinal study found NSBB as an independent risk factor for future PVT development irrespective of its effect over portal blood flow velocity or heart rate [16]. This finding was corroborated by a meta-analysis that found an increased 4.6-fold risk for PVT development in patients under NSBB [20]. Yet, the link between NSBB and PVT development may not be direct (through an effect on splanchnic hemodynamics), but indirect, as a reflection of more severe degree of portal hypertension through presence of large esophageal varices as an indication for NSBB administration. Robust and prospective data are still necessary before establishing a causal relationship of NSBB with PVT development.

**Hypercoagulability** In cirrhosis, pro- and anti-hemostatic drivers are altered, which results in an enhanced platelet-vessel wall interaction and platelet activation [21, 22]; an enhanced potential to generate thrombin [21, 23]; a disturbed fibrinolysis [21]; a modified structure and function of the fibrin clot [24]; and increased levels of procoagulant microparticles carrying tissue factor [25]. Altogether, these changes confer a state of rebalanced coagulation or even a procoagulant state [21] (discussed in details in Chap. 17). However, specific studies directly addressing the relationship of these factors to PVT development are still lacking. Decreased protein C [4, 26] or antithrombin levels [4] and increased D-dimer levels [4] have been associated with an increased risk for subsequent PVT development. The other available studies of retrospective or cross-sectional design, have analyzed risk factors determined at the time of the diagnosis of the thrombotic event [27–30]. When considering inherited thrombophilia, only Factor V Leiden [31, 32] and MTHFR mutations [33] have been recognized to be associated with an increased tendency to develop PVT. Conflicting results exist when considering the role of prothrombin G20210A mutation and PVT, as a previous meta-analysis failed to confirm an association [31], while a more recent one displayed exactly the opposite [32], reflecting different methodological approaches when choosing the studies to enroll. Still, current guidelines recommend considering the screening of underlying inherited thrombophilic conditions [7, 10], even though we consider that, in the absence of robust data, the search of these inherited factors is not mandatory. Myeloproliferative neoplasias are a known risk factor for PVT development in patients without cirrhosis, and JAK-2 V617F mutation may be present in up to 16% [34] to 31% [35] of such patients. A case-control study showed that 10% of patients with cirrhosis and PVT similarly harbored the JAK-2 V617F mutation in contrast with none of the patients without PVT [35]. These still unconfirmed results must be seen with caution as few patients were enrolled. In non-cirrhotic patients with JAK-2 V617F negative myeloproliferative neoplasia, calreticulin mutations may be present in up to 31% of patients with PVT [36], but corresponding data in patients with cirrhosis are lacking. Antiphospholipid antibodies have been found in patients with cirrhosis and with an increased prevalence according to the degree of liver failure [37]. However, their role in the development of PVT has not been documented yet [38].

**Endothelial Damage**  Even though endothelial activation predisposing to thrombosis has been documented in other vascular beds and is an attractive hypothesis, it has never been confirmed, to date, to be related to PVT. Inflammation and increased endothelial permeability is at the basis of vascular endothelial growth factor-mediated angiogenesis and related cofactor to portosystemic collaterals development [39, 40]. Endotoxemia, resulting from bacterial translocation occurs in proportion to the severity of portal hypertension and degree of liver insufficiency, being more severe at the level of the portal circulation than in the systemic circulation [41]. Endotoxins promote not only a von Willebrand factor (vWf) release from endothelial cells and related increased factor VIII [42], but also the up-regulation of tissue factor leading to factor VII activation and associated coagulation cascade activation [41, 43]. From the above, endothelial damage may, therefore, promote and aggravate portal hypertension and portosystemic collateral formation by inducing angiogenesis (both known to be triggers of PVT development), as it may also promote the activation of coagulation cascade via the inflammatory cascade leading, by this mean, to PVT. Such relationship between endotoxemia, inflammation and PVT has already been proposed as an attractive explanation to the observed clinical and laboratory data [43]. Recently, increased levels of IL-6 and lymphopenia were shown related to PVT development independently of markers of portal hypertension, reinforcing the idea of the role of inflammation and endothelial activation in the pathogenesis of PVT [44].

# Natural History

**PVT Outcome Without Anticoagulation**  By contrast with early studies in which no resolution of PVT was seen in patients without anticoagulation treatment [1], recent longitudinal studies report portal vein recanalization in up to 45–70% of the patients [6, 18, 45], aggravation in only 7% to 34% [18, 45], and recurrence in 19–21% of the patients [6, 18], as confirmed in a recent meta-analysis [46]. In cirrhosis, therefore, PVT is rather a dynamic process. Also, PVT is more often partial than complete [6, 18, 47], which ultimately translates into higher recanalization rates.

**Role of PVT in decompensation and progression of liver disease** PVT has been widely considered to play a role in the progression (and decompensation) of underlying liver disease. At the time of LT, ascites and gastrointestinal bleeding are more frequent in patients with PVT than in those without [48]. A more advanced liver disease was reported in patients with, than in patients without PVT [49]. Such a causal relationship could theoretically be associated to decreased liver perfusion with portal blood, which would result in parenchymal atrophy leading to further increase in portal hypertension and worsening of liver dysfunction [50]. However, these conclusions were drawn from cross-sectional studies where thrombosis was documented at the time of the liver decompensation, which leaves open the question of what occurred first. Recent longitudinal studies have provided data that support the opposite view. Luca et al. found no relationship between the development of PVT and hepatic decompensation, irrespective of PVT progression along time or not [45]. Moreover, in patients wait-listed for LT with PVT compared to those without PVT, upper gastrointestinal bleeding, worsening of ascites, spontaneous bacterial peritonitis or encephalopathy aggravation were not more frequent either at the time of listing or during the waiting period [51]. Furthermore, in a study enrolling 1243 Child A and B patients, PVT and liver decompensation were shown to share baseline risk factors (i.e. medium or large esophageal varices and prolonged prothrombin time), while PVT development did not influenced the progression or the decompensation of liver disease [6].

**Impact of PVT on survival** PVT could not be shown to alter survival in patients not candidates to LT or on the waiting list for LT [15, 18, 51, 52]. Remarkably PVT has been linked to a decreased mortality on the waiting list, [53], the interpretation of which will require further analysis of the interaction with anticoagulation therapy as there is preliminary evidence that anticoagulation may impact survival positively [26]. In recipients of liver transplant with prior PVT however, early-survival decreases compared to those without PVT [52, 54, 55]. The impact on post-LT survival may be related to higher degrees of PVT occlusion [1, 8], and also to longer operative times, higher transfusion requirements and rates of reoperation, longer intensive care and hospital stays and the particular surgical technics used for clot removal and alternative vascular reconstructions [8, 56, 57].

## Treatment

**Anticoagulation therapy** In patients with PVT without cirrhosis, anticoagulation therapy is the mainstay of treatment [10] as discussed in section "Epidemiology, Diagnosis and Classification", Chap. 17. In cirrhosis, some considerations shall be taken into account before considering anticoagulation therapy. First, as mentioned above, PVT in cirrhosis is a dynamic process with a possible spontaneous recanalization in more than half of the patients; second, PVT likely does not induce liver decompensation; third, PVT has no impact on survival in patients besides the LT setting. Therefore, there is no matter for an indication of anticoagulation therapy except in the context of patients listed for LT. However, this concept may change in the near future, as evidence of an improvement in survival in patients with PVT under anticoagulation therapy has been recently demonstrated in a meta-analysis enrolling 1696 cirrhotic patients, without significant increase in bleeding risk [58]. Yet, this advantage needs to be viewed with caution, as it may not be applicable to all patients regardless of the severity of the disease. In patients undergoing LT, the immediate goal is to avoid portal vein thrombus extension or to decrease its size in order to facilitate liver transplantation [7, 10]. However, even in this setting, the efficacy and safety of anticoagulation therapy must be discussed. Robust studies accessing the efficacy of anticoagulation on PVT in cirrhosis are lacking. Most of them were conducted with a small number of patients and with some heterogeneity concerning the type of anticoagulant agent used. In a series of 19 patients listed for LT with PVT in whom nadroparin followed by acenocoumarol was used, 8 patients (42%) had complete resolution of the thrombus (7 of them had partial PVT before anticoagulation was started) while only 1 patient (5%) had PVT extension [1]. Another longitudinal prospective study comparing 35 patients treated with nadroparin to 21 untreated patients showed significantly less progression of the thrombus in the former (15%) compared to the latter (71%). Sixty-three percent of the treated patients achieved some degree of recanalization and 36% had a complete PVT resolution [59]. Patients with thrombus extension to the splenic vein, those with previous gastrointestinal bleeding and with estimated thrombus duration of at least 6 months were less likely to recanalize [59]. The largest available study, which enrolled 55 patients given either low molecular weight heparin or vitamin K antagonists, showed an overall improvement of PVT in 60% of patients including 45% with complete recanalization [60]. Globally, around 50% of the patients who under anticoagulation achieved complete recanalization and 2/3 some degree of repermeabilization (partial or complete) [46, 61]. Importantly, when anticoagulation is stopped, PVT relapses in 40% of the patients [60], a reason why, in patients listed for LT, once started, anticoagulation treatment shall be maintained at least until the surgical procedure. Reluctance to the use of anticoagulant therapy in cirrhosis is related to the perceived risk of bleeding. It is now clear that patients with cirrhosis bleed from portal hypertension complications and not from hemostatic abnormalities. Anticoagulant therapy may be safely used in patients with cirrhosis and PVT as either no bleeding complications or only minor bleeding events have been reported [46, 61]. Remarkably, two recent meta-analysis have shown a decreased incidence of variceal bleeding in patients under anticoagulation therapy compared to those without [46, 62]. However, a platelet count below $50 \times 10^9$/L has been identified as a risk factor for bleeding from any site in patients with cirrhosis and PVT receiving anticoagulation [60]. Available options for anticoagulant agents are discussed elsewhere.

**Transjugular intrahepatic shunt (TIPS)** The complications of portal hypertension refractory to usual therapy have been the most common indications for TIPS placement in patients with cirrhosis and PVT [7]. In studies addressing TIPS procedure as a modality for PVT treatment, the main indication was usually not PVT itself, but a previous episode of bleeding or refractory ascites. TIPS placement displays a high rate of success, with 74% of the patients achieving complete and 84% complete or partial recanalization, as documented in a recent meta-analysis [63]. In patients with cirrhosis undergoing TIPS placement (irrespective of the indication), there was no difference in rebleeding, recurrence of ascites or hepatic encephalopathy, as well as short- and long-term survival between those with PVT and those without [63, 64]. TIPS dysfunction was found to be remarkably less frequent when placing a covered stent [65]. Among five patients that underwent TIPS placement after thrombus extension on anticoagulation therapy, 3 showed stability, 1 completely reverted and 1 died (TIPS placement failed) [59]. These limited data suggest that TIPS could be used as a rescue therapy when PVT does not resolve with standard anticoagulation therapy. TIPS insertion prior to LT is increasingly used in patients with PVT [55]. However, TIPS is still not recommended as a standard treatment for PVT in cirrhosis but to be considered individually and by experienced teams [10].

## Conclusion

As PVT in cirrhosis is a common event in the course of the disease, awareness shall be raised for this entity, which is multifactorial in origin. Once diagnosed and outside the liver transplant setting, anticoagulation treatment is not mandatory mainly due to the fact that (1) PVT is a dynamic entity, often resolving without any directed therapy and that (2) it is not currently recognized to affect the outcome (decompensation or survival). A different scenario is seen in patients undergoing liver transplantation, as, once diagnosed, PVT may affect not only the eligibility to surgery but also impact survival after transplantation. In this context, anticoagulation therapy shall be started and patients regularly monitored.

## References


1. Francoz C, Belghiti J, Vilgrain V, Sommacale D, Paradis V, Condat B, et al. Splanchnic vein thrombosis in candidates for liver transplantation: usefulness of screening and anticoagulation. Gut. 2005;54(5):691–7.
2. Manzanet G, Sanjuan F, Orbis P, Lopez R, Moya A, Juan M, et al. Liver transplantation in patients with portal vein thrombosis. Liver Transplant. 2001;7(2):125–31.
3. Gayowski TJ, Marino IR, Doyle HR, Echeverri L, Mieles L, Todo S, et al. A high incidence of native portal vein thrombosis in veterans undergoing liver transplantation. J Surg Res. 1996;60(2):333–8.
4. Zocco MA, Di Stasio E, De Cristofaro R, Novi M, Ainora ME, Ponziani F, et al. Thrombotic risk factors in patients with liver cirrhosis: correlation with MELD scoring system and portal vein thrombosis development. J Hepatol. 2009;51(4):682–9.

5. Abdel-Razik A, Mousa N, Elhelaly R, Tawfik A. De-novo portal vein thrombosis in liver cirrhosis: risk factors and correlation with the model for end-stage liver disease scoring system. Eur J Gastroenterol Hepatol. 2015;27(5):585–92.
6. Nery F, Chevret S, Condat B, de Raucourt E, Boudaoud L, Rautou PE, et al. Causes and consequences of portal vein thrombosis in 1,243 patients with cirrhosis: results of a longitudinal study. Hepatology. 2015;61(2):660–7.
7. de Franchis R, Baveno VIF. Expanding consensus in portal hypertension: report of the Baveno VI consensus workshop: stratifying risk and individualizing care for portal hypertension. J Hepatol. 2015;63(3):743–52.
8. Yerdel MA, Gunson B, Mirza D, Karayalcin K, Olliff S, Buckels J, et al. Portal vein thrombosis in adults undergoing liver transplantation: risk factors, screening, management, and outcome. Transplantation. 2000;69(9):1873–81.
9. Rafailidis V, Fang C, Yusuf GT, Huang DY, Sidhu PS. Contrast-enhanced ultrasound (CEUS) of the abdominal vasculature. Abdominal Radiol. 2018;43(4):934–47.
10. European Association for the Study of the Liver. Electronic address EEE. EASL clinical practice guidelines: vascular diseases of the liver. J Hepatol. 2016;64(1):179–202.
11. Sarin SK, Philips CA, Kamath PS, Choudhury A, Maruyama H, Nery FG, et al. Toward a comprehensive new classification of portal vein thrombosis in patients with cirrhosis. Gastroenterology. 2016;151(4):574–7. e3
12. Bagot CN, Arya R. Virchow and his triad: a question of attribution. Br J Haematol. 2008;143(2):180–90.
13. Zironi G, Gaiani S, Fenyves D, Rigamonti A, Bolondi L, Barbara L. Value of measurement of mean portal flow velocity by Doppler flowmetry in the diagnosis of portal hypertension. J Hepatol. 1992;16(3):298–303.
14. Lutz HH, Gassler N, Tischendorf FW, Trautwein C, Tischendorf JJ. Doppler ultrasound of hepatic blood flow for noninvasive evaluation of liver fibrosis compared with liver biopsy and transient elastography. Dig Dis Sci. 2012;57(8):2222–30.
15. Stine JG, Wang J, Shah PM, Argo CK, Intagliata N, Uflacker A, et al. Decreased portal vein velocity is predictive of the development of portal vein thrombosis: a matched case-control study. Liver Int. 2018;38(1):94–101.
16. Nery F, Correia S, Macedo C, Gandara J, Lopes V, Valadares D, et al. Nonselective beta-blockers and the risk of portal vein thrombosis in patients with cirrhosis: results of a prospective longitudinal study. Aliment Pharmacol Ther. 2019;
17. Chen H, Trilok G, Wang F, Qi X, Xiao J, Yang C. A single hospital study on portal vein thrombosis in cirrhotic patients – clinical characteristics & risk factors. Indian J Med Res. 2014;139(2):260–6.
18. Maruyama H, Okugawa H, Takahashi M, Yokosuka O. De novo portal vein thrombosis in virus-related cirrhosis: predictive factors and long-term outcomes. Am J Gastroenterol. 2013;108(4):568–74.
19. Qi XS, Bai M, Fan DM. Nonselective beta-blockers may induce development of portal vein thrombosis in cirrhosis. World J Gastroenterol. 2014;20(32):11463–6.
20. Xu X, Guo X, De Stefano V, Silva-Junior G, Goyal H, Bai Z, et al. Nonselective beta-blockers and development of portal vein thrombosis in liver cirrhosis: a systematic review and meta-analysis. Hepatol Int. 2019;13(4):468–81.
21. Tripodi A, Primignani M, Mannucci PM, Caldwell SH. Changing concepts of cirrhotic coagulopathy. Am J Gastroenterol. 2017;112(2):274–81.
22. Raparelli V, Basili S, Carnevale R, Napoleone L, Del Ben M, Nocella C, et al. Low-grade endotoxemia and platelet activation in cirrhosis. Hepatology. 2017;65(2):571–81.
23. Groeneveld D, Porte RJ, Lisman T. Thrombomodulin-modified thrombin generation testing detects a hypercoagulable state in patients with cirrhosis regardless of the exact experimental conditions. Thromb Res. 2014;134(3):753–6.
24. Lisman T, Ariens RA. Alterations in fibrin structure in patients with liver diseases. Semin Thromb Hemost. 2016;42(4):389–96.

25. Rautou PE, Vion AC, Luyendyk JP, Mackman N. Circulating microparticle tissue factor activity is increased in patients with cirrhosis. Hepatology. 2014;60(5):1793–5.
26. Villa E, Camma C, Marietta M, Luongo M, Critelli R, Colopi S, et al. Enoxaparin prevents portal vein thrombosis and liver decompensation in patients with advanced cirrhosis. Gastroenterology. 2012;143(5):1253–60 e1–4.
27. Martinelli I, Primignani M, Aghemo A, Reati R, Bucciarelli P, Fabris F, et al. High levels of factor VIII and risk of extra-hepatic portal vein obstruction. J Hepatol. 2009;50(5):916–22.
28. Zhang D, Hao J, Yang N. Protein C and D-dimer are related to portal vein thrombosis in patients with liver cirrhosis. J Gastroenterol Hepatol. 2010;25(1):116–21.
29. Zhang DL, Hao JY, Yang N. Value of D-dimer and protein S for diagnosis of portal vein thrombosis in patients with liver cirrhosis. J Int Med Res. 2013;41(3):664–72.
30. Singhal A, Karachristos A, Bromberg M, Daly E, Maloo M, Jain AK. Hypercoagulability in end-stage liver disease: prevalence and its correlation with severity of liver disease and portal vein thrombosis. Clin Appl Thrombosis/Hemostasis. 2012;18(6):594–8.
31. Qi X, Ren W, De Stefano V, Fan D. Associations of coagulation factor V Leiden and prothrombin G20210A mutations with Budd-Chiari syndrome and portal vein thrombosis: a systematic review and meta-analysis. Clin Gastroenterol Hepatol. 2014;12(11):1801–12. e7
32. Ma SD, Wang J, Bezinover D, Kadry Z, Northup PG, Stine JG. Inherited thrombophilia and portal vein thrombosis in cirrhosis: a systematic review and meta-analysis. Res Pract Thromb Haemostasis. 2019;3(4):658–67.
33. Qi X, Yang Z, De Stefano V, Fan D. Methylenetetrahydrofolate reductase C677T gene mutation and hyperhomocysteinemia in Budd-Chiari syndrome and portal vein thrombosis: a systematic review and meta-analysis of observational studies. Hepatol Res. 2014;44(14):E480–98.
34. Plessier A, Darwish-Murad S, Hernandez-Guerra M, Consigny Y, Fabris F, Trebicka J, et al. Acute portal vein thrombosis unrelated to cirrhosis: a prospective multicenter follow-up study. Hepatology. 2010;51(1):210–8.
35. Saugel B, Lee M, Feichtinger S, Hapfelmeier A, Schmid RM, Siveke JT. Thrombophilic factor analysis in cirrhotic patients with portal vein thrombosis. J Thromb Thrombolysis. 2015;40(1):54–60.
36. Li M, De Stefano V, Song T, Zhou X, Guo Z, Zhu J, et al. Prevalence of CALR mutations in splanchnic vein thrombosis: a systematic review and meta-analysis. Thromb Res. 2018;167:96–103.
37. Perney P, Biron-Andreani C, Joomaye Z, Fabbro-Peray P, Quenet F, Schved JF, et al. Antiphospholipid antibodies in alcoholic liver disease are influenced by histological damage but not by alcohol consumption. Lupus. 2000;9(6):451–5.
38. Qi X, De Stefano V, Su C, Bai M, Guo X, Fan D. Associations of antiphospholipid antibodies with splanchnic vein thrombosis: a systematic review with meta-analysis. Medicine. 2015;94(4):e496.
39. Iwakiri Y. Endothelial dysfunction in the regulation of cirrhosis and portal hypertension. Liver Int. 2012;32(2):199–213.
40. Greuter T, Shah VH. Hepatic sinusoids in liver injury, inflammation, and fibrosis: new pathophysiological insights. J Gastroenterol. 2016;51(6):511–9.
41. Violi F, Ferro D. Clotting activation and hyperfibrinolysis in cirrhosis: implication for bleeding and thrombosis. Semin Thromb Hemost. 2013;39(4):426–33.
42. Carnevale R, Raparelli V, Nocella C, Bartimoccia S, Novo M, Severino A, et al. Gut-derived endotoxin stimulates factor VIII secretion from endothelial cells. Implications for hypercoagulability in cirrhosis. J Hepatol. 2017;67(5):950–6.
43. Violi F, Lip GY, Cangemi R. Endotoxemia as a trigger of thrombosis in cirrhosis. Haematologica. 2016;101(4):e162–3.
44. Nery F, Carneiro P, Correia S, Macedo C, Gandara J, Lopes V, Valadares D, Ferreira S, Oliveira J, Teixeira Gomes M, Miranda HP, Rautou PE, Valla D. Systemic inflammation as a risk factor for portal vein thrombosis in cirrhosis: a prospective longitudinal study. Eur J Gastroenterol Hepatol. 2020 Nov 17.

45. Luca A, Caruso S, Milazzo M, Marrone G, Mamone G, Crino F, et al. Natural course of extrahepatic nonmalignant partial portal vein thrombosis in patients with cirrhosis. Radiology. 2012;265(1):124–32.
46. Loffredo L, Pastori D, Farcomeni A, Violi F. Effects of anticoagulants in patients with cirrhosis and portal vein thrombosis: A systematic review and meta-analysis. Gastroenterology. 2017;153(2):480–7. e1
47. Francoz C, Valla D, Durand F. Portal vein thrombosis, cirrhosis, and liver transplantation. J Hepatol. 2012;57(1):203–12.
48. Nonami T, Yokoyama I, Iwatsuki S, Starzl TE. The incidence of portal vein thrombosis at liver transplantation. Hepatology. 1992;16(5):1195–8.
49. Amitrano L, Guardascione MA, Brancaccio V, Margaglione M, Manguso F, Iannaccone L, et al. Risk factors and clinical presentation of portal vein thrombosis in patients with liver cirrhosis. J Hepatol. 2004;40(5):736–41.
50. Wanless IR, Wong F, Blendis LM, Greig P, Heathcote EJ, Levy G. Hepatic and portal vein thrombosis in cirrhosis: possible role in development of parenchymal extinction and portal hypertension. Hepatology. 1995;21(5):1238–47.
51. John BV, Konjeti R, Aggarwal A, Lopez R, Atreja A, Miller C, et al. Impact of untreated portal vein thrombosis on pre and post liver transplant outcomes in cirrhosis. Ann Hepatol. 2013;12(6):952–8.
52. Englesbe MJ, Schaubel DE, Cai S, Guidinger MK, Merion RM. Portal vein thrombosis and liver transplant survival benefit. Liver Transplant. 2010;16(8):999–1005.
53. Berry K, Taylor J, Liou IW, Ioannou GN. Portal vein thrombosis is not associated with increased mortality among patients with cirrhosis. Clin Gastroenterol. 2015;13(3):585–93.
54. Ghabril M, Agarwal S, Lacerda M, Chalasani N, Kwo P, Tector AJ. Portal vein thrombosis is a risk factor for poor early outcomes after liver transplantation: analysis of risk factors and outcomes for portal vein thrombosis in waitlisted patients. Transplantation. 2016;100(1):126–33.
55. Montenovo M, Rahnemai-Azar A, Reyes J, Perkins J. Clinical impact and risk factors of portal vein thrombosis for patients on wait list for liver transplant. Exp Clin Transplant. 2017;
56. Lendoire J, Raffin G, Cejas N, Duek F, Barros Schelotto P, Trigo P, et al. Liver transplantation in adult patients with portal vein thrombosis: risk factors, management and outcome. HPB. 2007;9(5):352–6.
57. Ponziani FR, Zocco MA, Senzolo M, Pompili M, Gasbarrini A, Avolio AW. Portal vein thrombosis and liver transplantation: implications for waiting list period, surgical approach, early and late follow-up. Transplant Rev. 2014;28(2):92–101.
58. Wang LGX, Xu X, De Stefano V, Plessier A, Ferreira CN, Qi X. Anticoagulation favors thrombus recanalization and survival in patients with liver cirrhosis and portal vein thrombosis: results of a meta-analysis. Adv Ther. 2021;38(1):495–520.
59. Senzolo MTMS, Rossetto V, Burra P, Cillo U, Boccagni P, et al. Prospective evaluation of anticoagulation and transjugular intrahepatic portosystemic shunt for the management of portal vein thrombosis in cirrhosis. Liver Int. 2012;32(6):919–27.
60. Delgado MG, Seijo S, Yepes I, Achecar L, Catalina MV, Garcia-Criado A, et al. Efficacy and safety of anticoagulation on patients with cirrhosis and portal vein thrombosis. Clin Gastroenterol Hepatol. 2012;10(7):776–83.
61. Chen H, Turon F, Hernandez-Gea V, Fuster J, Garcia-Criado A, Barrufet M, et al. Nontumoral portal vein thrombosis in patients awaiting liver transplantation. Liver Transplant. 2016;22(3):352–65.
62. Ghazaleh SB, Aburayyan K, Nehme C, Patel D, Khader Y, Sharma S, Aziz M, Abdel AY, Hammad T, Nawras A. Efficacy and safety of anticoagulation in non-malignant portal vein thrombosis in patients with liver cirrhosis: a systematic review and meta-analysis. Ann Gastroenterol. 2021;34(1):104–10.
63. Valentin N, Korrapati P, Constantino J, Young A, Weisberg I. The role of transjugular intrahepatic portosystemic shunt in the management of portal vein thrombosis: a systematic review and meta-analysis. Eur J Gastroenterol Hepatol. 2018.

64. Merola J, Fortune BE, Deng Y, Ciarleglio M, Amirbekian S, Chaudhary N, et al. Transjugular intrahepatic portosystemic shunt creation for cirrhotic portal hypertension is well tolerated among patients with portal vein thrombosis. Eur J Gastroenterol Hepatol. 2018;30(6):668–75.
65. Luca A, Miraglia R, Caruso S, Milazzo M, Sapere C, Maruzzelli L, et al. Short- and long-term effects of the transjugular intrahepatic portosystemic shunt on portal vein thrombosis in patients with cirrhosis. Gut. 2011;60(6):846–52.

# Chapter 9
# Porto-Sinusoidal Vascular Disorder

Susana G. Rodrigues, Matteo Montani, and Andrea De Gottardi

## Introduction

Idiopathic non-cirrhotic portal hypertension includes a heterogeneous group of vascular liver diseases that may lead to portal hypertension in the absence of parenchymal cirrhotic nodules [1]. It corresponds to a variety of histopathologic entities and that have been referred to as hepatoportal sclerosis, non-cirrhotic portal fibrosis, nodular regenerative hyperplasia or incomplete septal fibrosis/cirrhosis [2]. Until very recently, there were no conclusive diagnostic methods or characteristic histopathologic findings available for diagnosing idiopathic non-cirrhotic portal hypertension, which was thus made after excluding all other possible causes of liver disease. The pathophysiology of idiopathic non-cirrhotic portal hypertension is still poorly understood and therapy restricted to the manifestations of portal hypertension. Idiopathic non-cirrhotic portal hypertension has gained increased attention over the last two decades in parallel to the increased use of immunosuppressive drugs for autoimmune and hematological disorders, and to the increased prevalence of treated HIV infection, all conditions etiologically linked to idiopathic non-cirrhotic portal hypertension [3, 4]. Increased awareness and widespread use of liver elastography for fibrosis assessment have permitted diagnosis in patients in whom prominent

S. G. Rodrigues
Hepatology, University Clinic for Visceral Medicine and Surgery, Bern, Switzerland

Department of Biomedical Research, University of Bern, Bern, Switzerland

M. Montani
Institute of Pathology, University of Bern, Bern, Switzerland
e-mail: matteo.montani@pathology.unibe.ch

A. De Gottardi (✉)
Servizio di Gastroenterologia e Epatologia, Ente Ospedaliero Cantonale, Lugano, Switzerland

Università della Svizzera Italiana, Lugano, Switzerland
e-mail: andrea.degottardi@eoc.ch

© Springer Nature Switzerland AG 2022
D. Valla et al. (eds.), *Vascular Disorders of the Liver*,
https://doi.org/10.1007/978-3-030-82988-9_9

features of portal hypertension contrast with low liver stiffness [5]. In some patients with inconspicuous clinical features of portal hypertension, the diagnosis is made after detecting specific liver lesions at biopsy. Patients with extrahepatic splanchnic venous thrombosis may have idiopathic non-cirrhotic portal hypertension as an underlying condition. Last but not least, the previous definition –based on ruling out causes for cirrhosis—has excluded from specific attention patients with non-cirrhotic portal hypertension when concomitant causes for liver disease were present (e.g. hepatitis C, or alcohol consumption or metabolic syndrome).

The complexity and unclear pathogenesis of the entity so called idiopathic non-cirrhotic portal hypertension prompted the Vascular Liver Disease Interest Group (VALDIG) to organize a multidisciplinary conference in February 2017. Experts in vascular liver disease assembled to discuss the definition and terminology of portal vascular lesions, as well as the pathogenesis, causes, diagnostic workup, and treatment of idiopathic non-cirrhotic portal hypertension. The term *porto-sinusoidal vascular disorder* was proposed as a denomination for an entity incorporating various vascular liver disease based on clear criteria [6]. This chapter aims to clarify the new denomination of porto-sinusoidal vascular disorder as well as to provide a comprehensive view of its pathophysiology, diagnosis and treatment.


## Definition: Past and Present

According to the previous definition, idiopathic non-cirrhotic portal hypertension was characterized by direct and/or indirect signs of portal hypertension, including mild increase in hepatic venous pressure gradient, esophageal varices, non-malignant ascites, splenomegaly or hypersplenism, portosystemic collaterals, and the absence of cirrhosis on liver biopsy. Additionally, all other causes of chronic liver disease leading to cirrhotic and non-cirrhotic portal hypertension (sarcoidosis, schistosomiasis) and portal or hepatic vein thrombosis had to be excluded. This previous definition of idiopathic non-cirrhotic portal hypertension included the histopathologic entities previously known as obliterative portal venopathy, hepatoportal sclerosis, nodular regenerative hyperplasia, non-cirrhotic portal fibrosis and incomplete septal cirrhosis.

However, several key limitations to this definition were addressed in the 2017 VALDIG conference. First, this definition may be too restrictive because in early stages of disease, lesions can be present while significant portal hypertension has not yet developed or will not develop. Corresponding cases would be erroneously excluded. Second, the previous definition excludes any thrombosis of hepatic or portal venous systems; therefore, patients who develop portal vein thrombosis as a complication of their underlying intrahepatic vascular liver disease would similarly be erroneously excluded. Last, the previous definition did not allow for the presence of concomitant liver diseases, although it is well-known that some common diseases such as viral hepatitis, HIV infection or alcoholic or non-alcoholic fatty liver disease can concur with vascular liver disease.

The term *porto-sinusoidal vascular disorder* (PSVD) was developed to group together several conditions that, despite diverse pathophysiology, are characterized by lesions in the sinusoids and small-sized portal veins. This new denomination encompasses the whole spectrum of the disease spanning idiopathic non-cirrhotic portal hypertension, obliterative portal venopathy, incomplete septal cirrhosis and nodular regenerative hyperplasia [6]. The main components of this definition include the absence of histological cirrhosis and the detection of histological findings (Fig. 9.1), with or without portal hypertension.

In contrast with the criteria of the previous definition, the presence of causes for liver disease (i.e. alcohol misuse, metabolic syndrome, or viral hepatitis) does not exclude PSVD, *if* liver biopsy shows specific findings indicative of PSVD. In such overlapping cases, the relative contribution of PSVD and parenchymal liver disease to the development or degree of severity of portal hypertension remains an open question.

Similar to the previous definition, conditions affecting the hepatic veins or specific diseases that have been well characterized as causing microvascular disease such as sarcoidosis or congenital hepatic fibrosis are excluded (Box 9.1). Sinusoidal obstruction syndrome, which occurs after hematopoietic stem cell transplantation, is characterized by specific criteria and is not included in PSVD. Although extrahepatic portal vein thrombosis can cause, per se, non-cirrhotic portal hypertension, itis does not constitute an exclusion criteria, *if* liver biopsy shows specific findings indicative of PSVD. This is justified by its most frequent secondary occurrence in PSVD patients.

Overall, this new denomination is intended to clarify and facilitate diagnosis. From a research perspective, this inclusive definition is expected to facilitate

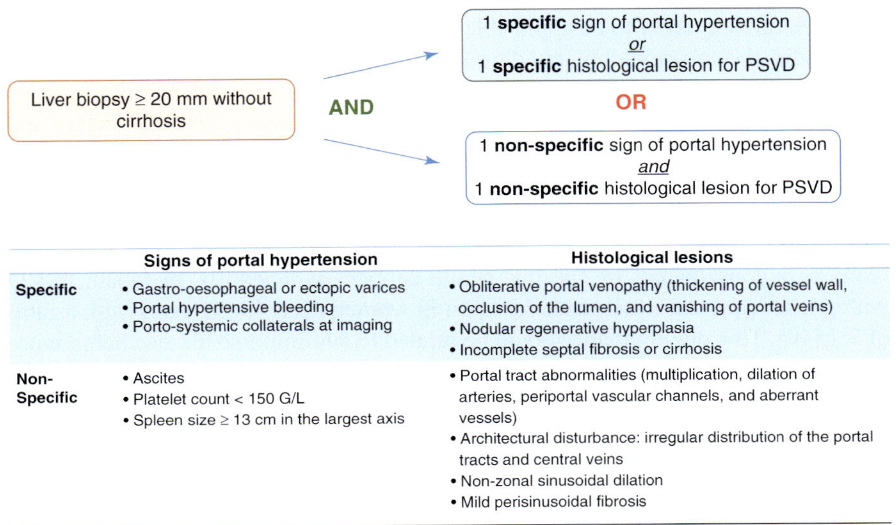


| | Signs of portal hypertension | Histological lesions |
|---|---|---|
| **Specific** | • Gastro-oesophageal or ectopic varices<br>• Portal hypertensive bleeding<br>• Porto-systemic collaterals at imaging | • Obliterative portal venopathy (thickening of vessel wall, occlusion of the lumen, and vanishing of portal veins)<br>• Nodular regenerative hyperplasia<br>• Incomplete septal fibrosis or cirrhosis |
| **Non-Specific** | • Ascites<br>• Platelet count < 150 G/L<br>• Spleen size ≥ 13 cm in the largest axis | • Portal tract abnormalities (multiplication, dilation of arteries, periportal vascular channels, and aberrant vessels)<br>• Architectural disturbance: irregular distribution of the portal tracts and central veins<br>• Non-zonal sinusoidal dilation<br>• Mild perisinusoidal fibrosis |

**Fig. 9.1**  Porto-sinusoidal vascular disorder (PSVD) definition

studieson this condition, by providing uniform criteria. On the other hand, it may be argued that these new criteria and terms may be overly simplistic and decrease precision to define a complex disease, and eventually introduce bias for studies that otherwise would not be concentrated on the same disease. It will therefore be important to gather further experience with this denomination and refine the definition accordingly.

> **Box 9.1 Conditions Excluded from the PSVD Definition**
> - Chronic cholestatic diseases
> - Tumoral liver infiltration
> - Budd-Chiari syndrome or hepatic venous outflow obstruction
> - Sarcoidosis
> - Hepatic schistosomiasis diagnosed on liver biopsy
> - Sinusoidal obstruction syndrome
> - Heart failure or Fontan surgery
> - Hereditary hemorrhagic telangiectasia
> - Abernethy syndrome
> - Congenital hepatic fibrosis

## Epidemiology

The overall prevalence of PSVD worldwide is unknown. Prevalence and denominations have differed according to geographic areas. Therefore, the new denomination was elaborated in order to be applicable independent of location.

In India, the corresponding condition was known as non-cirrhotic portal fibrosis. The prevalence in this area, although decreasing, is still high, accounting in some studies for 34% of all cases of portal hypertension [7]. Socioeconomic stature and sanitary/hygiene conditions have been suggested to be associated with its development. Males aged 30–49 years have been predominantly affected [8].

In Japan, the corresponding condition was denominated idiopathic portal hypertension. The prevalence of PSVD has dramatically shrunk during the last 4 decades, likely as a consequence of national health services policies [9]. In Japan, PSVD with portal hypertension is most common in women aged 40–59 years with a ratio of 2:1 [10]. This predominance could be related to autoimmune disease being more common in women than in men and to hormonal factors related to pregnancies and premenopausal age [11].

In Europe, PSVD appears to be rare, accounting for a lower proportion of cases of portal hypertension than reported in India or Japan. In France, nodular regenerative hyperplasia was found 4% of liver biopsies performed for various reasons [12]. The condition was found to predominantly affect men in France and UK (3:1) [13, 14]. In the U.S.A. and Canada, this prevalence was 3–7%; men aged 60–69 years were predominantly affected [15–17].

## Etiology: Associated Conditions

Causes have not been fully elucidated, yet. However, PVSD is associated with rare conditions in 43–58% of patients. These varied conditions can be categorized as drug exposure, immunological, coagulation disorders, infectious and congenital or familial defects (Box 9.2), [4, 18, 19]. Several of these conditions can be simultaneously present in occasional patients.

---

**Box 9.2 Conditions Associated with Porto-Snusoidal Vascular Disorder**
**Drug/toxin exposure**

- Didanosine
- Azathioprine, 6-Mercaptopurine
- Tioguanine
- Oxaliplatin
- Arsenic/vinylchloride
- Irradiation

**Immunological disorders**

- Common variable immune deficiency (significant hypogammaglobulinaemia & bacterial infections)
- Autoimmune hepatitis
- Systemic lupus erythematosus
- Scleroderma
- Rheumatoid arthritis
- HIV
- Celiac disease
- POEMS syndrome
- Autoimmune thyroiditis
- Multiple sclerosis

**Hemocoagulative disorders**

- Aplastic anaemia
- Myeloproliferative disorder
- Hodgkin's lymphoma
- Multiple myeloma
- Protein C or S deficiency
- Factor II or V gene mutation
- Antiphospholipid syndrome
- ADAMTS13 deficiency
- MTHFR deficiency

**Infectious**

- Repeated gastrointestinal infections (*E. coli*)

**Congenital, genetic or familial**

- Turner's syndrome
- Adams-Oliver syndrome
- *TERT* mutations
- Cystic fibrosis
- Familial cases
- KCNN3 mutation
- Noonan & Adams

## *Drug Exposure*

Older age and cumulative exposure to didanosine and stavudine were shown to be independent predictors for the development of nodular regenerative hyperplasia in patients with HIV infection [20]. The overall prevalence of HIV infection in PSVD patients was4% in a Dutch study [4]. Mallet et al. reported a significantly lower protein S activity in patients with HIV infection and nodular regenerative hyperplasia than in controls, but the unifying factor of PSVD in HIV patients was previous drug exposure [21]. Didanosine and stavudine currently being no longer used, if their responsibility is real, a decrease in the prevalence of PSVD among HIV infected patients is to be expected over the next decades.

PVSD has also been related to prior exposure to immunosuppressive or antineoplastic agents (in particular azathioprine and oxaliplatin) as well as to numerous other drugs [22].

## *Immunological Disorders*

Immune disorders, including acquired and congenital immune deficiencies and autoimmune diseases, have been detected in 10% of PSVD patients [23]. Conversely, PSVD has been found in up to 84% of patients with common variable immune deficiency [24], hyper-IgM syndrome, primary antibody-deficiency syndromes such as Bruton's disease [25], and in Felty's syndrome [26].

In patients with inflammatory bowel disease, the prevalence of PSVD was reported to be 6% [27]. However, it is difficult to decipher whether PVSD is mainly linked to the underlying inflammatory bowel disease or to azathioprine exposure. Adult celiac disease has also been associated with PSVD [13]. It has been proposed that the sinusoidal changes found in patients with conditions of disordered immunity, are related to intrasinusoidal cytotoxic T lymphocytes, granulomas, causing portal vein or sinusoidal endothelitis. This concept is in line with an over expression of lymphocyte activation genes in blood samples from PSVD patients [28, 29].

## *Coagulation Disorders*

There is evidence that micro-thrombosis and platelet aggregation contribute to the development of PSVD [10, 30]. In fact, thickening or occlusion and obliteration of portal vein venules detected at liver biopsy, is generally regarded as indicating previous thrombosis. Moreover, prothrombotic conditions such as protein C deficiency have been associated with a higher risk of PSVD [31]. Portal vein thrombosis is relatively common in these patients further pointing at a procoagulant tendency in these patients. Future studies should elucidate the prevalence and impact of prothrombotic risk factors in PSVD.

## *Infections*

Epidemiological studies have shown a relationship between low hygienic living conditions and PSVD, which has been interpreted as supporting a role for infections. Such a mechanism, however, could not be reproduced in experimental models [32]. Intra-abdominal infections may serve as a trigger for PSVD through recurrent small to medium portal branch occlusion [33, 34].

## *Congenital and Hereditary Disorders*

Porto-sinusoidal vascular disorder has been linked to genetic disorders such as Adams-Oliver syndrome, Turner's syndrome, familial obliterative portal venopathy, and cystic fibrosis [35–37].

In hereditary studies, familial aggregation has been found regarding PSVD and HLA-DR3 [38] and mutations in the telomerase gene complex [39]. Interestingly, a link between didanosine exposure in HIV patients and PSVD has been associated with certain single nucleotide polymorphisms of genes involved in the purine metabolic pathway [40]. Whole exome sequencing in families affected with PSVD led to the discovery of various mutations, but independent validation in other cohorts is still lacking [41, 42].

## Clinical Presentation and Features

### *PSVD with Portal Hypertension*

In higher income countries, patients with portal hypertension and PSVD are mainly middle-aged men. Patients with PSVD and portal hypertension are usually asymptomatic. In most cases, liver synthesis function is maintained and in about 80%, there is a slight increase (<2 time upper limit of normal) in liver biochemistry values, alanine aminotransferase or alkaline phosphatase. Some are detected through noninvasive methods with thrombocytopenia generally around 100 G/L, splenomegaly or an irregular liver aspect on ultrasound. Most patients have serum albumin and bilirubin levels within the normal range and prothrombin time slightly decreased, which aids in distinguishing them from those with cirrhosis. On the other hand, some patients develop complications of portal hypertension mostly variceal bleeding, which is the initial manifestation in around 20–40%, whereas ascites and encephalopathy are uncommon presenting manifestations in comparison.

One study examining the natural history of patients with idiopathic non-cirrhotic portal hypertension reported that large varices were found at initial presentation in two-thirds of the patients with PSVD and portal hypertension, or developed in 20% of patients within an average of 10 years of diagnosis [19]. Over time, PSVD patients with portal hypertension can develop ascites in 20–50% with a precipitant factor identified in the majority of cases and usually transient [18, 19]. Within 5 years of diagnosis, portal vein thrombosis develops in around a third of patients, but is completely obstructive (i.e. occupying more than 80% of the vessel lumen) in only a third of these [4, 18, 19]. The risk of thrombosis is increased in patients with a history of bleeding and with associated conditions, namely HIV infection. In cases of thrombosis and concomitant PSVD, hepatic venous pressure gradient measurement is particularly important to determine whether the origin of portal hypertension is pre-hepatic or sinusoidal. The latter could potentially indicate the insertion of a transjugular intrahepatic portosystemic shunt with portal vein recanalization (Fig. 9.2).

Regarding longer-term prognosis, one study with 69 patients showed minimal changes in markers of liver function in these patients, suggesting that PSVD is stable [18]. Patients can develop portopulmonary hypertension, hepatopulmonary syndrome, and liver regenerative nodules, but the precise risk factors leading to these complications are currently unidentified.

Concerning mortality, presence of ascites, age, and associated diseases are known risk factors [4]. Previous published series have demonstrated that the mortality can reach 15–20% after an 8-year follow-up period [4, 18, 19, 43]. The referral rate for liver transplantation (5–37%) appears to be very variable depending on the assessment of the risk of progression to end-stage liver disease.

## *PSVD Without Portal Hypertension*

Abnormal liver tests of unknown cause and without any signs of portal hypertension (splenomegaly, gastro-esophageal varices, portosystemic collaterals, ascites, or hepatic encephalopathy) could represent a pre-clinical stage of disease [18, 44] which may be followed by the development of manifest signs of portal hypertension [18]. Indeed, it appears that the prevalence of PSVD without portal hypertension is higher than previously thought (19% of cases with cryptogenic liver disease).

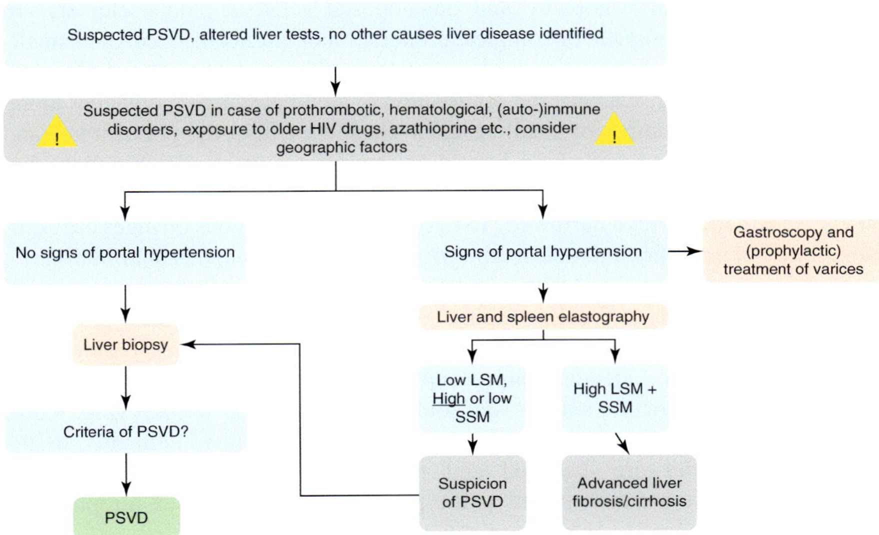


**Fig. 9.2** Diagnostic flowchart of porto-sinusoidal vascular disorder with and without portal hypertension. Abbreviations: *PSVD* porto-sinusoidal vascular disorder, *HIV* human immunodeficiency virus, *NRH* nodular regenerative hyperplasia, *EGD* esophagogastroduodenoscopy, *EVL* endoscopic variceal ligation, *LSM* liver stiffness measurement, *SSM* spleen stiffness measurement, *PH* portal hypertension

Moreover, the authors hypothesized that the presence of slightly impaired liver function tests, a higher rate of prothrombotic conditions, and immune diseases were likely to contribute in progressing to portal hypertension [18]. The diagnosis is established on specific findings at liver biopsy performed in asymptomatic patients with slight changes in liver biochemistry (Box 9.1).

Given the lack of longitudinal studies analyzing patients with PSVD without portal hypertension, there is currently insufficient data to clarify the natural history and risk factors of this form of the disease.

## Histopathological Findings

Liver biopsy for a diagnosis of PSVD can be considered in a variety of settings, including altered liver biochemistry of unknown cause, signs of portal hypertension without liver dysfunction, abnormal ultrasound findings, or portal hypertension with a low liver stiffness level. From a histological point of view there is an important diversity of lesions among patients that remains currently unexplained.

Obliterative portal venopathy, nodular regenerative hyperplasia, and incomplete septal cirrhosis are specific enough to be regarded as diagnostic for PSVD even in the absence of other clinical, laboratory or imaging alterations (Figs. 9.1 and 9.2).

Obliterative portal venopathy and hepatoportal sclerosis/phlebosclerosis are characterized by incomplete or complete obliteration of mainly medium- and small-sized intrahepatic portal vein branches with or without thickening of the wall (Fig. 9.3a). Moreover, scarring and obliteration of small portal vein branches along with an increased number of small vascular channels within the portal tracts and incomplete thin fibrous septa have been described. It is important to highlight that the portal vein branch is not always obliterated or absent (venopenia), as it can still be visible although with a narrowed [15]. Although portal venous changes are common, they can be difficult to detect atbiopsydue to a heterogeneous distribution.

Nodular regenerative hyperplasia is defined by lobular transformation into small nodules, with diffuse or focal nodular regeneration with architectural distortion, dilated sinusoids in areas of atrophy, increased number of venous profiles, and incomplete septa, i.e., slender fibrous septa originating from a portal tract that blindly ends in the lobule, and perisinusoidal and perivenular fibrosis (Fig. 9.3b). These nodules are generally lighter in tone and less well-defined compared to cirrhosis. The lobules are distorted and replaced by nodules of hyperplastic hepatocytes. These are surrounded at the periphery by compressed atrophic cell

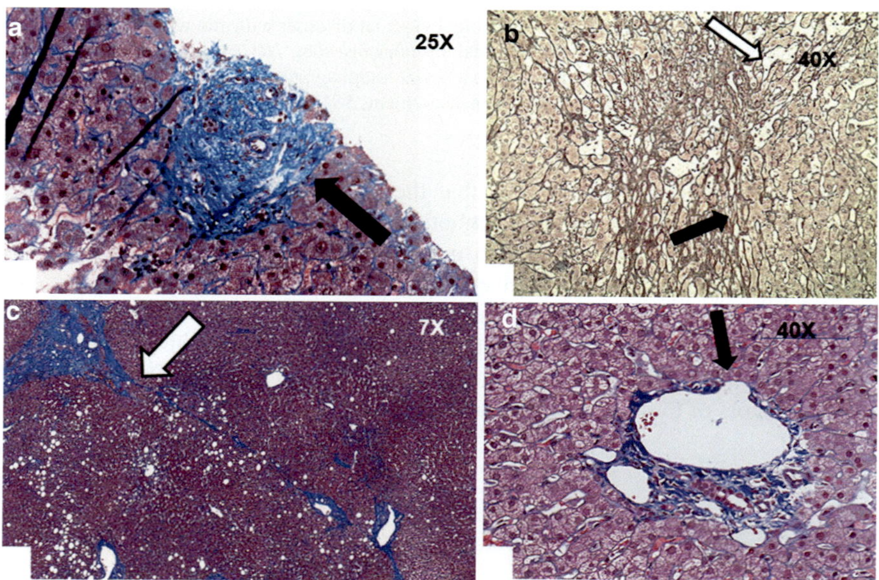

**Fig. 9.3** Histological findings of porto-sinusoidal vascular disorder. (**a**) Obliterative venopathy, section from a liver biopsy with CAB staining. Small portal tracts are sclerotic, and devoid of normal veins (indicated with arrow). (**b**) Nodular regenerative hyperplasia, section from a liver biopsy with argentic reticulin stain. Small nodules of hyperplasic hepatocytes (black arrow) in a non-fibrous parenchyma predominantly around portal tracts and sinusoidal dilatation (white arrow); (**c**) Incomplete septal fibrosis, section from a liver biopsy with CAB staining, Portal tracts are enlarged and prolonged by incomplete thin (white arrow) and blind-ended septa in a non-cirrhotic parenchyma; (**d**) thin-walled vessels prolapsing from the portal tract into the paraportal area, section from a liver biopsy with CAB staining

plates and a condensed reticulin network, but without significant fibrosis. Portal tract remnants, small portal tracts wherein the lumen of the bile duct or artery is smaller than adjacent hepatocytes, with inconspicuous or sometimes absent portal vein branches can be found. Reticulin staining is required for diagnosis, although the diagnosis is generally demanding and requires expert and experienced histopathologists [45].

Diffuse and poorly demarcated nodules and slender fibrous septa which span into the parenchyma without connection with other portal tracts or venules illustrates incomplete septal fibrosis (Fig. 9.3c). Isolated collagen bundles within the parenchyma are associated with disturbed vascular relationships and can be linked with incomplete septal fibrosis. In fact, these lesions were described in a period when cirrhosis was thought to have an irreversible progressive course, without the prospect of regression. Recent advances in chronic liver disease have clearly shown that hepatic architecture is in constant remodeling as a response to tissue damage and repair. Actually, incomplete septal fibrosis may derive from cirrhosis that had regressed [17]. Vascular lesions induced by cirrhosis may still be evident for many years after fibrosis regression and may explain the persistence of portal hypertension. It is still unclear how such vascular changes and subsequent portal hypertension evolve over time.

In addition, these specific findings, are frequently associated with other changes including fine perforated septa, isolated thick collagen fibers, thin periportal fibrous spikes, portal tract remnants aberrant thin-walled vessels prolapsing from the portal tract into the para portal area(Fig. 9.3d), regions of sinusoidal dilation orpeliosis, and prominent arteries or artery multiplication [46, 47]. The common link between these lesions is their location within the porto-sinusoidal area.


## Auxiliary Diagnostic Methods

### *Imaging*

Patients with PSVD and portal hypertension present signs indicative of the latter including splenomegaly and porto-systemic collaterals. In patients without portal hypertension, particular imaging features may be present although not specific for portal hypertension. Such features include an increased hepatic artery diameter, although also common in patients with cirrhosis. Hypertrophy of segments IV and I and atrophy of remaining segments, aids in distinguishing PSVD or portal vein thrombosis from cirrhosis where by contrast, there is atrophy of segment IV and hypertrophy of segment I. The increase in size of segments IV and I and atrophy of surrounding segments is related to an impaired flow in the portal vein leading to hypertrophy of the central part of the liver and atrophy of the periphery [48, 49]. Furthermore, in comparison with patients with cirrhosis, patients with PSVD have more frequently a reduced caliber, an occlusive thrombosis or a lack of visibility of intrahepatic portal vein branches and focal nodular hyperplasia-like nodules [49].

The presence of thrombosis of portal veins is currently not an exclusion criterion for a diagnosis of non-cirrhotic portal hypertension because patients with PSVD may develop secondary portal vein thrombosis.

## *Elastography*

In the last decade, the widespread implementation of liver and spleen elastography has aided in distinguishing among patients with clinically evident portal hypertension those with or without liver cirrhosis. Actually, patients with PSVD usually have liver stiffness values much lower than the cutoffs for clinically significant portal hypertension in cirrhosis, and spleen to liver stiffness ratio higher than in other liver diseases [50, 51].

Current data of elastography in PSVD are relatively limited. Reported liver stiffness values range between 8.4 and 11.3 kPa; which is higher than in patients with portal vein thrombosis without PVSD (6.4–8.4 kPa) and significantly lower than in patients with cirrhosis [5, 51]. Although elastography promises to be most useful in evaluating for PVSD patients with portal hypertension, the data being still limited, liver biopsy remains the basis for diagnosis.

## *Hepatic Venous Pressure Gradient Measurement and Hepatic Venography*

Hepatic venous pressure gradient measurement allows for documenting PSVD inpatients with signs of obvious portal hypertension. The majority of patients have a portal pressure gradient below 10 mm Hg, the cutoff for so-called clinically significant portal hypertension, despite signs of obvious portal hypertension. Additionally, in patients with PSVD, the hepatic venography performed during the portal pressure assessment commonly shows large hepatic veno-venous communications, a finding thus far incompletely understood [51].

## Special Considerations

### *Focal Liver Lesions*

Hepatocellular nodules can develop in PSVD patients, as they do in other vascular liver diseases, although less commonly than in patients with Budd-Chiari syndrome [52]. These nodules are generally benign, being for the most part focal nodular hyperplasia-like, and rarely adenomas. These nodules are considered to develop because of a distorted local blood perfusion combining enhanced arterialization and decreased portal venous perfusion, in addition to other probable hormonal and gender-related factors. Development or progression to hepatocellular carcinoma appears to be very rare [53, 54].

## *Pregnancy*

Pregnancy, *per se*, is not a recognized risk factor for PSVD. From a practical aspect, pregnancy desire should be addressed routinely in patients with PSVD, as about 15% of patients with PSVD are women of childbearing age, rendering reproductive issues particularly relevant [55–57]. It is paramount that liver disease remains stable before considering pregnancy.

Three small retrospective series including 40 women reported variceal bleeding in 15% of cases. Terlipressin is contraindicated during pregnancy. Low molecular weight heparin use was associated with post-partum genital bleeding; no deaths were observed. Nevertheless, in patients with PSVD with previous portal vein thrombosis, low molecular weight heparin can be safely used and a 24-hour interruption is recommended before delivery, ideally vaginal whenever possible [55, 57–60]. Ten to 25% of the pregnancies in these series resulted in fetal loss.

Primary and secondary prophylaxis for variceal bleeding should by routinely started, following the rules recommended for patients with liver cirrhosis. There is currently no evidence supporting primary prophylaxis of thrombosis with anticoagulation in pregnant women with PSVD.

## *Non-hepatic Abdominal Surgery*

A retrospective VALDIG study, including 47 patients with PSVD and portal hypertension, reported portal hypertension-related complications in 30% of patients within 3 months post-op; these were more common in those with extrahepatic comorbidities. In patients with preserved renal function, 6-month survival was very good [61]. No information is available regarding patients with PSVD without portal hypertension.

## Management

### *Medical*

#### Anticoagulation

The rationale for the use of anticoagulation in the setting of PSVD, even in the absence of portal vein thrombosis, includes several arguments. One of most common denominators of PSVD is thickening, narrowing or obliteration of intrahepatic portal venules. Such a narrowing is thought to produce an ischemic atrophy of the hepatocytes, as seen in nodular regenerative hyperplasia. Among explanted livers, portal venules were found to be obliterated in 100%, and large portal veins in 67% [18]. Portal vein thrombosisoccursin 13–45% of PSVD patients during follow-up [4, 18, 43, 62]. Whether the increased risk of splanchnic thrombosis is related with local venule endothelial factors or mechanical causes related to blood stasis and portal hypertension, or a combination of all these factors, remains unknown [63]. Last, patients with PSVD commonly have underlying disorders associated with an increased risk of thrombosis (0–18%) [4, 14, 18, 19].

Moreover, inpatients with non-cirrhotic portal hypertension secondary to portal vein thrombosis, recanalization occurs in less than half of those treated with early anticoagulation [19, 64]. Such poor outcomes might be avoided with prophylactic anticoagulation in PSVD patients at risk for portal vein thrombosis.

Notwithstanding the justification for anticoagulation, randomized trials are required to assess the benefit risk ratio of prophylactic anticoagulation in patients of PSVD. Anticoagulation therapy is currently recommended for patients with high-risk prothrombotic disorders or those developing portal vein thromboses [65].

## Treatment of Portal Hypertension

The incidence and risk factors for progression of portal hypertension in PSVD patientsarestill unclear so that no preventive therapy can currently be recommended [18, 66].

In patients with PSVD and portal hypertension, current practice guidelines propose treating varices following the recommendations elaborated for patients with cirrhosis [65]. The effectiveness of this approach has been demonstrated [19, 67]. The cornerstone of therapy is beta-blockers, either carvedilol and propranolol, and endoscopic variceal ligation.

In situations where drug exposure or associated conditions exist, drug cessation or disease directed therapy could theoretically improve the outcomes of PSVD, although uncertain. The optimal strategy and interval to screen for portal hypertension signs such as varices is currently undefined.

## *Transjugular Intrahepatic Porto-Systemic Shunt*

Transjugular intrahepatic portosystemic shunts can be an effective treatment option in patients with PSVD and complications of portal hypertension such as variceal bleeding and refractory ascites. A multicenter study of 41 patients with PSVD and portal hypertension described a comparable outcome to that of patients with cirrhosis and similar liver function. Normal kidney function and the absence of severe extrahepatic comorbidities were prognostic factors for a better outcome [68].

## *Surgery*

Based on limited data, the overall outcome of PVSD patients with portal hypertension treated with abdominal surgical appears to be favorable [61, 69]. Portosystemic shunting or splenectomy have been mainly reported in adults or children from India and Turkey [32, 61, 69–72]. In most patients, porto-systemic surgical shunts and splenectomies were performed in patients with either complications related to portal hypertension or symptoms caused be splenomegaly [32]. Although shunt surgery was effective in reducing portal hypertension and no operative mortality was described, delayed morbidity was frequent, occurring in 20–50% of patients [69–72]. Variceal rebleeding (10%), ascites and hepatic encephalopathy (up to 18% of cases) were the most frequently reported complications [70, 71]. This data highlights an important rate of complications in PSVD with portal hypertension treated surgically with shunt. In cases of severe hypersplenism, partial splenic embolization and splenectomy have been performed, but given the risks related to it, it must be only considered in rare, individual cases with symptomatic hypersplenism [68, 73].

Scarce reported data has demonstrated that survival of PSVD patients after liver transplantation is favorable [57]. Post-transplant (recurrent) PSVD has been reported, although its incidence is unclear [2].

## *Current and Future Perspectives in Translational and Clinical Research*

### Translational

There are currently some animal models that reproduce human PSVD. Among these are models replicating nodular regenerative hyperplasia and venous occlusion. Vascular embolization animal models using microspheres of dextran and serum bovine albumin, surgical models after splenic extraction and models with direct injection of bacteria into the portal vein did not accurately create PSVD [74–76]. Genetic models, namely *NOTCH1* knockout mice replicated all of the histological findings of nodular regenerative hyperplasia and portal hypertension [77, 78]. JAK1 (IL-6–JAK–STAT pathway) mutated mice induces a phenotype similar to autoimmune disease with histological signs of nodular regenerative hyperplasia [79]. Rats fed selenium-rich diet also generated nodular regenerative hyperplasia with portal hypertension [80]. Although promising, until now, no specific therapies have been tested in animal models.

### Clinical

The establishment of a new terminology to combine vascular liver diseases affecting the porto-sinusoidal area and its wide dissemination will allow for a better understanding of the epidemiology of the disease. Furthermore, cohort studies with patients with PSVD will advance knowledge of this condition and possibly help answer fundamental questions. It remains to be clarified why some patients develop portal hypertension while others remain asymptomatic. It is also unknown which is the best method to diagnose clinically significant portal hypertension considering that portal pressure gradient is not accurate in these patients, and at what intervals should they be screened. Additionally, it is obscure how PSVD should be defined histologically in patients with PSVD and concomitant liver diseases of other etiologies and what its relative impact is.

Lastly, the inclusion of patients under the terminology of PSVD will also facilitate the development of multicenter clinical trials testing the effect of directed therapy such as anticoagulation.

## Conclusions

The establishment of the new denomination aimed to cover a heterogeneous group of conditions and develop clear diagnostic criteria. Liver biopsy remains fundamental for diagnosis. The implementation of the term *porto-sinusoidal vascular disorder* is key to facilitate multicenter, collaborative cohort studies to address the critical questions regarding this entity.

## References


1. European Association for the Study of the Liver. EASL clinical practice guidelines: vascular diseases of the liver. J Hepatol. 2016;64(1):179–202.
2. Schouten JN, Garcia-Pagan JC, Valla DC, Janssen HL. Idiopathic noncirrhotic portal hypertension. Hepatology. 2011;54(3):1071–81.
3. Chang PE, Miquel R, Blanco JL, Laguno M, Bruguera M, Abraldes JG, et al. Idiopathic portal hypertension in patients with HIV infection treated with highly active antiretroviral therapy. Am J Gastroenterol. 2009;104(7):1707–14.
4. Schouten JN, Van der Ende ME, Koeter T, Rossing HH, Komuta M, Verheij J, et al. Risk factors and outcome of HIV-associated idiopathic noncirrhotic portal hypertension. Aliment Pharmacol Ther. 2012;36(9):875–85.
5. Vuppalanchi R, Mathur K, Pyko M, Samala N, Chalasani N. Liver stiffness measurements in patients with noncirrhotic portal hypertension-the devil is in the details. Hepatology. 2018;68(6):2438–40.
6. De Gottardi A, Rautou PE, Schouten J, Rubbia-Brandt L, Leebeek F, Trebicka J, et al. Porto-sinusoidal vascular disease: proposal and description of a novel entity. Lancet Gastroenterol Hepatol. 2019;4(5):399–411.
7. Dhiman RK, Chawla Y, Vasishta RK, Kakkar N, Dilawari JB, Trehan MS, et al. Non-cirrhotic portal fibrosis (idiopathic portal hypertension): experience with 151 patients and a review of the literature. J Gastroenterol Hepatol. 2002;17(1):6–16.
8. Mukta V, Panicker LC, Sivamani K, Goel A, Basu D, Dhanapathi H. Non-cirrhotic portal fibrosis at a tertiary care Centre in South India. Trop Dr. 2017;47(1):26–30.

9. Imai FKK, Komaba M. Interim report on IPH survey. In: Futagawa S, editor. Report of the research committee on aberrant portal hemodynamics 1992. Tokyo: Ministry of Health and Welfare; 1993. p. 107–10.

10. Murai Y, Ohfuji S, Fukushima W, Tamakoshi A, Yamaguchi S, Hashizume M, et al. Prognostic factors in patients with idiopathic portal hypertension: two Japanese nationwide epidemiological surveys in 1999 and 2005. Hepatol Res. 2012;42(12):1211–20.

11. Saito K, Nakanuma Y, Takegoshi K, Ohta G, Obata Y, Okuda K, et al. Non-specific immunological abnormalities and association of autoimmune diseases in idiopathic portal hypertension. A study by questionnaire. Hepato-Gastroenterology. 1993;40(2):163–6.

12. Barge S, Grando V, Nault JC, Broudin C, Beaugrand M, Ganne-Carrie N, et al. Prevalence and clinical significance of nodular regenerative hyperplasia in liver biopsies. Liver Int: Official Journal of the International Association for the Study of the Liver. 2016;36(7):1059–66.

13. Eapen CE, Nightingale P, Hubscher SG, Lane PJ, Plant T, Velissaris D, et al. Non-cirrhotic intrahepatic portal hypertension: associated gut diseases and prognostic factors. Dig Dis Sci. 2011;56(1):227–35.

14. Hillaire S, Bonte E, Denninger MH, Casadevall N, Cadranel JF, Lebrec D, et al. Idiopathic non-cirrhotic intrahepatic portal hypertension in the west: a re-evaluation in 28 patients. Gut. 2002;51(2):275–80.

15. Mikkelsen WP, Edmondson HA, Peters RL, Redeker AG, Reynolds TB. Extra- and intrahepatic portal hypertension without cirrhosis (hepatoportal sclerosis). Ann Surg. 1965;162(4):602–20.

16. Villeneuve JP, Huet PM, Joly JG, Marleau D, Cote J, Legare A, et al. Idiopathic portal hypertension. Am J Med. 1976;61(4):459–64.

17. Wanless IR, Nakashima E, Sherman M. Regression of human cirrhosis. Morphologic features and the genesis of incomplete septal cirrhosis. Arch Pathol Lab Med. 2000;124(11):1599–607.

18. Cazals-Hatem D, Hillaire S, Rudler M, Plessier A, Paradis V, Condat B, et al. Obliterative portal venopathy: portal hypertension is not always present at diagnosis. J Hepatol. 2011;54(3):455–61.

19. Siramolpiwat S, Seijo S, Miquel R, Berzigotti A, Garcia-Criado A, Darnell A, et al. Idiopathic portal hypertension: natural history and long-term outcome. Hepatology. 2014;59(6):2276–85.

20. Cotte L, Benet T, Billioud C, Miailhes P, Scoazec JY, Ferry T, et al. The role of nucleoside and nucleotide analogues in nodular regenerative hyperplasia in HIV-infected patients: a case control study. J Hepatol. 2011;54(3):489–96.

21. Mallet VO, Varthaman A, Lasne D, Viard JP, Gouya H, Borgel D, et al. Acquired protein S deficiency leads to obliterative portal venopathy and to compensatory nodular regenerative hyperplasia in HIV-infected patients. AIDS. 2009;23(12):1511–8.

22. Ghabril M, Vuppalanchi R. Drug-induced nodular regenerative hyperplasia. Semin Liver Dis. 2014;34(2):240–5.

23. Zuo C, Chumbalkar V, Ells PF, Bonville DJ, Lee H. Prevalence of histological features of idiopathic noncirrhotic portal hypertension in general population: a retrospective study of incidental liver biopsies. Hepatol Int. 2017;11(5):452–60.

24. Pulvirenti F, Pentassuglio I, Milito C, Valente M, De Santis A, Conti V, et al. Idiopathic non cirrhotic portal hypertension and spleno-portal axis abnormalities in patients with severe primary antibody deficiencies. J Immunol Res. 2014;2014:672458.

25. Malamut G, Ziol M, Suarez F, Beaugrand M, Viallard JF, Lascaux AS, et al. Nodular regenerative hyperplasia: the main liver disease in patients with primary hypogammaglobulinemia and hepatic abnormalities. J Hepatol. 2008;48(1):74–82.

26. Stock H, Kadry Z, Smith JP. Surgical management of portal hypertension in Felty's syndrome: a case report and literature review. J Hepatol. 2009;50(4):831–5.

27. Seinen ML, van Asseldonk DP, de Boer NK, Bouma G, van Nieuwkerk CM, Mulder CJ, et al. Nodular regenerative hyperplasia of the liver in patients with IBD treated with allopurinol-Thiopurine combination therapy. Inflamm Bowel Dis. 2017;23(3):448–52.

28. Kotani K, Kawabe J, Morikawa H, Akahoshi T, Hashizume M, Shiomi S. Comprehensive screening of gene function and networks by DNA microarray analysis in Japanese patients with idiopathic portal hypertension. Mediat Inflamm. 2015;2015:349215.
29. Yamaguchi N, Tokushige K, Haruta I, Yamauchi K, Hayashi N. Analysis of adhesion molecules in patients with idiopathic portal hypertension. J Gastroenterol Hepatol. 1999;14(4):364–9.
30. Holmes E, Wijeyesekera A, Taylor-Robinson SD, Nicholson JK. The promise of metabolic phenotyping in gastroenterology and hepatology. Nat Rev Gastroenterol Hepatol. 2015;12(8):458–71.
31. Nayak NC. Idiopathic portal hypertension (noncirrhotic portal fibrosis), thrombosis in portal venous system and protein C deficiency. Hepatology. 1989;10(5):902.
32. Khanna R, Sarin SK. Non-cirrhotic portal hypertension – diagnosis and management. J Hepatol. 2014;60(2):421–41.
33. Omanwar S, Rizvi MR, Kathayat R, Sharma BK, Pandey GK, Alam MA, et al. A rabbit model of non-cirrhotic portal hypertension by repeated injections of E.coli through indwelling cannulation of the gastrosplenic vein. Hepatobiliary Pancreat Dis Int: HBPD INT. 2004;3(3):417–22.
34. Sarin SK, Kumar A. Noncirrhotic portal hypertension. Clin Liver Dis. 2006;10(3):627–51.
35. Besmond C, Valla D, Hubert L, Poirier K, Grosse B, Guettier C, et al. Mutations in the novel gene FOPV are associated with familial autosomal dominant and non-familial obliterative portal venopathy. Liver Int: Official Journal of the International Association for the Study of the Liver. 2018;38(2):358–64.
36. Girard M, Amiel J, Fabre M, Pariente D, Lyonnet S, Jacquemin E. Adams-Oliver syndrome and hepatoportal sclerosis: occasional association or common mechanism? Am J Med Genet A. 2005;135(2):186–9.
37. Roulot D, Degott C, Chazouilleres O, Oberti F, Cales P, Carbonell N, et al. Vascular involvement of the liver in Turner's syndrome. Hepatology. 2004;39(1):239–47.
38. Sarin SK, Mehra NK, Agarwal A, Malhotra V, Anand BS, Taneja V. Familial aggregation in noncirrhotic portal fibrosis: a report of four families. Am J Gastroenterol. 1987;82(11):1130–3.
39. Calado RT, Regal JA, Kleiner DE, Schrump DS, Peterson NR, Pons V, et al. A spectrum of severe familial liver disorders associate with telomerase mutations. PLoS One. 2009;4(11):e7926.
40. Vispo E, Cevik M, Rockstroh JK, Barreiro P, Nelson M, Scourfield A, et al. Genetic determinants of idiopathic noncirrhotic portal hypertension in HIV-infected patients. Clin Infect Dis. 2013;56(8):1117–22.
41. Koot BG, Alders M, Verheij J, Beuers U, Cobben JM. A de novo mutation in KCNN3 associated with autosomal dominant idiopathic non-cirrhotic portal hypertension. J Hepatol. 2016;64(4):974–7.
42. Vilarinho S, Sari S, Yilmaz G, Stiegler AL, Boggon TJ, Jain D, et al. Recurrent recessive mutation in deoxyguanosine kinase causes idiopathic noncirrhotic portal hypertension. Hepatology. 2016;63(6):1977–86.
43. Hollande C, Mallet V, Darbeda S, Vallet-Pichard A, Fontaine H, Verkarre V, et al. Impact of Obliterative portal Venopathy associated with human immunodeficiency virus. Medicine. 2016;95(11):e3081.
44. Guido M, Sarcognato S, Sonzogni A, Luca MG, Senzolo M, Fagiuoli S, et al. Obliterative portal venopathy without portal hypertension: an underestimated condition. Liver Int: Official Journal of the International Association for the Study of the Liver. 2016;36(3):454–60.
45. Jharap B, van Asseldonk DP, de Boer NK, Bedossa P, Diebold J, Jonker AM, et al. Diagnosing nodular regenerative hyperplasia of the liver is thwarted by low Interobserver agreement. PLoS One. 2015;10(6):e0120299.
46. Guido M, Sarcognato S, Sacchi D, Colloredo G. Pathology of idiopathic non-cirrhotic portal hypertension. Virchows Archiv: An International Journal of Pathology. 2018;473(1):23–31.
47. Nakanuma Y, Hoso M, Sasaki M, Terada T, Katayanagi K, Nonomura A, et al. Histopathology of the liver in non-cirrhotic portal hypertension of unknown aetiology. Histopathology. 1996;28(3):195–204.

48. Arora A, Sarin SK. Multimodality imaging of primary extrahepatic portal vein obstruction (EHPVO): what every radiologist should know. Br J Radiol. 2015;88(1052):20150008.
49. Glatard AS, Hillaire S, d'Assignies G, Cazals-Hatem D, Plessier A, Valla DC, et al. Obliterative portal venopathy: findings at CT imaging. Radiology. 2012;263(3):741–50.
50. Berzigotti A. Non-invasive evaluation of portal hypertension using ultrasound elastography. J Hepatol. 2017;67(2):399–411.
51. Seijo S, Reverter E, Miquel R, Berzigotti A, Abraldes JG, Bosch J, et al. Role of hepatic vein catheterisation and transient elastography in the diagnosis of idiopathic portal hypertension. Dig Liver Dis: Official Journal of the Italian Society of Gastroenterology and the Italian Association for the Study of the Liver. 2012;44(10):855–60.
52. Moucari R, Rautou PE, Cazals-Hatem D, Geara A, Bureau C, Consigny Y, et al. Hepatocellular carcinoma in Budd-Chiari syndrome: characteristics and risk factors. Gut. 2008;57(6):828–35.
53. Montenovo MI, Jalikis FG, Yeh M, Reyes JD. Progression of hepatic adenoma to carcinoma in the setting of Hepatoportal sclerosis in HIV patient: case report and review of the literature. Case Rep Hepatol. 2016;2016:1732069.
54. Sempoux C, Paradis V, Komuta M, Wee A, Calderaro J, Balabaud C, et al. Hepatocellular nodules expressing markers of hepatocellular adenomas in Budd-Chiari syndrome and other rare hepatic vascular disorders. J Hepatol. 2015;63(5):1173–80.
55. Andrade F, Shukla A, Bureau C, Senzolo M, D'Alteroche L, Heurgue A, et al. Pregnancy in idiopathic non-cirrhotic portal hypertension: a multicentric study on maternal and fetal management and outcome. J Hepatol. 2018;69(6):1242–9.
56. Bissonnette J, Durand F, de Raucourt E, Ceccaldi PF, Plessier A, Valla D, et al. Pregnancy and vascular liver disease. J Clin Exp Hepatol. 2015;5(1):41–50.
57. Krasinskas AM, Eghtesad B, Kamath PS, Demetris AJ, Abraham SC. Liver transplantation for severe intrahepatic noncirrhotic portal hypertension. Liver Transpl: Official Publication of the American Association for the Study of Liver Diseases and the International Liver Transplantation Society. 2005;11(6):627–34. discussion 10-1
58. Aggarwal N, Sawhney H, Vasishta K, Dhiman RK, Chawla Y. Non-cirrhotic portal hypertension in pregnancy. Int J Gynaecol Obstet. 2001;72(1):1–7.
59. Henriksson P, Westerlund E, Wallen H, Brandt L, Hovatta O, Ekbom A. Incidence of pulmonary and venous thromboembolism in pregnancies after in vitro fertilisation: cross sectional study. BMJ. 2013;346:e8632.
60. Sumana G, Dadhwal V, Deka D, Mittal S. Non-cirrhotic portal hypertension and pregnancy outcome. J Obstet Gynaecol Res. 2008;34(5):801–4.
61. Elkrief L, Ferrusquia-Acosta J, Payance A, Moga L, Tellez L, Praktiknjo M, et al. Abdominal surgery in patients with idiopathic noncirrhotic portal hypertension: a multicenter retrospective study. Hepatology. 2019;70(3):911–24.
62. Matsutani S, Maruyama H, Akiike T, Kobayashi S, Yoshizumi H, Okugawa H, et al. Study of portal vein thrombosis in patients with idiopathic portal hypertension in Japan. Liver Int: Official Journal of the International Association for the Study of the Liver. 2005;25(5):978–83.
63. Rajekar H, Vasishta RK, Chawla YK, Dhiman RK. Noncirrhotic portal hypertension. J Clin Exp Hepatol. 2011;1(2):94–108.
64. Plessier A, Darwish-Murad S, Hernandez-Guerra M, Consigny Y, Fabris F, Trebicka J, et al. Acute portal vein thrombosis unrelated to cirrhosis: a prospective multicenter follow-up study. Hepatology. 2010;51(1):210–8.
65. de Franchis R, Baveno VIF. Expanding consensus in portal hypertension: report of the Baveno VI consensus workshop: stratifying risk and individualizing care for portal hypertension. J Hepatol. 2015;63(3):743–52.
66. Elkrief L, Rautou PE. Idiopathic non-cirrhotic portal hypertension: the tip of the obliterative portal venopathies iceberg? Liver I: Official Journal of the International Association for the Study of the Liver. 2016;36(3):325–7.

67. Sarin SK, Gupta N, Jha SK, Agrawal A, Mishra SR, Sharma BC, et al. Equal efficacy of endoscopic variceal ligation and propranolol in preventing variceal bleeding in patients with noncirrhotic portal hypertension. Gastroenterology. 2010;139(4):1238–45.
68. Bissonnette J, Garcia-Pagan JC, Albillos A, Turon F, Ferreira C, Tellez L, et al. Role of the transjugular intrahepatic portosystemic shunt in the management of severe complications of portal hypertension in idiopathic noncirrhotic portal hypertension. Hepatology. 2016;64(1):224–31.
69. Sharma BC, Singh RP, Chawla YK, Narasimhan KL, Rao KL, Mitra SK, et al. Effect of shunt surgery on spleen size, portal pressure and oesophageal varices in patients with non-cirrhotic portal hypertension. J Gastroenterol Hepatol. 1997;12(8):582–4.
70. Karagul S, Yagci MA, Tardu A, Ertugrul I, Kirmizi S, Sumer F, et al. Portosystemic shunt surgery in patients with idiopathic noncirrhotic portal hypertension. Ann Transplant. 2016;21:317–20.
71. Mitra SK, Rao KL, Narasimhan KL, Dilawari JB, Batra YK, Chawla Y, et al. Side-to-side lienorenal shunt without splenectomy in noncirrhotic portal hypertension in children. J Pediatric Surg. 1993;28(3):398–401. discussion-2
72. Pal S, Radhakrishna P, Sahni P, Pande GK, Nundy S, Chattopadhyay TK. Prophylactic surgery in non-cirrhotic portal fibrosis:is it worthwhile? Indian J Gastroenterol: Official Journal of the Indian Society of Gastroenterology. 2005;24(6):239–42.
73. Hirota S, Ichikawa S, Matsumoto S, Motohara T, Fukuda T, Yoshikawa T. Interventional radiologic treatment for idiopathic portal hypertension. Cardiovasc Intervent Radiol. 1999;22(4):311–4.
74. Albini B, Ito S, Brentjens J, Andres G. Splenomegaly and immune complex splenitis in rabbits with experimentally induced chronic serum sickness: immunopathological findings. J Reticuloendothel Soc. 1983;34(6):485–500.
75. Kathayat R, Pandey GK, Malhotra V, Omanwar S, Sharma BK, Sarin SK. Rabbit model of non-cirrhotic portal fibrosis with repeated immunosensitization by rabbit splenic extract. J Gastroenterol Hepatol. 2002;17(12):1312–6.
76. Komeichi H, Katsuta Y, Aramaki T, Okumura H. A new experimental animal model of portal hypertension. Intrahepatic portal obstruction by injecting DEAE-cross-linked dextran microspheres into the portal vein in the rabbit. Nihon Ika Daigaku zasshi. 1991;58(3):273–84.
77. Croquelois A, Blindenbacher A, Terracciano L, Wang X, Langer I, Radtke F, et al. Inducible inactivation of Notch1 causes nodular regenerative hyperplasia in mice. Hepatology. 2005;41(3):487–96.
78. Dubuisson L, Boussarie L, Bedin CA, Balabaud C, Bioulac-Sage P. Transformation of sinusoids into capillaries in a rat model of selenium-induced nodular regenerative hyperplasia: an immunolight and immunoelectron microscopic study. Hepatology. 1995;21(3):805–14.
79. McEntee MF, Wright KN, Wanless I, DeVovo R, Schneider JF, Shull R. Noncirrhotic portal hypertension and nodular regenerative hyperplasia of the liver in dogs with mucopolysaccharidosis type I. Hepatology. 1998;28(2):385–90.
80. Nielsen H, Binder V, Daugharty H, Svehag SE. Circulating immune complexes in ulcerative colitis. I. Correlation to disease activity. Clin Exp Immunol. 1978;31(1):72–80.

# Chapter 10
# Sinusoidal Obstruction Syndrome/Hepatic Veno-Occlusive Disease

**Vincent T. Ho, Nancy A. Kernan, Enric Carreras, and Paul G. Richardson**

## Introduction

Sinusoidal obstruction syndrome (SOS), also known as hepatic veno-occlusive disease (VOD), is a potentially life-threatening complication that occurs mainly after myeloablative hematopoietic cell transplantation (HCT) but can occur after reduced-intensity HCT [1] and following chemotherapy or immunoconjugate therapy [2–5].


V. T. Ho
Dana-Farber Cancer Institute, Harvard Medical School, Boston, MA, USA
e-mail: Vincent_Ho@dfci.harvard.edu

N. A. Kernan
Pediatric BMT Service, Memorial Sloan Kettering Cancer Center, New York, NY, USA
e-mail: kernann@MSKCC.ORG

E. Carreras
Barcelona Endothelium Team, Josep Carreras Leukaemia Research Institute, Hospital Clinic/University of Barcelona Campus, Barcelona, Spain
e-mail: enric.carreras@fcarreras.es

P. G. Richardson (✉)
Jerome Lipper Multiple Myeloma Center, Dana-Farber Cancer Institute, Harvard Medical School, Boston, MA, USA

Dana-Farber Cancer Institute, Jerome Lipper Multiple Myeloma Center, Boston, MA, USA
e-mail: Paul_Richardson@dfci.harvard.edu



© Springer Nature Switzerland AG 2022

143

D. Valla et al. (eds.), *Vascular Disorders of the Liver*,
https://doi.org/10.1007/978-3-030-82988-9_10

## Disease State

### *Incidence*

The incidence of SOS/VOD varies based on the type of transplant, the intensity of the conditioning regimen, the presence of risk factors, and the clinical diagnostic criteria used (Seattle or Baltimore). Recent estimates indicate an incidence of 10–15% after allogeneic HCT with a myeloablative conditioning regimen and < 5% after autologous HCT or allogeneic HCT with reduced-intensity conditioning [1, 6, 7]. One pooled analysis reported a mean incidence of 13.7% [8]. In a single-center study of 845 allogeneic HCTs performed between January 1985 and July 2008, the cumulativeincidence of SOS/VOD was reported to be 13.8% using the Seattle criteria and 8.8% using the Baltimore criteria [1]. This study also showed that the rate of SOS/VOD decreased significantly during the periods between 1985 to 1998 versus 1997 to 2008 ($P = 0.01$), likely due in part to the introduction of reduced-intensity conditioning.

Assuming a 5% to 10% incidence of SOS/VOD and more than 68,000 first-time HCTs (47% allogeneic; 53% autologous) performed worldwide in 2012, one would expect about 3500 to 7000 new cases of VOD per year [9]. Mortality may be greater than 80% for patients with severe SOS/VOD, which has been traditionally defined by multi-organ dysfunction (MOD; including its more severe form, multi-organ failure [MOF]) [8]. Similar findings were reported by Carreras et al. [2011] with myeloablative conditioning regimens, previous liver disease, poor performance status, and mismatcheddonors as the variables having the greatest impact on SOS/VOD development [1]. In children, the incidence is between 22% and 30%, 2-to three-fold higher than in adults [10–13].

Outside the transplant setting, SOS/VOD has been reported after chemotherapy, such as cyclophosphamide, cytarabine, vincristine, methotrexate, thioguanine, and especially with the calicheamicin-containing immunoconjugatesinotuzumaband gemtuzumabozogamicin [5, 14]. In the phase 3 trial of inotuzumabvs standard chemotherapy in patients with relapsed/refractory acute lymphoblastic leukemia, the incidence of SOS/VOD was 13% in the inotuzumabmonotherapy group vs < 1% in the standard chemotherapy group [5]. Studies that included patients who developed SOS/VOD following nontransplant chemotherapy have reported anSOS/VOD incidence of 7–12% [15, 16].

### *Pathophysiology*

The functional changes associated with SOS/VOD during HCT are believed to begin with toxic injury to the sinusoidal endothelial cells and hepatocytes in zone 3 of the liver acinus. This damage can be caused by the chemotherapy or radiotherapy used in the conditioning regimen, cytokines and endogenous microbial products released from damaged tissue, drugs used during HCT, and potentially alloreactivity associated with the engraftment process itself. *In vivo* studies in rats have determined that intense and sustained physiological activation of sinusoidal endothelial cells impairs the ability of these cells to regulate thrombo-fibrinolytic balance followed by reduced nitric oxide production and increased levels of matrix metalloproteinase [17]. The resulting damage to the sinusoidal endothelium opens gaps in the sinusoidal barrier, permitting the extravasation of red blood cells, leukocytes, and cellular and extracellular debris into the space of Disse beneath the endothelial cells, and the dissection of the endothelial lining. The sloughed sinusoidal lining cells also embolize downstream and obstruct sinusoidal flow (Fig. 10.1) [18].

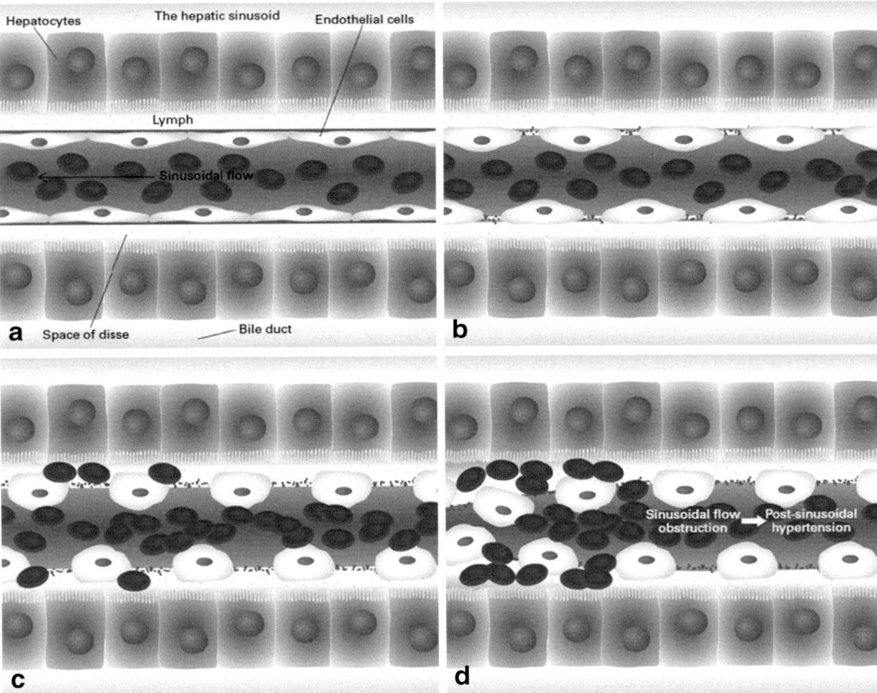


**Fig. 10.1** Pathogenesis of SOS/VOD. Sinusoidal obstruction syndrome pathogenesis. (**a**) Normal hepatic sinusoid; (**b**) sinusoidal endothelial cells demaged during conditioning round favoring the appearance of gaps in the sinusoidal barrier; (**c**) RBCs, leucocytes and celluar debris penetrate into the space of Disse detaching the endothelial linging; (**d**) the sloughed sinusoidal lining cells embolize downstream and obstruct the sinusoidal flow (sinusoidal obstruction syndrome). Adapted from 'The role of the endothelium in the short-tern complications of hematopoietic SCT' by E Carreras and M Diaz-Ricart [2]. Figure "Sinusoidal obstruction syndrome pathogenesis" from Mohty M, Malard F, Abecassis M, et al. Sinusoidal obstruction syndrome/veno-occlusive disease: current situation and perspectives-a position statement from the European Society for Blood and Marrow Transplantation (EBMT). *Bone Marrow Transplant.* 2015;50(6):781–789. This figure is licensed under a Creative Commons Attribution-Non Commercial-No Derivatives 4.0 International License (CC BY-NC-ND 4.0; http://creativecommons.org/licenses/by-nc-nd/4.0/). No changes were made to the original figure

In addition, compressed sinusoidal vessels, thickening of the subintimal zone and narrowing of the lumen, platelet activation, and fibrin-related aggregates further reduce sinusoidal flow and increase the potential for complete sinusoidal occlusion. These hemodynamic events combine to cause progressive post-sinusoidal portal hypertension, worsening liver dysfunction, ascites, and may eventually result in MOD and death [1, 8, 19]. Other mediators of SOS/VOD pathogenesis may include pro-inflammatory, pro-thrombotic, and pro-apoptotic influences on sinusoidal endothelial cells [6].

Following HCT conditioning, endothelial damage increases von Willebrand factor and platelet adhesion, both associated with a prothrombotic state, particularly in the allogeneic setting [20]. Further, unlike in an autologous setting, pro-inflammatory and pro-apoptotic changes on epithelial cells continue to increase in the allogeneic HCT setting, suggesting that alloreactivity could contribute to endothelial damage after conditioning [21, 22].

## Risk Factors

A good understanding of the risk factors for SOS/VOD is critical for prophylaxis or early treatment [23]. Risk factors may be related to the pre-transplant condition, the transplant itself, a pre-existing hepatic condition, the type of disease being transplanted, or individual patient characteristics and health. Risk factors for these categories are listed Table 10.1.

# Diagnosis

## Early Diagnosis

A timely diagnosis of SOS/VOD is of critical importance, given the availability of defibrotide as an approved therapeutic option with favorable tolerability. Several studies support the importance of early identification and treatment before progression of SOS/VOD [16, 26–31].

### Early Markers

Clinical signs of SOS/VOD incorporated into traditional Seattle and Baltimore criteria for SOS/VOD diagnosis include fluid retention and ascites, edema, jaundice (serum bilirubin >2 mg/dl), weight gain (>2% and $\geq$ 5%, respectively), and painful hepatomegaly before day +21 after HCT [32–34]. Potential limitations of these criteria are that they are less applicable in pediatrics or later onset (>day +21) SOS/

**Table 10.1** Traditional risk factors for SOS/VOD

| Pre-transplantation related | Transplantation related |
|---|---|
| • Prior abdominal radiation [23]<br>• Previous stem cell transplantation [23]<br>• Prior treatment with gemtuzumabozogamicin [23] or inotuzumabozogamicin [7]<br>• Impaired pulmonary function [23]<br>• Infection/antibiotic/antiviral use [23] (sepsis, vancomycin during cytoreductive therapy, pre-transplantation acyclovir) [10, 24]<br>• Ferritin levels >1000 ng/mL [23]<br>• Bilirubin >26 μmol/L before BMT [23] | • Allogeneic HCT > autologous HCT [6, 23]<br>• Unrelated/HLA-mismatched donor [6, 7, 23]<br>• High-dose busulfan with a second alkylator conditioning [6, 7, 25]<br>• High-dose total body irradiation conditioning [23]<br>• GVHD prophylaxis including combinations of sirolimus, methotrexate and cyclosporine [23]<br>• Non-T-cell-depleted graft [6, 23]<br>• Second myeloablative HCT [6] |
| *Disease related* | |
| • Activated protein C resistance [6, 7]<br>• Thalassemia [6, 7]<br>• Deficit of AT IIIor t-PA [6]<br>• Hemophagocyticlymphohistiocytosis [6]<br>• Osteopetrosis [6] | |
| *Hepatic related* | *Patient related* |
| • Transaminase >2.5 × ULN [6, 7]<br>• Cirrhosis [6, 7]<br>• Hepaticfibrosis [6, 7]<br>• History of viral hepatitis B or C [6]<br>• Abdominal or hepatic irradiation [7]<br>• Use of hepatotoxic drugs (chemotherapeutic agents, thiopurines, pyrrolizidine alkaloids) [7]<br>• Iron overload [7] | • Older > younger (in adult patients) [6, 7, 25]<br>• Female receiving norethisterone [6, 7]<br>• Karnofsky score < 90% [6, 7, 25]<br>• Gene polymorphism (GSTM1, GSMTT1, heparanase) [6, 7, 25]<br>• Advanced disease (beyond second CR or relapse) [6, 7, 25]<br>• Metabolic syndrome [6, 7] |
| *Specific pediatric related* | |
| • Hemophagocyticlymphohistiocytosis, [a]adrenoleukodystrophy, osteopetrosis [6]<br>• High-dose chemotherapy and autologous HCT in neuroblastoma [6]<br>• Young age (<1–2 years) [6]<br>• Low weight [6]<br>• Juvenile myelomonocytic chronic leukemia [6]<br>• Interval between diagnosis of malignancy and transplantation >12 months [23]<br>• Deteriorated health status within 30 days before transplantation [23] | |

Abbreviations: *AT III* antithrombin III, *BMT* bone marrow transplant, *CR* complete response, *GSTM1* glutathione S-transferase mu 1, *GSTT1* glutathione S-transferase theta 1, *GVHD* graft-versus-host disease, *HCT* hematopoietic cell transplantation, *SOS/VOD* sinusoidal obstruction syndrome/veno-occlusive disease, *t-PA* tissue plasminogen activator, *ULN* upper limit of normal
[a]Can occur in adults

VOD where hyperbilirubinemia is often less prominent and could be a late event. Roeker and colleagues recently assessed early clinical parameters in a cohort of more than 200 cases of SOS/VOD after myeloablative conditioning regimen HCT and found that in the 7 days prior to SOS/VOD diagnosis, patients with SOS/VOD are more likely to be refractory to platelet transfusion, and have higher serum creatinine levels and increased serum trough levels of calcineurin inhibitors compared to patients without SOS/VOD [35]. The development of SOS/VOD usually peaks around day +12 after HCT [36], but later onset can be seen in cases associated with sirolimus use and in adults receiving conditioning regimens that include two or more alkylators. Onset beyond day +30 may occur in 15% to 20% of children [13].

Although definitive benefits remain inconclusive, magnetic resonance imaging and gray-scale and color Doppler ultrasonography have been used for accurate assessment of liver size, the presence of ascites [13], thickening of the gallbladder wall [37] and absence/presence of vascular flow and flow direction [38]. With the new pediatric EBMT guidelines, baseline ultrasound imaging might become mandatory for children [39]. Elastography is a non-invasive imaging modality that maps the elastic properties and stiffness of soft tissue and may be a reasonable strategy to evaluate the presence of portal hypertension based on a liver stiffness value >21 kPa [38, 40, 41]. Serialultrasoundelastographymay also hold the potential for helping clinicians predict early onset of SOS/VOD. Several techniques have been developed using ultrasound, including strain imaging methods that rely on internal or external compression stimuli and shear wave imaging that relies on ultrasound generated shear-wave stimuli [42]. Post-graft ultrasound and Doppler examinations (flow recorded in the paraumbilical vein) have a prognostic significance according to the grade of SOS/VOD [43]. Laboratory findings associated with SOS/VOD include elevated aminotransferases, hyperbilirubinemia, prolonged prothrombin time, and signs of decreased synthetic function (e.g., low albumin and decreased coagulation factors, such as Factor VII) [6, 44].

## Hemodynamic Study of the Liver

The most accurate method of confirming SOS/VOD diagnosis and evaluating disease severity is measurement of hepatic venous gradient pressure (HVPG) through the jugular vein. HVPG is defined as the difference between wedged and free hepatic venous pressure and has an excellent correlation with portal vein pressure [45]. When performed by an expert hemodynamist, this procedure carries a low risk when only venous pressure is measured. However, the risk associated with this procedure increases notably if trans venous biopsies of the liver are obtained [46]. A HVPG of ≥10 mmHg in a patient without previous liver disease is seen almost exclusively in cases of SOS/VOD [45, 46]. HVPG also has prognostic value (patients with a HVPG of >15 mmHg rarely survive) and can help to monitor the effectiveness of treatment [45].

## Biopsy

In adults, trans jugular liver biopsy is an effective technique to establish the diagnosis of SOS/VOD [46, 47]. This approach is recommended over a percutaneous biopsy to reduce the risk of bleeding and problems associated with ascites and coagulopathy [48]. Liver biopsy is particularly useful for patients in whom the diagnosis of SOS/VOD is unclear based on standard clinical and laboratory diagnostic criteria, and/or if there is a need to exclude other diagnoses such as infection, graft-vs-host disease (GVHD), drug-induced liver injury, nonalcoholic steatohepatitis, or a combination of hepatic disorders [23, 49]. Trans jugular liver biopsy is not recommended for use in children [50].

## *Baltimore and Seattle Criteria*

The Baltimore, Seattle, and modified Seattle criteria were developed to diagnose SOS/VOD clinically without the need for a liver biopsy, based on clinical signs and symptoms of SOS/VOD rather than on the histopathology of disease [32, 33]. The 3 criteria differ in the number and magnitude of clinical features required for a positive diagnosis and in the time of assessment after HCT. For example, the Baltimore criteria require elevated bilirubin at diagnosis, while the modified Seattle criteria do not have this as a requirement. The original Seattle criteria lacked specificity with respect to bilirubin and weight gain (Table 10.2).

## *European Society for Blood and Marrow Transplantation (EBMT)*

New diagnostic and severity criteria for SOS/VOD were proposed by the EBMT for adults in 2016 [7] and for children in 2018 [13].

**Table 10.2** SOS/VOD Criteria

| |
|---|
| *Baltimore* [32] |
| Serum bilirubin >34 µmol/L (>2 mg/dL) within 21 days of transplantation AND ≥ 2 of the following:<br> • Painful hepatomegaly<br> • >5% weight gain from baseline<br> • Ascites |
| *Seattle* [24] |
| Development of ≥2 of the following before day 30 after transplantation<br> • Jaundice<br> • Hepatomegaly with right upper quadrant pain<br> • Ascites and/or unexplained weight gain |
| *Modified Seattle* [33] |
| Occurrence of ≥2 of the following within 20 days of transplantation<br> • Serum bilirubin>34 µmol/L (>2 mg/dL)<br> • Hepatomegaly with right upper quadrant pain<br> • >2% weight gain from baseline due to fluid retention |

Abbreviations: *HCT* hematopoietic cell transplantation, *SOS/VOD* sinusoidal obstruction syndrome/veno-occlusive disease

## Adults

In adults, the EBMT has established new diagnostic criteria for SOS/VOD in the first 21 days after HCT and for late-onset SOS/VOD (Table 10.3), in which the presence of hyperbilirubinemia is no longer mandatory.

## Children

The EBMT also set new criteria for diagnosing SOS/VOD in children (Table 10.4), as significant differences exist between adults and children in terms of incidence and presentation. Hyperbilirubinemia in children is frequently either absent, preexisting, or found only in advanced-stage SOS/VOD. Thus, bilirubin >2 mg/dL is not a mandatory diagnostic criterion in children [51]. Instead, the EBMT criteria include a bilirubin level elevated from an individual baseline on 3 consecutive days, after the exclusion of competing causes, as a possible criterion.

There are challenges in the diagnosis of SOS/VOD in children. Trans jugular liver biopsy is difficult to perform and should be used with caution in patients with profound thrombocytopenia [45, 46]. Despite its limitations, such as day-to-day variability in findings and the need to transport the child to the radiology department for assessment, ultrasoundis recommended to support the diagnosis [13, 52]. The Baltimore criteria are not applicable to anicteric SOS/VOD, which is seen in up to 30% of pediatric patients, and the modified Seattle criteria may lead to early or

**Table 10.3** 2016 EBMT adult criteria for SOS/VOD[a]

| Classic SOS/VOD | Late-onset SOS/VOD |
| --- | --- |
| In the first 21 days after HCT | >21 days after HCT |
| Bilirubin ≥2 mg/dL and 2 of the following criteria must be present:<br>• Painful hepatomegaly<br>• Weight gain >5%<br>• Ascites | Classic SOS/VOD beyond day 21 OR<br>Histologically proven SOS/VODOR<br>Two or more of the following criteria must be present:<br>• Bilirubin ≥2 mg/dL (or 34 μmol/L)<br>• Painful hepatomegaly<br>• Weight gain >5%<br>• Ascites<br>AND<br>Hemodynamic or/and ultrasound evidence of SOS/VOD |

Abbreviations: *HCT* hematopoietic cell transplantation, *SOS/VOD* sinusoidal obstruction syndrome/veno-occlusive disease. These symptoms/signs should not be attributable to other causes
Table ("New EBMT criteria for SOS/VOD diagnosis in adults") from Mohty M, Malard F, Abecassis M, et al. Revised diagnosis and severity criteria for sinusoidal obstruction syndrome/veno-occlusive disease in adult patients: a new classification from the European Society for Blood and Marrow Transplantation. *Bone Marrow Transplant.* 2016;51(7):906–912. This table is licensed under a Creative Commons Attribution-NonCommercial-No Derivatives 4.0 International License (CC BY-NC-ND 4.0; http://creativecommons.org/licenses/by-nc-nd/4.0/). No changes were made to the original table
[a]After the exclusion of competing causes

**Table 10.4**  2018 EBMT child criteria for SOS/VOD

| |
|---|
| No limitation for time of onset of SOS/VOD |
| The presence of two or more of the following with the exclusion of other potential differential diagnoses:<br>• Unexplained consumptive and transfusion-refractory thrombocytopenia ($\geq$1 weight-adjusted platelet substitution/day to maintain institutional transfusion guidelines)<br>• Otherwise unexplained weight gain on 3 consecutive days despite the use of diuretics or a weight gain >5% above baseline value<br>• Hepatomegaly (best if confirmed by imaging) above baseline value[a]<br>• Ascites (best if confirmed by imaging) above baseline value[a]<br>• Rising bilirubin from a baseline value on 3 consecutive days or bilirubin $\geq$2 mg/dL within 72 h |

Abbreviations: *SOS/VOD* sinusoidal obstruction syndrome/veno-occlusive disease

Table ("EBMT diagnostic criteria for hepatic SOS/VOD in children") from Corbacioglu S, Carreras E, Ansari M, et al. Diagnosis and severity criteria for sinusoidal obstruction syndrome/veno-occlusive disease in pediatric patients: a new classification from the European society for blood and marrow transplantation. *Bone Marrow Transplant.* 2018;53(2):138–145. Table is licensed under a Creative Commons Attribution 4.0 International License (CC BY 4.0; http://creativecommons.org/licenses/by/4.0/)

[a]Suggested: imaging (ultrasonography, computed tomography, or magnetic resonance imaging) immediately before HCT to determine baseline value for both hepatomegaly and ascites

over-diagnosed SOS/VOD in the presence of fluid overload [13, 51, 53]. In 2017, the HCT Committee of Pediatric Acute Lung Injury and Sepsis Investigators (PALISI) established a set of supportive care guidelines for the management of suspected SOS/VOD in children and adolescents in the presence of increasing weight gain, hepatomegaly, ascites, increased need of platelet transfusions, and/or hyperbilirubinemia [52].

## Assessing Severity

The EBMT prospectively classifies SOS/VOD as mild, moderate, severe, or very severe [7, 13]; however, SOS/VOD is unpredictable and vigilance for signs of progression must be maintained. Using the Common Terminology Criteria for Adverse Events (CTCAE) grading system, the EBMT proposed criteria for grading of SOS/VOD severity in adults based on key signs and symptoms and the kinetics of their onset (Table 10.5). These severity criteria should be analyzed at the same time that the diagnosis of SOS/VOD is established using the clinical criteria mentioned above.

The EBMT [13] criteria for assessing severity in children are also based on the CTCAE grading scale but are tailored to signs and symptoms noted in children. In addition, liver and pulmonary function, coagulation, central nervous system, ascites, and persistent refractory thrombocytopenia also are assessed (Table 10.6). Elevated transaminases are not usually found in the early stages of SOS/VOD but may reflect advanced-stage disease. Elevated glutamate dehydrogenase may also be considered a reliable measure of severity. Presence of two or more of the elevated liver function tests is categorized as very severe SOS/VOD.

**Table 10.5** 2016 EBMT criteria for severity grading of suspected SOS/VOD in adults[a]

|  | Mild[b] | Moderate[b] | Severe | Very Severe-MOD/MOF[c] |
|---|---|---|---|---|
| Time since first clinical symptoms of SOS/VOD[d] | >7 days | 5–7 days | <4 days | Anytime |
| Bilirubin (mg/dL) | ≥2 and < 3 | ≥3 and < 5 | ≥5 and < 8 | ≥8 |
| Bilirubin (µmol/L) | ≥34 and < 51 | ≥51 and < 85 | ≥85 and < 136 | ≥136 |
| Bilirubin kinetics |  |  | Doubling within 48 h |  |
| Transaminases | ≤2 × normal | >2 and ≤ 5 × normal | >5 and ≤ 8 × normal | >8 × normal |
| Weight increase | <5% | ≥5% and < 10% | ≥5% and < 10% | ≥10% |
| Renal function | <1.2 × baseline at transplant | ≥1.2 and < 1.5 × baseline at transplant | ≥1.5 and < 2 × baseline at transplant | ≥2 × baseline at transplant or other signs of MOD/MOF |

Note: Renal failure is defined as creatinemia ≥2 times the baseline at transplant, or creatinine clearance ≤50% level at transplant, or dialysis

Abbreviations: *EBMT* European Society for Blood and Marrow Transplantation, *MOD* multi-organ dysfunction, *MOF* multi-organ failure, *SOS/VOD* sinusoidal obstruction syndrome/veno-occlusive disease

Table ("New EBMT criteria for SOS/VOD diagnosis in adults") from Mohty M, Malard F, Abecassis M, et al. Revised diagnosis and severity criteria for sinusoidal obstruction syndrome/veno-occlusive disease in adult patients: a new classification from the European Society for Blood and Marrow Transplantation. *Bone Marrow Transplant.* 2016;51(7):906–912. This table is licensed under a Creative Commons Attribution-NonCommercial-No Derivatives 4.0 International License (CC BY-NC-ND 4.0; http://creativecommons.org/licenses/by-nc-nd/4.0/). No changes were made to the original table

[a]Patients belong to the category that fulfills 2 or more criteria. If patients fulfill 2 or more criteria in 2 different categories, they must be classified in the most severe category. Patients with weight increase ≥5% and < 10% are considered by default as having severe SOS/VOD; however, if patients do not fulfill other criteria for severe SOS/VOD, weight increase ≥5% and < 10% is therefore considered as a criterion for moderate SOS/VOD

[b]In the case of presence of 2 or more risk factors for SOS/VOD, patients should be in the upper grade

[c]Patients with multi-organ dysfunction must be classified as very severe

[d]Time from the date when the first signs/symptoms of SOS/VOD began to appear (retrospectively determined) and the date when the symptoms fulfilled SOS/VOD diagnostic criteria

# Treatment

## *Non-pharmacologic Prevention*

SOS/VOD risk can be reduced by considering the potential interaction of the patient's reversible risk factors, such as reducing iron overload, treating active viral hepatitis, and allowing abnormal liver tests to normalize before starting conditioning therapy [54]. Transplant-related risk factors, especially in regards to the conditioning agents, dose intensity, and type of GVHD prophylaxis, also may be modified to

**Table 10.6**  2018EBMT criteria for severity grading of suspected SOS/VOD in children[a]

|  | Mild1 | Moderate2 | Severe3 | Very severe MOD/MOF4 |
|---|---|---|---|---|
| LFT[b] (ALT, AST, GLDH) | ≤2 × normal | >2 and ≤ 5 × normal | >5 | >5 |
| Persistent RT[b] | <3 days | 3–7 Days | >7 days | >7 days |
| Bilirubin[b,c] (mg/dL; μmol/L) | <2; <34 | <2; <34 | ≥2; ≥34 | ≥2; ≥34 |
| Ascites[b] | Minimal | Moderate | Necessity for paracentesis (external drainage) | Necessity for paracentesis (external drainage) |
| Bilirubin kinetics |  |  |  | Doubling within 48 h |
| Coagulation | Normal | Normal | Impaired coagulation | Impaired coagulation with need for replacement of coagulation factors |
| Renal function GFR (mL/min) | 89–60 | 59–30 | 29–15 | <15 (renal failure) |
| Pulmonary function (oxygen requirement) | <2 L/min | >2 L/min | Invasive pulmonary ventilation (including CPAP) | Invasive pulmonary ventilation (including CPAP) |
| CNS | Normal | Normal | Normal | New onset cognitive impairment |

Abbreviations: *ALT* alanine transaminase, *AST* aspartate transaminase, *CNS* central nervous system, *CPAP* continuous positive airway pressure, *CTCAE* Common Terminology Criteria for Adverse Events, *GFR* glomerular filtration rate, *GLDH* glutamate dehydrogenase, *LFT* liver function test, *MOD/MOF* multi-organ dysfunction/multi-organ failure, *RT* refractory thrombocytopenia, *SOS/VOD* sinusoidal obstruction syndrome/veno-occlusive disease
Table "EBMT criteria for grading the severity of suspected hepatic SOS/VOD in children" from Corbacioglu S, Carreras E, Ansari M, et al. Diagnosis and severity criteria for sinusoidal obstruction syndrome/veno-occlusive disease in pediatric patients: a new classification from the European society for blood and marrow transplantation. *Bone Marrow Transplant.* 2018;53(2):138–145. Table is licensed under a Creative Commons Attribution 4.0 International License (CC BY 4.0; http://creativecommons.org/licenses/by/4.0/).
[a]If patient fulfills criteria in different categories they must be classified in the most severe category. In addition, the kinetics of the evolution of cumulative symptoms within 48 h predicts severe disease
[b]Presence of ≥2 of these criteria qualifies for an upgrade to level 4 (very severe SOS/VOD)
[c]Excluding pre-existent hyperbilirubinemia due to primary disease

mitigate the risk of SOS/VOD [25]. The use of reduced-intensity conditioning, reduced toxicity myeloablative conditioning regimen by combining intravenous busulfan (BU) and fludarabine instead of double alkylating regimens [55–57], and/or a change in the order of the drugs, e.g., cyclophosphamide (CY)/BU instead of BU/CY [58] may decrease the incidence of SOS/VOD and should be considered in elderly patients and in heavily pretreated adult patients or those with comorbidities.

At-risk patients, such as those undergoing a second myeloablative HCT, those with pre-existing liver disease or prior radiation, or those treated with gemtuzumabozogamicin or inotuzumabozogamicin, should be considered for preventive measures, as well as children with high risk diseases like adrenoleukodystrophy, lymphohistiocytosis, or osteopetrosis. Splitting the dose of gemtuzumabozogamicin is recommended to possibly decrease SOS/VOD risk [25, 54]. Patients receiving inotuzumab should be limited to 2 cycles, if feasible, and use of dual alkylator conditioning regimen should be avoided if possible [59]. Efforts must be made to avoid any hepatotoxic concomitant drug in the peri-transplant period [60].

Efforts also should be made to reduce the risk of the alloreactive phenomena. Donors with the maximum degree of human leukocyte antigen compatibility should be sought, and the use of *in vivo* or *ex vivo* T-cell depletion should be considered in unrelated or mismatched settings [61, 62]. Finally, it is necessary to consider the nature of the GVHD prophylaxis. In particular, sirolimus-based GVHD prophylaxis in conjunction with a calcineurin inhibitor is associated with higher incidence of SOS/VOD after allogeneic HCT [59] and especially when used together with tacrolimus and methotrexate [63].

## Supportive Care

Treatment of SOD/VOD is largely symptomatic and supportive; however, because of the variable nature of SOS/VOD, all patients should be managed and monitored in the inpatient setting, with strict attention to total body fluid balance, daily weights, hepatorenal parameters, monitoring for bleeding and infections, and vigilance for development of MOD, which is the hallmark of severe SOS/VOD.

Careful use of diuretics is designed to minimize extracellular fluid overload without worsening renal function. Given the propensity for sodium avid fluid retention in SOS/VOD, sodium restriction and the avoidance of hepato- and nephrotoxic drugs are key in the management paradigm. Oxygen supplementation to minimize liver ischemia, analgesia, therapeutic paracentesis, thoracentesis, and hemodialysis/hemofiltration maybe required to achieve comfort, alleviate volume overload and temporize complications of acute renal dysfunction [25, 64]. SOS/VOD with MOD often requires transfer to an intensive care unit for close monitoring and management [23].

## Pharmacotherapy

### Prevention

At present, no drugs are approved for prophylaxis of SOS/VOD. The data for prophylactic use of ursodeoxycholic acid (UDCA) are inconclusive. Although some studies have shown that it decreases the incidence of VOD [64–67] the evidence is of low to very low quality [68]. Despite that, UDCA is usually recommended in HCT, as all studies show a lower liver toxicity, GVHD incidence and severity, and treatment-related mortality among patients receiving this prophylaxis. Prophylactic use of defibrotide has shown encouraging results in several studies [69, 70], including a prospective Phase 3 study in children [12]. A large international randomized trial (NCT02851407) of prophylactic use of defibrotide for SOS/VOD is currently ongoing in adult and pediatric patients post-HCT. The prophylactic use of defibrotide also may be helpful in patients undergoing autologous transplantation using high-risk conditioning regimens [54]. Although results are inconclusive [71], heparin remains in use for prevention in some centers; however, it is associated with bleeding risk. Other agents such as low molecular weight heparin, antithrombin III, prostaglandin E1, and pentoxifylline have proven to be ineffective or the study results inconclusive [25]. Recently, in a retrospective study of post-HCT pediatric patients with at least one risk factor for SOS/VOD from 2007 to 2016 at Showa University Fujigaoka Hospital (n = 19), no cases of SOS/VOD developed in 8 patients who received recombinant thrombomodulin with UDCA and low-molecular-weight heparin (LMWH) as prophylaxis for SOS/VOD, while 3 cases developed in the control group of 11 patients who received only UDCA and LMWH [72].

## *Treatment*

### General

Unfractionated heparin and LMWH appeared to be effective in some trials [73–75] but not in others [71, 76], and are not recommended in light of the significant risk of hemorrhage [54]. High-dose methylprednisolone may be beneficial in adults with mild to moderate SOS/VOD [77], but caution is recommended due to a risk of infection [54]. Methylprednisolone has been used in combination with defibrotide for treatment of SOS/VOD [29, 78]; also, 1 of the authors (NAK) has observed effective treatment with methylprednisolone in patients who develop SOS/VOD while on prophylactic defibrotide. Tissue plasminogen activator is no longer recommended for the treatment of SOS/VOD because of a high incidence of hemorrhagic complications in patients with MOD [79]. Other treatments used with limited evidence of success include prostaglandin E1 andantithrombin III [25]. A recent retrospective survey in Japan examining data from 65 patients between 1999 and 2011 found similar efficacy rates between recombinant thrombomodulin (n = 41; Day +100 overall survival rate, 48%; Day +100 complete response rate, 54%) and defibrotide (n = 24; Day +100 overall survival rate, 50%; Day +100 complete response rate, 50%) [80].

### Defibrotide

To-date, the only approved treatment for SOS/VOD is defibrotide. Defibrotide is approved to treat severe hepatic SOS/VOD post-HCT in patients aged >1 month in the European Union [81], and to treat SOS/VOD with renal or pulmonary dysfunction post-HCT in the United States [82] and Canada [83]. The recommended dosage of defibrotide for adult and pediatric patients is 6.25 mg/kg every 6 h administered over 2 h by intravenous infusion. It is recommended that defibrotide be administered for a minimum of 21 days and until signs and symptoms of SOS/VOD have resolved, up to a maximum of 60 days. Defibrotide is not recommended for patients with active bleeding or those receiving systemic anticoagulants or fibrinolytic therapy and it is advised that all patients be monitored for signs of bleeding.

Defibrotide is a polydisperse mixture of predominantly single-stranded polydeoxyribonucleotidesodium salts [84, 85]. It has been shown to maintain endothelial cell integrity and to have fibrinolytic, antithrombotic, and anti-inflammatory actions. *In vitro*, defibrotide protects endothelial cells from chemotherapy-induced apoptosis [86]. In addition, defibrotide inhibits heparinase activity, thus protecting heparan sulfate proteoglycans, a key component of the extracellular matrix and basement membranes [87, 88]. In human macro- and microvascular endothelial cells, defibrotide prevented increased von Willebrand Factor expression and endothelial cell matrix reactivity toward platelets induced by exposure to sera from patients with GVHD [89, 90]. Defibrotide also modulated lipopolysaccharide-induced changes in micro- and macrovascular endothelial cells, preventing increases in plasminogen activator inhibitor-1 expression and enhancing tissue plasminogen activator antigen expression, leading to an overall increase in fibrinolytic activity [84]; a similar increase in fibrinolytic activity was seen in defibrotide-treated patients [91]. Defibrotide reduced platelet adhesion and aggregate formation in humans [92] and inhibited platelet activation *in vitro* [93]. Defibrotide has been shown to decrease the presence of pro-inflammatory factors, such as IL-6, thromboxane A2, leukotriene B4, tissue necrosis factor, and reactive oxygen species in endothelial cells [94, 95]. In a mouse model of GVHD, prophylactic administration of defibrotide reduced pro-inflammatory mediators and promoted anti-inflammatory factors, compared with control mice [96].

Defibrotide efficacy and safety were first suggested in a compassionate use program [97] followed by a Phase 2 trial [28] in SOS/VOD patients with MOD following HCT. Complete response and Day +100 survival rates were promising in both studies. In a Phase 3 trial of patients with SOS/VOD and advanced MOF, defibrotide was associated with significant improvement in Day +100 survival (38.2% vs 25.0%; $P = 0.0109$) and complete response rates (25.5% vs 12.5%; $P = 0.0160$) compared with historical controls [98]. In an expanded-access protocol (T-IND), the efficacy and safety of defibrotide was consistent with previous studies. The large number of patients in the T-IND (n = 1137) allowed for evaluation of defibrotide in multiple subpopulations, including comparisons between adult (>16 years) and pediatric patients, patients with allogeneic and autologous transplants, patients with SOS/VOD onset ≤21 days and > 21 days post-HCT, patients with post-HCTSOS/VOD with and without MOD, and patients with non transplant-associated SOS/VOD with and without MOD [16, 31]. Patient subgroups without MOD had higher survival rates than those with MOD (Fig. 10.2).

**Fig. 10.2** Kaplan-meier estimated survival of patients with SOS/VOD following HCT (**a**) or nontransplant-associated chemotherapy (**b**) and Treated with Defibrotide. (**a**) Day + 100 Post-HCT (**b**) Day + 70 Post-nontransplant chemotherapy. Figure "Kaplan-Meier estimated survival to Day +100 by MOD status" (panel A) from Kernan NA, Grupp S, Smith AR, et al. Final results from a defibrotide treatment-IND study for patients with hepatic veno-occlusive disease/sinusoidal obstruction syndrome. *Br J Haematol.* 2018;181(6):816–827. Figure "Kaplan-Meier survival plot to Day +70" (panel B) from Kernan NA, Richardson PG, Smith AR, et al. Defibrotide for the treatment of hepatic veno-occlusive disease/sinusoidal obstruction syndrome following nontransplant-associated chemotherapy: Final results from a post hoc analysis of data from an expanded-access program. *Pediatr Blood Cancer.* 2018;65(10):e27269. Both figures are licensed under a Creative Commons Attribution-NonCommercial 4.0 International License (CC BY-NC 4.0; https://creative-commons.org/licenses/by-nc/4.0/). No changes were made to the original figures

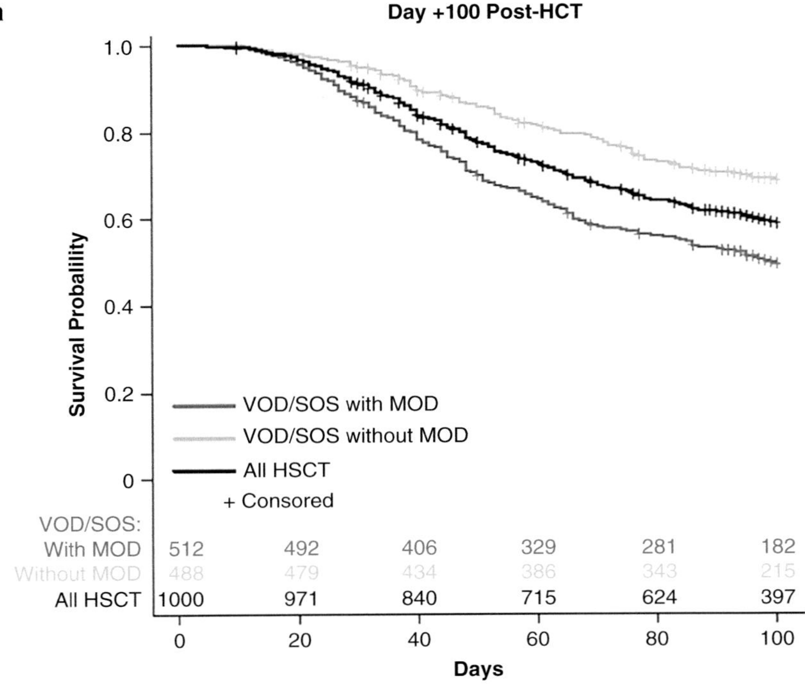
a
Day +100 Post-HCT
Survival Probalility
VOD/SOS with MOD
VOD/SOS without MOD
All HSCT
+ Consored
VOD/SOS:
With MOD 512 492 406 329 281 182
Without MOD 488 479 434 386 343 215
All HSCT 1000 971 840 715 624 397
0 20 40 60 80 100
Days

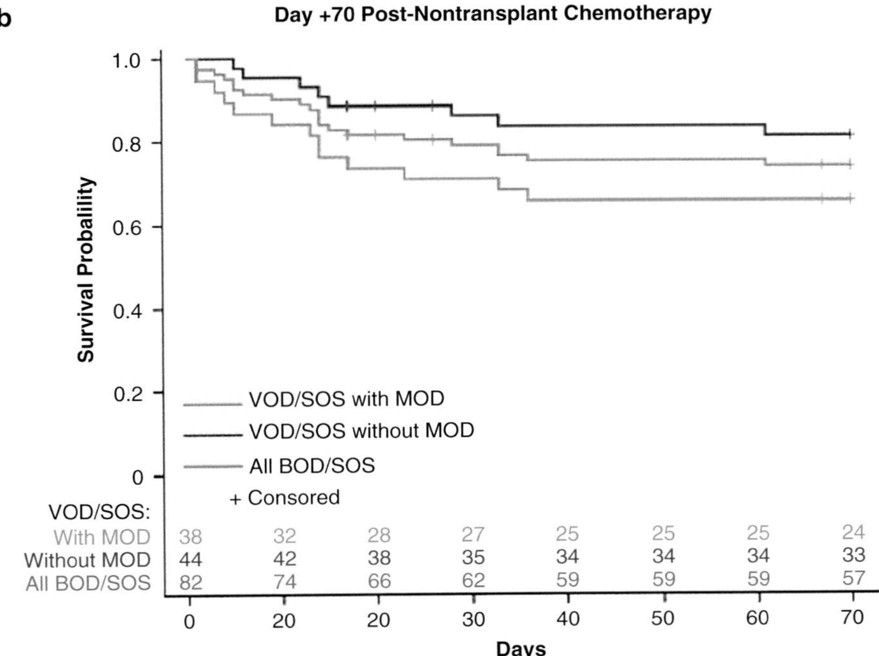
b
Day +70 Post-Nontransplant Chemotherapy
Survival Probability
VOD/SOS with MOD
VOD/SOS without MOD
All BOD/SOS
+ Consored
VOD/SOS:
With MOD 38 32 28 27 25 25 25 24
Without MOD 44 42 38 35 34 34 34 33
All BOD/SOS 82 74 66 62 59 59 59 57
0 20 20 30 40 50 60 70
Days

In addition, data from the T-IND showed that earlier initiation of defibrotide treatment was associated with higher Day +100 survival ($P < 0.001$; Cochran-Armitage test for trend) [31]. Taken together, these data emphasize the importance of prompt initiation of defibrotide treatment, further supporting its efficacy in the setting of SOS/VOD, and in particular its use for established disease, as well as preemptively in high-risk patients.

In summary, SOS/VOD remains a serious and potentially fatal condition after HCT that requires ongoing vigilance to achieve earlier diagnosis and intervention. Promising future directions include defibrotide prophylaxis for SOS/VOD in adults and pediatric patients post-HCT, and prophylaxis and treatment of SOS/VOD with recombinant thrombomodulin. Ongoing research in ultrasound radiography, clinical and chemical biomarkers should improve our ability to identify and prognosticate this disease early in its course, and to promote earlier intervention to improve treatment outcomes.

**Acknowledgements** Writing and editorial assistance was provided by Maria B Vinall of The Curry Rockefeller Group, LLC, Tarrytown, NY, USA, which was funded by Jazz Pharmaceuticals, Inc., Palo Alto, CA, USA.

# References


1. Carreras E, Diaz-Beya M, Rosinol L, Martinez C, Fernandez-Aviles F, Rovira M. The incidence of veno-occlusive disease following allogeneic hematopoietic stem cell transplantation has diminished and the outcome improved over the last decade. Biol Blood Marrow Transplant. 2011;17(11):1713–20.
2. Bearman SI. The syndrome of hepatic veno-occlusive disease after marrow transplantation. Blood. 1995;85(11):3005–20.
3. Wadleigh M, Richardson PG, Zahrieh D, et al. Prior gemtuzumab ozogamicin exposure significantly increases the risk of veno-occlusive disease in patients who undergo myeloablative allogeneic stem cell transplantation. Blood. 2003;102(5):1578–82.
4. Battipaglia G, Labopin M, Candoni A, et al. Risk of sinusoidal obstruction syndrome in allogeneic stem cell transplantation after prior gemtuzumab ozogamicin treatment: a retrospective study from the acute leukemia working party of the EBMT. Bone Marrow Transplant. 2017;52(4):592–9.
5. Kantarjian HM, DeAngelo DJ, Advani AS, et al. Hepatic adverse event profile of inotuzumab ozogamicin in adult patients with relapsed or refractory acute lymphoblastic leukaemia: results from the open-label, randomised, phase 3 INO-VATE study. Lancet Haematol. 2017;4(8):e387–98.
6. Mohty M, Malard F, Abecassis M, et al. Sinusoidal obstruction syndrome/veno-occlusive disease: current situation and perspectives-a position statement from the European Society for Blood and Marrow Transplantation (EBMT). Bone Marrow Transplant. 2015;50(6):781–9.
7. Mohty M, Malard F, Abecassis M, et al. Revised diagnosis and severity criteria for sinusoidal obstruction syndrome/veno-occlusive disease in adult patients: a new classification from the European Society for Blood and Marrow Transplantation. Bone Marrow Transplant. 2016;51(7):906–12.
8. Coppell JA, Richardson PG, Soiffer R, et al. Hepatic veno-occlusive disease following stem cell transplantation: incidence, clinical course, and outcome. Biol Blood Marrow Transplant. 2010;16(2):157–68.

9. Niederwieser D, Baldomero H, Szer J, et al. Hematopoietic stem cell transplantation activity worldwide in 2012 and a SWOT analysis of the worldwide network for blood and marrow transplantation group including the global survey. Bone Marrow Transplant. 2016;51(6):778–85.

10. Barker CC, Butzner JD, Anderson RA, Brant R, Sauve RS. Incidence, survival and risk factors for the development of veno-occlusive disease in pediatric hematopoietic stem cell transplant recipients. Bone Marrow Transplant. 2003;32(1):79–87.

11. Cesaro S, Pillon M, Talenti E, et al. A prospective survey on incidence, risk factors and therapy of hepatic veno-occlusive disease in children after hematopoietic stem cell transplantation. Haematologica. 2005;90(10):1396–404.

12. Corbacioglu S, Cesaro S, Faraci M, et al. Defibrotide for prophylaxis of hepatic veno-occlusive disease in paediatric haemopoietic stem-cell transplantation: an open-label, phase 3, randomised controlled trial. Lancet. 2012;379(9823):1301–9.

13. Corbacioglu S, Carreras E, Ansari M, et al. Diagnosis and severity criteria for sinusoidal obstruction syndrome/veno-occlusive disease in pediatric patients: a new classification from the European society for blood and marrow transplantation. Bone Marrow Transplant. 2018;53(2):138–45.

14. Robinson SM, Wilson CH, Burt AD, Manas DM, White SA. Chemotherapy-associated liver injury in patients with colorectal liver metastases: a systematic review and meta-analysis. Ann Surg Oncol. 2012;19(13):4287–99.

15. Corbacioglu S, Carreras E, Mohty M, et al. Defibrotide for the treatment of hepatic veno-occlusive disease: final results from the international compassionate-use program. Biol Blood Marrow Transplant. 2016;22(10):1874–82.

16. Kernan NA, Richardson PG, Smith AR, et al. Defibrotide for the treatment of hepatic veno-occlusive disease/sinusoidal obstruction syndrome following nontransplant-associated chemotherapy: final results from a post hoc analysis of data from an expanded-access program. Pediatr Blood Cancer. 2018;65(10):e27269.

17. DeLeve LD, Wang X, Kanel GC, et al. Decreased hepatic nitric oxide production contributes to the development of rat sinusoidal obstruction syndrome. Hepatology. 2003;38(4):900–8.

18. Carreras E, Diaz-Ricart M. The role of the endothelium in the short-term complications of hematopoietic SCT. Bone Marrow Transplant. 2011;46(12):1495–502.

19. Carreras E, Bertz H, Arcese W, et al. Incidence and outcome of hepatic veno-occlusive disease after blood or marrow transplantation: a prospective cohort study of the European Group for Blood and Marrow Transplantation. European Group for Blood and Marrow Transplantation Chronic Leukemia Working Party. Blood. 1998;92(10):3599–604.

20. Palomo M, Diaz-Ricart M, Carbo C, et al. Endothelial dysfunction after hematopoietic stem cell transplantation: role of the conditioning regimen and the type of transplantation. Biol Blood Marrow Transplant. 2010;16(7):985–93.

21. Cooke KR, Jannin A, Ho V. The contribution of endothelial activation and injury to end-organ toxicity following allogeneic hematopoietic stem cell transplantation. Biol Blood Marrow Transplant. 2008;14(1 Suppl 1):23–32.

22. Palomo M, Diaz-Ricart M, Carbo C, et al. The release of soluble factors contributing to endothelial activation and damage after hematopoietic stem cell transplantation is not limited to the allogeneic setting and involves several pathogenic mechanisms. Biol Blood Marrow Transplant. 2009;15(5):537–46.

23. Dalle JH, Giralt SA. Hepatic veno-occlusive disease after hematopoietic stem cell transplantation: risk factors and stratification, prophylaxis, and treatment. Biol Blood Marrow Transplant. 2016;22(3):400–9.

24. McDonald GB, Sharma P, Matthews DE, Shulman HM, Thomas ED. Venocclusive disease of the liver after bone marrow transplantation: diagnosis, incidence, and predisposing factors. Hepatology. 1984;4(1):116–22.

25. Carreras E. How I manage sinusoidal obstruction syndrome after haematopoietic cell transplantation. Br J Haematol. 2015;168(4):481–91.

26. Corbacioglu S, Greil J, Peters C, et al. Defibrotide in the treatment of children with veno-occlusive disease (VOD): a retrospective multicentre study demonstrates therapeutic efficacy upon early intervention. Bone Marrow Transplant. 2004;33(2):189–95.

27. Cheuk DK, Wang P, Lee TL, et al. Risk factors and mortality predictors of hepatic veno-occlusive disease after pediatric hematopoietic stem cell transplantation. Bone Marrow Transplant. 2007;40(10):935–44.

28. Richardson PG, Soiffer RJ, Antin JH, et al. Defibrotide for the treatment of severe hepatic veno-occlusive disease and multiorgan failure after stem cell transplantation: a multicenter, randomized, dose-finding trial. Biol Blood Marrow Transplant. 2010;16(7):1005–17.

29. Myers KC, Lawrence J, Marsh RA, Davies SM, Jodele S. High-dose methylprednisolone for veno-occlusive disease of the liver in pediatric hematopoietic stem cell transplantation recipients. Biol Blood Marrow Transplant. 2013;19(3):500–3.

30. Richardson PG, Smith AR, Triplett BM, et al. Earlier defibrotide initiation post-diagnosis of veno-occlusive disease/sinusoidal obstruction syndrome improves day +100 survival following haematopoietic stem cell transplantation. Br J Haematol. 2017;178(1):112–8.

31. Kernan NA, Grupp S, Smith AR, et al. Final results from a defibrotide treatment-IND study for patients with hepatic veno-occlusive disease/sinusoidal obstruction syndrome. Br J Haematol. 2018;181(6):816–27.

32. Jones RJ, Lee KS, Beschorner WE, et al. Venoocclusive disease of the liver following bone marrow transplantation. Transplantation. 1987;44(6):778–83.

33. McDonald GB, Hinds MS, Fisher LD, et al. Veno-occlusive disease of the liver and multiorgan failure after bone marrow transplantation: a cohort study of 355 patients. Ann Intern Med. 1993;118(4):255–67.

34. Carreras E. Veno-occlusive disease of the liver after hemopoietic cell transplantation. Eur J Haematol. 2000;64(5):281–91.

35. Roeker LE, Kim HT, Glotzbecker B, et al. Early clinical predictors of hepatic veno-occlusive disease/sinusoidal obstruction syndrome after myeloablative stem cell transplantation. Biol Blood Marrow Transplant. 2019;25(1):137–44.

36. Carreras E, Rosinol L, Terol MJ, et al. Veno-occlusive disease of the liver after high-dose cytoreductive therapy with busulfan and melphalan for autologous blood stem cell transplantation in multiple myeloma patients. Biol Blood Marrow Transplant. 2007;13(12):1448–54.

37. Nicolau C, Bru C, Carreras E, et al. Sonographic diagnosis and hemodynamic correlation in veno-occlusive disease of the liver. J Ultrasound Med. 1993;12(8):437–40.

38. Chan SS, Colecchia A, Duarte RF, Bonifazi F, Ravaioli F, Bourhis JH. Imaging in hepatic Veno-occlusive disease/sinusoidal obstruction syndrome. Biol Blood Marrow Transplant. 2020;26(10):1770–9.

39. Dietrich CF, Trenker C, Fontanilla T, et al. New ultrasound techniques challenge the diagnosis of sinusoidal obstruction syndrome. Ultrasound Med Biol. 2018;44(11):2171–82.

40. Colecchia A, Marasco G, Ravaioli F, et al. Usefulness of liver stiffness measurement in predicting hepatic veno-occlusive disease development in patients who undergo HSCT. Bone Marrow Transplant. 2017;52(3):494–7.

41. Reddivalla N, Robinson AL, Reid KJ, et al. Using liver elastography to diagnose sinusoidal obstruction syndrome in pediatric patients undergoing hematopoetic stem cell transplant. Bone Marrow Transplant. 2018;55(3):523–30.

42. Sigrist RMS, Liau J, Kaffas AE, Chammas MC, Willmann JK. Ultrasound elastography: review of techniques and clinical applications. Theranostics. 2017;7(5):1303–29.

43. Lassau N, Auperin A, Leclere J, Bennaceur A, Valteau-Couanet D, Hartmann O. Prognostic value of doppler-ultrasonography in hepatic veno-occlusive disease. Transplantation. 2002;74(1):60–6.

44. Chao N. How I treat sinusoidal obstruction syndrome. Blood. 2014;123(26):4023–6.

45. Carreras E, Granena A, Navasa M, et al. Transjugular liver biopsy in BMT. Bone Marrow Transplant. 1993;11(1):21–6.

46. Shulman HM, Gooley T, Dudley MD, et al. Utility of transvenous liver biopsies and wedged hepatic venous pressure measurements in sixty marrow transplant recipients. Transplantation. 1995;59(7):1015–22.

47. Carreras E, Granena A, Navasa M, et al. On the reliability of clinical criteria for the diagnosis of hepatic veno-occlusive disease. Ann Hematol. 1993;66(2):77–80.

48. Ahmed O, Ward TJ, Lungren MP, et al. Assessing the risk of hemorrhagic complication following transjugular liver biopsy in bone marrow transplantation recipients. J Vasc Interv Radiol. 2016;27(4):551–7.
49. Ruggiu M, Bedossa P, Rautou PE, et al. Utility and safety of liver biopsy in patients with undetermined liver blood test anomalies after allogeneic hematopoietic stem cell transplantation: a monocentric retrospective cohort study. Biol Blood Marrow Transplant. 2018;24(12):2523–31.
50. Oshrine B, Lehmann LE, Duncan CN. Safety and utility of liver biopsy after pediatric hematopoietic stem cell transplantation. J Pediatr Hematol Oncol. 2011;33(3):e92–7.
51. Myers KC, Dandoy C, El-Bietar J, Davies SM, Jodele S. Veno-occlusive disease of the liver in the absence of elevation in bilirubin in pediatric patients after hematopoietic stem cell transplantation. Biol Blood Marrow Transplant. 2015;21(2):379–81.
52. Bajwa RPS, Mahadeo KM, Taragin BH, et al. Consensus report by pediatric acute lung injury and sepsis investigators and pediatric blood and marrow transplantation consortium joint working committees: supportive care guidelines for management of veno-occlusive disease in children and adolescents, part 1: focus on investigations, prophylaxis, and specific treatment. Biol Blood Marrow Transplant. 2017;23(11):1817–25.
53. Naples JC, Skeens MA, Auletta J, et al. Anicteric veno-occlusive disease after hematopoietic stem cell transplantation in children. Bone Marrow Transplant. 2016;51(1):135–7.
54. Dignan FL, Wynn RF, Hadzic N, et al. BCSH/BSBMT guideline: diagnosis and management of veno-occlusive disease (sinusoidal obstruction syndrome) following haematopoietic stem cell transplantation. Br J Haematol. 2013;163(4):444–57.
55. de Lima M, Couriel D, Thall PF, et al. Once-daily intravenous busulfan and fludarabine: clinical and pharmacokinetic results of a myeloablative, reduced-toxicity conditioning regimen for allogeneic stem cell transplantation in AML and MDS. Blood. 2004;104(3):857–64.
56. Daly A, Savoie ML, Geddes M, et al. Fludarabine, busulfan, antithymocyte globulin, and total body irradiation for pretransplantation conditioning in acute lymphoblastic leukemia: excellent outcomes in all but older patients with comorbidities. Biol Blood Marrow Transplant. 2012;18(12):1921–6.
57. Nagler A, Labopin M, Berger R, et al. Allogeneic hematopoietic SCT for adults AML using i.v. BU in the conditioning regimen: outcomes and risk factors for the occurrence of hepatic sinusoidal obstructive syndrome. Bone Marrow Transplant. 2014;49(5):628–33.
58. Cantoni N, Gerull S, Heim D, et al. Order of application and liver toxicity in patients given BU and CY containing conditioning regimens for allogeneic hematopoietic SCT. Bone Marrow Transplant. 2011;46(3):344–9.
59. Kebriaei P, Cutler C, de Lima M, et al. Management of important adverse events associated with inotuzumab ozogamicin: expert panel review. Bone Marrow Transplant. 2018;53(4):449–56.
60. Hagglund H, Remberger M, Klaesson S, Lonnqvist B, Ljungman P, Ringden O. Norethisterone treatment, a major risk-factor for veno-occlusive disease in the liver after allogeneic bone marrow transplantation. Blood. 1998;92(12):4568–72.
61. Soiffer RJ, Dear K, Rabinowe SN, et al. Hepatic dysfunction following T-cell-depleted allogeneic bone marrow transplantation. Transplantation. 1991;52(6):1014–9.
62. Moscardo F, Urbano-Ispizua A, Sanz GF, et al. Positive selection for CD34+ reduces the incidence and severity of veno-occlusive disease of the liver after HLA-identical sibling allogeneic peripheral blood stem cell transplantation. Exp Hematol. 2003;31(6):545–50.
63. Cutler C, Stevenson K, Kim HT, et al. Sirolimus is associated with veno-occlusive disease of the liver after myeloablative allogeneic stem cell transplantation. Blood. 2008;112(12):4425–31.
64. Ruutu T, Eriksson B, Remes K, et al. Ursodeoxycholic acid for the prevention of hepatic complications in allogeneic stem cell transplantation. Blood. 2002;100(6):1977–83.
65. Essell JH, Thompson JM, Harman GS, et al. Pilot trial of prophylactic ursodiol to decrease the incidence of veno-occlusive disease of the liver in allogeneic bone marrow transplant patients. Bone Marrow Transplant. 1992;10(4):367–72.
66. Essell JH, Schroeder MT, Harman GS, et al. Ursodiol prophylaxis against hepatic complications of allogeneic bone marrow transplantation. A randomized, double-blind, placebo-controlled trial. Ann Intern Med. 1998;128(12 Pt 1):975–81.

67. Ohashi K, Tanabe J, Watanabe R, et al. The Japanese multicenter open randomized trial of ursodeoxycholic acid prophylaxis for hepatic veno-occlusive disease after stem cell transplantation. Am J Hematol. 2000;64(1):32–8.

68. Cheuk DK, Chiang AK, Ha SY, Chan GC. Interventions for prophylaxis of hepatic veno-occlusive disease in people undergoing haematopoietic stem cell transplantation. Cochrane Database Syst Rev. 2015;5:CD009311.

69. Chalandon Y, Roosnek E, Mermillod B, et al. Prevention of veno-occlusive disease with defibrotide after allogeneic stem cell transplantation. Biol Blood Marrow Transplant. 2004;10(5):347–54.

70. Dignan F, Gujral D, Ethell M, et al. Prophylactic defibrotide in allogeneic stem cell transplantation: minimal morbidity and zero mortality from veno-occlusive disease. Bone Marrow Transplant. 2007;40(1):79–82.

71. Imran H, Tleyjeh IM, Zirakzadeh A, Rodriguez V, Khan SP. Use of prophylactic anticoagulation and the risk of hepatic veno-occlusive disease in patients undergoing hematopoietic stem cell transplantation: a systematic review and meta-analysis. Bone Marrow Transplant. 2006;37(7):677–86.

72. Yamamoto S, Toyama D, Sugishita Y, et al. Prophylactic recombinant thrombomodulin treatment prevents hepatic sinusoidal obstruction syndrome in high-risk pediatric patients that undergo hematopoietic stem cell transplants. Pediatr Transplant. 2018;22(7):e13269.

73. Attal M, Huguet F, Rubie H, et al. Prevention of hepatic veno-occlusive disease after bone marrow transplantation by continuous infusion of low-dose heparin: a prospective, randomized trial. Blood. 1992;79(11):2834–40.

74. Or R, Nagler A, Shpilberg O, et al. Low molecular weight heparin for the prevention of veno-occlusive disease of the liver in bone marrow transplantation patients. Transplantation. 1996;61(7):1067–71.

75. Simon M, Hahn T, Ford LA, et al. Retrospective multivariate analysis of hepatic veno-occlusive disease after blood or marrow transplantation: possible beneficial use of low molecular weight heparin. Bone Marrow Transplant. 2001;27(6):627–33.

76. Marsa-Vila L, Gorin NC, Laporte JP, et al. Prophylactic heparin does not prevent liver veno-occlusive disease following autologous bone marrow transplantation. Eur J Haematol. 1991;47(5):346–54.

77. Al Beihany A, Al Omar H, Sahovic E, et al. Successful treatment of hepatic veno-occlusive disease after myeloablative allogeneic hematopoietic stem cell transplantation by early administration of a short course of methylprednisolone. Bone Marrow Transplant. 2008;41(3):287–91.

78. Gloude NJ, Jodele S, Teusink-Cross A, et al. Combination of high-dose methylprednisolone and defibrotide for Veno-occlusive disease in pediatric hematopoietic stem cell transplant recipients. Biol Blood Marrow Transplant. 2018;24(1):91–5.

79. Bearman SI, Lee JL, Baron AE, McDonald GB. Treatment of hepatic venocclusive disease with recombinant human tissue plasminogen activator and heparin in 42 marrow transplant patients. Blood. 1997;89(5):1501–6.

80. Yakushijin K, Ikezoe T, Ohwada C, et al. Clinical effects of recombinant thrombomodulin and defibrotide on sinusoidal obstruction syndrome after allogeneic hematopoietic stem cell transplantation. Bone Marrow Transplant. 2019;54(5):674–80.

81. Gentium SRL. Defitelio 80 mg/mL summary of product characteristics EU; 2016.

82. Pharmaceuticals J. Defitelio (defibrotide sodium): prescribing information; 2016.

83. Pharmaceuticals J. Product monograph including patient medication information Defitelio™ defibrotide sodium; 2017.

84. Falanga A, Vignoli A, Marchetti M, Barbui T. Defibrotide reduces procoagulant activity and increases fibrinolytic properties of endothelial cells. Leukemia. 2003;17(8):1636–42.

85. Echart CL, Graziadio B, Somaini S, et al. The fibrinolytic mechanism of defibrotide: effect of defibrotide on plasmin activity. Blood Coagul Fibrinolysis. 2009;20(8):627–34.

86. Eissner G, Multhoff G, Gerbitz A, et al. Fludarabine induces apoptosis, activation, and allogenicity in human endothelial and epithelial cells: protective effect of defibrotide. Blood. 2002;100(1):334–40.

87. Barash U, Lapidot M, Zohar Y, et al. Involvement of heparanase in the pathogenesis of mesothelioma: basic aspects and clinical applications. J Natl Cancer Inst. 2018;110(10):1102–14.
88. Hallmann R, Horn N, Selg M, Wendler O, Pausch F, Sorokin LM. Expression and function of laminins in the embryonic and mature vasculature. Physiol Rev. 2005;85(3):979–1000.
89. Palomo M, Diaz-Ricart M, Rovira M, Escolar G, Carreras E. Defibrotide prevents the activation of macrovascular and microvascular endothelia caused by soluble factors released to blood by autologous hematopoietic stem cell transplantation. Biol Blood Marrow Transplant. 2011;17(4):497–506.
90. Martinez-Sanchez J, Hamelmann H, Palomo M, et al. Acute graft-vs-host disease-associated endothelial activation in vitro is prevented by defibrotide. Front Immunol. 2019;10:2339.
91. Falanga A, Marchetti M, Vignoli A, Barbui T. Changes in fibrinolysis, coagulation and endothelium activation in patients given defibrotide for hematopoietic stem cell transplant-associated veno-occlusive disease. Thromb Haemost. 1999;Suppl:A529.
92. Ulutin ON, Balkuv-Ulutin S, Bezer-Goker B, et al. Effect of defibrotide on platelet function. Semin Thromb Hemost. 1996;22(Suppl 1):21–4.
93. Evangelista V, Piccardoni P, de Gaetano G, Cerletti C. Defibrotide inhibits platelet activation by cathepsin G released from stimulated polymorphonuclear leukocytes. Thromb Haemost. 1992;67(6):660–4.
94. Pescador R, Capuzzi L, Mantovani M, Fulgenzi A, Ferrero ME. Defibrotide: properties and clinical use of an old/new drug. Vasc Pharmacol. 2013;59(1–2):1–10.
95. Palomo M, Mir E, Rovira M, Escolar G, Carreras E, Diaz-Ricart M. What is going on between defibrotide and endothelial cells? Snapshots reveal the hot spots of their romance. Blood. 2016;127(13):1719–27.
96. García-Bernal D, Palomo M, Martínez CM, et al. Defibrotide inhibits donor leukocyte endothelial interactions and protects against acute graft-versus-host disease. J Cell Mol Med. 2020;24:8031–44.
97. Richardson PG, Elias AD, Krishnan A, et al. Treatment of severe veno-occlusive disease with defibrotide: compassionate use results in response without significant toxicity in a high-risk population. Blood. 1998;92(3):737–44.
98. Richardson PG, Riches ML, Kernan NA, et al. Phase 3 trial of defibrotide for the treatment of severe veno-occlusive disease and multi-organ failure. Blood. 2016;127(13):1656–65.

# Chapter 11
# Sinusoidal Dilatation and Peliosis Hepatis

Loretta L. Jophlin, Vijay H. Shah, and Douglas A. Simonetto

## Normal Hepatic Sinusoids

Healthy hepatic sinusoids are capillary-sized (7–15 μm) [1] endothelial-lined blood vessels where oxygen-rich arterial blood and nutrient-rich portal blood merge within the healthy liver. Oxygenated blood is carried to the sinusoids via branches of the hepatic arteries whereas portal blood reaches the sinusoids via branches of the portal vein. Blood from both sources converge within the sinusoids, which are arranged similar to spokes of a wheel with cords of hepatocytes running parallel to them. The terminal end of each sinusoid empties into the central vein. The central vein resides in the center of each hepatic lobule, the repeating functional unit of the liver containing the liver parenchyma, bile ducts and all previously mentioned vascular structures. Sinusoids differ from typical capillaries as sinusoidal endothelial cells harbor clusters of fenestra, each measuring 150–175 nm [2], within the flattened ends of their cellular processes. These fenestrated areas are termed "sieve-plates" and allow for the size-restricted passage of particulates to the sub endothelial space of Disse. Likewise, size-restricted material can pass from the space of Disse via the fenestra into the sinusoids for systemic delivery. As such, the sinusoids function as a size-restricted, bidirectional sieve within the liver. Sinusoidal endothelial cells also have high endocytic and exocytic potential and can serve as a direct port of entry and export for molecules and pathogens to the liver. The space of Disse

L. L. Jophlin
University of Louisville, Louisville, Kentucky, USA
e-mail: loretta.jophlin@uoflhealth.org

V. H. Shah · D. A. Simonetto (✉)
Mayo Clinic, Rochester, MN, USA

University of Louisville, Louisville, Kentucky, USA

Department of Medicine, Mayo Clinic, Rochester, USA
e-mail: Shah.vijay@mayo.edu; simonetto.douglas@mayo.edu

© Springer Nature Switzerland AG 2022
D. Valla et al. (eds.), *Vascular Disorders of the Liver*,
https://doi.org/10.1007/978-3-030-82988-9_11

resides adjacent to the hepatic parenchyma composed predominantly of hepatocytes, functional liver cells responsible for bile production, protein synthesis, glucose homeostasis, and metabolism of drugs and toxins. Within the space of Disse also reside contractile, vitamin A-laden hepatic stellate cells, which are responsible for retinoid storage and extracellular matrix production in response to liver injury. As the conduit between the space of Disse and the systemic circulation, the hepatic sinusoids are integral for maintaining hepatic homeostasis.

## Sinusoidal Pressure and Compression

The tonicity of blood flow in hepatic sinusoids is regulated by factors proximal to, distal to and within (or adjacent to) the sinusoid. The sinusoid itself is the lowest pressure space within the liver (~6 mmHg) [3] and its pressure can be measured indirectly by performing a wedged hepatic venous pressure [4]. When sinusoidal outflow is impaired, pressure within the sinusoids increases. When this pressure exceeds the free hepatic venous pressure by greater than 6 mmHg, sequelae of portal hypertension may manifest with the development of ascites and portosystemic shunts including esophageal varices [5]. When the etiology of increased sinusoidal pressure exists within the liver, with *constriction* rather than dilatation of the sinusoids, the resultant portal hypertension is classified as **sinusoidal portal hypertension**. In the setting of liver injury, this scenario can arise from the contraction of sinusoidal endothelial cells and hepatic stellate cells, secondary to increases in local vasoconstrictors, such as endothelin-1, and decreases in vasodilators, such as nitrous oxide [6]. Acute inflammation leading to sinusoidal plugging with inflammatory cells [1] or hepatocyte injury resulting in swelling of adjacent liver parenchyma can also slow the flow within sinusoids leading to sinusoidal portal hypertension. When acute, sinusoidal portal hypertension and its sequelae can be reversed upon cessation of the insult and subsequent hepatic recovery [6]. The accumulation of extracellular matrix fibers produced by transdifferentiated hepatic stellate cells in response to viral hepatitis C infection, excessive alcohol use and non-alcoholic fatty liver disease (the three most common etiologies of cirrhosis) can also impair sinusoidal blood flow, generally in a less reversible manner, and as such sinusoidal portal hypertension is the most common type of portal hypertension. Portal hypertension can also result from disease processes outside of the sinusoids (**pre- or post-sinusoidal portal hypertension**) and may yield distortion or *dilatation* of the sinusoids. Sinusoidal dilatation, however, can exist with or without concomitant portal hypertension as described below.

## Classifications of Sinusoidal Distortion

Abnormal architecture of hepatic sinusoids can be classified as idiopathic (without identifiable etiology) or acquired (secondary to an identified insult or condition). Both idiopathic and acquired sinusoidal abnormalities can first manifest during human development *in utero* (congenital) or can manifest after birth throughout the course of the human lifespan (adult-onset). Adult-onset abnormalities are generally secondary to conditions causing hepatic outflow obstruction or exposure to drugs or infections which damage the sinusoidal endothelium. In addition to the causes of sinusoidal portal hypertension described above, dozens of secondary causes of sinusoidal architecture disruption are known and herein we focus our discussion on the architectural manifestations and etiologies of sinusoidal dilatation (Table 11.1) and peliosis(Table 11.2). Lastly, we identify capillarization (also referred to as defenestration), the loss of fenestra from sinusoidal endothelial cells, as a unique type of sinusoidal architectural disruption. This process can be secondary to hepatic fibrosis [7], toxin exposure [8] or normal aging [9].

Microscopically, sinusoidal disruptions can be classified as pan acinar or zonal. Pan acinar disruptions affect all sinusoids regardless of location in the hepatic

**Table 11.1** Conditions associated with sinusoidal dilatation

| Outflow obstruction | Non-obstructive |
| --- | --- |
| Cardiac pathology<br>  Right-sided heart failure<br>  Valvular heart disease<br>  Constrictive pericarditis | Antiphospholipid syndrome |
| Budd-chiari syndrome<br>  Hepatic vein<br>    Thrombosis/compression<br>  Inferior vena cava<br>    Thrombosis/compression | Drugs<br>  Anabolic steroids<br>  Azathioprine<br>  Oral contraceptives<br>  Oxaliplatin-based chemotherapy |
| Sinusoidal obstruction syndrome | Congenital absence of the portal vein |
| Hepatic veno-occlusive disease with immunodeficiency | Extrahepatic malignancy<br>  Renal cell carcinoma<br>  Hodgkin's lymphoma<br>  Pseudo papillary tumor |
| Sickle cell anemia | Infections<br>  Pyelonephritis<br>  Pneumonia<br>  Septicemia<br>  Brucellosis<br>  Pulmonary tuberculosis |
|  | Inflammatory conditions<br>  Sarcoidosis<br>  Inflammatory bowel disease<br>  Rheumatoid arthritis<br>  Still disease<br>  Pancreatitis<br>  Castleman's disease |
|  | Portal vein thrombosis |
|  | Post-operative states<br>  Gastric bypass<br>  Cholecystectomy<br>  Splenectomy<br>  Liver transplant (allograft) |

**Table 11.2** Conditions associated with peliosis hepatis

| Drug exposures | Infections | Malignancies | Other |
| --- | --- | --- | --- |
| Azathioprine | Bartonellosis | Colon cancer | Immunocompromised state |
| Methotrexate | HIV/AIDS | Hodgkin's disease | Post-organ transplant |
| Oral contraceptives/anabolic steroids | Syphilis | Prostate cancer | Pregnancy |
| Tamoxifen | Tuberculosis | Seminoma | |
| Vitamin A | | | |

lobule. Zonal disruptions can affect the portion of the sinusoids closer to feeding tributaries near the portal triad (zone 1), near the mid sinusoid (zone 2) or closer to the central vein (zone 3) [10]. Macroscopically, sinusoidal dilatation may be focal (affecting small portions of a hepatic lobe), lobar (affecting one entire hepatic lobe) or pan-hepatic (affecting the entire liver). The pattern is generally dependent on the etiology. Likewise, peliosis may be focal, lobar or pan-hepatic [11].

## Sinusoidal Dilatation

### *Features of Sinusoidal Dilatation*

Hepatic sinusoidal dilatation is the non-physiologic architectural disruption and enlargement of the hepatic sinusoidal lumen beyond its normal size of 7–15 μm, noting that sinusoids are physiologically larger towards zone 3 of the hepatic lobule [12]. When present, both pan-acinar and zonal sinusoidal dilatation can be readily seen on low power light microscopy. Radiographically, on magnetic resonance imaging or contrast-enhanced computed tomography, a heterogeneous enhancement pattern of the liver parenchyma may be seen as a consequence of altered hemodynamics, locally or throughout the liver [13]. Focal or lobar areas of sinusoidal dilatation may be missed on a random liver biopsy. Likewise, mild foci of sinusoidal dilatation may not be detected with imaging. If liver function tests are abnormal in the setting of sinusoidal dilatation, they are typically in a cholestatic pattern [14].

## Etiologies of Sinusoidal Dilatation

### *Outflow Obstruction*

Most often, sinusoidal dilatation is caused by impaired hepatic venous outflow [14, 15]. Sinusoidal dilatation from outflow obstruction is usually limited to zone 3 microscopically [15] with alternating areas of red blood cell extravasation and parenchyma extinction giving the liver a gross "nutmeg" appearance. The most common causes of outflow obstruction resulting in sinusoidal dilatation are listed in Table 11.1 and described in detail below.

## Cardiac Conditions

Disease processes resulting in increased right ventricular pressure, such as ventricular heart failure, valvular heart disease, restrictive cardiomyopathy and pericardial disease can result in congestion of all vessels proximal to the inferior vena cava. As a result, passive venous congestion occurs throughout the entire liver. Decreased outflow of the central veins and sinusoids results in their dilatation and engorgement with blood. The subsequent state is one of congestive hepatopathy and can result in hepatomegaly and post-sinusoidal portal hypertension with sequelae including ascites and the development of gastroesophageal varices. Patients may experience right upper quadrant pain and show aberrant liver function tests. Longstanding passive congestion can lead to hepatic fibrosis, nodular regenerative hyperplasia (NRH) and, in severe cases, cardiac cirrhosis; however the clinical course in regards to liver manifestations for patients with chronic heart failure is highly heterogeneous [16]. Sinusoidal dilatation and congestion may be seen with mild or early cardiac dysfunction. As the cardiac diseases progresses however, hepatic NRH may result in sinusoidal compression and collapse [17].

## Budd-Chiari syndrome

Budd-Chiari syndrome is a hepatic outflow disorder occurring in the setting of narrowing or obstruction(usually from thrombosis) of the inferior vena cava or hepatic veins. It can occur in an acute, subacute or chronic manner and may be an indication for liver transplantation in select patients [18]. Grossly, the liver becomes enlarged and patients may experience right upper quadrant pain, ascites and liver failure. Microscopically, there is engorgement of the central veins with zone 3 sinusoidal dilatation [17]. Further hepatic architectural disruption including NRH and fibrosis can follow and physiologic sequelae are similar to those seen in cardiac etiologies of venous outflow obstruction.

## Sinusoidal Obstruction Syndrome

Sinusoidal obstruction syndrome (SOS), previously known as venoocclusive disease (VOD), is a condition manifested by sinusoidal architectural disruption secondary to sinusoidal or central vein endothelial cell injury. Numerous injurious culprits have been identified to trigger SOS including accidental ingestions of products containing pyrrolizidine alkaloids [19], conditioning regimens for hematopoietic stem cell transplantation as well as chemotherapeutic agents utilized outside of the realm of stem cell transplantation such as oxaliplatin [20]. Other rarer etiologies include an autosomal recessive condition of veno-occlusive disease with immunodeficiency (VODI) described in the pediatric population [21]. Following transplantation, liver allografts, with presumably normal pre-transplant sinusoidal architecture, can also sustain sinusoidal endothelial injury resulting in SOS [22, 23]. Microscopic analysis has revealed that a component of the pathophysiological mechanism of SOS is the detachment of vascular endothelial cells leading to plugging and subsequent dilation of the sinusoids with extravasation of red blood cells into the space of Disse [24]. Sequelae of portal hypertension emanating from the level of the sinusoids can ensue and in severe cases, liver failure may occur. Ursodeoxycholic acid (UDCA), a naturally occurring bile salt, is often employed prophylactically to protect against SOS when high-risk chemotherapeutic regimens are administered. While the mechanism of its protective effect is incompletely understood, it is believed that UDCA replaces hepatotoxic bile salts which may promote endothelial injury [25]. Treatment of mild SOS is supportive however for moderate-severe cases, Defibrotide, an oligonucleotide agent which protects endothelial cells and modifies the balance of thrombosis and fibrinolysis within hepatic venules and sinusoids, may be considered [26]. Additionally, transjugular intrahepatic portosystemic shunt has been undertaken successfully to relieve the sequelae of portal hypertension in select patients with SOS [27].

## Sickle Cell Anemia

Similar to SOS, sickle cell anemia can lead to sinusoidal dilatation due to the sluggish or frank mechanical blockage of sinusoids by misshapen, sickle-shaped erythrocytes. Passive congestion and iron overload from repeated blood transfusions can lead to NRH and hepatic fibrosis respectively with concomitant sequelae of portal hypertension [15, 28].

## *Non-Obstructive Sinusoidal Dilatation*

### Isolated (Benign) Sinusoidal Dilatation

Data from large case series on the subject have found that approximately 18–33% of patients with sinusoidal dilatation on liver biopsy show no underlying sinusoidal, central venous or post-hepatic vessel outflow obstruction [14, 15] (Table 11.1). Prehepatic vascular disease appear to be a common association in one case series with portal vein thrombosis and congenital absence of portal vein noted [15]. Inflammatory and infectious disorders including granulomatous hepatitis, Still disease, rheumatoid arthritis, pyelonephritis and inflammatory bowel disease have also been associated with sinusoidal dilatation, possibly secondary to increased circulating levels of vasodilatory molecules [29]. Oncologic conditions arising outside of the liver including renal cell carcinoma and Hodgkin's lymphoma (not previously treated with chemotherapy or stem cell transplant) were also documented as comorbid conditions in patients with sinusoidal dilatation [14, 15]. Sinusoidal dilatation may also be associated with antiphospholipid syndrome [30], oral contraceptives [31] and azathioprine [32] though the mechanisms of these culprits remain unclear. Patients in the postoperative state from gastric bypass surgery, cholecystectomy and splenectomy have also been noted to develop sinusoidal dilatation of unclear significance [14, 15].

## Sinusoidal Dilatation Associated with Idiopathic Non-Cirrhotic Portal Hypertension

Non-isolated sinusoidal dilatation often occurs in concert with NRH in the setting of idiopathic non-cirrhotic portal hypertension (INCPH). In recognition of the pathophysiologic mechanism of INCPH relative to the hepatic microvasculature, it has recently been renamed porto-sinusoidal vascular disease [33]. Sinusoidal dilatation can be viewed as a feature of INCPH as 95% of patients with INCPH show some sinusoidal dilatation on their biopsies [29]. Evidence suggesting that isolated sinusoidal dilatation may herald forthcoming INCPH was reported in a study of post-liver transplant patients finding that sinusoidal dilatation was seen in80% of allografts which eventually developed NRH [34] in the absence of overt large vessel vascular abnormalities. Mild or imperceptible post-transplant vascular alterations or sinusoidal endothelial injury from reperfusion may contribute to the development of NRH and subsequent INCPH in this population [22]. As such, sinusoidal dilatation may be a precursor for NRH [15] in the transplant allograft and its presence on liver biopsy should trigger investigation for subtle vascular problems, that if corrected, could halt the development of NRH and INCPH [35].

In addition to the post-transplant state, several diseases, infections and toxins are associated with both sinusoidal dilatation and INCPH [14, 32, 33] and could suggest a continuum of disease progression. In other words, a liver with predominant, non-physiologic sinusoidal dilatation may represent a substrate primed for the development of INCPH. As such, the management of sinusoidal dilatation first involves recognition that bland sinusoidal dilatation on liver biopsy may be secondary to obstructive microvasculopathy from damaged sinusoidal endothelium. Second, the finding of sinusoidal dilatation should prompt an investigation for culprit diseases, infections, drugs and toxins, that if treated or avoided, could avert the progression of sinusoidal dilatation to INCPH.

## Peliosis Hepatis

Peliosis hepatis is hepatic sinusoidal disruption manifested by blood filled cavities throughout the liver, larger than those seen in cases of sinusoidal dilatation (ranging from 2mm to 3cm in diameter). The pattern of these cavities may be random throughout the liver or may be localized to a single lobe. There are two morphological types of peliosis: phlebectatic and parenchymal. In phlebectatic peliosis, the sinusoidal endothelium remains continuous and intact, and as such, this type may be considered a form of massive sinusoidal dilatation. In parenchymal peliosis, the sinusoidal architecture is disrupted and blood enters the parenchymal space. Radiographically, peliosis can have a highly variable appearance [36] and may often mimic hepatocellular carcinoma or hepatic metastases [37], however peliosis hepatis is known to be is ometabolic on PET-CT scan [38]. Nonetheless, liver biopsy is frequently undertaken demonstrating benign tissue [39]. Given the risk of hemorrhage with percutaneous intervention in the setting of peliosis hepatis [40], contrast enhanced ultrasound may prove helpful when there remains a diagnostic dilemma [41]. While some cases are idiopathic and deemed congenital, there are several known etiologies of acquired peliosis listed in Table 11.2 and described below.

## Etiologies of Peliosis

### *Infection*

Systemic bacterial infections with showering of bacteria into the circulation can cause bacillary peliosis, with microabcesses arising in the liver in a miliary pattern. Localized inflammatory response, followed by parenchymal cell loss via necrosis and apoptosis, leave large empty spaces which communicate with the sinusoids and result in blood-filled pools within the liver. The most cited form of miliary peliosis is in association with *Bartonella* sp. bloodstream infection(Bartonellosis) [42, 43], however disseminated tuberculosis [44] and syphilis [45] have also been implicated. Human immunodeficiency virus and acquired immunodeficiency syndrome predisposing to immunocompromised states with concomitant bacillary infections are often reported in association with peliosis hepatis [43].

### *Malignancy*

Numerous case reports have shown an association of peliosis hepatis with extrahepatic malignancies. Typically, liver imaging suggestive of metastatic disease leads to more extensive workup that subsequently shows peliosis hepatis without cancer involvement [46]. Prostate cancer [47], Hodgkin's lymphoma [48] and seminoma [49] have been described in association with hepatic peliosis. The pathophysiology of peliosis hepatis in such scenarios may be related to ectopic hormone production by the tumor.

## *Drug exposure*

Azathioprine is commonly implicated in hepatotoxicity and has been well documented to associate with peliosis hepatis [50]. Causality has been difficult to determine as often thiopurine analogs are taken with steroids which have also been associated with the development of peliosis hepatis [51]. Anabolic steroids [52, 53], endogenously produced steroids from tumors [54], pregnancy [55], oral contraceptives [56, 57] and tamoxifen [58] have all been linked to the development of peliosis hepatis suggesting that the underlying pathophysiology can be hormonally driven. Up to 20% of post-renal transplant patients develop biopsy-proven peliosis hepatis [59] however given the frequent use of thiopurine analogs and steroids in this population it cannot be concluded that the renal transplant itself is responsible for hepatic sinusoidal architectural changes.

## Management of Peliosis Hepatis

The management of peliosis hepatis is typically aimed at its sequelae. Treatment must be undertaken to avert catastrophic hepatic rupture in extensive peliosis hepatis arising from steroid hormone excess [52, 60, 61]. Hepatic artery embolization [62], partial hepatectomy [63], or orthotopic liver transplant [64] may be considered when large portions of the liver are affected by peliosis. No validated predictors of progression or rupture have been yet identified. When peliosis is secondary to a pharmacologic culprit, avoidance of the insulting agent is advised. Resolution of peliosis has been documented upon cessation of implicated medications [65]. Likewise, appropriate antibiotic therapy for bacillary peliosis can lead to radiographic resolution of peliotic lesions [36].

## Conclusions

Sinusoidal dilatation and peliosis hepatis are architectural disruptions of the hepatic sinusoid with a wide range of etiologies and sequelae. Sinusoidal dilatation in the absence of overt hepatic venous outflow abnormalities may represent silent microvasculopathy and should be considered as an early warning for the eventual development of INCPH. Thus, its diagnosis warrants further investigation for culprit diseases, infections and toxins. For peliosis hepatis, exposure to steroids and infections are commons culprit etiologies which can be avoided or treated, respectively. When peliosis hepatisis limited and idiopathic, management is typically expectant. In extreme cases, peliosislesions may be life threatening, requiring urgent vascular or surgical interventions including liver transplant.

# References


1. Vollmar B, Menger MD. The hepatic microcirculation: mechanistic contributions and therapeutic targets in liver injury and repair. Physiol Rev. 2009;89:1269–339.
2. Braet F, Wisse E. Structural and functional aspects of liver sinusoidal endothelial cell fenestrae: a review. Comp Hepatol. 2002;1:1.
3. Mitzner W. Hepatic outflow resistance, sinusoid pressure, and the vascular waterfall. Am J Physiol. 1974;227:513–9.
4. Groszmann RJ, Wongcharatrawee S. The hepatic venous pressure gradient: anything worth doing should be done right. Hepatology. 2004;39:280–2.
5. Bosch J, Abraldes JG, Berzigotti A, et al. The clinical use of HVPG measurements in chronic liver disease. Nat Rev Gastroenterol Hepatol. 2009;6:573–82.
6. Rockey DC. Hepatic blood flow regulation by stellate cells in normal and injured liver. Semin Liver Dis. 2001;21:337–49.
7. DeLeve LD. Liver sinusoidal endothelial cells in hepatic fibrosis. Hepatology. 2015;61:1740–6.
8. Straub AC, Stolz DB, Ross MA, et al. Arsenic stimulates sinusoidal endothelial cell capillarization and vessel remodeling in mouse liver. Hepatology. 2007;45:205–12.
9. Le Couteur DG, Fraser R, Cogger VC, et al. Hepatic pseudocapillarisation and atherosclerosis in ageing. Lancet. 2002;359:1612–5.
10. Bruguera M, Aranguibel F, Ros E, et al. Incidence and clinical significance of sinusoidal dilatation in liver biopsies. Gastroenterology. 1978;75:474–8.
11. Crocetti D, Palmieri A, Pedulla G, et al. Peliosis hepatis: personal experience and literature review. World J Gastroenterol. 2015;21:13188–94.
12. Miller DL, Zanolli CS, Gumucio JJ. Quantitative morphology of the sinusoids of the hepatic acinus. Quantimet analysis of rat liver. Gastroenterology. 1979;76:965–9.
13. Furlan A, Minervini MI, Borhani AA, et al. Hepatic sinusoidal dilatation: a review of causes with imaging-pathologic correlation. Semin Ultrasound CT MR. 2016;37:525–32.
14. Sunjaya DB, Ramos GP, Braga Neto MB, et al. Isolated hepatic non-obstructive sinusoidal dilatation, 20-year single center experience. World J Hepatol. 2018;10:417–24.
15. Kakar S, Kamath PS, Burgart LJ. Sinusoidal dilatation and congestion in liver biopsy: is it always due to venous outflow impairment? Arch Pathol Lab Med. 2004;128:901–4.
16. Louie CY, Pham MX, Daugherty TJ, et al. The liver in heart failure: a biopsy and explant series of the histopathologic and laboratory findings with a particular focus on pre-cardiac transplant evaluation. Mod Pathol. 2015;28:932–43.
17. Gonzalez RS, Gilger MA, Huh WJ, et al. The spectrum of histologic findings in hepatic outflow obstruction. Arch Pathol Lab Med. 2017;141:98–103.
18. Hidaka M, Eguchi S. Budd-Chiari syndrome: Focus on surgical treatment. Hepatol Res. 2017;47:142–8.
19. Rubbia-Brandt L. Sinusoidal obstruction syndrome. Clin Liver Dis. 2010;14:651–68.
20. Fan CQ, Crawford JM. Sinusoidal obstruction syndrome (hepatic veno-occlusive disease). J Clin Exp Hepatol. 2014;4:332–46.
21. Wang T, Ong P, Roscioli T, et al. Hepatic veno-occlusive disease with immunodeficiency (VODI): first reported case in the U.S. and identification of a unique mutation in Sp110. Clin Immunol. 2012;145:102–7.
22. Bakshi N, Rastogi A, Pamecha V, et al. Sinusoidal dilatation and congestion in post-transplant liver biopsies from patients presenting with transaminitis. J Clin Pathol. 2020; https://doi.org/10.1136/jclinpath-2020-206870.
23. Peralta C, Jimenez-Castro MB, Gracia-Sancho J. Hepatic ischemia and reperfusion injury: effects on the liver sinusoidal milieu. J Hepatol. 2013;59:1094–106.
24. Vreuls CP, Driessen A, Olde Damink SW, et al. Sinusoidal obstruction syndrome (SOS): A light and electron microscopy study in human liver. Micron. 2016;84:17–22.
25. Cheuk DK, Chiang AK, Ha SY, et al. Interventions for prophylaxis of hepatic veno-occlusive disease in people undergoing haematopoietic stem cell transplantation. Cochrane Database Syst Rev. 2015;(5):CD009311.

26. Richardson P, Aggarwal S, Topaloglu O, et al. Systematic review of defibrotide studies in the treatment of veno-occlusive disease/sinusoidal obstruction syndrome (VOD/SOS). Bone Marrow Transplant. 2019;54:1951–62.
27. Campos-Varela I, Castells L, Dopazo C, et al. Transjugular intrahepatic portosystemic shunt for the treatment of sinusoidal obstruction syndrome in a liver transplant recipient and review of the literature. Liver Transpl. 2012;18:201–5.
28. Zakaria N, Knisely A, Portmann B, et al. Acute sickle cell hepatopathy represents a potential contraindication for percutaneous liver biopsy. Blood. 2003;101:101–3.
29. Marzano C, Cazals-Hatem D, Rautou PE, et al. The significance of nonobstructive sinusoidal dilatation of the liver: Impaired portal perfusion or inflammatory reaction syndrome. Hepatology. 2015;62:956–63.
30. Saadoun D, Cazals-Hatem D, Denninger MH, et al. Association of idiopathic hepatic sinusoidal dilatation with the immunological features of the antiphospholipid syndrome. Gut. 2004;53:1516–9.
31. Balazs M. Sinusoidal dilatation of the liver in patients on oral contraceptives. Electron microscopical study of 14 cases. Exp Pathol. 1988;35:231–7.
32. Gerlag PG, Lobatto S, Driessen WM, et al. Hepatic sinusoidal dilatation with portal hypertension during azathioprine treatment after kidney transplantation. J Hepatol. 1985;1:339–48.
33. De Gottardi A, Rautou PE, Schouten J, et al. Porto-sinusoidal vascular disease: proposal and description of a novel entity. Lancet Gastroenterol Hepatol. 2019;4:399–411.
34. Devarbhavi H, Abraham S, Kamath PS. Significance of nodular regenerative hyperplasia occurring de novo following liver transplantation. Liver Transpl. 2007;13:1552–6.
35. Krasinskas A. The significance of nodular regenerative hyperplasia in the transplanted liver. Liver Transpl. 2007;13:1496–7.
36. Iannaccone R, Federle MP, Brancatelli G, et al. Peliosis hepatis: spectrum of imaging findings. AJR Am J Roentgenol. 2006;187:W43–52.
37. Iwata T, Adachi K, Takahashi M. Peliosis hepatis mimicking malignant hypervascular tumors. J Gastrointest Surg. 2017;21:1095–8.
38. Seo M, Lee SH, Han S, et al. Peliosis hepatis shows isometabolism on (18)F-FDG PET/CT: two case reports. Nucl Med Mol Imaging. 2014;48:309–12.
39. Levin D, Hod N, Anconina R, et al. Peliosis hepatis simulating metastatic liver disease on FDG PET/CT. Clin Nucl Med. 2018;43:e234–6.
40. Cohen GS, Ball DS, Boyd-Kranis R, et al. Peliosis hepatis mimicking hepatic abscess: fatal outcome following percutaneous drainage. J Vasc Interv Radiol. 1994;5:643–5.
41. Loizides A, Glodny B, Zoller H, et al. Contrast enhanced ultrasound of a rare case of Peliosis hepatis. Med Ultrason. 2017;19:114–6.
42. Relman DA, Falkow S, LeBoit PE, et al. The organism causing bacillary angiomatosis, peliosis hepatis, and fever and bacteremia in immunocompromised patients. N Engl J Med. 1991;324:1514.
43. Mohle-Boetani JC, Koehler JE, Berger TG, et al. Bacillary angiomatosis and bacillary peliosis in patients infected with human immunodeficiency virus: clinical characteristics in a case-control study. Clin Infect Dis. 1996;22:794–800.
44. Sanz-Canalejas L, Gomez-Mampaso E, Canton-Moreno R, et al. Peliosis hepatis due to disseminated tuberculosis in a patient with AIDS. Infection. 2014;42:185–9.
45. Chen JF, Chen WX, Zhang HY, et al. Peliosis and gummatous syphilis of the liver: a case report. World J Gastroenterol. 2008;14:1961–3.
46. Wannesson L, Chigrinova E, Raditchkova M, et al. Peliosis hepatis in cancer patients mimicking infection and metastases. Onkologie. 2009;32:54–6.
47. Hidaka H, Ohbu M, Nakazawa T, et al. Peliosis hepatis disseminated rapidly throughout the liver in a patient with prostate cancer: a case report. J Med Case Rep. 2015;9:194.
48. Kleger A, Bommer M, Kunze M, et al. First reported case of disease: peliosis hepatis as cardinal symptom of Hodgkin's lymphoma. Oncologist. 2009;14:1088–94.
49. Engel P, Jacobsen GK. An unusual case of retroperitoneal seminoma and fatal peliosis of the liver. Histopathology. 1993;22:379–82.
50. Calabrese E, Hanauer SB. Assessment of non-cirrhotic portal hypertension associated with thiopurine therapy in inflammatory bowel disease. J Crohns Colitis. 2011;5:48–53.

51. Lorcerie B, Grobost O, Lalu-Fraisse A, et al. Peliosis hepatis in dermatomyositis treated with azathioprine and corticoids. Rev Med Interne. 1990;11:25–8.
52. Ishak KG. Hepatic lesions caused by anabolic and contraceptive steroids. Semin Liver Dis. 1981;1:116–28.
53. Naeim F, Copper PH, Semion AA. Peliosis hepatis. Possible etiologic role of anabolic steroids. Arch Pathol. 1973;95:284–5.
54. Willen H, Willen R, Gad A, et al. Peliosis hepatis as a result of endogenous steroid hormone production. Virchows Arch A Pathol Anat Histol. 1979;383:233–40.
55. Cimbanassi S, Aseni P, Mariani A, et al. Spontaneous hepatic rupture during pregnancy in a patient with peliosis hepatis. Ann Hepatol. 2015;14:553–8.
56. Lockhat D, Katz SS, Lisbona R, et al. Oral contraceptives and liver disease. Can Med Assoc J. 1981;124:993–9.
57. Perarnau JM, Bacq Y. Hepatic vascular involvement related to pregnancy, oral contraceptives, and estrogen replacement therapy. Semin Liver Dis. 2008;28:315–27.
58. Loomus GN, Aneja P, Bota RA. A case of peliosis hepatis in association with tamoxifen therapy. Am J Clin Pathol. 1983;80:881–3.
59. Yu CY, Chang LC, Chen LW, et al. Peliosis hepatis complicated by portal hypertension following renal transplantation. World J Gastroenterol. 2014;20:2420–5.
60. Choi SK, Jin JS, Cho SG, et al. Spontaneous liver rupture in a patient with peliosis hepatis: a case report. World J Gastroenterol. 2009;15:5493–7.
61. Spormann H, Willgeroth C, Tautenhahn P. Peliosis hepatis with liver rupture. Zentralbl Allg Pathol. 1985;130:545–50.
62. Suzuki S, Suzuki H, Mochida Y, et al. Liver hemorrhage due to idiopathic peliosis hepatis successfully treated with hepatic artery embolization. Int Surg. 2011;96:310–5.
63. Pan W, Hong HJ, Chen YL, et al. Surgical treatment of a patient with peliosis hepatis: a case report. World J Gastroenterol. 2013;19:2578–82.
64. Hyodo M, Mogensen AM, Larsen PN, et al. Idiopathic extensive peliosis hepatis treated with liver transplantation. J Hepatobiliary Pancreat Surg. 2004;11:371–4.
65. Kim SB, Kim DK, Byun SJ, et al. Peliosis hepatis presenting with massive hepatomegaly in a patient with idiopathic thrombocytopenic purpura. Clin Mol Hepatol. 2015;21:387–92.

# Chapter 12
# Hypoxic Hepatitis

Hongqun Liu, Ki Tae Yoon, and Samuel S. Lee

## Introduction

All organs including the liver depend on the heart for adequate perfusion. Thus, cardiovascular dysfunction of diverse etiologies can result in hepatopathy due to either inadequate perfusion/ischemia (so-called 'forward failure') or passive congestion ('backward failure'), or a combination of these two factors. Both types of cardiac-origin hepatopathy comprise the syndrome that the French call 'foie cardiaque' [1, 2]. Indeed, it has been suggested that this elegant French term be adopted by the international community to recognize that much of the pioneering work in 'foie cardique' is found in the Francophone literature [3].

Forward failure hepatopathy also comprises syndromes with names such as shock liver or hypoxic hepatitis. Histological patterns in hypoxic hepatitis have been recognized for more than a century. Centrilobularor zone 3 necrosis was first noted in 1901 based on 1190 autopsies [4]. In 1979, Bynum and colleagues noted the same pattern of necrosis in 7 patients with cardiac failure; these patients had no evidence of viral or drug injury. These authors further retrospectively reviewed 15 liver biopsies and noted that all patients with notable (>5 times the upper limit of normal, ULN) transaminase elevations had centrilobular necrosis. They termed this entity (centrilobular necrosis + hypertransaminasemia) as 'hypoxic hepatitis' (HH) [5]. The underlying conditions that lead to HH include cardiovascular dysfunction, respiratory failure and septic shock. HH occurs in very sick patients; itis not

H. Liu · S. S. Lee (✉)
Liver Unit, Cumming School of Medicine, University of Calgary, Calgary, Canada
e-mail: hliu@ucalgary.ca; samlee@ucalgary.ca

K. T. Yoon
Division of Gastroenterology, Pusan National University Yangsan Hospital, Yangsan, South Korea
e-mail: ktyoon@pusan.ac.kr

© Springer Nature Switzerland AG 2022
D. Valla et al. (eds.), *Vascular Disorders of the Liver*,
https://doi.org/10.1007/978-3-030-82988-9_12

uncommon in patients in intensive care units (ICU) and such patients usually have poorer outcomes compared to those without HH. Hypoxic hepatitis heralds a high mortality rate.

Congestive hepatopathy arises due to different etiologies such as cardiac valvular disease, cardiomyopathy, myocardial infarction and other acute or chronic heart diseases. Patients with congestive hepatopathy have elevated central venous pressure, with resultant increased resistance of blood outflow through the hepatic veins [6] (Fig. 12.1).

The definition of congestive hepatopathy is also inconsistent in the literature. Hilscher and Lightsey defined congestive hepatopathy as a chronic passive congestion of the liver underlying heart failure [7, 8]. We believe that congestive hepatopathy should be classified into three types, (1) acute: symptoms less than 2 weeks duration and no prior cardiac disease; (2) chronic: known, compensated cardiac disease; and (3) acute on chronic: prior cardiac disease with acute decompensation over the preceding 2 weeks [6].

This chapter concentrates on hypoxic hepatitis of which 50% is due to acute cardiac failure/dysfunction [9]. However, many cases of hypoxic hepatitis are caused by not purely forward or backward failure, but a combination of these two factors.

## Definition

The definition of hypoxic hepatitis, also referred to in the literature as "ischemic hepatitis" or "shock liver," is diverse. The basic concept is an acute hepatic injury manifested histologically as centrilobular or zone 3 liver cell necrosis, due to

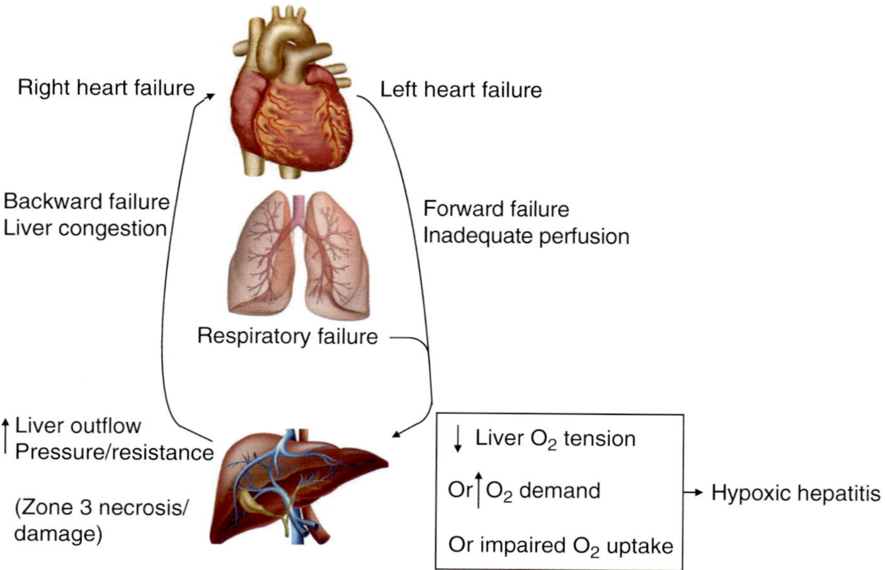


**Fig. 12.1** Pathogenic mechanisms of hypoxic hepatitis

insufficient oxygen delivery/uptake to/by the hepatocytes [9]. The suggested diagnostic criteria include 3 conditions: (1) a compatible clinical setting, such as cardiac or respiratory failure; (2) abrupt, significant but transient elevations of serum aminotransferase levels [7, 9]; and (3) exclusion of other causes of hepatocellular necrosis, such as viral hepatitis or drug-induced liver injury [7, 9, 10]. To date, the most frequently used diagnostic method is the serum aminotransferase levels [11]. However, there is no universally accepted cut-off value of transaminase elevation that would be diagnostic for HH. There is wide variability in the literature with some advocating a cut-off value>5 times [9] the upper limit of normal (ULN), and others>10 times ULN [7]. Some investigators have even advocated using a cut-off aminotransferase value of >20 times ULN [12].

Tamiyama and colleagues suggested that transaminase elevations exceeding 2.5 times the baseline within 24 h of admission could be a diagnostic method for defining HH [13]. However, this definition may be imprecise because the patient's baseline aminotransferases will be crucially affected by the degree of liver injury at time of admission, i.e., how far along the disease course the patient presents to hospital.

Most studies used the three criteria above to diagnose hypoxic hepatitis. Liver biopsy is not required for the HH diagnosis [2, 9, 11]. However, if the diagnosis is in doubt, liver biopsy is useful for definitive diagnosis [14]. It will show the typical appearance of zone 3 necrosis and collapse. A typical HH liver is shown in Fig. 12.2.

The term "ischemic hepatitis" has in the past been used interchangeably with hypoxic hepatitis. In patients with toxic/septic shock, oxygen delivery is not reduced, but rather the increased tissue oxygen requirement unbalances the oxygen supply/demand relationship. Thus, another mechanism that causes hypoxic

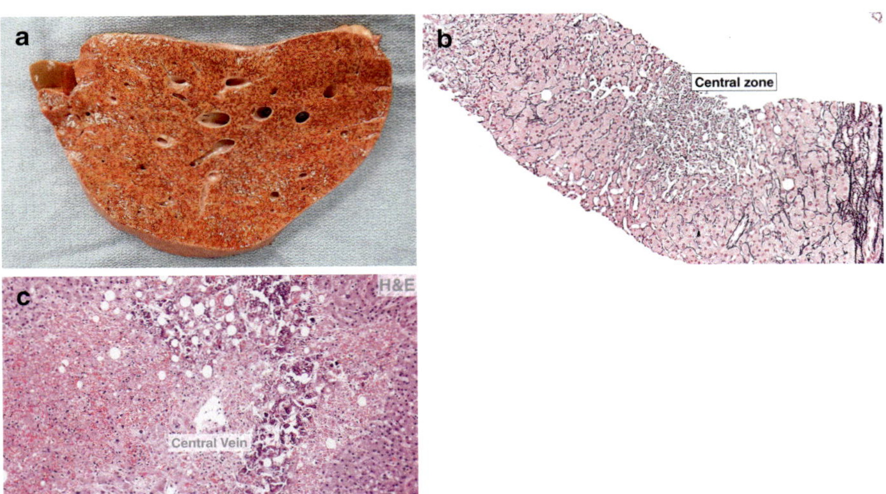


**Fig. 12.2** Liver tissue in a case of hypoxic hepatitis. (**a**) Autopsy specimen showing the classical 'nutmeg liver' pattern of a 75-year old male with acute MI and chronic congestive heart failure. (photo courtesy of Dr. Adrian Box, Histopathology Dept, Calgary Laboratory Services). (**b**) Reticulin stain showing zone 3 collapse/necrosis. (courtesy of Drs Ksenia Chezar and Konstantin Koro, Histopathology Dept, Calgary Laboratory Services). (**c**) H&E stain showing zone 3 necrosis and apoptosis. (courtesy of Drs K. Chezar and K. Koro)

hepatitis is that the liver is unable to use oxygen properly. Another term, "shock liver" is also improper because only 50% of HH patients experience a shock state [15].

In HH due to acute or chronic respiratory failure, liver hypoxia is mainly due to severe hypoxemia. Therefore, 'hypoxic hepatitis' should replace the terms "shock liver" or "ischemic hepatitis" and be the preferred term for this entity [12].

## Epidemiology

The incidence of HH is not completely clear. The large variability in the literature is due to numerous factors including divergent diagnostic criteria and nature of the studied population. Most studies have examined critically-ill patients admitted to intensive care units. Tapper et al. performed a meta-analysis, that included 1782 cases and found that the HH rate is 0.2% of total hospital admissions, 2.5% of ICU admissions and 40% of those with aminotransferase levels>10 times ULN. The HH rate is 78% of those who had an acute cardiac event and 23% for those with sepsis [16].

Because the majority of the HH cases are in a ICU setting, it is useful to know the frequency of HH in ICU patients. However, the reported incidence of HH in ICU patients is variable. One of the reasons for the inconsistency is the definition cut-off value of aminotransferases. The study of Aboelsoud et al. reported HH in 1.5% of ICU patients, but their transaminase definition cut-off was ≥20 ULN [17]. The incidence in the study of Tapper and coworkers is 2.5%, but their transaminase cut-off value was 10 ULN [16], Van Den Broecke used transaminases>5 ULN as the cut-off value, and the incidence in their study is 4% [9]. However, the diagnostic rate is not always inversely correlated to the cut-off value of transaminases. Fuhrmann and coworkers used 20-fold ULN transaminase as part of the diagnostic criteria, and reported a HH rate in their ICU cohort was 11% (118/1066) [18] which is the highest reported rate in the literature.

## Pathophysiology

Hypoxic hepatitis is due to insufficient liver oxygenation which causes liver hypoxia and tissue necrosis. There are 3 mechanisms of HH: (1) right heart failure (backward failure); (2) left heart failure or respiratory failure which results in decreased perfusion and/or insufficient oxygen supply to the liver (forward failure) and (3) an unbalanced hepatic oxygen supply/demand relationship. About 70–83% of HH patients have reduced cardiac function and 13–32% of HH patients have septic shock [19].

Hepatic blood flow accounts for about 25% of the cardiac output [20] and the liver oxygen consumption accounts for about 20% of whole-body oxygen consumption [21]. The liver, in contrast to other organs, has two afferent blood supplies, from the hepatic artery and portal vein. The dual blood supply maintains adequate liver perfusion in many different situations. Hepatic artery blood flow is regulated by variety of factors including nerves and blood-borne factors reaching the arterial resistance sites. The portal venous system is dependent on mesenteric circulation and the gradient between portal and hepatic venous pressures.

Blood from the hepatic artery contributes to approximately 20–25% of the total liver blood flow; the remainder is supplied by the portal vein [22]. The arterial blood is rich in oxygen and approximately 50% of oxygen consumed in the liver is from arterial blood. The portal vein has no valve and is a low pressure/low resistance vessel. Besides the rich content of nutritive elements, portal venous blood is only partially oxygen-desaturated and thus supplies the other half of the liver's oxygen supply [20].

According to Rapaport's acinar concept of microvascular anatomy, there are 3 zones in the liver lobule. Zone 1 has the highest oxygen tension as the hepatic arterioles and portal venules flow into this zone. Blood then flows through the sinusoids (zone 2) and into zone 3 (drained by the terminal hepatic vein or central vein). Thus zone 3 enjoys the lowest oxygen tension and consequently is the most vulnerable to hypoxemia.

The oxygen delivery to most organs depends on the regulation of blood perfusion. However, the total blood flow to the liver is relatively fixed. Despite this, the liver is relatively well-protected from ischemic injury through at least three mechanisms [21]. Firstly, it has the dual blood supply from both an arterial and venous system, so it has a 'backup' vascular system in case of disruption in blood flow. Secondly, the sinusoids are highly permeable which increases the oxygen diffusion ability to the hepatocytes. It is estimated that up to 90% of the oxygen is extracted [23]. Thirdly, hepatic arterioles dilate when portal vein blood flow is decreased, the so-called "hepatic arterial buffer response" [24]. The mechanism underlying the buffer response is mediated through the vasodilator adenosine [24]. Normally, portal blood flow quickly washes away local endogenous adenosine produced in the hepatic arterial resistance site. If portal flow diminishes, this allows accumulation of the local adenosine concentration around arteriolar resistance sites, leading to arterial dilation [24].

Because of the complexity of liver circulation, the pathophysiology of hypoxic hepatitis is also complicated. Lightsey and Rockey proposed a "two-hit" theory [7]. The first hit is decreased blood supply, typically because of right-sided heart failure which elevates hepatic vein pressure and reduces the pressure gradient between portal and hepatic venous (backward failure). This decreases the blood supply and places the liver at risk for hypoxic injury. The second hit is the systemic hypotension resulting from acute cardiac, circulatory, or respiratory failure (forward failure). Thus, the simplified two-hit hypothesis is a sequential combination of backward, then forward failure.

See to and colleagues compared HH patients with nonhepatic trauma patients whose systolic pressures were lower than 75 mmHg. They suggested that hypotension *per se* does not cause HH. In their study, blood pressure was undetectable for prolonged periods of time in several patients; one patient even had no pulse for more than 30 minutes. However, these nonhepatic trauma patients had normal serum aminotransferase levels throughout their hospital stay [25]. Another scenario that decreases the liver blood supply in patients in ICU is the administration of vasoconstrictors such as catecholamines. Norepinephrine and epinephrine divert blood flow away from the mesenteric circulation and thus decrease microcirculatory blood flow in the gastrointestinal tract which results in reduction of portal venous flow [26]. Furthermore, catecholamines may deteriorate hepatocellular function via induction of inflammation [27].

Besides the decreased oxygen supply to the liver, the increased oxygen consumption of the hepatocytes and inability of the liver to extract oxygen also likely play a role. In septic shock-related hypoxic hepatitis, the hyperthermia increases oxygen consumption and the liver oxygen uptake is low [28]. The mechanism underlying the inability of the liver to extract oxygen in septic patients remains unclear. Endotoxins and proinflammatory cytokines may affect the cellular metabolism and microcirculatory function. Oxygen metabolism is also disturbed in mitochondria of hepatocytes. Septic shock damages the mitochondria and decreases ATP production [29]. The increased oxygen demand at the hepatocyte level combined with the disturbance of ATP production can induce hepatocyte death.

Although HH can afflict persons with no pre-existing liver disease, the presence of any chronic hepatopathy, particularly cirrhosis, is likely to exacerbate the clinical features and severity of hypoxic hepatitis. This is because the liver microcirculation in cirrhosis is already significantly deranged, making the cirrhotic liver more susceptible to injury from even relatively modest cardiorespiratory perturbations. In particular, the Wanless 'extinction' hypothesis of cirrhosis contends that much of the parenchymal damage is caused by micro thrombi and severe distortion of the micro- and eventually, macro-vasculature [30]. Moreover, there are significant perturbations of oxygen metabolism in the cirrhotic patient. Moreau and colleagues showed that cirrhotic patients seem to have a latent ischemic state, similar to patients with septic shock: increasing oxygen delivery to these patients results in increased oxygen uptake, as if the tissues are 'starved' of oxygen [31]. The response of the normal person to increased oxygen delivery would be unchanged oxygen uptake.

Several studies confirm that the cirrhotic liver is more prone to HH than normal livers [13, 15, 18]. For example, in the study of Fuhrmann and colleagues, of 1066 consecutive ICU admissions, HH was found in 118 patients (11%), but cirrhosis was present in only 6% of the 948 without HH whereas it was present in 14% of those with HH [18].

## Clinical Manifestations

The majority of HH patients are older. Chang et al. reported a mean age of 61.9 ± 16.6 years [32]; See to et al. noted a mean age of 51 ± 17 [25]. A meta-analysis showed a mean age of 64.2 years (95% confidence interval, 61.4–66.9)

[16]. Males are more affected than females. Aboelsoud et al. reported that 58% of their cases are male; this percentage is 57% in Chang's study [32], 67% in Henrion's study [12], 71% in Seeto's report [25], and 60% in Van Den Broecke's study. The only outlier is the series of Taylor and co-workers who reported a 67% female preponderance [33].

Since HH is found in critically ill patients, the co-morbidities include heart failure, chronic respiratory failure and septic shock or other serious states of hemodynamic instability [17]. Clinical presentations are dominated by the underlying conditions. Heart failure manifests as lower cardiac output and hypotension (systolic blood pressure < 90 mmHg [34, 35]). Patients with right ventricular failure may have dyspnea, tender hepatomegaly, ankle edema, and hepatojugular reflux [12] and right upper abdominal pain because of the congested and enlarged liver [36]. Chest x-ray shows pulmonary edema in left ventricular failure. Respiratory failure causes severe hypoxemia. Depending on etiology of respiratory failure, patients may present with occupational respiratory diseases such as silicosis and coal-miner pneumoconiosis, others may have chronic obstructive pulmonary disease (COPD) [37] and *cor pulmonale* [38]. Severe hepatocellular hypoxia may also be caused by significant obstructive sleep apnea [39, 40].

Septic shock manifests itself as infection or positive blood culture plus more than two of the following symptoms: (1). (temperature > 38 °C) or hypothermia (temperature < 36 °C); (2). tachycardia (heart rate > 90/min), (3). tachypnea (respiratory rate > 20/min) or hyperventilation ($PaCO_2$ < 32 mmHg), and (4). White blood cell count>12,000 or < 4000/$mm^3$ or > 10% immature forms. Sepsis-induced hypotension is refractory to treatment: adequate fluid resuscitation or vasopressor may not increase blood pressure [41]. Encephalopathy is not uncommon in HH patients. The encephalopathy may be due to hyperammonemia [42] and/or cerebral malperfusion [36].

The liver injury markers such as AST, ALT, lactate dehydrogenase *(LDH)*, and prothrombin time-international normalized ratio (INR) show sudden and significant increases following the hypoxicinsult to the liver. Among these markers, AST is the most obvious and useful marker for the diagnosis of HH. It is estimated that 57% of the patients with extreme elevations of serum AST (>1000 U/L) have HH [16]. Moreover, our study showed that patients with acute cardiac dysfunction, the aminotransferases were correlated strongly and positively with the right-sided cardiac and hepatic venous pressures; patients with centrilobular and periportal damage had higher HVPGs [6].

## Diagnosis

The diagnosis of HH is based on three widely accepted criteria: (1) compatible clinical setting, such as heart failure, circulatory or respiratory failure; (2) sudden, significant, but transient rise in plasma aminotransferase levels [7, 9]; and (3) exclusion of other causes of hepatocellular necrosis, especially viral hepatitis or drug-induced hepatopathy [7, 9, 10].

A characteristic liver enzyme pattern of HH is that AST is higher than ALT at the onset of the disease, and after reaching peak value, AST declines faster than ALT. Thus, the ratio of AST/ALT is reversed from >1 to <1 within 3 days. This quick rise and subsequent fall in aminotransferases and reversal of the AST/ALT ratio in a compatible clinical setting should raise a suspicion of HH. Aboelsoud and colleagues [17] documented typical patterns of liver chemistry elevations in their cohort of 565 ptatients with HH (Fig. 12.3). The definition cutoff value of AST is not universally settled (from 5 to 20 times ULN). Van Den Broecke and colleagues proposed that AST/ALT, INR and creatinine comprise a triad of biochemical abnormalities that may suggest the HH diagnosis [9].

HH is usually a clinical diagnosis in practice. When the diagnosis is not clear, liver biopsy may be necessary to demonstrate the characteristic pattern of zone 3 necrosis [23].

The differential diagnosis of very high serum transaminase includes viral hepatitis, toxin- or drug-induced hepatitis, autoimmune hepatitis, or liver trauma. In patients with viral hepatitis, the high serum transaminase levels decrease slowly because the virus is a sustained pathogenic factor; high serum transaminase levels are decreased faster in the patients with HH and toxin- or drug-induced disease if the insult factors are eliminated. The patients with toxin or drug-induced liver injury have the history of inciting agent usage. Autoimmune hepatitis is usually accompanied by characteristic patterns of abnormal autoantibodies such as anti-smooth muscle and anti-nuclear antibodies as well as pronounced hypergamma-globulinemia. Moreover, an increase in INR, serum creatinine and LDH support HH diagnosis [43].

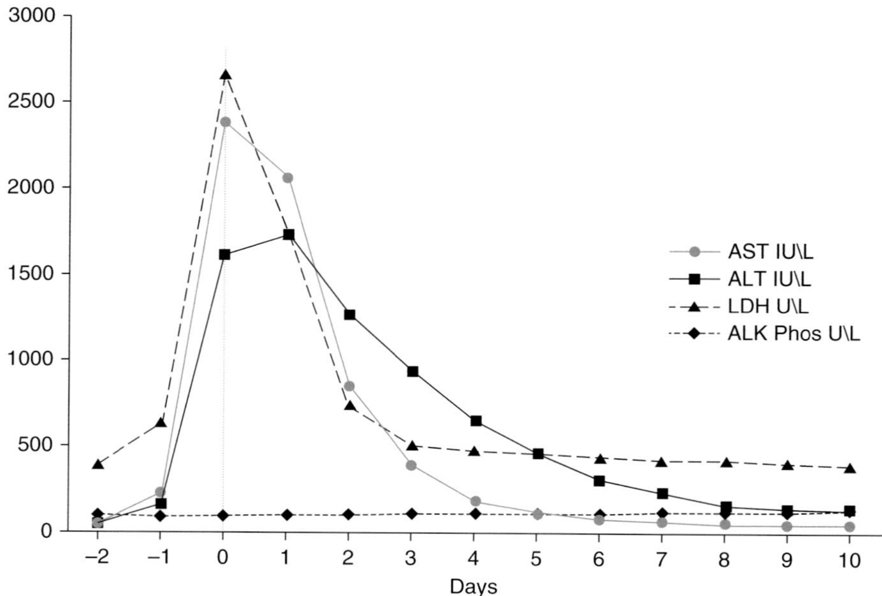


**Fig. 12.3** Pattern of liver biochemistry tests in patients with hypoxic hepatitis (reproduced from reference 17; Aboelsoud M et al.)

## Management

There is no randomized controlled clinical trial of HH management. Therefore, suggested management according to our literature review is based on expert opinion and logical presumptions.

HH should be treated with cardiorespiratory support in an intensive-care setting. Optimization of oxygenation and mechanical ventilation are the mainstays of such ICU care. Since HH is due to different conditions such as cardio-circulatory failure, respiratory dysfunction and septic shock, it follows that management must primarily be directed to resolution or treatment of the underlying or precipitating condition. Heart disease such as acute myocardial infarction should be treated accordingly, such as anti-platelet therapy, thrombolysis, heparin and primary angioplasty [36].

The treatment of patients with septic shock starts with appropriate antibiotic therapy. Hemodynamic treatment should include the optimization of volume with isotonic saline to increase the central venous pressure to 8–12 mmHg. Norepinephrine should be used to adjust the mean arterial pressure to 65 mmHg and above. Positive inotropic agents should be used if the cardiac output is low. The goal of hemodynamic resuscitation is to keep the urinary output higher than 0.5 mL/ kg/h [44].

HH often is complicated with abnormal glucose metabolism, hypoglycemia or hyperglycemia. Hypoglycemia was defined as blood glucos level<40 mg/ dL. Fuhrmann et al. found that 14% of HH patients developed spontaneous hypoglycemia (glucose 31 ± 8 mg/dL). These patients need continuous glucose infusions to maintain the blood glucose level in the normal range [41]. Gitlin and Serio found that 6 out of 9 patients in their study had abnormal serum glucose levels, 3 of whom required insulin therapy [45]. The rational management goal of hyperglycemia control should aim for glucose<150 mg/dl [36].

Hyperammonemia is another metabolic abnormality in patients with HH [42]. However, the exact pathogenic role of hyperammonemia in encephalopathy in HH patients remains unclear because encephalopathy may also result from sepsis or cerebral malperfusion. That said, many authorities advocate measures to reduce hyperammonemia in hypoxic hepatitis. There is some controversy on this point. Acharya and coworkers showed in a randomized controlled study that the hypoammonemic drug L-ornithine L-aspartate (LOLA) does not benefit HH patients with acute liver failure [46]. The application of agents reducing blood ammonia in HH patients need further study. Molecular Adsorbents Recirculatory System (MARS) is designed to remove protein-bound and water-soluble toxic metabolites from the blood stream. Drolz and colleagues reported a case of a patient with severe HH successfully treated with MARS [19].

## Prognosis

HH is associated with poor outcome, the overall mortality after the onset is about 50–60% in one month [19]. Some markers, such as AST, LDH, INR [41], jaundice, and arterial ammonia etc., predict the poor outcomes. The peak AST levels are associated with the severity of illness scores (The Simplified Acute Physiology *Score,* SAPS-II); patient with higher peak AST level has a higher illness scores and the scale of AST increase is significantly correlated with 28-day mortality [9]. New onset of jaundice during HH is correlated with an increased frequency of complications for the patients who survived the acute event of HH. (54% with jaundice versus 35% without jaundice; P < 0.05), especially infections, renal and GI complications. Compared to patients without jaundice, one-year survival rate is significantly lower in those with jaundice (8% vs 25%, P < 0.05) [47]. Drolz et al. found that arterial ammonia levels at admission were independently associated with hepatic encephalopathy (p < 0.01) and peak arterial ammonia concentration is an independent predictor of 28-day mortality in patients with HH [42]. Another study demonstrated that a hyperphosphatemia at admission and more advanced encephalopathy (3/4) are independent and significant predictors of poor outcomes in weeks of HH onset [33]. Unmeasured anions are indices of metabolic acidosis. The strong ion gap (SIG) is a quantitative measure of unmeasured anions. SIG values are positively correlated with AST and ALT. The elevated Unmeasured anions may indicate tissue damage in HH patients and are associated with mortality [48]. All the above indices represent the liver damage. Indocyanine green plasma disappearance rate (ICG-PDR) represents the functional liver mass. Horvatits and coworkers compared the diagnostic accuracies of sequential organ failure assessment (SOFA), arterial serum lactate, AST levels, INR and ICG-PDR. They found that in patients with HH, ICG-PDR is the best predictor of 28-day mortality [49].

## Conclusion

Hypoxic hepatitis is not uncommon in intensive care units. It has a high mortality rate, approximately 50% within the first month. The diagnosis is based on a triad: underlying clinical condition, sudden and sharp, transient rise in plasma transaminase levels, and exclusion of other causes of hepatocellular necrosis. Management strategies focus on treating the underlying condition and trying to prevent the complications.

## References


1. Tricot R, Benhamou JP, Guillemot R. Urbanczyk a: [hemodynamics of the cardiac liver]. Pathol Biol. 1962;10:1361–4.
2. Mirouze D, Michel H. The liver in heart failure (author's transl). Gastroenterol Clin Biol. 1982;6(2):143–7.
3. Lee SS. 'Foie cardiaque': a new name for an old syndrome? Liver Int. 2008;28(6):755–6.
4. Mallory FB. Necroses of the liver. J Med Res. 1901;6(1):264–80.
5. Bynum TE, Boitnott JK, Maddrey WC. Ischemic hepatitis. Dig Dis Sci. 1979;24(2):129–35.

6. Myers RP, Cerini R, Sayegh R, Moreau R, Degott C, Lebrec D, Lee SS. Cardiac hepatopathy: clinical, hemodynamic, and histologic characteristics and correlations. Hepatology. 2003;37(2):393–400.
7. Lightsey JM, Rockey DC. Current concepts in ischemic hepatitis. Curr Opin Gastroenterol. 2017;33(3):158–63.
8. Hilscher MSW. Congestive hepatopathy. Clin Liver Dis. 2016;8(1):68–71.
9. Van den Broecke A, Van Coile L, Decruyenaere A, Colpaert K, Benoit D, Van Vlierberghe H, Decruyenaere J. Epidemiology, causes, evolution and outcome in a single-center cohort of 1116 critically ill patients with hypoxic hepatitis. Ann Intensive Care. 2018;8(1):15.
10. Ciobanu AO, Gherasim L. Ischemic hepatitis – Intercorrelated pathology. Maedica (Buchar). 2018;13(1):5–11.
11. Jung C, Fuernau G, Eitel I, Desch S, Schuler G, Kelm M, Adams V, Thiele H. Incidence, laboratory detection and prognostic relevance of hypoxic hepatitis in cardiogenic shock. Clin Res Cardiol. 2017;106(5):341–9.
12. Henrion J, Schapira M, Luwaert R, Colin L, Delannoy A, Heller FR. Hypoxic hepatitis: clinical and hemodynamic study in 142 consecutive cases. Medicine (Baltimore). 2003;82(6):392–406.
13. Kamiyama T, Miyakawa H, Tajiri K, Marumo F, Sato C. Ischemic hepatitis in cirrhosis. Clinical features and prognostic implications. J Clin Gastroenterol. 1996;22(2):126–30.
14. Henrion J, Schapira M, Heller FR. Ischemic hepatitis: the need for precise criteria. J Clin Gastroenterol. 1996;23(4):305.
15. Henrion J. Hypoxic hepatitis. Liver Int. 2012;32(7):1039–52.
16. Tapper EB, Sengupta N, Bonder A. The incidence and outcomes of ischemic hepatitis: a systematic review with meta-analysis. Am J Med. 2015;128(12):1314–21.
17. Aboelsoud MM, Javaid AI, Al-Qadi MO, Lewis JH. Hypoxic hepatitis – its biochemical profile, causes and risk factors of mortality in critically-ill patients: a cohort study of 565 patients. J Crit Care. 2017;41:9–15.
18. Fuhrmann V, Kneidinger N, Herkner H, Heinz G, Nikfardjam M, Bojic A, Schellongowski P, Angermayr B, Schoniger-Hekele M, Madl C, et al. Impact of hypoxic hepatitis on mortality in the intensive care unit. Intensive Care Med. 2011;37(8):1302–10.
19. Drolz A, Saxa R, Scherzer T, Fuhrmann V. Extracorporeal artificial liver support in hypoxic liver injury. Liver Int. 2011;31(Suppl 3):19–23.
20. Eipel C, Abshagen K, Vollmar B. Regulation of hepatic blood flow: the hepatic arterial buffer response revisited. World J Gastroenterol. 2010;16(48):6046–57.
21. Vollmar B, Menger MD. The hepatic microcirculation: mechanistic contributions and therapeutic targets in liver injury and repair. Physiol Rev. 2009;89(4):1269–339.
22. Vernon H, Kasi A. Anatomy, abdomen, liver. Treasure Island, FL: StatPearls; 2018.
23. Waseem N, Chen PH. Hypoxic hepatitis: a review and clinical update. J Clin Transl Hepatol. 2016;4(3):263–8.
24. Lautt WW. Mechanism and role of intrinsic regulation of hepatic arterial blood flow: hepatic arterial buffer response. Am J Phys. 1985;249(5 Pt 1):G549–56.
25. Seeto RK, Fenn B, Rockey DC. Ischemic hepatitis: clinical presentation and pathogenesis. Am J Med. 2000;109(2):109–13.
26. Krejci V, Hiltebrand LB, Sigurdsson GH. Effects of epinephrine, norepinephrine, and phenylephrine on microcirculatory blood flow in the gastrointestinal tract in sepsis. Crit Care Med. 2006;34(5):1456–63.
27. Aninat C, Seguin P, Descheemaeker PN, Morel F, Malledant Y, Guillouzo A. Catecholamines induce an inflammatory response in human hepatocytes. Crit Care Med. 2008;36(3):848–54.
28. Edwards JD. Oxygen transport in cardiogenic and septic shock. Crit Care Med. 1991;19(5):658–63.
29. Rudiger A, Singer M. Mechanisms of sepsis-induced cardiac dysfunction. Crit Care Med. 2007;35(6):1599–608.
30. Wanless IR, Wong F, Blendis LM, Greig P, Heathcote EJ, Levy G. Hepatic and portal vein thrombosis in cirrhosis: possible role in development of parenchymal extinction and portal hypertension. Hepatology. 1995;21(5):1238–47.

31. Moreau R, Lee SS, Soupison T, Roche-Sicot J, Sicot C. Abnormal tissue oxygenation in patients with cirrhosis and liver failure. J Hepatol. 1988;7(1):98–105.
32. Chang PE, Goh BG, Ekstrom V, Ong ML, Tan CK. Low serum albumin predicts early mortality in patients with severe hypoxic hepatitis. World J Hepatol. 2017;9(22):959–66.
33. Taylor RM, Tujios S, Jinjuvadia K, Davern T, Shaikh OS, Han S, Chung RT, Lee WM, Fontana RJ. Short and long-term outcomes in patients with acute liver failure due to ischemic hepatitis. Dig Dis Sci. 2012;57(3):777–85.
34. Mohacsi P, Meier B. Hypoxic hepatitis in patients with cardiac failure. J Hepatol. 1994;21(5):693–5.
35. Henrion J, Descamps O, Luwaert R, Schapira M, Parfonry A, Heller F. Hypoxic hepatitis in patients with cardiac failure: incidence in a coronary care unit and measurement of hepatic blood flow. J Hepatol. 1994;21(5):696–703.
36. Fuhrmann V, Jager B, Zubkova A, Drolz A. Hypoxic hepatitis – epidemiology, pathophysiology and clinical management. Wien Klin Wochenschr. 2010;122(5–6):129–39.
37. Henrion J, Minette P, Colin L, Schapira M, Delannoy A, Heller FR. Hypoxic hepatitis caused by acute exacerbation of chronic respiratory failure: a case-controlled, hemodynamic study of 17 consecutive cases. Hepatology. 1999;29(2):427–33.
38. Ucgun I, Ozakyol A, Metintas M, Moral H, Orman A, Bal C, Yildirim H. Relationship between hypoxic hepatitis and cor pulmonale in patients treated in the respiratory ICU. Int J Clin Pract. 2005;59(11):1295–300.
39. Mathurin P, Durand F, Ganne N, Mollo JL, Lebrec D, Degott C, Erlinger S, Benhamou JP, Bernuau J. Ischemic hepatitis due to obstructive sleep apnea. Gastroenterology. 1995;109(5):1682–4.
40. Henrion J, Colin L, Schapira M, Heller FR. Hypoxic hepatitis caused by severe hypoxemia from obstructive sleep apnea. J Clin Gastroenterol. 1997;24(4):245–9.
41. Fuhrmann V, Kneidinger N, Herkner H, Heinz G, Nikfardjam M, Bojic A, Schellongowski P, Angermayr B, Kitzberger R, Warszawska J, et al. Hypoxic hepatitis: underlying conditions and risk factors for mortality in critically ill patients. Intensive Care Med. 2009;35(8):1397–405.
42. Drolz A, Jager B, Wewalka M, Saxa R, Horvatits T, Roedl K, Perkmann T, Zauner C, Kramer L, Ferenci P, et al. Clinical impact of arterial ammonia levels in ICU patients with different liver diseases. Intensive Care Med. 2013;39(7):1227–37.
43. Trilok G, Qing YC, Li-Jun X. Hypoxic hepatitis: a challenging diagnosis. Hepatol Int. 2012;6(4):663–9.
44. Raurich JM, Perez O, Llompart-Pou JA, Ibanez J, Ayestaran I, Perez-Barcena J. Incidence and outcome of ischemic hepatitis complicating septic shock. Hepatol Res. 2009;39(7):700–5.
45. Gitlin N, Serio KM. Ischemic hepatitis: widening horizons. Am J Gastroenterol. 1992;87(7):831–6.
46. Acharya SK, Bhatia V, Sreenivas V, Khanal S, Panda SK. Efficacy of L-ornithine L-aspartate in acute liver failure: a double-blind, randomized, placebo-controlled study. Gastroenterology. 2009;136(7):2159–68.
47. Jager B, Drolz A, Michl B, Schellongowski P, Bojic A, Nikfardjam M, Zauner C, Heinz G, Trauner M, Fuhrmann V. Jaundice increases the rate of complications and one-year mortality in patients with hypoxic hepatitis. Hepatology. 2012;56(6):2297–304.
48. Kneidinger N, Funk GC, Lindner G, Drolz A, Schenk P, Fuhrmann V. Unmeasured anions are associated with short-term mortality in patients with hypoxic hepatitis. Wien Klin Wochenschr. 2013;125(15–16):474–80.
49. Horvatits T, Kneidinger N, Drolz A, Roedl K, Rutter K, Kluge S, Trauner M, Fuhrmann V. Prognostic impact of ICG-PDR in patients with hypoxic hepatitis. Ann Intensive Care. 2015;5(1):47.

# Chapter 13
# Congestive Cardiac Hepatopathy


**Luis Téllez, Enrique Rodríguez-Santiago, María Jesús del Cerro, and Agustín Albillos**


## Introduction

Congestive cardiac hepatopathy appears in patients with a failing heart and spans a broad spectrum of clinical situations that share two pathophysiological scenarios: a rise in pressure transmitted to the hepatic veins due to inefficient liver drainage, and a reduced oxygen supply due to low cardiac output [1]. While this liver disease can occur in all forms of heart failure, it is more frequent in chronic states in which there is severe right heart dysfunction. The impact of hepatic dysfunction on the prognosis of adults with heart disease varies according to the clinical scenario so it is essential to distinguish three different situations: (1) patients with chronic congestive heart failure, (2) patients with congenital malformations and abnormal hemodynamic changes after surgical palliation, especially patients who have undergone Fontan surgery, and (3) patients with acute heart failure and rapid hemodynamic derangement where so-called hypoxic hepatits may occur. In acute and chronic congestive heart failure, the liver is usually a mere spectator of the precarious hemodynamic situation and prognosis is mainly driven by the course of the heart disease. In contrast, in adolescents and adults with certain congenital heart malformations, the liver complications such as ascites, esophagealvariceal bleeding, and even hepatocellular carcinoma can determine the prognosis [2].


L. Téllez · E. Rodríguez-Santiago · A. Albillos (✉)
Department of Gastroenterology and Hepatology, Hospital Universitario Ramón y Cajal, Universidad de Alcalá, Instituto Ramón y Cajal de Investigación Sanitaria (IRYCIS), Centro de Investigación Biomédica en Red de Enfermedades Hepáticas y Digestivas (CIBERehd), Instituto de Salud Carlos III, Madrid, Spain
e-mail: luis.tellez@salud.madrid.org; agustin.albillos@uah.es

M.-J. del Cerro
Department of Pediatric Cardiology and Congenital Heart Disease, Hospital Universitario Ramón y Cajal, Instituto Ramón y Cajal de Investigación Sanitaria, Universidad de Alcalá, Madrid, Spain



© Springer Nature Switzerland AG 2022
D. Valla et al. (eds.), *Vascular Disorders of the Liver*,
https://doi.org/10.1007/978-3-030-82988-9_13

## The Liver in Chronic Congestive Heart Failure

Any cause of right-sided cardiac failure may result in transmission of central venous pressure directly from the heart to the hepatic sinusoids. Some causes are relatively frequent, such as severe tricuspid stenosis/regurgitation, pulmonary arterial hypertension or cor pulmonale. Other less common causes are constrictive pericarditis or end-stage cardiomyopathy [3].

### *Epidemiology*

The burden of congestive cardiac hepatopathy is unknown as no epidemiological studies have been performed so far. This could be due to the lack of a recognized definition of the syndrome and the great heterogeneity of its etiologies. However, given the high prevalence of valvular and non-valvular cardiovascular disease and the survival improvement registered in Europe in patients with cardiac hepatopathy, this form of liver disease is probably frequent but underdiagnosed [3].

### *Mechanism of Liver Injury*

The key point in the pathophysiology of congestive cardiac hepatopathy is a disturbance in the liver's vascular supply and drainage. Elevated systemic venous pressure leads to inefficient liver blood drainage, determining a state of chronic passive congestion. This pressure is easily transmitted to the hepatic veins, which lack self-regulating flow capacity, and from there to the small hepatic venules. Sinusoidal congestion and subsequent dilation of fenestrations promote blood hyperfiltration, causing protein-rich edema and bleeding into the Disse space. Perisinusoidal edema, more evident in zone 3 of the lobule, hinders the diffusion of oxygen to the hepatocytes, promoting hepatocellular necrosis and atrophy [4]. In addition, mechanical tension also plays an important role by inducing a phenotypic change in the endothelial cells and enabling the activation of hepatic stellate cells and fibroblasts. Similar to other causes of liver fibrosis, TGF-β and other autocrine profibrogenic molecules play a central driving role in the fibrogenic process [5, 6]. It is also likely that other mechanisms such as intrahepatic microthrombosis contribute to the vascular changes that occur in congestive liver disease [7].

It is unlikely, however, that chronic venous congestion alone in the long run leads to advanced liver damage [8], since no correlations have ever been found between right atrial pressure and the extent of hepatocellular injury in patients with congestive heart failure. Moreover, the increased vulnerability of patients with congestive heart disease to acute episodes of hypoxic hepatitis is a clue that chronically reduced liver inflow must be another factor contributing to liver damage in this setting (**Fig. 13.1**) [9].

## *Histological Changes*

Visually, the liver is usually enlarged and reddish purple, with prominent hepatic veins. Sinusoidal dilation and hemorrhagic necrosis around centrilobular veins are the earliest parenchymal changes [10–12]. Biliary thrombi and ductular reaction could be present due to canaliculi de formation [13]. If the patient survives and heart failure persists, liver damage progresses and the hepatocytes of zone 3 are replaced by reticulin and collagen, forming fibrous bands that emerge from the centrilobular veins (cardiac sclerosis). Finally, extensive bridges of centrilobular fibrosis associated with regenerative nodules may appear in patients with advanced liver disease [14]. Noticeably, periportal inflammation is usually minimal or absent.

## *Clinical Manifestations*

Congestive cardiac hepatopathy is often clinically silent, and usually diagnosed through routine liver function tests, while the signs and symptoms of heart failure are predominant. Patients with chronic hepatic congestion may complain of discomfort in the upper right quadrant of the abdomen, due to stretching of the capsule of the enlarged liver. Early satiety, nausea and anorexia are reported by some patients [15]. More severe abdominal pain has been described in cases of constrictive pericarditis

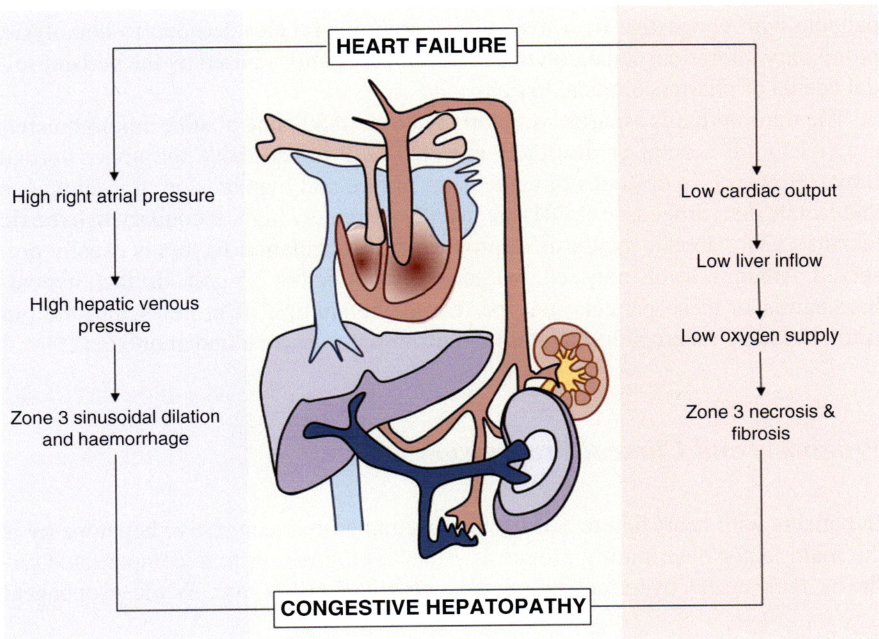


**Fig. 13.1**  Mechanisms of the hepatic damage in congestive hepatopathy

and acute cardiac tamponade [16]. In patients with congestive liver disease, the liver edge is easily palpable, hard, smooth and tender. When tricuspid regurgitation is present, the liver becomes pulsatile and this systolic pulsation can be palpated if the abdomen is explored bimanually [17]. Hepatojugular reflux is easily identified after applying compression over the liver and has been related to short-term mortality since it is a sign of persistent congestion [18]. Mild jaundice is common yet deeper jaundice is rare, though may occur at the end of an episode of hypoxic hepatitis [9]. Ascites is usually more related to heart failure than liver damage. The ascitic fluid is rich in proteins, similar to the one observed in other situations of obstructed hepatic venous outflow such as Budd-Chiari syndrome [19]. Differentiating the cause of ascites, heart failure or liver disease can be challenging in patients experiencing their first episode of ascites, a situation in which serum biomarkers, such as pro-BNP, can be of help [20]. Although patients usually develop splenomegaly, the presence of esophageal varices and variceal bleeding is exceptional.

## Laboratory Findings

Primary laboratory findings in congestive hepatopathy are elevated serum cholestasis markers, including bilirubin, alkaline phosphatase, and $\gamma$-glutamyl-transpeptidase (GGT) [21–23]. Hyperbilirubinemia, present in up to 70% of patients, is mostly unconjugated and rarely exceeds 3 mg/dL. Although part of the excess bilirubin is due to direct liver damage (hepatocellular necrosis in zone 3), it is known that in patients with congestive liver disease bilirubin can be elevated due to hemolysis, pulmonary infarction, canaliculi obstruction/deformation caused by the perisinusoidal edema or pharmacological toxicity.

The transaminases aspartate aminotransferase (AST) and alanine aminotransferase (ALT) are normal or discretely elevated (2–3 times above the upper normal limit). However, in episodes of acute heart failure and hypotension, transaminases and lactate dehydrogenase (LDH) are usually extremely high, secondary to hypoxic hepatitis [24]. Hepatic synthesis of proteins and coagulation factors is usually preserved. Albumin levels may fall, but generally not below 2.5 g/dL. In fact, hypoalbuminemia in these patients may be due to the spilling of proteins into the gut (protein-losing enteropathy) and/or malnutrition due to wear and anorexia [25].

## Prognosis and Clinical Progression

In patients with heart failure, cardiac disease rather than congestive hepatopathy is the main factor determining prognosis. Hence, progression to decompensated cirrhosis with portal hypertension-related complications is rare. While esophageal varices can be present, variceal bleeding is infrequent, and variceal screening not recommended. Similarly, overt hepatic encephalopathy is unlikely although serum ammonia levels are usually elevated [26]. In fact, in cases of encephalopathy, causes other than the liver should be first ruled out, such as hypoxia, hypercapnia or electrolyte abnormalities.

## *Treatment*

The cornerstone of therapy for congestive hepatopathy in adults is treatment of the underlying heart disease. Ascites is usually well controlled with high doses of loop and/or antialdosterone diuretics. However, in patients with chronic advanced heart failure with ascites and renal insufficiency, large-volume paracentesis might be useful to correct fluid loss and improve renal function [27]. Further, in cases of severe ascites or when diuretics are contraindicated, repeated high volume paracentesis can be an effective alternative since transjugular intrahepatic portosystemic shunting (TIPS) is not recommended [28, 29]. Although we lack specific studies in this particular population, if more than 5 liters of ascites is removed, albumin infusion could be advisable to reduce the incidence of hypotension and hyponatremia. While for decades hepatic dysfunction has been considered a hypocoagulant state and the use of anticoagulants is discouraged, more recent evidence does not support this attitude [30]. Hepatotoxic drugs, such as amiodarone, should be used with caution and the dosage of antiarrhythmics significantly metabolized in the liver adjusted in consequence.

## The Liver in Congenital Cardiac Disease

In Europe, we currently face an estimated prevalence of ~2.3 million adults with congenital cardiac disease [2]. The remarkably improved survival of patients with repaired congenital heart defects has meant that increasing numbers of adult patients are at risk of congestive hepatopathy. These adult patients have a much greater risk of complications related to the liver with a true impact on prognosis than patients in whom heart failure arises in adulthood. While the entity most clearly associated with liver damage is the single ventricle physiology that occurs after the Fontan palliation, other congenital heart diseases listed in **Table 13.1** can also cause severe liver injury (**Fig. 13.2**) [31]. Finally, it should be highlighted that patients with congenital cardiac disease can feature additional risk factors for chronic liver disease unrelated to congestive hepatopathy, such as blood-borne hepatitis C virus infection or treatment with hepatotoxic antiarrhythmic agents (e.g., amiodarone) [32, 33].

**Table 13.1** Main congenital cardiac diseases leading to liver damage

| **"Right-sided" failure** |
| --- |
| Single-ventricle physiology after Fontan surgery |
| Dextro-transposition of the great arteries after atrial switch repair (Mustard, Senning procedure) |
| Eisenmenger syndrome |
| Repaired tetralogy of Fallot with pulmonary regurgitation |
| Ebstein's anomaly |
| Pulmonary stenosis/pulmonary regurgitation |
| Secundum atrial septal defect with pulmonary stenosis or pulmonary hypertension |
| Partial atrioventricular septal defect with tricuspid regurgitation and/or pulmonary hypertension |
| **"Left-sided" failure** |
| Left ventricular outflow tract obstruction/coarctation of the aorta |
| Repaired complete atrioventricular septal defect with residual regurgiation or left ventricular outflow obstruction |

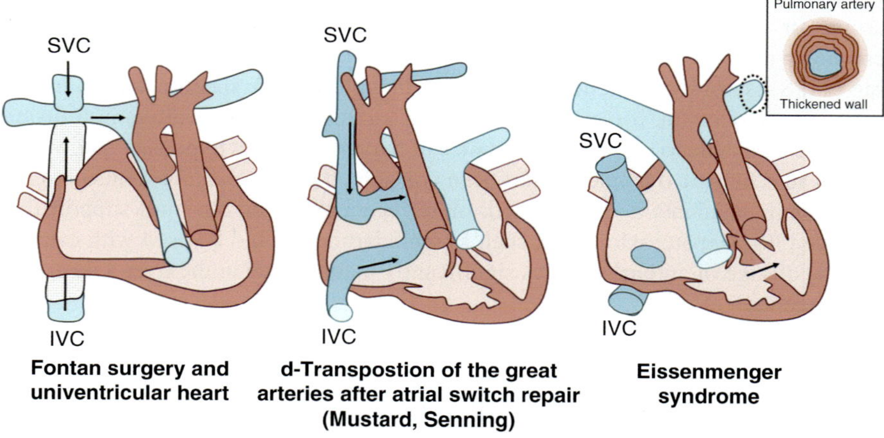


**Fig. 13.2** Main congenital cardiac situations related to liver injury

## *Fontan-Associated Liver Disease (FALD)*

Fontan surgery is the final stage of surgical treatment for diverse cyanotic congenital cardiac malformations associated with a functionally univentricular heart. The common characteristic of these cardiac defects is the mixing of desaturated blood from the caval veins and oxigenated blood from the pulmonary veins in a single ventricular pump [34]. Fontan circulation is a palliative strategy that aims to restore a double circulation system to avoid cyanosis, but at the expense of chronic increase in central venous pressure and low cardiac output (**Fig. 13.3**).

As shown in **Fig. 13.4**, atriopulmonary and bi-cavopulmonary are the two major variants of the diversion technique. The atriopulmonary anastomosis is the original Fontan procedure, which converts the right atrium into a pumping channel that conducts the blood from the inferior and superior cava veins to the pulmonary artery [35]. In the more recent bi-cavopulmonary anastomosis procedure, the inferior vena cava is connected by an artificial intra or extracardiac conduit to the pulmonary arteries.

## Fontan Circulation

The normal cardiovascular system is based on two circuits, pulmonary and systemic, which are driven by two synchronized heart pumps, the right and left ventricles (**Fig. 13.5**). In univentricular heart congenital malformations, there is mixing of desaturated and oxygenated blood in a common ventricle. After Fontan surgery, the single or remaining ventricle is used as a systemic pump and both caval veins are directly connected to the pulmonary arteries. The immediate consequence is the development of a gradient of pressure between the caval veins and left atrium, as the main mechanism that passively drives deoxygenated blood from the systemic veins to the pulmonary vasculature, and finally to the left atrium. However, this new circulatory system is not perfect and pulmonary artery input impedance hinders venous return through the pulmonary bed and leads to chronic venous congestion and systemic low cardiac output (**Fig. 13.1**). Reduced pulmonary wall strain and adverse

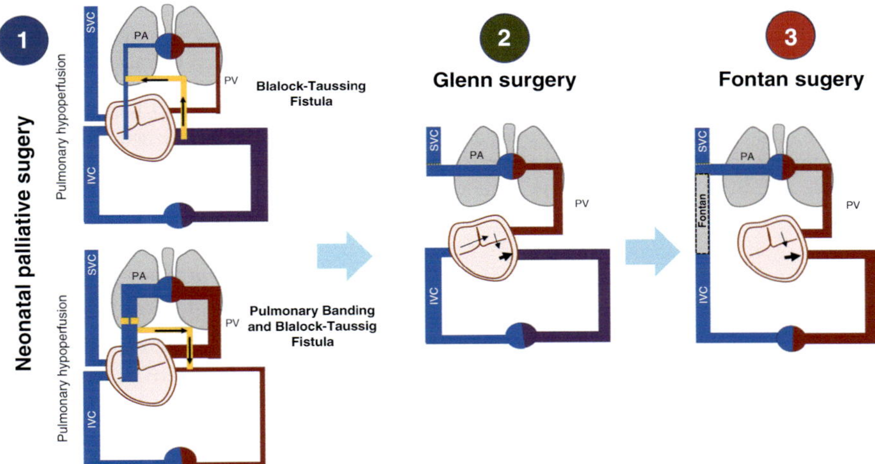


**Fig. 13.3** Surgical treatment for univentricular cardiac malformations. (1) First stage (neonatal palliation): This surgery is performed to guarantee an adequate pulmonary and systemic perfusion provisionally. In some cases, as in patients with double left ventricular inlet, the high pulmonary inflow requires banding of the pulmonary artery. In others, blood hardly reaches the lungs, and the circuit needs surgical fistulas between the aorta and the pulmonary arteries (Blalock-Taussig fistula). (2) Second stage (Glenn surgery): This surgery is performed to partially restore the pulmonary flow from the systemic venous return, connecting the superior vena cava to the pulmonary artery. (3) Third stage (Fontan surgery): At this surgical stage, the inferior vena cava is also anastomosed to the pulmonary artery, so all systemic venous return reaches passively the pulmonary circulation, due to the pressure gradient between caval veins and the right atrium without the participation of a subpulmonary pumping ventricle. In this way, pulmonary and systemic circulation are separated, which eliminates mixing of venous and arterial blood and cyanosis. *SVC* Superior vena cava, *IVC* Inferior vena cava, *PA* Pulmonary artery, *PV* Pulmonary vein

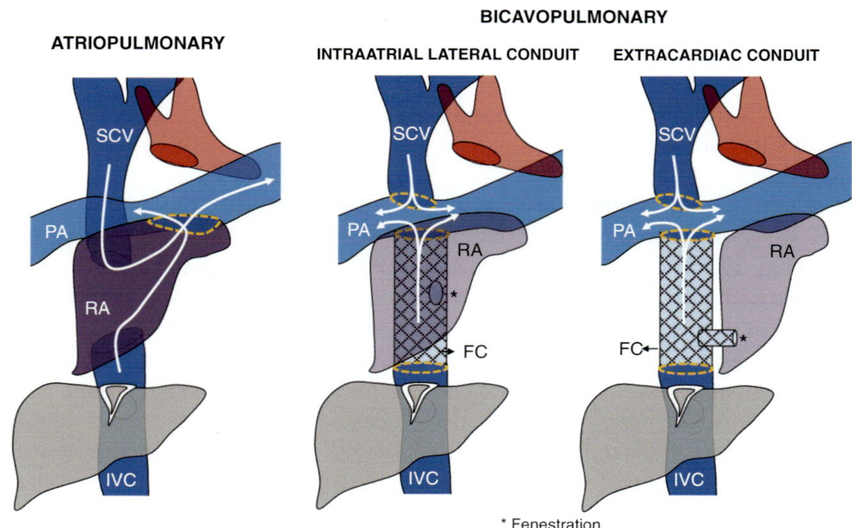



**Fig. 13.4** Major variants of Fontan surgery. Atriopulmonary Fontan (left): superior and inferior cava drain to the right atrium, that is connected to the pulmonary artery. Intraatrial lateral conduit (middle): superior vena cava drains directly to the right pulmonary artery, and the inferiorvena cava is connected through an intraatrial tunnel to the right pulmonary artery. Extracardiac conduit (right): superior vena cava connected directly to the right pulmonary artery, and the inferiorvena cava connected to the right pulmonary arterya through an extracardiac conduit. In both modalities, a fenestration can be left open between the tunnel/conduit and the left atrium to decrease the central venous pressure and maintain higher cardiac output at the expense of mild cyanosis (Fenestrated Fontan). *SVC* Superior vena cava, *IVC* Inferior vena cava, *PA* Pulmonary artery, *PV* Pulmonary vein, *RA* Right atrium, *FC* Fontan Conduit

vessel remodeling in the non-pulsatile Fontan circulation lead to increased intimal fibrosis, disrupted endothelial integrity and loss of vascular smoth muscle cells. All changes together lead to progressively increased pulmonary vascular resistance, formation of systemic venous collaterals, and development of cyanosis. Hence, the volume load into the single ventricle becomes markedly reduced resulting in decreased cardiac output. "Fontan failure" is the term used for this hemodynamic breakdown in the long-term, which is clinically characterized by multi-system organ dysfunction (**Table 13.3**). When Fontan failure occurs, only cardiac transplantation can completely reverse this situation. Fenestration of the Fontan conduit allows some of the deoxygenated caval blood to be derived directly from the systemic venous return to the left atrium, which results in cardiac output improvement at the expense of worsening cyanosis [36].

Finally, in some patients, Fontan failure can develop abruptly in the context of an acute cardiopulmonary event, such as atrial arrhythmia, pulmonary thromboembolism or thrombosis/stenosis of the Fontan conduit, that unbalances a previously balanced system. The treatment of these local complications or reversal of cardiac arrhythmia can also improve the hemodynamic situation [37, 38].

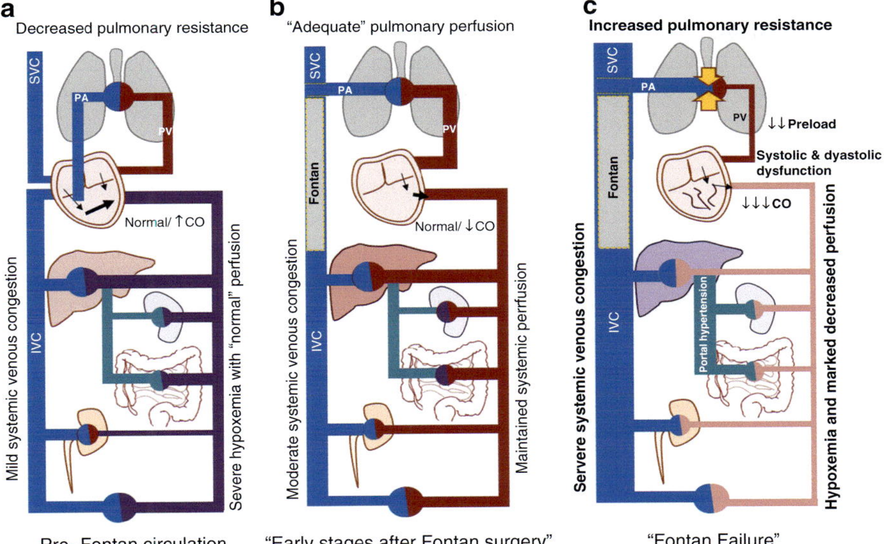



**Fig. 13.5** Fontan circulation and "Fontan Failure". "Pre-Fontan circulation" is characterized by an imbalance between oxygenated and non-oxygenated blood that mixes in the single ventricle, which results in severe hypoxemia that cannot be maintained in the long term. In patients with an "operative Fontan circulation" systemic venous pressure progressively increases, but the pulmonary microcirculation is able to maintain an adequate trans pulmonary gradient that guarantees preload and keeps cardiac output normal. Finally, in patients with "Fontan failure", systemic venous hypertension is maximum and the highly increased pulmonary vascular resistance hinders that blood reaches the heart and cardiac output drops. *SVC* superior vena cava, *IVC* inferior vena cava, *CO* Cardiac output, *PA* Pulmonary artery, *PV* Pulmonary veins

## Pathophysiology of FALD

Liver damage is one of the most significant complications of Fontan failure, and is more frequent than in other forms of heart failure. FALD shares some of the mechanisms described in **Fig. 13.1** for cardiac congestive hepatopathy, but its pathogenesis is much more complex and it has a multifactorial origin. In contrast to most of the right-sided cardiac hepatopathies in which venous congestion and low cardiac output are the consequence of ventricular or valve dysfunction, these are not the main factors of FALD. Here, the key element is the Fontan circuit pathophysiology itself, that causes both liver congestion and is chemia related to low cardiac output. We could state that what keeps the patient alive puts the liver at risk: *"the cure of the heart is the hurt of the liver"* (**Fig. 13.6**):

1. Liver congestion. Fontan surgery worsens the systemic venous congestion already present in patients with univentricular congenital heart disease. In parallel with the failure of the Fontan circuit in the long-term, systemic congestion further increases, liver drainage is compromised, and portal pressure rises.

Moreover, the maintained sinusoidal hypertension promotes the mechanical activation of hepatic stellate cells, resulting in tissue fibrosis [7]. The technique-dependent flow characteristics of the Fontan connection in each patient, which determines different grades of impedance for blood to egress from the liver, partly explains individual differences in liver damage.

2. Hypoxia and hepatic ischemia. From birth, a large number of hemodynamic insults appear cumulatively. During the neonatal period, patients invariably present hemodynamic instability that can result in altered hepatic perfusion. In the first years of life, before completing the Fontan surgery, systemic hypoxemia and cyanosis are constantly present. Further acute hypoxic liver injury is possible simultaneously with cardiac surgeries. Finally, over time, up to 25% of Fontan surgery patients can develop severe systolic and diastolic dysfunction with reduced cardiac output and an inability to increase this output in response to metabolic demands [36]. This precarious hemodynamic situation is usually long-time maintained, so the liver is subjected to a permanent hypoxic state.

3. Prothrombotic state. Thromboembolic events are a constant feature in Fontan patients. Recent reports suggest that the prothrombotic state is not only related to the anatomical and functional characteristics of Fontan circulation [39]. Indeed, Fontan patients show a hypercoagulability state featuring low levels of antithrombin III, thrombomodulin, alpha2-antiplasmin and C and S proteins, and high levels of thrombin-antithrombin complex, similar to that observed in

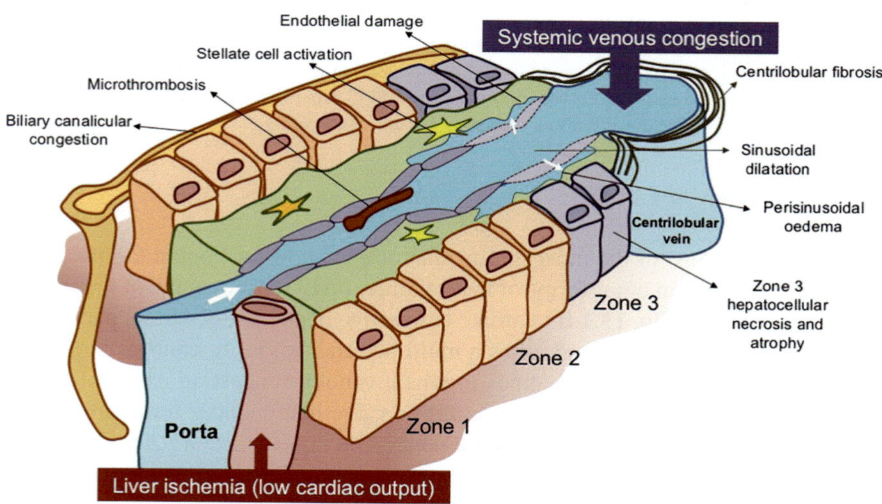


**Fig. 13.6** Pathophysiology of Fontan-associated liver disease. Systemic venous hypertension secondary to Fontan surgery results in a decreased hepatic venous drainage, with sinusoidal dilatation and hypertension of the sinusoids and leakage of fluid to the Disse space. Mechanical stress induces a phenotypic change in sinusoidal endothelial cells with production of mediators, such as TGF-β, that activate autocrine stellate cells and promote fibrosis. Hypoxia, perisinusoidal edema and fibrosis will eventually lead to hepatocyte parenchymal necrosis, more evident in zone 3

cirrhosis [40, 41]. Although the exact cause of these alterations of the coagulation system are unknown, it has been proposed liver damage, sustained hypoxemia and endothelial damage as possible mechanisms. In Fontan patients, hypercoagulability has two major consequences that can directly lead to liver damage. First, "circuit thrombosis" (e.g. inferior vena cava, Fontan conduit, pulmonary arteries or right/left atrium) may develop in one third of Fontan patients, leading to further impairment of systemic and liver venous drainage. Second, intrahepatic micro thrombosis, a well-known mechanism of vascular liver injury, becomes more relevant than in other forms of cardiac hepatopathy and can accelerate liver damage. Indeed, mechanical strain secondary to blood stasis and thrombosis of the sinusoids were the main promoters of liver fibrosis in a mouse model of congestive hepatopathy through partial ligation of the inferior vena cava [7]. In this model, a course of warfarin improved liver fibrosis opening the gate for new therapeutic strategies for FALD.

**Natural History of FALD**

Liver damage is universal after Fontan surgery and, in most patients, develops slowly and silently without overt clinical features. Liver function is usually preserved for many years and the first manifestation of FALD frequently coincides with dysfunction of another organ, such as protein-losing enteropathy suggestive of Fontan failure (**Table 13.2**), or a decline in functional class [42]. Liver disease in the Fontan circulation involves three main stages: sinusoidal dilatation without fibrosis, mild-moderate fibrosis without portal hypertension and advanced fibrosis with portal hypertension [34]. The **first stage** starts even before Fontan surgery and continues into the following few years [43]. Clinical findings are similar to those previously described in congestive hepatopathy secondary to right heart failure, including painful hepatomegaly in half of the cases, mild indirect hyperbilirubinemia and increased GGT due to perisinusoidal edema [44]. The **second stage** occurs around 5–10 years after Fontan surgery and is characterized by perisinusoidal fibrosis, regenerative nodules and hepatocellular necrosis, which can beaggravated if cardiac output further decreases. This stage is potentially reversible if the patient undergoes heart transplantation [45]. Finally, the **third stage** is clinically indistinguishable from other forms of end-stage liver disease. In consequence, patients might show manifestations of liver insufficiency, such as hypoalbuminemia, prolonged coagulation time and low platelet count, and others of portal hypertension, such as ascites, variceal haemorrhage or encephalopathy. At this stage, there is an increased, though not well quantified, risk of hepatocellular carcinoma.

It is important to highlight that, as stated before, FALD is not a primary liver disease and its progression depends on the proper functioning and hemodynamic progression of the Fontan circulation. A large number of variables, listed in **Table 13.3** have been associated with an increased risk of liver damage. Among them, time since Fontan surgery is the main risk factor for FALD, probably reflecting the failure of the Fontan circulation that develops in most patients over time. Hence,

**Table 13.2** Multi-system organ dysfunction in "Fontan failure"

| Organ/system | Complication | Mechanism | Clinical Findings |
|---|---|---|---|
| Lungs | Veno-venous/atrial shunts | Caval veins-left atrium gradient -passive circulation | Cyanosis, dyspnea, hypoxia, exercise intolerance |
| | Plastic bronchitis | ↓ Lymphatic return | |
| | Chylothorax | ↓ Lymphatic return | |
| | Thromboembolism | Hypercoagulability | |
| | Pulmonary hypertensive vascular disease | Endothelial dysfunction (non-pulsatile flow) Pulmonary artery hypoplasia Chronic thromboembolism | |
| Kidneys | Proteinuria | Hyperfiltration due to systemic venous hypertension | Edema, ascites |
| | Kidney injury (acute/chronic) | Ischemia due to ↓ cardiac output | Dyspnea, oliguria |
| Bowel | Protein-losing enteropathy | ↓ Lymphatic return Splanchnic venous congestion Systemic and local inflammation Hormonal activation | Malnutrition, edema, ascites, diarrhea |
| Liver | Chronic liver disease | Liver congestion Ischemia due to ↓↓ cardiac output | Ascites, varices, encephalopathy, hepatocarcinoma |
| Brain | Cerebrovascular disease | Cardioembolism Ischemia due to ↓↓ cardiac output Congenital brain abnormalities | Decreased executive skills |
| Heart | Bradi- and tachy-arrhythmia | Atrial and ventricular remodeling | Hemodynamic instability |
| | Ventricular dysfunction | Activation of neurohormonal systems | Dyspnea, exercise intolerance |
| Vascular system | Varicosities | Venous hypertension ↓ lymphatic return | Edema, varicose veins |

whereas the risk of FALD is low within the first five years after surgery, it increases by nine-fold after 15 years [46].

## Serological Biomarkers of FALD

Classic serum markers such as AST, ALT and bilirubin correlate poorly with liver fibrosis in Fontan patients. In small case series, a platelet count <150,000/μL, which is associated with portal hypertension, may correlate with fibrosis stage on biopsy. Controversial results have suggested a relationship between GGT and alkaline phosphatase, markers of canalicular congestion, with liver fibrosis [43]. Low serum albumin could indicate liver damage, but it can also result from protein-losing enteropathy, which is another frequent complication in Fontan patients that usually coexists with severe liver fibrosis [42].

**Table 13.3** Risk factors for liver damage in Fontan circulation

| Related to the hemodynamic situation |
| --- |
| ↓ Cardiac output |
| ↑ Pulmonary capillary pressure |
| ↑ Central venous pressure |
| ↓ Mixed venous oxygen saturation |
| **Related to the surgery** |
| Pulmonary atresia as surgery precipitant |
| Surgical technique (atriopulmonary variant) |
| Absence of conduit fenestration |
| Fontan conduit stenosis/thrombosis |
| Time since Fontan surgery |
| **Related to cardiopulmonary events** |
| Cardiac arrhythmia |
| Sinus node dysfunction |
| Systolic ventricular dysfunction |
| Intracardiac thrombosis |
| Pulmonary thromboembolism |
| **Others** |
| Viral hepatitis |
| Exposure to hepatotoxic drugs (e.g. amiodarone) |

The different clinical, analytical and radiological methods developed in recent years to diagnose and stratify liver fibrosis have not yet been specifically validated against liver biopsy in Fontan patients. Non-invasive signs of liver damage (nodular liver surface, edema, splenomegaly, ascites and collateral veins) and serological markers such as FibroSURE, hyaluronic acid levels, APRI, AST/ALT, Forns and FIB4, were tested in a cohort of 204 Fontan patients. The ability of all these markers to predict liver damage was at most moderate and for none of them did the area under the curve exceed 0.8 [46, 47]. This is not surprising, since some of these scores reflect liver necroinflammatory activity rather than fibrosis and/or have been validated in liver diseases of etiologies other than Fontan. Thus, we actually lack validated cut-off values of serological markers of FALD that can be recommended in clinical practice to facilitate clinical decision making, such as screening for esophageal varices, or the optimal timing for heart transplantation.

The model for end-stage liver disease excluding the international normalized ratio (MELD-XI) has been designed to overcome the main limitation of MELD in this population, namely an increased INR due to anticoagulation. The results of the only retrospective study including 79 Fontan patients seem to indicate good correlation of MELD-XI with liver elastography [45]. Moreover, in another cohort of 96 Fontan patients, a MELD-XI $\geq$19 was related to all-cause mortality and was also found valuable as a predictor of early and late mortality after cardiac transplantation [48, 49]. However, it should be noted that while MELD-XI seems to be useful as a predictor of cardiac morbimortality in this setting, its accuracy to predict hepatic outcomes is unknown.

## Radiological Findings in FALD

Among Fontan patients undergoing liver imaging (ultrasound, MRI or CT scan), the most frequent radiological findings are the heterogeneity of liver parenchyma, surface irregularity, segmental atrophy/hypertrophy, and small-sized nodules [50]. Although these findings are highly suggestive of advanced liver disease in other etiologies, there is minimal evidence correlating their presence to the fibrosis stage by biopsy or clinical hepatic decompensation in the Fontan population. In fact, heterogeneous hepatic enhancement, which seems to be due to passive hepatic congestion, is present in 67–90% of Fontan patients [51]. It has been proposed that reduced portal vein velocity, inverted portal flow and a monophasic pattern in the hepatic veins by Doppler ultrasound may reflect advanced liver damage [52]. In recent promising MRI studies, though not validated by liver biopsy, reduced hepatic micro perfusion was suggested to be related to liver fibrosis [53–55]. Today, we need to be cautious about relying only on imaging methods to diagnose severe fibrosis in Fontan patients.

## Liver Stiffness in FALD

The accuracy of elastography (transient elastography, shear wave, acoustic radiation force impulse and MR elastography) is not well established in Fontan patients, where congestion itself can increase stiffness [47]. In fact, Fontan surgery immediately increases liver stiffness to a mean value of 11.2 kPa, blunting the usefulness of elastography and outlining the need to set higher cut-offs for advanced liver disease in this population [56]. However, the longer the time elapsed from Fontan surgery, the greaterthe decrease in liver function estimated by MELD-XI and greater the liver stiffness, suggesting that in addition to congestion, fibrosis progressively contributes to liver stiffness [57, 58]. While we await further studies to establish the optimal cut-off for advanced FALD, today the main contribution of transient elastography is to rule out severe liver damage, as defined by a liver stiffness <15 kPa [59]. Other novel methods, such as shear-wave and MRI-elastography, have recently shown good correlation between liver stiffness and histology in small case-series [60].

## Hepatic Hemodynamics in FALD

As in other situations of post-sinusoidal portal hypertension due to obstructed hepatic venous outflow, free and wedged hepatic vein pressures are elevated and, in consequence, the hepatic venous pressure gradient (HVPG) is normal in most Fontan patients, even in those with ascites or esophageal varices [61, 62]. In patients with advanced fibrosis, portal hypertension must be due to an added sinusoidal component, since the frequent development of decompressive porto-systemic shunts. In fact, the numerous presence of fistulas between the hepatic and portal veins could be another source of underestimation of sinusoidal pressure [63, 64]. **Figure 13.7** presents the distinctive features of portal hypertension in FALD.

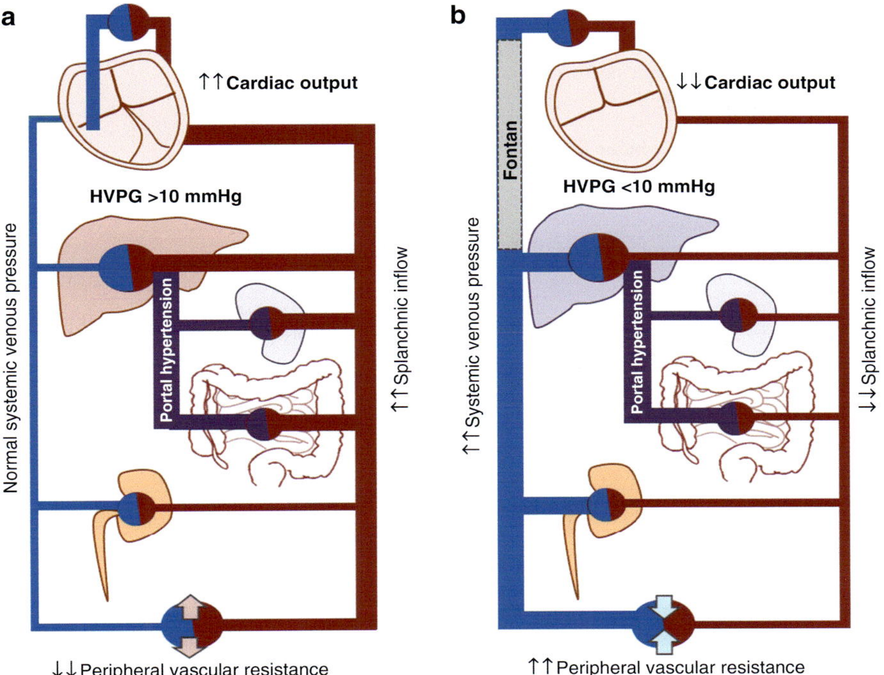



**Fig. 13.7** Systemic and splanchnic hemodynamics of portal hypertension in cirrhosis and in Fontan associated liver disease. (**a**) Cirrhosis. Portal hypertension due to cirrhosis is characterized by a hyperdynamic circulatory state with low systemic vascular resistance, high cardiac output, and increased splanchnic inflow. (**b**) Fontan associated liver disease. Portal hypertension due to severe fibrosis in advanced Fontan-associated liver disease is associated to high systemic venous pressures, and low cardiac output and splanchnic inflow. *HVPG* Hepatic vein pressure gradient

## Liver Biopsy in Fontan Patients

Liver biopsy remains the gold standard to establish the severity of FALD and to rule out other etiologies. **Table 13.4** describes the wide spectrum of histological abnormalities in the liver of Fontan patients. Sinusoidal dilation is the earliest parenchymal change, and it is usually more severe than in other congestive hepatopathies. In early stages of FALD fibrosis follows a predominantly perisinusoidal pattern instead of the centrilobular one observed in other forms of congestive hepatopathy. Periportal inflammation is usually minimal or absent, allowing a differential diagnosis with other liver disease etiologies [65]. A liver biopsy to diagnose and stage fibrosis has been recommended in all patients 10 years after Fontan surgery, to individualize follow-up and establish the need and timing of referral to an hepatologist [66]. The poor correlation between fibrosis stage and clinically relevant hepatic events in this setting and the absence of specific treatment available for these patients question the utility of protocolized liver biopsies in clinical practice [67]. Otherwise, liver biopsy is highly-advisable when the etiology of liver disease is uncertain and in candidates for heart and/or liver transplantation, and recommended in clinical research.

**Table 13.4** Histological features of Fontan-associated liver disease

| |
| --- |
| Sinusoidal dilatation |
| Centrolobular hemorrhagic necrosis |
| **Perisinusoidal fibrosis** |
| **Ductular reaction** |
| **Periportal and centrolobular fibrosis** |
| **Perivenular fibrous septa** |
| **Central fibrous bridges** |
| **Regenerative nodules** |
| **Absence/minimal portal inflammation, iron deposition, and steatosis** |

**Table 13.5** Differential diagnosis of hepatic nodules in Fontan patient

| Type of nodule | Dynamic imaging pattern (CT/MRI) | Histology |
| --- | --- | --- |
| Nodular focal Regenerative Hyperplasia- like | Multiple, small (<3 cm), hypervascular, with (less common) or without wash-out | Normal hepatocytes, mild ductular reaction, large dystrophic arteries, absence of central scar |
| Large Regenerative nodules | Hypervascular nodules without washout | Normal hepatocytes, No ductular reaction |
| Hepatocellular Adenoma | Hypervascular nodule With (more common) or without washout | Proliferation of sheets of well-differentiated hepatocytes, absence of portal triads or bile ducts |
| Hepatocellular carcinoma | Hypervascular nodule With (more common) or without washout | Cytologic atypia, pseudoacinar changes |

## Hepatic Nodules in FALD

Arterialized hepatic nodules are present in 17–48% of Fontan patients [68, 69]. The pattern of hepatic nodules in this setting is similar to that observed in Budd-Chiari and other vascular liver diseases, being typically multiple, hyper vascular, smaller than 3 cm, and located in the outer margins of the liver [51, 70–72]. The vascular origin of the nodules is suggested by their peripheral location, radiological behaviour and the observed correlation between their number and the degree of systemic venous hypertension. Indeed, nodules correspond to areas of focal regenerative hyperplasia, since they seem to represent an adverse adaptation of the parenchyma to the arterialization of the hepatic blood supply in response to hypoperfusion, secondary to portal venous flow deprivation. As such, these nodules are composed of normal hepatocytes, ductular reaction and large dystrophic arteries, without a central scar [73]. The prevalence of focal regenerative hyperplasia-like nodules increases with the severity of FALD and time elapsed since surgery [69], as do other less common nodules observed in these patients, such as large regenerative or neoplastic nodules, which makes the differential diagnosis more difficult (**Table 13.5**). Hepatocellular adenoma and its malignant transformation have rarely been reported in Fontan patients [74].

## Hepatocellular Carcinoma

The prevalence of hepatocellular carcinoma in Fontan patients based on case reports and short case series seems close to 5% [75–87]. The time elapsed since surgery is the strongest risk factor for the development of hepatocellular carcinoma [87]. Age at the time of hepatocelluar carcinoma diagnosis ranged from 12 to 52 years, and it can be developed in the absence of cirrhosis [88]. The diagnosis of neoplasia in patients with Fontan is challenging considering the high prevalence of different types of nodules in Fontan patients. Malignant nodules typically show hyper vascularity and delayed washout in dynamic imaging, and most (~70%) show elevated levels of serum alpha-fetoprotein [84]. The imaging features described are not pathognomonic of hepatocellular carcinoma, and hypervascularity and even washout can be present in non-malignant nodules, while washout may be absent in malignant ones [69, 86]. It should be considered that current diagnostic criteria for hepatocellular carcinoma in cirrhosis have not been specifically validated in other settings, and the characteristics described above are based on published cases mostly with advanced stage hepatocarcinoma. Collectively, these data mean that the diagnosis of hepatocellular carcinoma in Fontan patients requires histologic confirmation and cannot be based only on imaging [34]. Fine-needle aspiration/biopsy is advisable in hypervascular nodules showing delayed washout larger than 3 cm and/or associated with even minimal elevations in serum alpha-fetoprotein. In this scenario, the optimal imaging technique and surveillance interval are currently unknown. Based on the limited experience available and on our expert opinion, hepatocellular carcinoma screening should be started in all patients from 10 years after surgery [88]. Since periodic abdominal ultrasound has not yet been validated in this population, a proposed practical approach is a baseline CT/MRI and there after Doppler US every 6-months by an experienced operator. Hepatic MRI is also recommended when cardiac MRI is performed [34].

## Portal Hypertension-Related Complications after Fontan Surgery

Ascites is the most frequent form of hepatic decompensation with a prevalence ranging from 2 to 17% [68]. Noteworthy, ascites in Fontan patients can occur in the absence of advanced liver fibrosis and may be due to any of the causes listed in **Table 13.6**. The estimated prevalence of **esophageal varices** ranges from 19 to 43% [89]. Variceal bleeding has been reported, which highlights the need for screening when signs of advanced liver disease or portal hypertension are present [90]. To date, only three cases of **hepatic encephalopathy** have been described [91, 92].

**Table 13.6**  Causes of ascites in Fontan patients

| |
|---|
| "Fontan failure" |
| Stenosis/thrombosis of the Fontan conduit |
| Sinusoidal portal hypertension (advanced liver fibrosis) |
| Portal vein thrombosis |
| Hypoalbuminemia secondary to protein-losing enteropathy |

**Follow-up and Treatment of FALD**

Although there is a lack of robust evidence to establish firm recommendations for liver follow-up after surgery, detailedassessment of liver state is advisable in all Fontan patients [93]. In every patient, a complete etiological study is warranted to rule out primary liver disease as well as chronic viral hepatitis. Adequate seroprotection against hepatitis A and B virus must be guaranteed. Within the first 10 years of Fontan surgery, severe liver damage is exceptional in the absence of other complications suggesting Fontan failure. Hence, the determination of serum liver function parameters, a liver ultrasound and an elastography every 5 years may be sufficient to confirm the absence of liver damage. After 10 years, follow-up must be closer to achieve early diagnosis of focal liver lesions and/or signs of portal hypertension, as shown in **Table 13.7** [34].

Most liver complications usually respond to the treatments ordinarily used in patients with cirrhosis of any other etiology, with some special considerations. Ascites is easily mobilized with diuretics and optimization of hemodynamics [93]. Considering the low risk of variceal bleeding and the particular characteristics of this hemodynamic model of portal hypertension, primary prophylaxis is controversial. The use of non-selective adrenergic beta-blockers is not clear, since portal hypertension usually coexists with low cardiac index and portal venous inflow in Fontan patients. TIPS placement could be an option for refractory variceal bleeding in highly selected patients in whom the cardiac function is normal or only minimally impaired [90]. Finally, as in other cardiac hepatopathies, liver disease may improve and even normalize if cardiac function is restored by **heart transplantation** [94]. Considering the severity of heart and liver disease run in parallel and that some degree of liver damage is practically universal in Fontan patients, it becomes critical to identify patients who require an isolated heart transplant or a double heart and liver transplant. Based on small series, a double transplant is recommended in all patients with advanced liver fibrosis, with or without previous hepatic decompensation [95–97]. However, the choice of isolated heart or double transplantation should be tailored to each patient by a multidisciplinary team.


## *Liver Damage in Other Congenital Heart Diseases*


***Atrial and Ventricular Defects*** Atrial septal defects can lead to right atrium and right ventricular enlargement, complicated with tricuspid regurgitation when the tricuspid annulus becomes dilatated. When pulmonary hypertension occurs, the shunted flow usually reverses and cyanosis appears (Eisenmenger's syndrome). Hepatic congestion is frequent in unrepaired atrial and ventricular defects, but cirrhosis rarely develops [31].

**Table 13.7**  Follow-up recommendations for liver disease after Fontan surgery

| **Diagnosis of FALD** | | |
| --- | --- | --- |
| <10 years after Fontan surgery | HAV (IgG), HBV and HCV antibodies[a] and screening for autoimmune and metabolic liver disease. | Baseline |
| | Liver function parameters | Annual |
| | Doppler ultrasound | Every 5 years |
| | Elastography | Every 5 years |
| ≥10 years after Fontan surgery or "Fontan failure" | Liver function parameters<br>Alpha-fetoprotein<br>Doppler ultrasound<br>Elastography<br>Dynamic MRI/CT | Every 6 months<br>Every 6 months<br>Every 6 months<br>Baseline and annual<br>Baseline |
| Liver biopsy | Uncertain diagnosis and candidates for liver and/or heart transplantation | |
| **Screening for and diagnosis of hepatocellular carcinoma** | | |
| Doppler ultrasound | Every 6 months from 10 years after surgery[b] | |
| Dynamic MRI/CT | • ≥10 years after surgery (baseline)<br>• If "benign" nodules are present in the basal test (hypercapting in the arterial phase, without venous or late phase clearance, multiple, peripheral and with normal AFP) repeat at 3 months. If there is no suspicion of hepatocarcinoma, continue with semiannual ultrasound screening.<br>• If one or more nodules develop during follow-up.<br>• Hepatic MRI is recommended when cardiac MRI is performed. | |
| Biopsy/FNAB | Any nodule suggestive of hepatocellular carcinoma (venous phase clearance, growth or elevated AFP) requires histologic confirmation. | |
| **Esophagogastric varices screening** | | |
| Analytical, clinical, radiological or elastographic data of FALD | Basal upper digestive endoscopy<br>If no varices veins or these are small, watch every 1–3 years. | |

[a]Perform HAV, HCV and HBV ELISA (HBsAg, HBcAb and HBsAb) in all patients subjected to Fontan surgery. If not immunized, vaccination against HAV and HBV should be indicated and its efficacy tested with new serologies. 10 years after effective vaccination against HBV, levels of HBsAg should be determined and a new dose should be indicated if levels are <100 IU/L
[b]Will be advanced in those patients with "Fontan failure", Fontan's duct thrombosis or transitional elastography ≥15 kPa

***Ebstein's Malformation***  This is a congenital defect in which the septal and posterior leaflets of the tricuspid valve are displaced towards the apex of the right ventricle. Some degree right ventricle dysfunction is the rule, even after tricuspid valve repair. This anomaly is usually detected in childhood or adolescence, but liver disease secondary to systemic venous congestion could be the debut in undiagnosed cases [98].

***Tetralogy of Fallot*** This complex congenital defect (pulmonary stenosis, ventricular septal defect, right ventricular hypertrophy and overriding aorta) usually requires surgical treatment. Pulmonary and tricuspid regurgitation and right ventricular dysfunction are common complications, resulting in chronic liver congestion. Restrictive right ventricles can be less prone to dilatation, but cause higher pressures in the right atrium. Liver damage is less frequent in Fallot's than in other congenital cardiac diseases and surveillance is not universally indicated [99].

***Dextro-Transposition of the Great Arteries and Mustard Surgery*** In Mustard surgery, a baffle is employed to redirect blood flow through the superior and inferior cavalveins to the anatomic left ventricle, connected to the pulmonary arteries. The pulmonary venous blood is diverted through the right ventricle to the aorta. Right ventricular failure and secondary tricuspid regurgitation occur because the right ventricle is not prepared to work as a systemic pump. Only patients with severe dysfunction of the right ventricle or thrombosis/stenosis in the lower venous baffle can develop hepatic venous congestion, so in the absence of these complications, liver damage is very unlikely [100].

# References


1. Moller BM. Interactions of the heart and the liver. Eur Heart J. 2013;34:2804–11.
2. Moons P, Meijboom FJ, Baumgartner H, Trindade PT, Huyghe E, Kaemmerer H. ESC working group on grown-up congenital heart disease structure and activities of adult congenital heart disease programmes in Europe. Eur Heart J. 2010;31:1305–1.
3. Giallourakis CC, Rosenberg PM, Friedman LS. The liver in heart failure. Clin Liver Dis. 2002;6:947–67.
4. Greuter T, Shah VH. Hepatic sinusoids in liver injury, inflammation, and fibrosis: new pathophysiological insights. J Gastroenterol. 2016;51:511–9.
5. Safran AP, Schaffner F. Chronic passive congestion of the liver in man. Electron microscopic study of cell atrophy and intralobular fibrosis. Am J Pathol. 1967;50:447–63.
6. Wanless IR, Liu JJ, Butany J. Role of thrombosis in the pathogenesis of congestive hepatic fibrosis (cardiac cirrhosis). Hepatology. 1995;21:1232–7.
7. Simonetto DA, Yang H, Yin M, de Assuncao TM, Kwon JH, Hilscher M, et al. Chronic passive venous congestion drives hepatic fibrogenesis via sinusoidal thrombosis and mechanical forces. Hepatology. 2015;61:648–59.
8. Sherlock S. The liver in heart failure: relation of anatomical, functional and circulatory changes. Br Heart J. 1951;13:273–93.
9. Tapper EB, Sengupta N, Bonder A. The incidence and outcomes of ischemic hepatitis: a systematic review with meta-analysis. Am J Med. 2015;128:1314–21.
10. Koehne de Gonzalez AK, Lefkowitch JH. Heart disease and the liver: pathologic evaluation. Gastroenterol Clin N Am. 2017;46:421–35.
11. Louie CY, Pham MX, Daugherty TJ, et al. The liver in heart failure: a biopsy and explant series of the histopathologic and laboratory findings with a particular focus on pre-cardiac transplant evaluation. Mod Pathol. 2015;28:932–43.
12. Dai DF, Swanson PE, Krieger EV, et al. Congestive hepatic fibrosis score: a novel histologic assessment of clinical severity. Mod Pathol. 2014;27:1552–8.

13. Kakar S, Batts KP, Poterucha JJ, et al. Histologic changes mimicking biliary disease in liver biopsies with venous outflow impairment. Mod Pathol. 2004;17:874–8.

14. Wells ML, Venkatesh SK. Congestive hepatopathy. Abdom Radiol (NY). 2018;43:2037–51.

15. Khalid U, Favot M, Ubaid F. Pericardial tamponade masquerading as abdominal pain diagnosed by point-of-care ultrasonography. Clin Pract Cases Emerg Med. 2017;1:403–6.

16. Belzunegui T. Cardiac tamponade presenting as abdominal pain and being the initial manifestation of malignant disease: a case report. JMC. 2013;4:485–7.

17. Maisel AS, Atwood JE, Goldberg AL. Hepatojugular reflux: useful in the bedside diagnosis of tricuspid regurgitation. Ann Intern Med. 1984;101:871–2.

18. Omar HR, Gulin M. Clinical and prognostic significance of positive hepatojugular reflux on discharge in acute heart failure: insights from the ESCAPE trial. Biomed Res Int. 2017;2017:5734749.

19. Runyon BA. Cardiac ascites: a characterization. J Clin Gastroenterol. 1988;10:410–2.

20. Sheer TA, Joo E, Runyon BA. Usefulness of serum N-terminal-ProBNP in distinguishing ascites due to cirrhosis from ascites due to heart failure. J Clin Gastroenterol. 2010;44:e23–6.

21. Alvarez AM, Mukherjee D. Liver abnormalities in cardiac diseases and heart failure. Int J Angiol. 2011;20:135–42.

22. Samsky MD, Patel CB, DeWald TA, et al. Cardiohepatic interactions in heart failure: an overview and clinical implications. J Am Coll Cardiol. 2013;61:2397–405.

23. Poelzl G, Eberl C, Achrainer H, et al. Prevalence and prognostic significance of elevated gamma-glutamyltransferase in chronic heart failure. Circ Heart Fail. 2009;2:294–302.

24. Henrion J, Schapira M, Luwaert R, Colin L, Delannoy A, Heller FR. Hypoxic hepatitis: clinical and hemodynamic study in 142 consecutive cases. Medicine (Baltimore). 2003;82:392–406.

25. Arques S, Ambrosi P. Human serum albumin in the clinical syndrome of heart failure. J Card Fail. 2011;17:451–8.

26. Bessman AN, Evans JM. The blood ammonia in congestive heart failure. Am Heart J. 1955;50:715–9.

27. Mullens Z, Abrahams GS, Francis DO, Tylor RC, Starling WH. Tang. Prompt reduction in intra-abdominal pressure following mechanical fluid removal improves renal insufficiency in refractory decompensated heart failure. J Card Fail. 2008;14:508–14.

28. MacFadyen RN, Chuen NK, Davis RC. Loop diuretic therapy in left ventricular systolic dysfunction: has familiarity bred contempt for a critical but potentially nepthrotoxiccardio renal therapy? Eur J Heart Fail. 2010;12:649–52.

29. Verbrugge FH, Dupont M, Steels P, Grieten L, Malbrain M, Tang WH, et al. Abdominal contributions to cardiorenal dysfunction in congestive heart failure. J Am Coll Cardiol. 2013;62:485–95.

30. Tripodi A. Liver disease and hemostatic (Dys) function. Semin Thromb Hemost. 2015;41:462–7.

31. Asrani SK, Asrani NS, Freese DK, Phillips SD, Warnes CA, Heimbach J, et al. Congenital heart disease and the liver. Hepatology. 2012;56:1160–9.

32. Sung PS, Yoon SK. Amiodarone hepatotoxicity. Hepatology. 2012;55:325–6.

33. Wang A, Book WM, McConnell M, Lyle T, Rodby K, Mahle WT. Prevalence of hepatitis C infection in adult patients who underwent congenital heart surgery prior to screening in 1992. Am J Cardiol. 2007;100:1307–9.

34. Tellez L, Rodriguez-Santiago E, Albillos A. Fontan-associated liver disease: a review. Ann Hepatol. 2018;17:192–204.

35. Fontan F, Baudet E. Surgical repair of tricuspid atresia. Thorax. 1971;26:240–8.

36. Gewillig M, Brown SC. The Fontan circulation after 45 years: update in physiology. Heart Br. Card. Soc. 2016;102:1081–6.

37. Quinton E, Nightingale P, Hudsmith L, Thorne S, Marshall H, Clift P, et al. Prevalence of atrial tachyarrhythmia in adults after Fontan operation. Heart Br. Card. Soc. 2015;101:1672–7.

38. Balaji S, Gewillig M, Bull C, de Leval MR, Deanfield JE. Arrhythmias after the Fontan procedure. Comparison of total cavopulmonary connection and atriopulmonary connection. Circulation. 1991;84:III162–7.

39. Seipelt RG, Franke A, Vazquez-Jimenez JF, Hanarth P, von Bernuth G, Messmer BJ, et al. Thromboembolic complications after Fontan procedures: comparison of different therapeutic approaches. Ann Thorac Surg. 2002;74:556–62.

40. Johnson JA, Cetta F, Graham RP, Smyrk TC, Driscoll DJ, Phillips SD, et al. Identifying predictors of hepatic disease in patients after the Fontan operation: a postmortem analysis. J Thorac Cardiovasc Surg. 2013;146:140–5.

41. Faircloth JM, Roe O, Alsaied T, Palumbo JS, Vinks A, Veldtman GR. Intermediate term thrombotic risk in contemporary total cavo-pulmonary connection for single ventricle circulations. J Thromb Thrombolysis. 2017;44:275–80.

42. Rodriguez de Santiago E, Téllez L, Garrido-Lestache Rodríguez-Monte E, Garrido-Gómez E, Aguilera-Castro L, Álvarez-Fuente M, et al. Fontan protein-losing enteropathy is associated with advanced liver disease and proinflamatory intestinal and systemic state. Liver Int. 2020;40:638–45.

43. Wu FM, Jonas MM, Opotowsky AR, Harmon A, Raza R, Ukomadu C, et al. Portal and centrilobular hepatic fibrosis in Fontan circulation and clinical outcomes. J Heart Lung Transplant Off Publ Int Soc Heart Transplant. 2015;34:883–91.

44. Bae JM, Jeon TY, Kim JS, Kim S, Hwang SM, Yoo S-Y, et al. Fontan-associated liver disease: Spectrum of US findings. Eur J Radiol. 2016;85:850–6.

45. Evans WN, Acherman RJ, Ciccolo ML, Carrillo SA, Galindo A, Rothman A, et al. MELD-XI scores correlate with post-Fontan hepatic biopsy fibrosis scores. Pediatr Cardiol. 2016;37:1274–7.

46. Baek JS, Bae EJ, Ko JS, Kim GB, Kwon BS, Lee SY, et al. Late hepatic complications after Fontan operation; non-invasive markers of hepatic fibrosis and risk factors. Heart Br Card Soc. 2010;96:1750–5.

47. Munsterman ID, Duijnhouwer AL, Kendall TJ, Bronkhorst CM, Ronot M, van Wettere M, et al. The clinical spectrum of Fontan-associated liver disease: results from a prospective multimodality screening cohort. Eur Heart J. 2019;40:1057–68.

48. Assenza GE, Graham DA, Landzberg MJ, Valente AM, Singh MN, Bashir A, et al. MELD-XI score and cardiac mortality or transplantation after Fontan surgery. Heart. 2013;99:491–6.

49. Lemmer A, VanWagner LB, Ganger D. Assessment of advanced liver fibrosis and the risk for hepatic decompensation in patients with congestive hepatopathy. Hepatology. 2018 (in press).

50. Kutty SS, Peng Q, Danford DA, Fletcher SE, Perry D, Talmon GA, et al. Increased hepatic stiffness as consequence of high hepatic afterload in the Fontan circulation: a vascular Doppler and elastography study. Hepatology. 2014;59:251–60.

51. Wallihan DB, Podberesky DJ. Hepatic pathology after Fontan palliation: spectrum of imaging findings. Pediatr Radiol. 2013;43:330–8.

52. Camposilvan S, Milanesi O, Stellin G, Pettenazzo A, Zancan L, D'Antiga L. Liver and cardiac function in the long term after Fontan operation. Ann Thorac Surg. 2008;86:177–82.

53. Bulut OP, Romero R, Mahle WT, McConnell M, Braithwaite K, Shehata BM, et al. Magnetic resonance imaging identifies unsuspected liver abnormalities in patients after the Fontan procedure. J Pediatr. 2013;163:201–6.

54. Dijkstra H, Wolff D, van Melle JP, Bartelds B, Willems TP, Oudkerk M, et al. Disminished liver microperfusion in Fontan patients: a biexponential DWI study. PLoS One. 2017;12:e0173149.

55. Wolff D, van Melle JP, Dijkstra H, Bartelds B, Willems TP, Hillege H, et al. The Fontan circulation and the liver: a magnetic resonance diffusion-weighted imaging study. Int J Cardiol. 2016;202:595–600.

56. Deorsola L, Aidala E, Cascarano MT, Valori A, Agnoletti G, Pace NC. Liver stiffness modifications shortly after total cavopulmonary connection. Interact Cardiovasc Thorac Surg. 2016;23:513–8.

57. Wu FM, Opotowsky AR, Raza R, Harney S, Ukomadu C, Landzberg MJ, et al. Transient elastography may identify Fontan patients with unfavorable hemodynamics and advanced hepatic fibrosis. Congenit Heart Dis. 2014;9:438–47.
58. Kutty SS, Peng Q, Danford DA, Fletcher SE, Perry D, Talmon GA, et al. Increased hepatic stiffness as consequence of high hepatic afterload in the Fontan circulation: a vascular Doppler and elastography study. Hepatol Baltim Md. 2014;59:251–60.
59. Agnoletti G, Ferraro G, Bordese R, Marini D, Gala S, Bergamasco L, et al. Fontan circulation causes early, severe liver damage. Should we offer patients a tailored strategy? Int J Cardiol. 2016;209:60–5.
60. Poterucha JT, Johnson JN, Qureshi MY, O'Leary PW, Kamath PS, Lennon RJ, et al. Magnetic resonance elastography: a novel technique for the detection of hepatic fibrosis and hepatocellular carcinoma after the Fontan operation. Mayo Clin Proc. 2015;90:882–94.
61. Mori M, Hebson C, Shioda K, Elder RW, Kogon BE, Rodriguez FH, et al. Catheter-measured hemodynamics of adult Fontan circulation: associations with adverse event and end-organ dysfunctions. Congenit Heart Dis. 2016;11:589–97.
62. Kendall TJ, Stedman B, Hacking N, Haw M, Vettukattill JJ, Salmon AP, et al. Hepatic fibrosis and cirrhosis in the Fontan circulation: a detailed morphological study. J Clin Pathol. 2008;61:504–8.
63. Bosch J, Abraldes JG, Albillos A, Aracil C, Bañares R, Berzigotti A, et al. Hipertensión portal: recomendaciones para su evaluación y tratamiento. Gastroenterol Hepatol. 2012;35:421–50.
64. Guzeltas A, Tanidir IC, Saygi M. Major intrahpatic veno-venous fistula after Fontan operation treated by transcatheter implantation of amplatzer septal occluder through internal jugular vein. Braz J Cardiovasc Surg. 2016;31:174–7.
65. Kendall TJ, Stedman B, Hacking N, Haw M, Vettukattill JJ, Salmon AP, et al. Hepatic fibrosis and cirrhosis in the Fontan circulation: a detailed morphological study. J Clin Pathol. 2008;61:504–8.
66. Rychik J, Veldtman G, Rand E, Russo P, Rome JJ, Krok K, et al. The precarious state of the liver after a Fontan operation: summary of a multidisciplinary symposium. Pediatr Cardiol. 2012;33:1001–12.
67. Goldberg DJ, Surrey LF, Glatz AC, Dodds K, O'Byrne ML, Lin HC, et al. Hepatic fibrosis is universal following Fontan operation, and severity is associated with time from surgery: a liver biopsy and hemodynamic study. J Am Heart Assoc. 2017;6(5):e004809.
68. Asrani SK, Asrani NS, Freese DK, Phillips SD, Warnes CA, Heimbach J, et al. Congenital heart disease and the liver. Hepatology. 2012;56:1160–9.
69. Téllez L, Rodríguez de Santiago E, Mínguez B, Payance A, Clemente A, Baiges A, et al. Prevalence, features and predictive factors of liver nodules in Fontan surgery patients: the VALDIG Fonliver prospective cohort. J Hepatol. 2020;72:702–10.
70. Kiesewetter CH, Sheron N, Vettukattill JJ, Hacking N, Stedman B, Millward-Sadler H, et al. Hepatic changes in the failing Fontan circulation. Heart Br. Card. Soc. 2007;93:579–84.
71. Wu FM, Kogon B, Earing MG, Aboulhosn JA, Broberg CS, John AS, et al. Liver health in adults with Fontan circulation: a multicenter cross-sectional study. J Thorac Cardiovasc Surg. 2017;153:656–64.
72. Shimamatsu K, Wanless IR. Role of ischemia in causing apoptosis, atrophy, and nodular hyperplasia in human liver. Hepatol Baltim Md. 1997;26:343–50.
73. Sempoux C, Balabaud C, Paradis V, Bioulac-Sage P. Hepatocellular nodules in vascular liver diseases. Virchows Arch. 2018;473:33–44.
74. Ghaferi AA, Hutchins GM. Progression of liver pathology in patients undergoing the Fontan procedure: chronic passive congestion, cardiac cirrhosis, hepatic adenoma, and hepatocellular carcinoma. J Thorac Cardiovasc Surg. 2005;129:1348–52.
75. Saliba T, Dorkhom S, O'Reilly EM, Ludwig E, Gansukh B, Abou-Alfa GK. Hepatocellular carcinoma in two patients with cardiac cirrhosis. Eur J Gastroenterol Hepatol. 2010;22:889–91.

76. Asrani SK, Warnes CA, Kamath PS. Hepatocellular carcinoma after the Fontan procedure. N Engl J Med. 2013;368:1756–7.
77. Elder RW, Parekh S, Book WM. More on hepatocellular carcinoma after the Fontan procedure. N Engl J Med. 2013;369:490.
78. Takuma Y, Fukada Y, Iwadou S, Miyatake H, Uematsu S, Okamoto R, et al. Surgical resection for hepatocellular carcinoma with cardiac cirrhosis after the Fontan procedure. Intern Med Tokyo Jpn. 2016;55:3265–72.
79. Rajoriya N, Clift P, Thorne S, Hirschfield GM, Ferguson JW. A liver mass post-Fontan operation. QJM Mon J Assoc Physicians. 2014;107:571–2.
80. Weyker PD, Allen-John Webb C, Emond JC, Brentjens TE, Johnston TA. Anesthetic implications of extended right hepatectomy in a patient with Fontan physiology. Case Rep. 2014;2:99–101.
81. Kwon S, Scovel L, Yeh M, Dorsey D, Dembo G, Krieger EV, et al. Surgical management of hepatocellular carcinoma after Fontan procedure. J Gastrointest Oncol. 2015;6:E55–60.
82. Yamada K, Shinmoto H, Kawamura Y, Wakamatsu H, Kawauchi T, Soga S, et al. Transarterial embolization for pediatric hepatocellular carcinoma with cardiac cirrhosis. Pediatr Int Off J Jpn Pediatr Soc. 2015;57:766–70.
83. Oh C, Youn JK, Han J-W, Kim GB, Kim H-Y, Jung S-E. Hepatocellular carcinoma after the Fontan procedure in a 16-year-old girl: a case report. Medicine (Baltimore). 2016;95:e4823.
84. Conroy MR, Moe TG. Hepatocellular carcinoma in the adult Fontan patient. Cardiol Young. 2017;27:407–9.
85. Josephus Jitta D, Wagenaar LJ, Mulder BJM, Guichelaar M, Bouman D, van Melle JP. Three cases of hepatocellular carcinoma in Fontan patients: review of the literature and suggestions for hepatic screening. Int J Cardiol. 2016;206:21–6.
86. Wells ML, Hough DM, Fidler JL, Kamath PS, Poterucha JT, Venkatesh SK. Benign nodules in post-Fontan livers can show imaging features considered diagnostic for hepatocellular carcinoma. Abdom Radiol (NY). 2017;42:2623–31.
87. Nandwana SB, Olaiya B, Cox K, Sahu MP. Abdominal imaging surveillance in adult patients after Fontan procedure: risk of chronic liver disease and hepatocellular carcinoma. Curr Probl Diagn Radiol. 2018;47:19–22.
88. Rodríguez de Santiago E, Téllez L, Guerrero A, Albillos A. Hepatocellular carcinoma after Fontan surgery: a Systematic Review. Hepatol Res. 2020. In press.
89. Elder RW, McCabe NM, Hebson C, Veledar E, Romero R, Ford RM, et al. Features of portal hypertension are associated with major adverse events in Fontan patients: the VAST study. Int J Cardiol. 2013;168:3764–9.
90. Velpula M, Sheron N, Guha N, Salmon T, Hacking N, Veldtman GR. Direct measurement of Porto-systemic gradient in a failing Fontan circulation. Congenit Heart Dis. 2011;6:175–8.
91. Pundi K, Pundi KN, Kamath PS, Cetta F, Li Z, Poterucha JT, et al. Liver disease in patients after the Fontan operation. Am J Cardiol. 2016;117:456–60.
92. Koteda Y, Suda K, Kishimoto S, Iemura M. Portal-systemic encephalopathy after Fontan-type operation in patient with polysplenia syndrome. Eur J Cardio-Thorac Surg Off J Eur Asszoc Cardio-Thorac Surg. 2009;35:1083–5.
93. Hilscher MB, Johnson JN, Cetta F, Driscoll DJ, Poterucha JJ, Sanchez W, et al. Surveillance for liver complications after the Fontan procedure. Congenit Heart Dis. 2017;12:124–32.
94. Dichtl W, Vogel W, Dunst KM, Grander W, Alber HF, Frick M, et al. Cardiac hepatopathy before and after heart transplantation. Transpl Int Off J Eur Soc Organ Transplant. 2005;18:697–702.
95. Crespo-Leiro MG, Robles O, Paniagua MJ, Marzoa R, Naya C, Flores X, et al. Reversal of cardiac cirrhosis following orthotopic heart transplantation. Am J Transplant Off J Am Soc Transplant Am Soc Transpl Surg. 2008;8:1336–9.
96. D'Souza BA, Fuller S, Gleason LP, Hornsby N, Wald J, Krok K, et al. Single-center outcomes of combined heart and liver transplantation in the failing Fontan. Clin Transpl. 2017;31(3):e12892. https://doi.org/10.1111/ctr.12892.

97. Simpson KE, Pruitt E, Kirklin JK, Naftel DC, Singh RK, Edens RE, et al. Fontan patient survival after pediatric heart transplantation has improved in the current era. Ann Thorac Surg. 2017;103:1315–20.
98. De Vette LC, Brugts JJ, McGhie JS, Roos-Hesselink JW. Long-lasting symptoms and diagnostics in a patient with <u>unrecognizedright sided</u> heart failure: why listening to the heart is so important? World J Cardiol. 2014;26:345–8.
99. McCabe N, Farris AB, Hon H, Ford R, Book WM. Hepatocellular carcinoma in an adult with repaired tetralogy of Fallot. Congenit Heart Dis. 2013;8:139–44.
100. Patel S, Shah D, Chintala K, Karpawich PP. Atrial baffle problems following the mustard operation in children and young adults with dextro-transposition of the great arteries: the need for improved clinical detection in the current era. Congenit Heart Dis. 2011;6:466–74.

# Chapter 14
# Regenerative Nodules and Liver Tumors in Vascular Liver Diseases

Valerie Paradis and Aurélie Beaufrère

## Introduction

Hepatocellular nodules may occur either in a background normal liver or in the context of chronic liver diseases, including vascular liver diseases (VLD) [1, 2]. Although the relationship between hepatocellular nodules and VLD has long been recognized, their pathogenesis has been more recently deciphered [1]. Indeed, the pathogenesis of most of hepatocellular nodules associated with VLD has been linked to the imbalance between hepatic arterial and portal venous blood flow leading to an increased hepatic arterial inflow [3, 4].

Hepatocellular nodules have been firstly described in Budd-Chiari syndrome (BCS), Hereditary Hemorrhagic Telangiectasia (HHT), and congenital porto-systemic shunts (CPSS) [1, 2], and most cases have been reported in BCS [5–9]. Noteworthy, by contrast to other chronic liver diseases leading to cirrhosis, hepatocellular nodules associated with VLD correspond in the great majority of cases to benign hepatocellular nodules, either regenerative or neoplastic.

While the relationship between hepatocellular nodules and VLD is better described in imaging than in pathology [2, 6, 10], their radiological features are less characteristic yielding an accurate "noninvasive" diagnostic difficult. Indeed, the distinction between neoplastic, either benign (hepatocellular adenoma) or malignant

V. Paradis (✉) · A. Beaufrère
Department of Pathology, APHP Beaujon Hospital, Clichy, France

Université de Paris, Paris, France
e-mail: valerie.paradis@aphp.fr; aurelie.beaufrere@aphp.fr



D. Valla et al. (eds.), *Vascular Disorders of the Liver*,
https://doi.org/10.1007/978-3-030-82988-9_14

(hepatocellular carcinoma), and regenerative nodules is complex on imaging in VLD [2, 3]. Therefore, a liver biopsy is almost always required to characterize precisely the lesion and exclude malignancy [11, 12]. Nevertheless, definite diagnosis of nodules is based on a specialized multidisciplinary team, including clinicians, radiologists and pathologists, and leads in most of cases to a close follow-up [1].

In this chapter, we will first describe the main morphological features of the hepatocellular nodules developed in VLD and we will review the type of hepatocellular nodules according to the most common VLDs.

## Hepatocellular Nodules: A Wide Spectrum of Lesions

Both benign and malignant hepatocellular nodules can be observed in VLD. Dysplastic nodules will not be discussed in this chapter because of their low described association with VLD. Diffuse lesions like NRH are treated in Chap. 9. While benign hepatocellular nodules encompass a wide spectrum of lesions [large regenerative nodule (LRN), focal nodular hyperplasia (FNH) and hepatocellular adenoma (HCA)], malignant hepatocellular nodules correspond to hepatocellular carcinoma (HCC). The main histological features of each type of nodules observed in VLD are listed in Table 14.1.

### *Large Regenerative Nodules (LRN) (Fig. 14.1)*

### *Pathology*

LRN, also known as macro regenerative nodule or multi-acinar regenerative nodule, corresponds to a reactive hepatocellular nodule, mostly observed in cirrhotic liver [10, 13]. LRN measures commonly more than 0.5–1 cm in diameter (Fig. 14.1a). In practice, they are larger than the surrounding cirrhotic nodules. They are composed of normal looking hepatocytes without atypia arranged in one-to two-cell-thick plates (Fig. 14.1b). Portal tracts are present and reticulin framework is intact (Fig. 14.1c and d). No central scar and no ductular reaction are present [1, 14]. Their main differential diagnoses are dysplastic nodules (low grade) and in a lesser extent focal nodular hyperplasias [15].

### Imaging

LRN may be unique or multiple. With multi-phasic, contrast-enhanced CT nodules are enhanced homogeneously on the arterial phase and remained slightly hyperdense relative to liver parenchyma on the portal venous phase. On MRI, these lesions is hyper intense relative to liver parenchyma on the T1-weighted images and isointense or hypointense relative to liver parenchyma on T2-weighted images [16].

**Table 14.1** Main macroscopic and microscopic features of hepatocellular nodules observed in vascular liver disorders

|  | Macroscopic features | Microscopic features |
|---|---|---|
| Large regenerative nodule | Large nodule (amore than 1 cm) | Nodule composed of hepatocytes with normal or near-normal cytology, with plates one to two cells thick. Intact reticulin framework |
| Focal nodular hyperplasia | Well-circumscribed but not encapsulated lesion (a few mm to >10 cm in diameter), paler than the surrounding hepatic parenchyma and firm. Cut section: Central stellate scar surrounded by parenchymal nodules delimited by fibrous septa radiating from the scar | Central scar with radiating branches, together with variable size nodules made of normal hepatocytes Ductular reaction and large dystrophic arteries in the fibrous septa Absence of portal tract Intact reticulin framework GS map-like pattern |
| Hepatocellular adenoma | Soft and relatively uniform lesion (1 mm up to 20 cm in diameter) Areas of congestion, necrosis, hemorrhage or fibrosis possible | Proliferation of hepatocytes arranged in sheets and cords of one or two cells thick without cytological atypia No portal tract Preserved reticulin framework IHC classification in 5 sub-types |
| Hepatocellular carcinoma | Soft lesion sometimes encapsulated, often with areas of necrosis (1 cm in diameter up to an entire lobe) Colors: Tan or yellow, and green if they produce bile. | Proliferation of hepatocytes arranged in more than two-cells thick plates. Pseudo acinar changes can be present, cytological atypia: mild to high No portal tract, unpaired arteries Loss or disruption of reticulin framework IHC: Expression of Glypican 3, GS and HSP70 |

*GS* glutamine synthetase, *IHC* immunohistochemistry

## LRN in VLD

LRN is mostly observed in cirrhotic liver, whatever its etiology, including vascular diseases [1, 17]. That is why it was more frequently observed in BCS [8]. It has been also frequently described in HHT [18].

## *Focal Nodular Hyperplasia (FNH) (Fig. 14.2)*

### Pathology

FNH may be single (two-thirds of cases) or multiple, and can be of any size [1]. On gross examination, FNH is well-circumscribed but not encapsulated. It is firm and paler than the surrounding liver parenchyma. On cut section, a central stellate scar is in most cases present, which is surrounded by parenchymal nodules delimited by fibrous septa radiating from the scar (Fig. 14.3a).

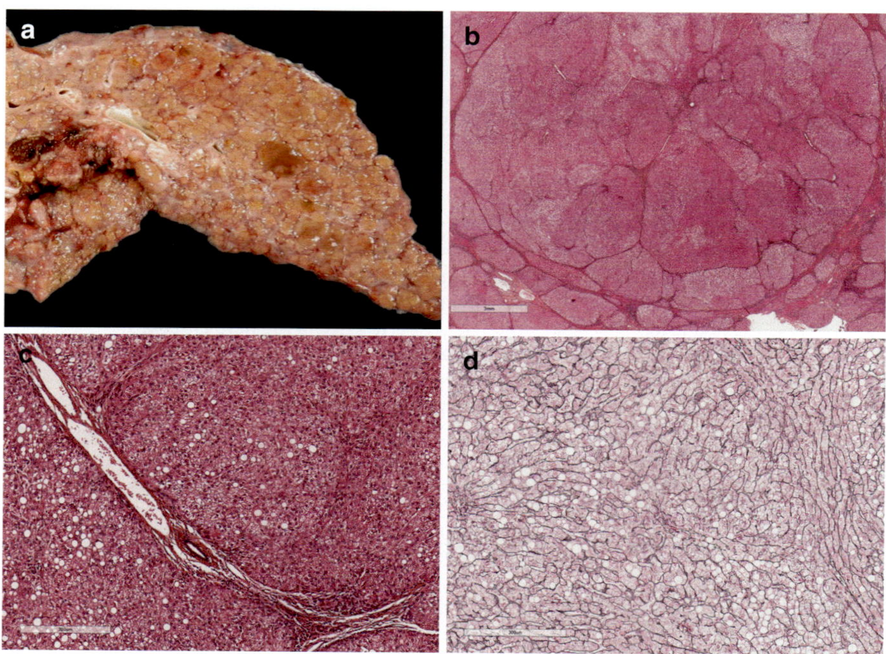

**Fig. 14.1** Large regenerative nodule (LRN). (**a**) Gross examination: large nodule contrasting with the surrounding liver parenchyma. (**b**) Microscopic examination: large nodule composed of hepatocytes organized in plates one to two cells thick. (**c**) Plates of hepatocytes with normal or near-normal cytology and portal tract. (**d**) Intact reticulin framework

On microscopic examination, the central scar presents radiating branches, together with variable size nodules made of normal hepatocytes (Fig. 14.3b). Ductular reaction is observed at the interface between the nodules and the fibrotic bands. The fibrous septa contain large dystrophic arteries without main bile duct or portal vein branch (Fig. 14.3c) [1, 19, 20].

A specific pattern of glutamine synthetase expression has been described in FNH, consisting of broad, anastomosing ('map-like') areas of positive hepatocytes, commonly centered on veins with broad bands usually at a distance from the fibrous septa (Fig. 14.3d). Indeed, FNH is specifically characterized by an activation of the beta-catenin pathway without beta-catenin mutation, leading to an increased expression of GLUL, the gene coding for GS. The 'map-like' positivity of hepatocytes for GS is never observed in the other types of hepatocellular nodules, and then constitutes a key diagnostic feature helpful in atypical FNH (i.e. lacking the central scar) and on biopsy in which all the morphological diagnostic features are not represented [19, 20].

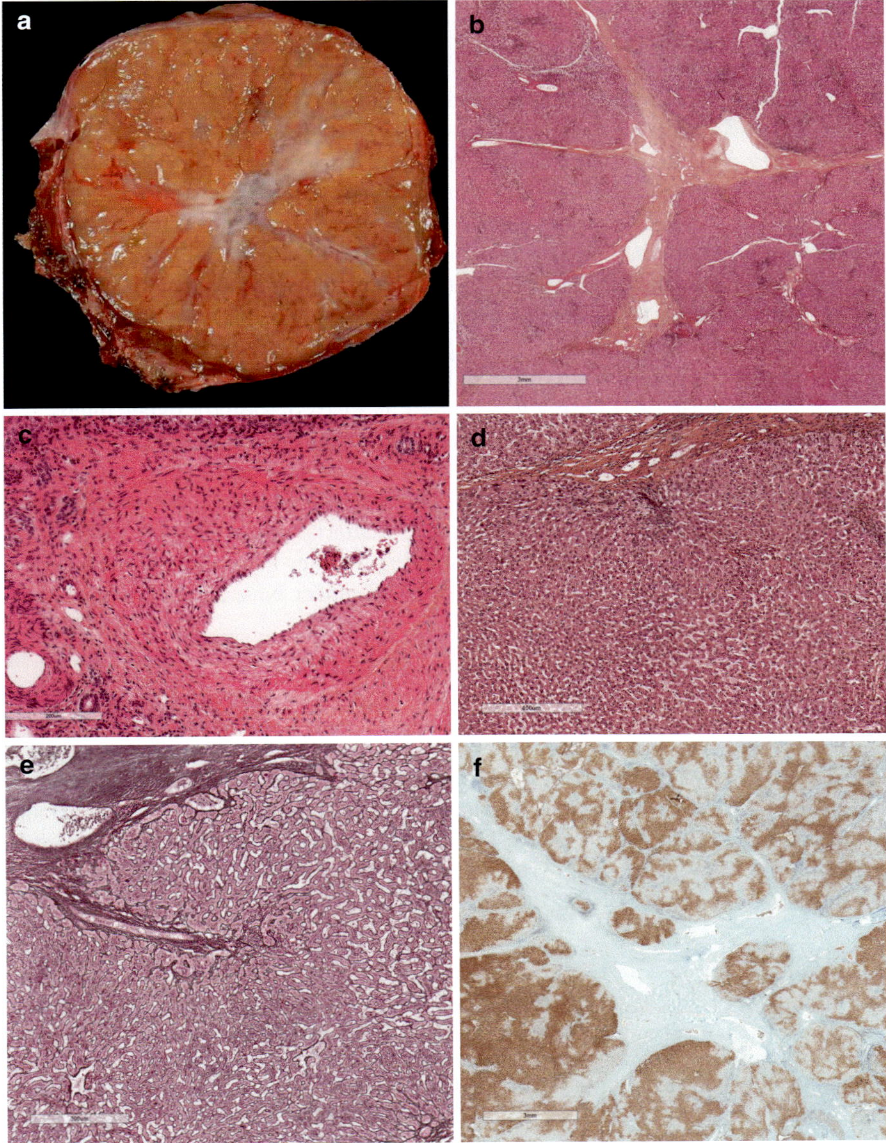

**Fig. 14.2** Focal nodular hyperplasia (FNH). (**a**) Gross examination: well-circumscribed nodule with central stellate scar surrounded by parenchymal nodules delimited by fibrous septa radiating from the scar. (**b**) Microscopic examination: central scar with radiating branches. (**c**) Large dystrophic artery in a fibrous septum. (**d**) Nodule made of normal-appearing hepatocytes. (**e**) Intact reticulin framework. (**f**) Glutamine synthetase immunostaining: map-like pattern

## Imaging

FNH is often typical and recognized by imaging technique in >80–90% of cases, except if small, lacking typical characteristics or with fatty infiltration [1]. At ultrasound, FNH is usually slightly hypoechoic or isoechoic, and may only be detected because they displace the surrounding vessels. Hypoechoic halo or lobulated contours are often observed. The central scar is difficult to visualize at US (20% of the cases). On CT scans, FNH spontaneously appears as a focal hypoattenuating mass. The central hypo attenuating scar is depicted in only one-third of the cases. At the arterial phase of contrast-enhanced CT, the lesion enhances rapidly in most cases. At the portal venous phase, the lesion is either iso- or slightly hyper-attenuating relative to normal liver. On MR imaging, there are five major criteria to assess a proper diagnosis: (1) lesion not different from the liver before contrast injection, i.e. iso- or hypo-intense on T1-weighted images and iso- or slightly hyper intense on T2-weighted images, (2) lesion homogeneity apart the central scar, (3) presence of a central scar, corresponding to a central hypo intense area on T1-weighted images, strongly hyperintense on T2-weighted images, and showing enhancement on delayed phase, (4) strong hyper enhancement at arterial phase without washout, (5) no capsule with lobulated aspect. These imaging findings in a patient with no underlying chronic liver disease or clinical history of cancer have a specificity close to 100% [2, 3].

## FNH in VLD

In the context of VLD, FNH are often multiple and of small size. Importantly, some hepatocellular nodules may show overlapping features between LRN and FNH and have been called FNH-like nodules. These nodules often do not show a real central scar but only thin fibrous septa with a more or less obvious ductular reaction [14]. FNH are frequently reported in BCS, CPSS and HHT [18, 21, 22].

**Fig. 14.3** Hepatocellular adenoma (HCA). (**a, b, c**) HNF1A inactivated adenoma: (**a**) gross examination: well circumscribed yellow red-brownish tumor, (**b**) microscopic examination: well differentiated hepatocellular proliferation with steatosis, (**c**) LFABP immunostaining: loss of LFABP expression. (**d, e, f**) Inflammatory adenoma, (**d**) Gross examination: yellow-brown tumor with area of hemorrhage, (**e**) well differentiated hepatocellular proliferation with sinusoidal dilatation and congestion, (**f**) SAA immunostaining: overexpression of SAA protein in the tumor cells. (**g, h, i**) β-catenin mutated (exon 3) adenoma: (**g**) gross examination: well circumscribed red-brownish tumor, (**h**) microscopic examination: hepatocellular proliferation with cytological atypia, (**i**) β-catenin immunostaining: nuclear and cytoplasmic expression of β-catenin in the tumor cells. (**j, k, l**) β-catenin mutated (exon 7 or 8) adenoma: (**j**) gross examination: Not well-limited red brownish tumor, (**k**) Reticulin stain: multifocal reticuln loss, (**l**) Glutamine synthetase immunostaining: heterogenous expression of glutamine synthetase. (**m, n, o**) Sonic Hedgehog adenoma: (**m**) gross examination: red-brownish nodule with large areas of hemorrhage, (**n**) microscopic examination: well differentiated hepatocellular proliferation with large areas of hemorrhage, (**o**) PGTDS immunostaining: expression of PGTDS in the tumor cells

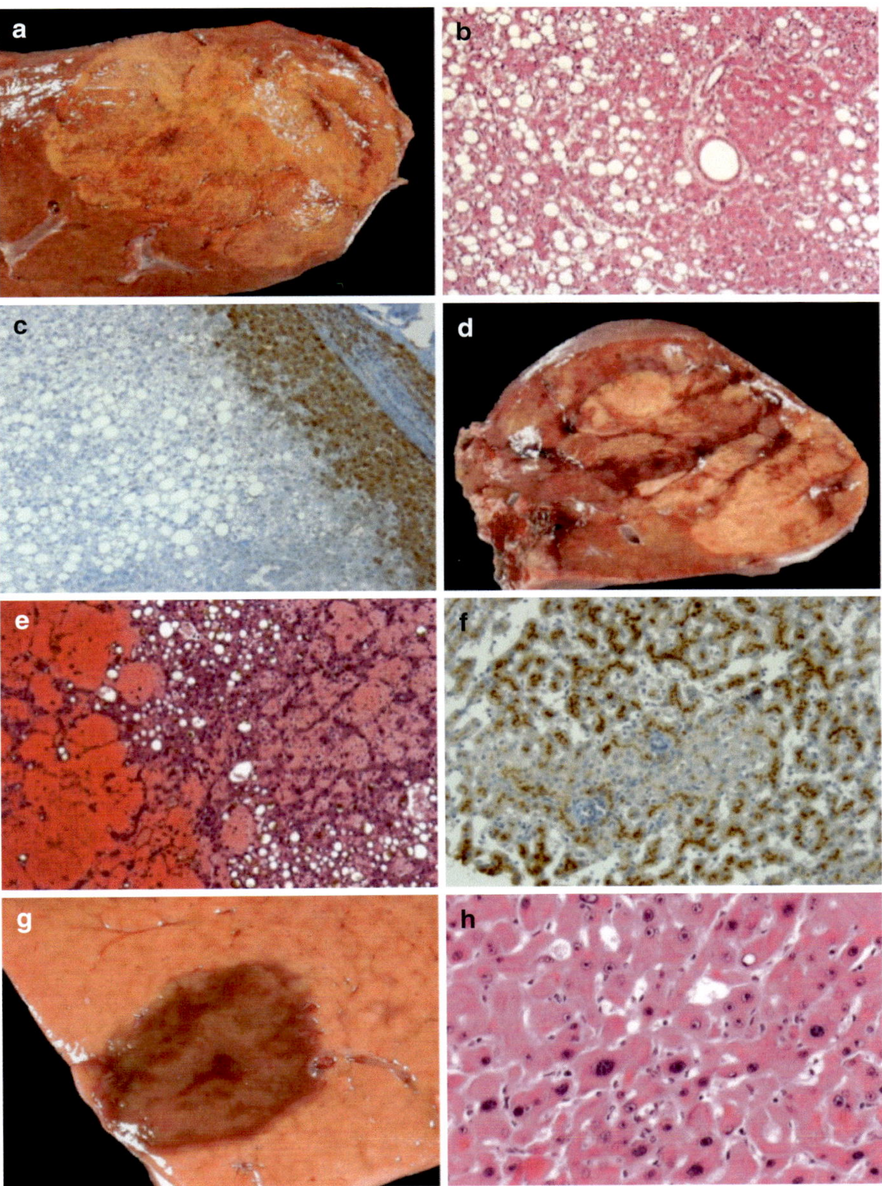

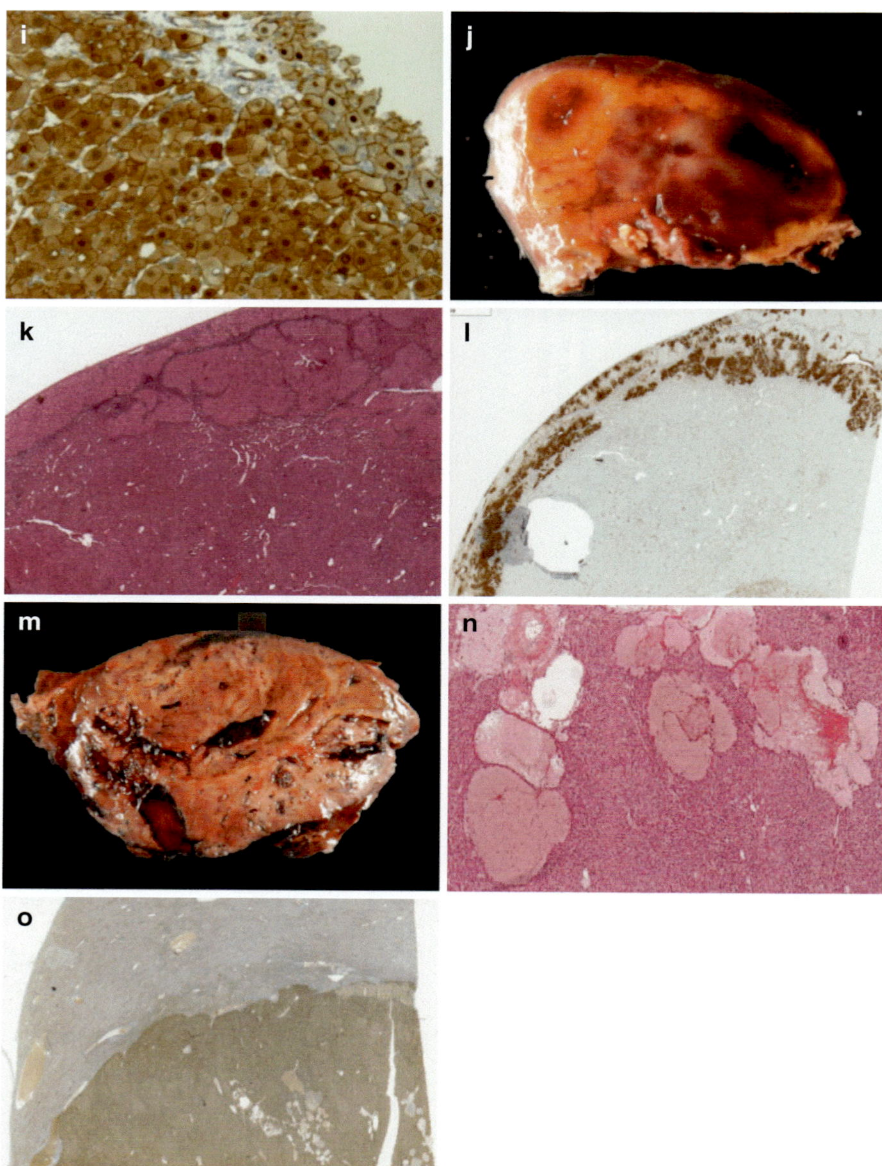

**Fig. 14.3** (continued)

## *Hepatocellular Adenoma (HCA) (Fig. 14.3)*

### Pathology

HCA may be unique or multiple, and their size is very variable, ranging from microscopic foci up to 30 cm [1]. On gross examination, the lesion may be well circumscribed or not, and can be difficult to distinguish from the surrounding parenchyma. HCA is soft and relatively uniform, although areas of congestion, necrosis, hemorrhage, or fibrosis can be observed. The color varies from yellow or tan to brown (Fig. 14.4a).

On microscopic examination, HCA corresponds to a proliferation of well-differentiated, usually bland-looking, hepatocytes arranged in sheets and cords composed of one or two cells, with a preserved reticulin framework and no portal tract (Fig. 14.4b and c). Since 2006, HCA define an heterogeneous group of neoplastic benign hepatocellular proliferations composed of different subtypes characterized by specific molecular alterations that are associated with morphological features, clinical settings and complications [1, 23–25]. The genotype-phenotype classification led to the description of 5 well-recognized subtypes based on morphological and immunophenotypical features, that are currently used in practice.

Hepatocyte Nuclear Factor 1A (HNF1A) Inactivated HCA (H-HCA)

The first group of HCAs is defined by HNF1A mutation in 30–40% of all HCAs. The gene defect was found to be somatic in 90% but germline in 10%. It occurs mostly in women taking oral contraception as well as MODY3. The main morphological hallmark of this subtype is the presence of steatosis, even though it could be of variable extent. The reticulin framework shows a pericellular pattern in which reticulin fibers can partially encircle small clusters of hepatocytes. Expression of liver fatty acid binding protein (LFABP) involved in lipid trafficking, is specifically absent in all H-HCA (always expressed in the normal liver), as a consequence of HNF1A inactivating mutation and serves as a translational marker to identify specifically this subtype [23, 24, 26].

Inflammatory HCA (IHCA)

The group of inflammatory HCAs accounts for 40% of all HCAs. The cardinal molecular feature of IHCAs is the activation of the JAK/STAT pathway, which may be related to various gene mutations, such as gp130 activating mutations in 65% of cases, STAT3 mutations in 5% of cases, and GNAS mutations in 5% of cases. It occurs mainly in women but also in men with high BMI and alcohol consumption. These HCAs show pseudo-portal tracts with inflammation, large arteries and ductular reaction, together with variable degrees of sinusoidal dilatation and congestion.

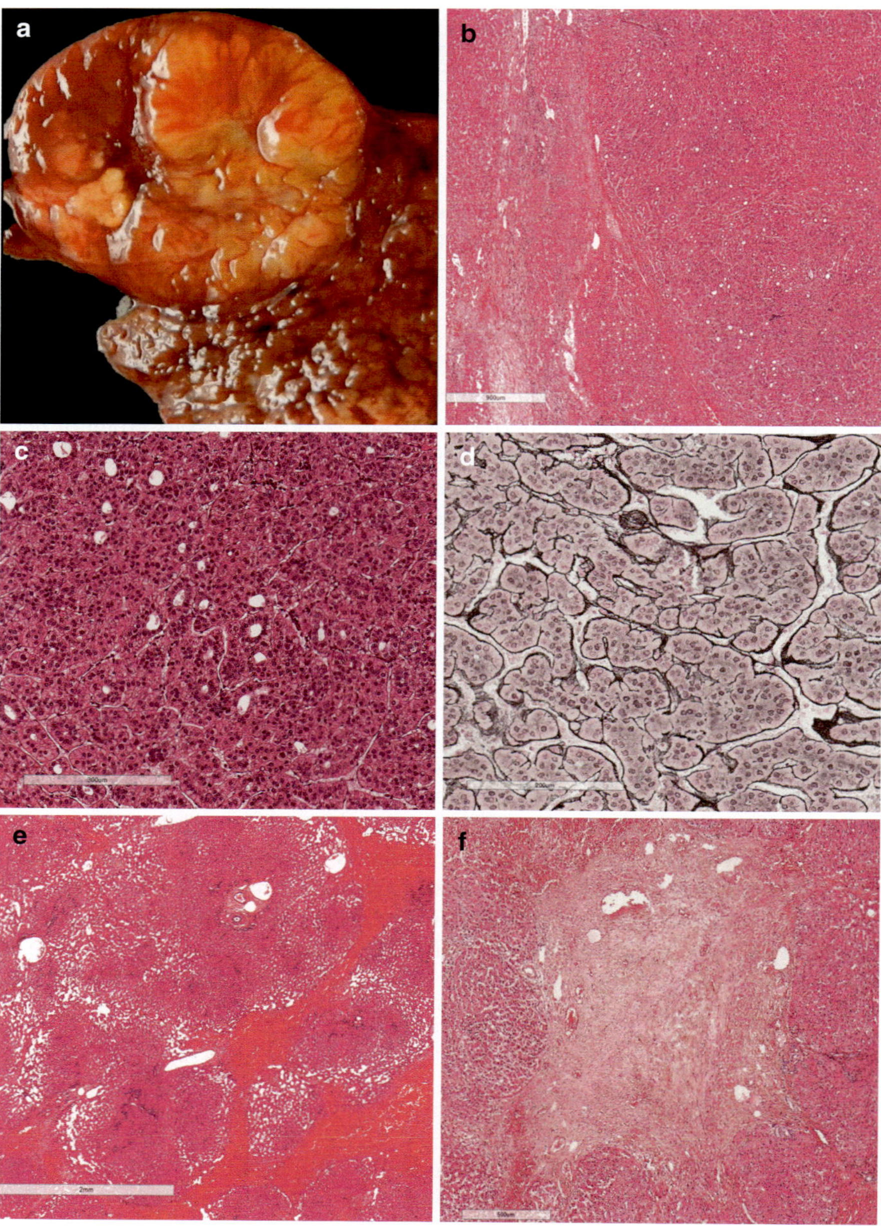

**Fig. 14.4** Well-differentiated HCC developed in Budd-Chiari syndrome. (**a**) Gross examination: Yellow encapsulated lesion, (**b**) Microscopic examination: proliferation of hepatocytes arranged in more than two-cells thick plates and with pseudo acinar changes, (**c**) Pseudo-glands and plates of hepatocytes with mild atypia and without portal tract, (**d**) Reticulin stain showing plates of more than two-cells thick, (**e**) Non tumoral liver: extensive fibrosis and marked sinusoidal dilatation, (**f**) Obliteration of a central vein

Steatosis may be present. IHCAs exhibit overexpression of inflammatory proteins, such as serum amyloid A (SAA) and C-reactive protein (CRP) by immunohisto-chemistry that represents the hallmark of this subtype [1, 23, 24].

## b-Catenin Mutated HCA (b-HCA) and b-Catenin Mutated Inflammatory HCA (b-IHCA)

b-catenin-mutated HCAs constitute approximately 10–15% of all HCAs. More than 10% of b-HCA are also inflammatory (b-IHCA). b-HCA occurs more often in men than the other sub-types and is more often associated with malignant transformation (). Different kinds of mutations or deletions (exons 3, 7 and 8) in the CTNNB1 gene coding for b-catenin have been reported, associated with different levels of b-catenin pathway activation. Cytological atypia, small-cell change, pseudo glandular/acinar architecture, and cholestasis may be observed. Reticulin loss may be focally described.

According to the b-catenin mutations, different patterns of GS may be observed. The most robust is the pattern associated with mutations and deletions of exon 3 (non S45) which is strong and diffuse. Additionally, aberrant nuclear b-catenin staining (the best specific marker but poorly sensitive) may be present. For all other mutations, b-catenin pathway is less activated and leads to mild to moderate staining with heterogeneous distribution. In b-IHCA, an expression of GS and SAA/CRP was observed [24, 27].

## Sonic Hedgehog HCA (shHCA)

This sub-group has been recently described by Nault et al. in 2017 [26] and constitute approximately 4% of HCA. It defined by a GLI1 overexpression due to a deletion leading to a fusion between *INHBE* and *GLI1*. These fusions activate constitutively the sonic hedgehog pathway into tumor hepatocytes. shHCAs occur more frequently in women and are associated with higher BMI and/or cumulative consumption of oral contraceptive. shHCAs have been associated with a high rate of histological but also clinical symptomatic bleeding [26]. No specific morphological features are described while prostaglandin D synthase (PTGDS) and argininosuccinate synthase 1 (ASS1) have been reported as overexpressed in shHCA. However, ASS1 may also be overexpressed in other HCA subtypes, almost exclusively in IHCA [28, 29].

## Unclassified HCA

The last group of HCA (<5% of all HCAs) is characterized by the lack of specific histological features without any specific molecular abnormality [24].

## Imaging

HCA demonstrates variable echogenicity on ultrasound and cannot readily be distinguished from other lesions. On computed tomography, and MRI HCAs were classically described as lesions different from FNH due to common presence of hemorrhage, necrosis, or fat. Actually, imaging and MRI in particular correspond to the different subtypes. Indeed, on MR, H-HCA are homogeneous and have a variable signal on T2-sequences: usually slightly hyper intense on non-fat suppressed sequence and iso-or hypo intense on T2-weighted fat suppressed sequence. The striking finding is a diffuse and homogeneous signal dropout on chemical shift T1-weighted sequences (93%) [30, 31]. In I-HCA, MR imaging shows a strong hyper intense signal on T2-weighted images either diffuse or as a rim-like band in the periphery of the lesion defined as the atoll sign [32]. b-HCA and unclassified HCA are less characteristic on imaging. They share findings of hepatocellular tumors (mainly arterial enhancement and portal or delayed wash-out) and may have heterogeneous content [30]. shHCA is a relatively new entity and its imaging features are yet not well-known.

## HCA in VLD

While HCAs have rarely been described in the context of VLD, they are frequently observed in BCS and CPPS, and, importantly, all sub-types may be seen [10].

## *Hepatocellular Carcinoma (HCC) (Fig. 14.4)*

### Pathology

On gross examination, the tumor may form a single mass or there may be multiple scattered discrete nodules. Some tumors form an expanding mass well demarcated from the surrounding liver, with or without a capsule, whereas others appear to infiltrate the surrounding liver tissue. HCCs can be variably tan or yellow and green. Satellite nodules and vascular invasion are common and constitute main histopronostic factors. On microscopic examination, HCC can have a highly variable appearance. Well-differentiated HCC can show overlapping features with HCA, and, in cirrhotic livers, with dysplastic nodules [14]. Diagnosis is based on (1) architectural criteria (enlarged hepatocytic plates ($\geq 2$), pseudo-glandular formations), (2) cytologic criteria (atypia such as small cell changes and nuclear pleomorphism), and presence of unpaired arteries. Reticulin staining is very useful, showing a loss or a fragmentation of the framework [14, 33, 34]. Immunostainings can be used, such as the combination of HSP70, glypican 3, and GS staining has been shown to help in differentiate HCC from high-grade dysplastic nodules in cirrhosis [35]. Glypican 3 is more reliable in less-differentiated HCC, being often negative in well-differentiated HCC [36].

## Imaging

CT and MRI are the most common modalities used for radiographic diagnosis of HCC. The criteria proposed by the American Association for the Study of Liver Diseases and EASL state that for tumors >1 cm in cirrhotic liver, biopsy is not necessary to confirm the diagnosis if classical features of HCC are seen on multiphasic contrast-enhanced CT or MRI. The classic features include non-rim arterial phase hyper enhancement followed by washout during the portal venous and/or delayed phases enhancement of the lesion in the arterial phase and washout in the venous phase [11, 37, 38].

## HCC in VLD

Most commonly, HCC arise in the context of chronic liver diseases, and are less frequently reported in the context of VLD [1, 2]. However, BCS, which may progress to advanced fibrosis and cirrhosis, is the main VLD associated with HCC [39]. HCC is rare in the other VLD. In this context, biopsy of the nodule is recommended as it often develops in a non-cirrhotic liver.

# Hepatocellular Nodules in Vascular Liver Diseases

Interestingly, the development of hepatocellular nodules is varying according to the type of VLD (Table 14.2). Globally, they correspond more frequently to benign rather to malignant hepatocellular proliferations.

**Table 14.2** Prevalence of liver nodules in vascular liver disorders

|  | NRH | LRN | FNH | HCA | HCC |
|---|---|---|---|---|---|
| Budd Chiari syndrome | Very frequent | Very frequent | Very frequent | Possible | Frequent |
| Congenital Porto-systemic shunts | Frequent | Not described | Very frequent | Possible | Rare |
| Porto-sinusoidal vascular disease | Very frequent | Rare | Frequent | Rare | Not described |
| Hereditary hemorraghic telangiectasia | Frequent | Frequent | Very frequent | Rare | Rare |
| Sinusoidal obstruction syndrome | Rare | Not described | Rare | Not described | Not described |
| Congenital hepatic fibrosis | Not described | Not described | Rare | Rare | Rare |

*NRH* nodular regenerative hyperplasia, *LRN* large regenerative nodule, *FNH* focal nodular hyperplasia, *HCA* hepatocellular adenoma, *HCC* hepatocellular carcinoma

## *Budd Chiari Syndrome (BCS) (Figs. 14.4 and 14.5)*

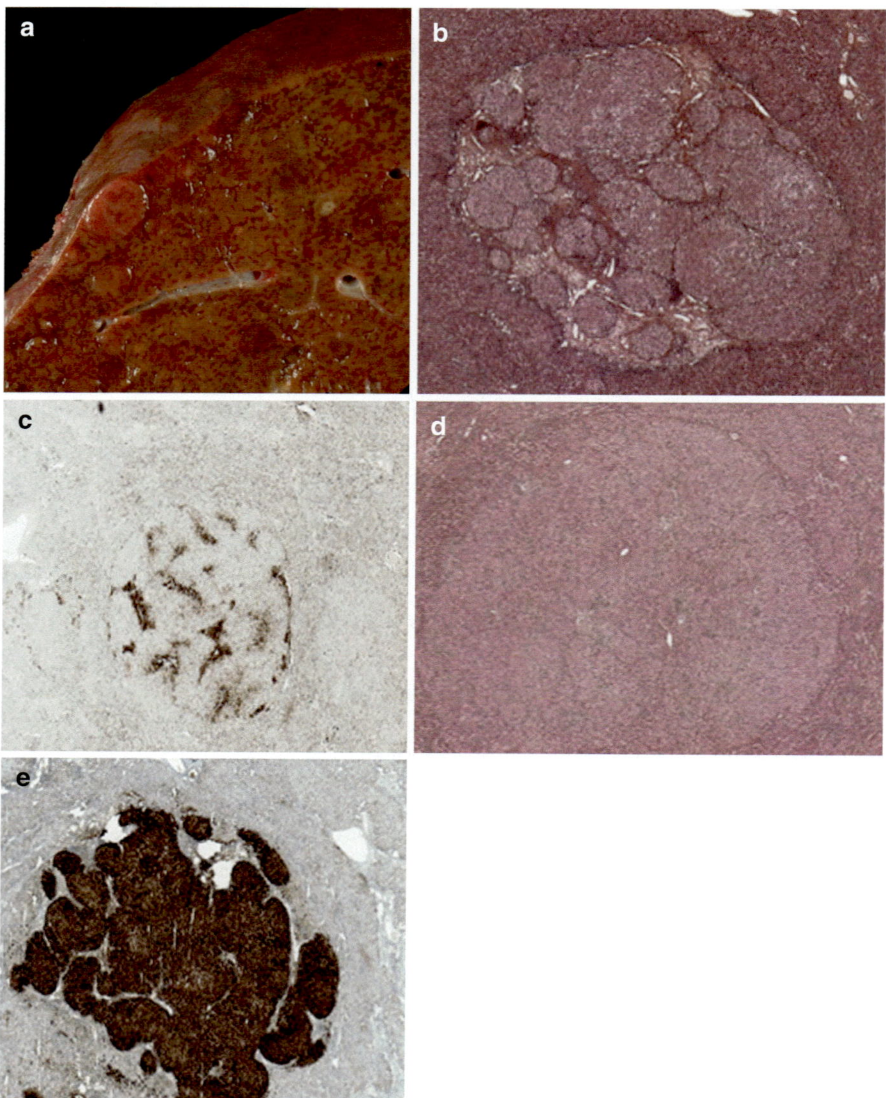

**Fig. 14.5** Focal nodular hyperplasia and β-catenin mutated adenoma developed in Budd-Chiari syndrome. (**a**) Gross examination: one well-circumscribed lesion paler than the surrounding hepatic parenchyma and one well-circumscribed brownish lesion. (**b**) Microscopic examination: variable size nodules made of normal hepatocytes delimited by fibrous septa containing large dystrophic arteries and ductular reaction. (**c**) Glutamine synthetase immunostaining: map-like pattern, (**d**) Microscopic examination: proliferation of hepatocytes arranged in sheets and cords of one or two cells thick, (**e**) Glutamine synthetase immunostaining: diffuse and intense expression

BCS is defined by an obstruction of the hepatic venous outflow tract. In short term, the early decrease of portal perfusion is responsible for the development of NRH or infarcts if complicated with large thrombi. An increase in arterial perfusion compensates impaired portal flow in chronic BCS, and then contributes to the development of benign regenerative nodule, corresponding mostly to LRN, FNH or FNH-like lesions [2, 8]. Nevertheless, HCAs are also reported in the literature including H-HCA, IHCA or b-HCA [10, 21]. The main issue regarding liver nodules in BCS concerns HCC. Indeed, HCC in BCS is relatively frequent with a variable prevalence observed between the different studies, ranging from 17% to 26% [6, 39, 40]. The diagnosis between FNH-like lesions and HCC remains difficult at imaging as both lesions are hyper vascular. Moreover, many FNH-like lesions show wash-out, which is explained by the congestive liver. Combination of criteria such as signal intensity on T1-, on T2, on diffusion, and on hepatobiliary phase is helpful [41]. Therefore, accurate diagnosis requires multidisciplinary approach including clinical, laboratory (AFP), and imaging work-up including MR imaging with hepatobiliary MR contrast agents. In case of doubt, a tumor biopsy may be performed however the diagnosis may be difficult in case of well-differentiated HCC [2].

## *Congenital Porto-Systemic Shunts (CPSS)*

In case of malformation of the splanchnic venous system, the splanchnic venous flow bypasses the liver and drains directly into the systemic venous circulation. The result of CPSS is the diversion of the blood flow to the systemic venous system, through an either complete or partial shunt of the portal blood from the liver [1, 42]. All types of hepatocellular nodules have been reported in CPSS and linked to the deprivation of the portal flow with increased arterial flow [43–45]. The majority of reported cases includes NRH, FNH and HCA with all subtypes described [10, 22, 46–49]. Importantly, regression of some hepatocellular nodules has been reported after closure of the shunt [50]. By contrast, HCA may also progress into HCC, particularly in cases of b-HCA and H-HCA without steatosis [10, 51, 52]. Finally, de novo HCC have been also described. Tumors in these cases were often large and well to moderately differentiated [53, 54].

## *Porto-sinusoidal Vascular Disease (PSVD) (Fig. 14.6)*

PSVD or obliterative portal venopathy is observed in patients with idiopathic noncirrhotic portal hypertension without extrahepatic portal vein obstruction. The disease is generally stable or progresses only slowly but does not evolve to cirrhosis [55–57]. The most common hepatocellular nodule observed in PSVD is NRH, followed by FNH-like [58, 59]. Rare cases of HCA have been reported while HCC has not been described so far [10, 59] [1].

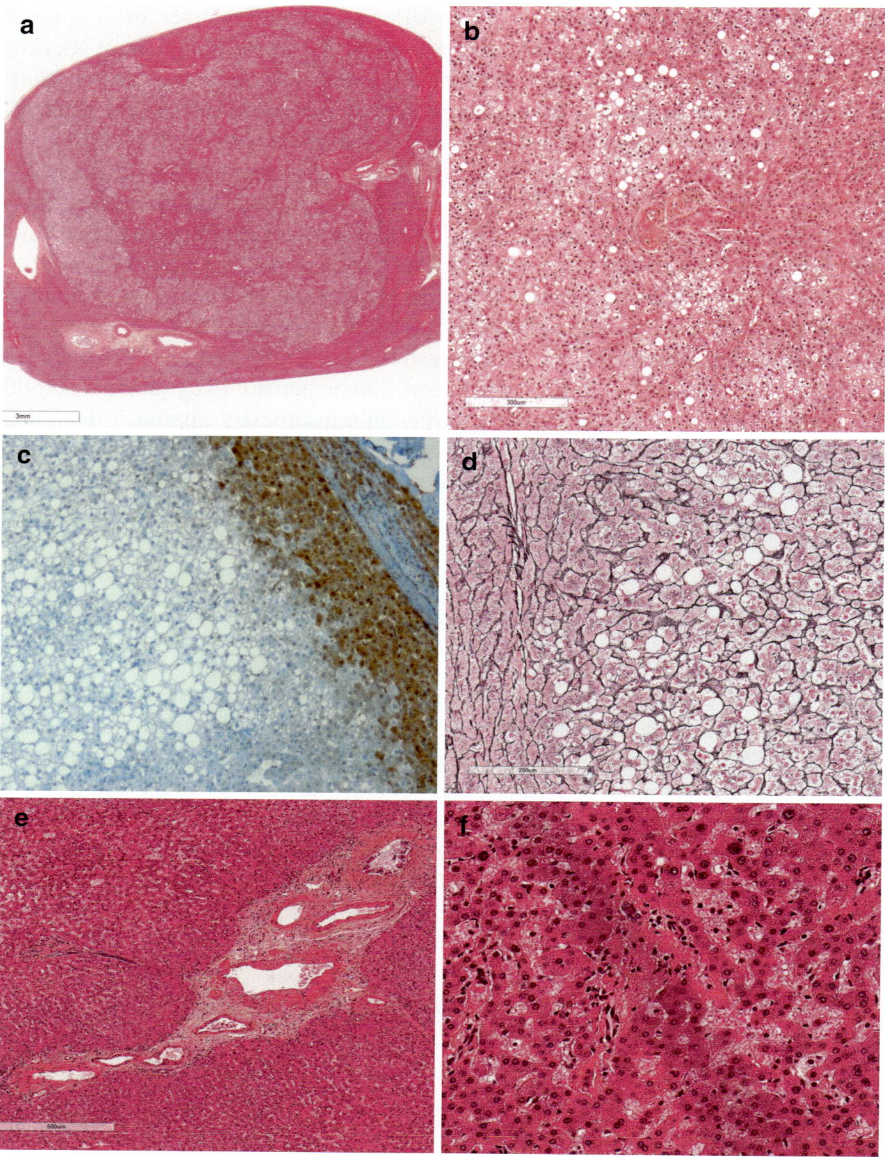

**Fig. 14.6** HNF1A inactivated adenoma developed in the context of porto-sinusoidal vascular disease. (**a**) Microscopic examination: proliferation of hepatocytes arranged in sheets and cords of one or two cells thick, (**b**) hepatocytes arranged in sheets and cords of one or two cells thick without cytological atypia and with steatosis and few unpaired arteries, (**c**) LFABP immunostaining: loss of expression of LFABP in the tumoral cells, (**d**) Intact reticulin framework, (**e**) Non-tumoral liver: Arterialization of large portal associated with sinusoidal dilatation, (**f**) Non-tumoral liver: Absence of portal vein in a small portal tract

## *Hereditary Hemorraghic Telangiectasia (HHT) (Fig. 14.7)*

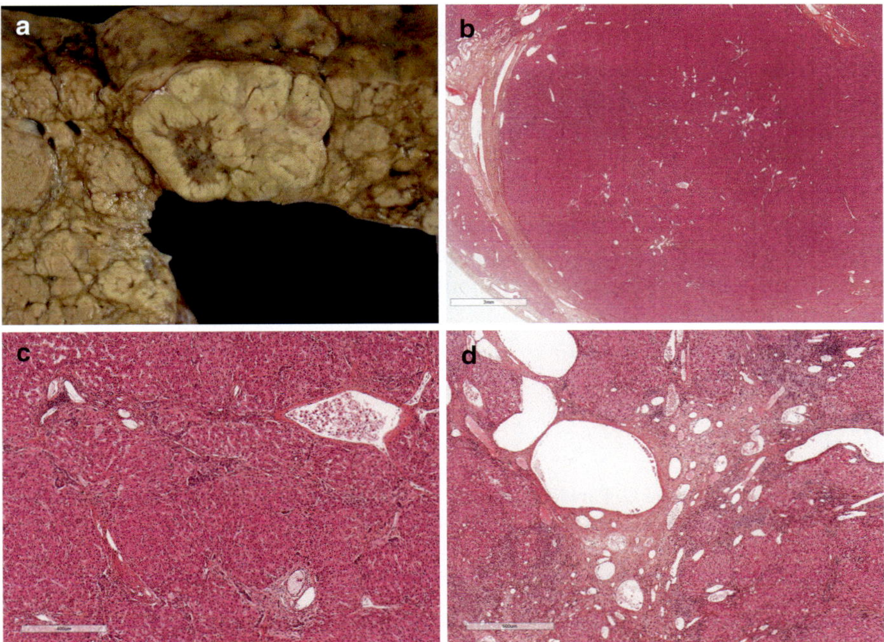

**Fig. 14.7** FNH-like nodule developed in hereditary hemorrhagic telangiectasia. (**a**) Gross examination: well-circumscribed nodule with fibrous change, (**b**) Microscopic examination: well circumscribed nodule of normal hepatocytes without central scar, (**c**) variable size nodules made of normal hepatocytes surrounded by fibrous septa with ductular reaction and dystrophic arteries. (**d**) Non-tumoral liver: vascular dilations involving sinusoids, veins and arteries

HHT is an autosomal dominant vascular disorder with molecular heterogeneity, characterized by hepatic involvement in HHT in up to 30% of cases, showing enlarged hepatic artery, hepatic aneurysm, intrahepatic telangiectasia and arteriovenous, arterioportal and portovenous shunts [60]. In HHT, an increase in the arterial flow is observed and may induce a nodular transformation of the liver parenchyma. Consequently, regenerative nodules, such as LRN, FNH and FNH-like lesions, are much more frequently observed. HCA and HCC have not been described in the literature [18, 61–65].

## *Sinusoidal Obstruction Syndrome (SOS)*

SOS is characterized by sinusoidal endothelium damage, with or without occlusion of the central vein, observed namely in the context of oxaliplatin chemotherapy. NRH may be frequently observed in SOS [66–68]. FNH is also rarely described in patients with chemotherapy but the link with SOS lesions is not yet known [69].

## *Congenital Hepatic Fibrosis (CHF)*

CHF is an autosomal recessive disease affecting primarily the hepatobiliary system and the kidneys, belonging to the group of fibro-polycystic diseases. Few cases of FNH, HCA and dysplastic nodules have been reported [70, 71]. Rare cases of HCC are described in the literature [72, 73].

**In conclusion,** Hepatocellular nodules in the context of VLD represent a real challenge for radiology and pathology. Indeed, imaging is less typical in this context, therefore a liver biopsy has often to be performed. The diagnosis on biopsy may be nevertheless difficult, particularly to distinguish HCA well-differentiated HCC. Actually, modern imaging techniques combined with tumor biopsy (providing a morphophenotypical analysis) significantly improve the classification of liver nodules.

# References


1. Sempoux C, Balabaud C, Paradis V, Bioulac-Sage P. Hepatocellular nodules in vascular liver diseases. Virchows Arch Int J Pathol. 2018 Jul;473(1):33–44.
2. Vilgrain V, Paradis V, Van Wettere M, Valla D, Ronot M, Rautou P-E. Benign and malignant hepatocellular lesions in patients with vascular liver diseases. Abdom Radiol N Y. 2018 Aug;43(8):1968–77.
3. Ronot M, Vilgrain V. Imaging of benign hepatocellular lesions: current concepts and recent updates. Clin Res Hepatol Gastroenterol. 2014 Dec;38(6):681–8.
4. Ueda T, Starkey J, Mori K, Fukunaga K, Shimofusa R, Motoori K, et al. A pictorial review of benign hepatocellular nodular lesions: comprehensive radiological assessment incorporating the concept of anomalous portal tract syndrome. J Hepato-Biliary-Pancreat Sci. 2011 May;18(3):386–96.
5. Tanaka M, Wanless IR. Pathology of the liver in Budd-Chiari syndrome: portal vein thrombosis and the histogenesis of veno-centric cirrhosis, veno-portal cirrhosis, and large regenerative nodules. Hepatol Baltim Md. 1998 Feb;27(2):488–96.
6. Vilgrain V, Lewin M, Vons C, Denys A, Valla D, Flejou JF, et al. Hepatic nodules in Budd-Chiari syndrome: imaging features. Radiology. 1999 Feb;210(2):443–50.
7. Zhou H, Wolff M, Pauleit D, Fischer HP, Pfeifer U. Multiple macroregenerative nodules in liver cirrhosis due to Budd-Chiari syndrome. Case reports and review of the literature. Hepato-Gastroenterology. 2000 Apr;47(32):522–7.
8. Cazals-Hatem D, Vilgrain V, Genin P, Denninger M-H, Durand F, Belghiti J, et al. Arterial and portal circulation and parenchymal changes in Budd-Chiari syndrome: a study in 17 explanted livers. Hepatol Baltim Md. 2003 Mar;37(3):510–9.
9. Brancatelli G, Federle MP, Grazioli L, Golfieri R, Lencioni R. Large regenerative nodules in Budd-Chiari syndrome and other vascular disorders of the liver: CT and MR imaging findings with clinicopathologic correlation. AJR Am J Roentgenol. 2002 Apr;178(4):877–83.
10. Sempoux C, Paradis V, Komuta M, Wee A, Calderaro J, Balabaud C, et al. Hepatocellular nodules expressing markers of hepatocellular adenomas in Budd-Chiari syndrome and other rare hepatic vascular disorders. J Hepatol. 2015 Nov;63(5):1173–80.
11. European Association for the Study of the Liver (EASL). EASL clinical practice guidelines on the management of benign liver tumours. J Hepatol. 2016;65(2):386–98.
12. Sannier A, Cazejust J, Lequoy M, Cervera P, Scatton O, Rosmorduc O, et al. Liver biopsy for diagnosis of presumed benign hepatocellular lesions lacking magnetic resonance imag-

ing diagnostic features of focal nodular hyperplasia. Liver Int Off J Int Assoc Study Liver. 2016;36(11):1668–76.
13. Hytiroglou P, Theise ND. Differential diagnosis of hepatocellular nodular lesions. Semin Diagn Pathol. 1998 Nov;15(4):285–99.
14. Hytiroglou P. Well-differentiated hepatocellular nodule: making a diagnosis on biopsy and resection specimens of patients with advanced stage chronic liver disease. Semin Diagn Pathol. 2017 Mar;34(2):138–45.
15. Hytiroglou P, Park YN, Krinsky G, Theise ND. Hepatic precancerous lesions and small hepatocellular carcinoma. Gastroenterol Clin N Am. 2007 Dec;36(4):867–87.
16. Ames JT, Federle MP, Chopra K. Distinguishing clinical and imaging features of nodular regenerative hyperplasia and large regenerative nodules of the liver. Clin Radiol. 2009 Dec;64(12):1190–5.
17. International Working Party. Terminology of nodular hepatocellular lesions. Hepatol Baltim Md. 1995 Sep;22(3):983–93.
18. Brenard R, Chapaux X, Deltenre P, Henrion J, De Maeght S, Horsmans Y, et al. Large spectrum of liver vascular lesions including high prevalence of focal nodular hyperplasia in patients with hereditary haemorrhagic telangiectasia: the Belgian registry based on 30 patients. Eur J Gastroenterol Hepatol. 2010 Oct;22(10):1253–9.
19. Rebouissou S, Couchy G, Libbrecht L, Balabaud C, Imbeaud S, Auffray C, et al. The beta-catenin pathway is activated in focal nodular hyperplasia but not in cirrhotic FNH-like nodules. J Hepatol. 2008 Jul;49(1):61–71.
20. Bioulac-Sage P, Laumonier H, Rullier A, Cubel G, Laurent C, Zucman-Rossi J, et al. Overexpression of glutamine synthetase in focal nodular hyperplasia: a novel easy diagnostic tool in surgical pathology. Liver Int Off J Int Assoc Study Liver. 2009 Mar;29(3):459–65.
21. Ibarrola C, Castellano VM, Colina F. Focal hyperplastic hepatocellular nodules in hepatic venous outflow obstruction: a clinicopathological study of four patients and 24 nodules. Histopathology. 2004 Feb;44(2):172–9.
22. Hao Y, Hong X, Zhao X. Congenital absence of the portal vein associated with focal nodular hyperplasia of the liver and congenital heart disease (Abernethy malformation): a case report and literature review. Oncol Lett. 2015 Feb;9(2):695–700.
23. Bioulac-Sage P, Sempoux C, Balabaud C. Hepatocellular adenoma: classification, variants and clinical relevance. Semin Diagn Pathol. 2017 Mar;34(2):112–25.
24. Nault J-C, Bioulac-Sage P, Zucman-Rossi J. Hepatocellular benign tumors-from molecular classification to personalized clinical care. Gastroenterology. 2013 May;144(5):888–902.
25. Rebouissou S, Franconi A, Calderaro J, Letouzé E, Imbeaud S, Pilati C, et al. Genotype-phenotype correlation of CTNNB1 mutations reveals different ß-catenin activity associated with liver tumor progression. Hepatol Baltim Md. 2016;64(6):2047–61.
26. Nault J-C, Couchy G, Balabaud C, Morcrette G, Caruso S, Blanc J-F, et al. Molecular classification of hepatocellular adenoma associates with risk factors, bleeding, and malignant transformation. Gastroenterology. 2017;152(4):880–894.e6.
27. Saldarriaga J, Bisig B, Couchy G, Castain C, Zucman-Rossi J, Balabaud C, et al. Focal β-catenin mutation identified on formalin-fixed and paraffin-embedded inflammatory hepatocellular adenomas. Histopathology. 2017 Dec;71(6):989–93.
28. Nault J-C, Couchy G, Caruso S, Meunier L, Caruana L, Letouzé E, et al. Argininosuccinate synthase 1 and periportal gene expression in sonic hedgehog hepatocellular adenomas. Hepatol Baltim Md. 2018;68(3):964–76.
29. Henriet E, Abou Hammoud A, Dupuy J-W, Dartigues B, Ezzoukry Z, Dugot-Senant N, et al. Argininosuccinate synthase 1 (ASS1): a marker of unclassified hepatocellular adenoma and high bleeding risk. Hepatol Baltim Md. 2017;66(6):2016–28.
30. Ronot M, Bahrami S, Calderaro J, Valla D-C, Bedossa P, Belghiti J, et al. Hepatocellular adenomas: accuracy of magnetic resonance imaging and liver biopsy in subtype classification. Hepatol Baltim Md. 2011 Apr;53(4):1182–91.
31. Laumonier H, Bioulac-Sage P, Laurent C, Zucman-Rossi J, Balabaud C, Trillaud H. Hepatocellular adenomas: magnetic resonance imaging features as a function of molecular pathological classification. Hepatol Baltim Md. 2008 Sep;48(3):808–18.

32. van Aalten SM, Thomeer MGJ, Terkivatan T, Dwarkasing RS, Verheij J, de Man RA, et al. Hepatocellular adenomas: correlation of MR imaging findings with pathologic subtype classification. Radiology. 2011 Oct;261(1):172–81.
33. Pittman ME, Brunt EM. Anatomic pathology of hepatocellular carcinoma: histopathology using classic and new diagnostic tools. Clin Liver Dis. 2015 May;19(2):239–59.
34. Agni RM. Diagnostic histopathology of hepatocellular carcinoma: a case-based review. Semin Diagn Pathol. 2017 Mar;34(2):126–37.
35. Di Tommaso L, Franchi G, Park YN, Fiamengo B, Destro A, Morenghi E, et al. Diagnostic value of HSP70, glypican 3, and glutamine synthetase in hepatocellular nodules in cirrhosis. Hepatol Baltim Md. 2007 Mar;45(3):725–34.
36. Shafizadeh N, Ferrell LD, Kakar S. Utility and limitations of glypican-3 expression for the diagnosis of hepatocellular carcinoma at both ends of the differentiation spectrum. Mod Pathol Off J U S Can Acad Pathol Inc. 2008 Aug;21(8):1011–8.
37. Bruix J, Sherman M. Practice guidelines committee, American Association for the Study of Liver Diseases. Management of hepatocellular carcinoma. Hepatol Baltim Md. 2005 Nov;42(5):1208–36.
38. Ronot M, Purcell Y, Vilgrain V. Hepatocellular carcinoma: current imaging modalities for diagnosis and prognosis. Dig Dis Sci. 2019 Mar 2;64(4):934–50.
39. Gwon D, Ko G-Y, Yoon H-K, Sung K-B, Kim JH, Lee SS, et al. Hepatocellular carcinoma associated with membranous obstruction of the inferior vena cava: incidence, characteristics, and risk factors and clinical efficacy of TACE. Radiology. 2010 Feb;254(2):617–26.
40. Ren W, Qi X, Yang Z, Han G, Fan D. Prevalence and risk factors of hepatocellular carcinoma in Budd-Chiari syndrome: a systematic review. Eur J Gastroenterol Hepatol. 2013 Jul;25(7):830–41.
41. Van Wettere M, Purcell Y, Bruno O, Payancé A, Plessier A, Rautou P-E, et al. Low specificity of washout to diagnose hepatocellular carcinoma in nodules showing arterial hyperenhancement in patients with Budd-Chiari syndrome. J Hepatol. 2019 Jan 14;70(6):1123–32.
42. Valla D-C, Cazals-Hatem D. Vascular liver diseases on the clinical side: definitions and diagnosis, new concepts. Virchows Arch Int J Pathol. 2018 Jul;473(1):3–13.
43. Kobayashi S, Matsui O, Gabata T, Sanada J, Koda W, Minami T, et al. Radiological and histopathological manifestations of hepatocellular nodular lesions concomitant with various congenital and acquired hepatic hemodynamic abnormalities. Jpn J Radiol. 2009 Feb;27(2):53–68.
44. Bernard O, Franchi-Abella S, Branchereau S, Pariente D, Gauthier F, Jacquemin E. Congenital portosystemic shunts in children: recognition, evaluation, and management. Semin Liver Dis. 2012 Nov;32(4):273–87.
45. Lisovsky M, Konstas AA, Misdraji J. Congenital extrahepatic portosystemic shunts (Abernethy malformation): a histopathologic evaluation. Am J Surg Pathol. 2011 Sep;35(9):1381–90.
46. Gülşen Z, Yiğit H, Demir P. Multiple regenerative nodular hyperplasia in the left infrarenal vena cava accompanied by Abernethy malformation. Surg Radiol Anat SRA. 2016 Apr;38(3):373–8.
47. Osorio MJ, Bonow A, Bond GJ, Rivera MR, Vaughan KG, Shah A, et al. Abernethy malformation complicated by hepatopulmonary syndrome and a liver mass successfully treated by liver transplantation. Pediatr Transplant. 2011 Nov;15(7):E149–51.
48. Sinakos E, Hytiroglou P, Chourmouzi D, Akriviadis E. Focal nodular hyperplasia in an individual with Abernethy malformation type 1b. Dig Liver Dis Off J Ital Soc Gastroenterol Ital Assoc Study Liver. 2015 Dec;47(12):1089.
49. Pupulim LF, Vullierme M-P, Paradis V, Valla D, Terraz S, Vilgrain V. Congenital portosystemic shunts associated with liver tumours. Clin Radiol. 2013 Jul;68(7):e362–9.
50. Franchi-Abella S, Branchereau S, Lambert V, Fabre M, Steimberg C, Losay J, et al. Complications of congenital portosystemic shunts in children: therapeutic options and outcomes. J Pediatr Gastroenterol Nutr. 2010 Sep;51(3):322–30.
51. Arrivé L, Zucman-Rossi J, Balladur P, Wendum D. Hepatocellular adenoma with malignant transformation in a patient with neonatal portal vein thrombosis. Hepatol Baltim Md. 2016;64(2):675–7.

52. Sorkin T, Strautnieks S, Foskett P, Peddu P, Thompson RJ, Heaton N, et al. Multiple β-catenin mutations in hepatocellular lesions arising in Abernethy malformation. Hum Pathol. 2016;53:153–8.
53. Benedict M, Rodriguez-Davalos M, Emre S, Walther Z, Morotti R. Congenital extrahepatic portosystemic shunt (Abernethy malformation type Ib) with associated hepatocellular carcinoma: case report and literature review. Pediatr Dev Pathol Off J Soc Pediatr Pathol Paediatr Pathol Soc. 2017 Aug;20(4):354–62.
54. Sharma R, Suddle A, Quaglia A, Peddu P, Karani J, Satyadas T, et al. Congenital extrahepatic portosystemic shunt complicated by the development of hepatocellular carcinoma. Hepatobiliary Pancreat Dis Int HBPD INT. 2015 Oct;14(5):552–7.
55. Cazals-Hatem D, Hillaire S, Rudler M, Plessier A, Paradis V, Condat B, et al. Obliterative portal venopathy: portal hypertension is not always present at diagnosis. J Hepatol. 2011 Mar;54(3):455–61.
56. Guido M, Sarcognato S, Sonzogni A, Lucà MG, Senzolo M, Fagiuoli S, et al. Obliterative portal venopathy without portal hypertension: an underestimated condition. Liver Int Off J Int Assoc Study Liver. 2016 Mar;36(3):454–60.
57. Lee H, Rehman AU, Fiel MI. Idiopathic noncirrhotic portal hypertension: an appraisal. J Pathol Transl Med. 2016 Jan;50(1):17–25.
58. Glatard A-S, Hillaire S, d'Assignies G, Cazals-Hatem D, Plessier A, Valla DC, et al. Obliterative portal venopathy: findings at CT imaging. Radiology. 2012 Jun;263(3):741–50.
59. Sugimoto K, Kondo F, Furuichi Y, Oshiro H, Nagao T, Saito K, et al. Focal nodular hyperplasia-like lesion of the liver with focal adenoma features associated with idiopathic portal hypertension. Hepatol Res Off J Jpn Soc Hepatol. 2014 Oct;44(10):E309–15.
60. Garcia-Tsao G, Korzenik JR, Young L, Henderson KJ, Jain D, Byrd B, et al. Liver disease in patients with hereditary hemorrhagic telangiectasia. N Engl J Med. 2000 Sep 28;343(13):931–6.
61. Wanless IR, Mawdsley C, Adams R. On the pathogenesis of focal nodular hyperplasia of the liver. Hepatol Baltim Md. 1985 Dec;5(6):1194–200.
62. Scardapane A, Ficco M, Sabbà C, Lorusso F, Moschetta M, Maggialetti N, et al. Hepatic nodular regenerative lesions in patients with hereditary haemorrhagic telangiectasia: computed tomography and magnetic resonance findings. Radiol Med (Torino). 2013 Feb;118(1):1–13.
63. Shimoyama Y, Kakizaki S, Katano A, Takakusaki S, Mizuide M, Ichikawa T, et al. Hereditary hemorrhagic telangiectasia with multiple hepatic and pulmonary nodular lesions. Clin J Gastroenterol. 2009 Apr;2(2):131–6.
64. Dissanayake R, Wickramarathne KPKYMDS, Seneviratne SN, Perera SN, Fernando MUJ, Wickramasinghe VP. Hereditary hemorrhagic telangiectasia, liver disease and elevated serum testosterone (Osler-weber-Rendu syndrome): a case report. BMC Res Notes. 2017 Jan 23;10(1):58.
65. Buscarini E, Gandolfi S, Alicante S, Londoni C, Manfredi G. Liver involvement in hereditary hemorrhagic telangiectasia. Abdom Radiol N Y. 2018 Aug;43(8):1920–30.
66. Viganò L, Rubbia-Brandt L, De Rosa G, Majno P, Langella S, Toso C, et al. Nodular regenerative hyperplasia in patients undergoing liver resection for colorectal metastases after chemotherapy: risk factors, preoperative assessment and clinical impact. Ann Surg Oncol. 2015 Dec;22(13):4149–57.
67. Hubert C, Sempoux C, Horsmans Y, Rahier J, Humblet Y, Machiels J-P, et al. Nodular regenerative hyperplasia: a deleterious consequence of chemotherapy for colorectal liver metastases? Liver Int Off J Int Assoc Study Liver. 2007 Sep;27(7):938–43.
68. Rubbia-Brandt L, Lauwers GY, Wang H, Majno PE, Tanabe K, Zhu AX, et al. Sinusoidal obstruction syndrome and nodular regenerative hyperplasia are frequent oxaliplatin-associated liver lesions and partially prevented by bevacizumab in patients with hepatic colorectal metastasis. Histopathology. 2010 Mar;56(4):430–9.
69. Furlan A, Brancatelli G, Dioguardi Burgio M, Grazioli L, Lee JM, Murmura E, et al. Focal nodular hyperplasia after treatment with Oxaliplatin: a multiinstitutional series of cases diagnosed at MRI. AJR Am J Roentgenol. 2018 Apr;210(4):775–9.

70. Paradis V, Bioulac-Sage P, Balabaud C. Congenital hepatic fibrosis with multiple HNF1α hepatocellular adenomas. Clin Res Hepatol Gastroenterol. 2014 Dec;38(6):e115–6.
71. Roncalli M, Maggioni M, Opocher E, Coggi G. Development of a high grade dysplastic nodule in a case of congenital hepatic fibrosis. Ital J Gastroenterol Hepatol. 1999 May;31(4):301–4.
72. Bauman ME, Pound DC, Ulbright TM. Hepatocellular carcinoma arising in congenital hepatic fibrosis. Am J Gastroenterol. 1994 Mar;89(3):450–1.
73. Hirosawa T, Morimoto N, Miura K, Ono K, Watanabe S, Fujieda T, et al. The successful treatment of hepatocellular carcinoma arising from congenital hepatic fibrosis using radiofrequency ablation under laparoscopy. Clin J Gastroenterol. 2019 Jan 7;12(3):223–30. https://doi.org/10.1007/s12328-018-00932-0.

# Chapter 15
# Pregnancy in Vascular Liver Disease

A. Payancé, Pierre-Emmanuel Rautou, and Dominique Valla

## Abbreviations

BCS     Budd Chiari syndrome
HTT     Hereditary hemorrhagic telangiectasia
TIPS    transjugular intrahepatic portosystemic shunt

Among patients with Budd Chiari syndrome (BCS), portal vein thrombosis and porto-sinusoidal vascular disease, women of childbearing age account for 50%, 20% and 15%, respectively [1–3]. The affected women in this age have gained a long life expectancy since anticoagulation therapy, followed in specific cases by transjugular intrahepatic portosystemic shunt (TIPS), angioplasty or liver transplantation have been applied. Indeed, with an appropriate management, five-year survival rate is currently above 90% for women with BCS or portal vein thrombosis, and 85% for porto-sinusoidal vascular disease [1, 2, 4]. It is therefore not surprising that affected women with a well-controlled disease express a desire for pregnancy.

A. Payancé · D. Valla
Service d'Hépatologie, DHU Unity, Pôle des Maladies de l'Appareil Digestif, Hôpital Beaujon, AP-HP, Clichy, France

Centre de Référence des Maladies Vasculaires du Foie, French Network for Rare Liver Diseases (FILFOIE), European Reference Network (ERN) 'Rare-Liver', Clichy, France
e-mail: audrey.payance@aphp.fr; dominique.valla@aphp.fr

P.-E. Rautou (✉)
Service d'Hépatologie, DHU Unity, Pôle des Maladies de l'Appareil Digestif, Hôpital Beaujon, AP-HP, Clichy, France

Centre de Référence des Maladies Vasculaires du Foie, French Network for Rare Liver Diseases (FILFOIE), European Reference Network (ERN) 'Rare-Liver', Clichy, France

Université de Paris, Centre de recherche sur l'inflammation, Paris, France
e-mail: pierre-emmanuel.rautou@inserm.fr

Recently reported clinical studies suggest that favorable pregnancy outcomes can be expected in women with vascular liver diseases. Currently therefore, pregnancy cannot be as systematically contraindicated in such women as it was in the past. However, a specific management is needed which requires a collaboration between several specialists, including hepatologists, hematologists and obstetrician-gynecologists. Management of pregnancy in women with vascular liver disease requires clarification of level of portal hypertension, and of patients' coagulation status. It is also important to take into account the consequences of circulation and coagulation changes in women with portal hypertension on the course of pregnancy or delivery, and on both mother and fetus outcomes.

In this chapter, we first summarize what it is known about coagulation and physiologic changes associated with pregnancy, and then we address (1) what are the outcomes of pregnancy in women with established vascular liver diseases, and (2) how to manage pregnancy, delivery and puerperium in these women.

## Pregnancy-Related Changes in Circulation and Coagulation

In healthy women, blood volume and cardiac output increase by 30–50% during the second and third trimesters of pregnancy, while heart rate increases, and arterial blood pressure decreases by 10% reaching its nadir between the 16th and 20th weeks of gestation [5, 6]. These changes are reminiscent of those in patients with portal hypertension, suggesting that an exacerbation of the latter might occur during pregnancy [7]. However, changes occurring in the portal circulation during a normal pregnancy in a healthy woman have been poorly characterized. Two studies dating back to the seventies suggested increased or unchanged total hepatic blood flow [5, 8]. In addition, pressure is exerted on the inferior vena cava by the pregnant uterus, and particularly so during the third trimester, which may impact on portal hemodynamics. However, portal hemodynamic data during pregnancy are scarce, in healthy women as well as in patients with portal hypertension. Most recent studies using arterial Doppler ultrasonography showed unchanged hepatic arterial blood flow [9].

In the general population, estimates of the incidence of pregnancy-associated venous thromboembolism (pulmonary embolism and/or deep vein thrombosis) range from 1 in 1000 to 1 in 2000 deliveries [9]. The risk of venous thromboembolism is five times higher during pregnancy and puerperium than in a non-pregnant woman. About two thirds of thrombosis episodes take place antepartum, while 40–60% of pulmonary embolism episodes occur 4–6 weeks postpartum [10]. Indeed, pregnancy is associated with a significant prothrombotic shift in the hemostatic system balance related to an increased level of coagulation factors (namely factor VII, factor X, and fibrinogen), a decreased level of certain natural anticoagulant (i.e. free protein S) and a decreased fibrinolytic potential (through an increase in plasminogen activator inhibitor type 1 level) [9].

# Outcomes of Pregnancy in Women with Vascular Liver Disease

## *Budd-Chiari Syndrome*

### Pregnancy and Post-Partum, a Risk Factor for Budd-Chiari Syndrome

In a recent systematic review with meta-analysis, BCS first manifesting during pregnancy or post-partum accounted for 0 to 21.5% of cases reported in 20 studies and the pooled proportion was 13.1% in women with BCS. The proportion varies with the area and also with the date of inception. Indeed, in studies carried out before 2000, the proportion ranged from 3.8 to 21.5% in India and from 2.6 to 7.7% in Europe [11]. A study conducted by the European Network for Vascular Disorders of the Liver (EN-Vie) between 2003 and 2005 recorded a proportion of 3.7% [2]. Such high proportions suggest that pregnancy might be a relatively common causal factor for BCS. Rautou and colleagues compared 7 women with a diagnosis of BCS made during pregnancy or post-partum and 36 women with BCS diagnosis before any pregnancy or at least 6 months after pregnancy. The proportion of primary protein S deficiency in women with BCS first manifesting during pregnancy or post-partum was significantly higher (66%) than in BCS women with BCS not revealed by pregnancy [12]. Furthermore, in a series of 237 pregnancies in 158 women with essential thrombocythemia, a high incidence of splanchnic vein thromboses was observed (13/237; 5.5%) [13]. Those data suggest that pregnancy is unlikely to cause BCS in the absence of an underlying prothrombotic condition. Out of a context of pregnancy, a combination of several prothrombotic disorders has been reported in 28% of patients with BCS. Therefore, women presenting with BCS during pregnancy or post-partum should be comprehensively investigated for other underlying prothrombotic risks factors [14].

### Budd-Chiari Syndrome Presenting During Pregnancy or Post-Partum

In surveys carried out in India between 1963 and 1991, women presenting with a yet unknown and untreated BCS during pregnancy had a poor outcome. In the latter surveys including women with BCS not adequately managed prior to conception, 54 pregnancies have been evaluated collectively and about 50% of women died within one year from the onset of their illness [15, 16].

### Pregnancy in a Patient with Previously Recognized Budd-Chiari Syndrome

The main data on maternal and fetal risks of pregnancy in women with previously documented and treated BCS have been reported in two European and one Indian retrospective series including 55 pregnancies in 36 patients [17–19].

These patients usually had a stable and relatively good condition. Indeed, management of these patients before conception had followed the stepwise strategy largely used in Europe including anticoagulation, management of portal hypertension, decompressive therapy (i.e. angioplasties with or without stenting, or TIPS) and treatment of underlying thrombotic disorders [20]. This allowed compensated disease at the time of conception for all women with a median time between diagnosis and conception of 57 to 60 months.

Reported fetal outcomes appear to be poorer than in a general population. Indeed, the reported rate of miscarriages or ectopic pregnancies before the 20th week of pregnancy was about 30%, higher than in a healthy female population of similar age since an estimated 11–20% of clinically recognized pregnancies result in spontaneous abortion [21]. On the other hand, after 20 weeks of pregnancy, 93% of children were healthy while 4 cases of fetal death *in utero* have been observed (including 3 in the Indian study). Prematurity rate between 32 and 36 weeks of pregnancy was high (3/40, data not available for the Indian study) but no morbidity-mortality was observed. No obviously higher rate of fetal malformations was observed in women with BCS than in the general population.

In these surveys, carried out between 1985 and 2015, no maternal death was reported during a total of 55 pregnancies with a follow up of more than 30 months [17–19]. Forty three pregnancies occurred on anticoagulation therapy and 24 pregnancies were performed while radiological decompressive interventions had been performed before conception. Liver related complications seem to be rare as only 4 women developed ascites or pulmonary hypertension. The seven hemorrhagic events occurred in patients receiving anticoagulation and were not related to portal hypertension. The majority of liver related events were pregnancy related, including a surprisingly high rate of intrahepatic cholestasis of pregnancy, especially in Indian women. In the study by Rautou et al., factor II gene mutation was significantly associated with a poor outcome (i.e., birth before 32 weeks of gestation and/or serious obstetrical complications) [18].

## *Portal Vein Thrombosis*

### Portal Vein Thrombosis Presenting During Pregnancy or Post-Partum

Recognition of portal vein thrombosis during pregnancy or postpartum has been reported in 0 to 4% of patients with portal vein thrombosis. By contrast with its impact on BCS development, pregnancy alone does not appear to constitute a significant risk factor for portal vein thrombosis [9].

### Pregnancy in Patients with Previously Recognized Portal Vein Thrombosis

Three large retrospective studies have assessed pregnancy outcomes and fetal risks in women with known portal vein thrombosis and have included a total of 104 pregnancies. At a first glance, the high rate of live birth (83%) among these 104 pregnancies with portal vein thrombosis is comparable to that in a general population. However, the rates of prematurity and fetal death in utero appear to be higher in women with portal vein thrombosis than in the general population. In one of the surveys, evaluating 45 pregnancies in 24 women with portal vein thrombosis, 58% of women delivered a live child at term. In this study, pregnancies reaching the 20th week of gestation ended with the birth of a live baby [22].

Considering maternal outcome, increased morbidity but no death has been reported. Although studies differ in terms of underlying prothrombotic conditions and anticoagulant therapy, they all suggest that anticoagulant therapy in such women is well tolerated [22–24]. Indeed, there was no bleeding related maternal death. Five women not treated with anticoagulation therapy had bleeding due to ruptured gastroesophageal varices (3 women had not received adequate prophylaxis for portal hypertension), 6 had gynaecological or parietal bleeding (mostly peripartum, including 1 patient on anticoagulation therapy). Among these 104 pregnancies, two thromboembolic events were reported and no case of intestinal ischemia or deep vein thrombosis was reported. A higher platelet count and a JAK2 V617F mutation were significantly associated with a complicated pregnancy (miscarriage, prematurity, severe obstetric complications, neonatal complications). These findings suggest that the underlying thrombotic conditions, particularly myeloproliferative neoplasia, could be a possible cause for unfavorable pregnancy outcome, e.g. due to thrombotic occlusion in the placental circulation [22].

## *Porto-Sinusoidal Vascular Disease*

Pregnancy outcomes in patients with porto-sinusoidal vascular disease were evaluated in a multicenter European study on 24 pregnancies in 16 patients. All women met recent criteria for a diagnosis of porto-sinusoidal vascular disease [4]. At conception, diagnosis was known and liver function was preserved since all patients had an international normalized ratio below 1.5 and a serum bilirubin level below 2 mg/dL. There was adequate prophylaxis of gastrointestinal bleeding at conception for 21/24 pregnancies (four women had a TIPS). Rate of pregnancy loss prior to 20 weeks of gestation (21% (95% CI 5%–37%)) appeared to be increased as compared with the general population, but close to that of women with portal vein thrombosis [21, 22]. There was also an increased rate of prematurity (50% (95% CI 27%–73%)).

Out of the 24 pregnancies, 6 had complications related to portal hypertension: 2 had increases in pre-existing ascites at conception, 1 an aggravation of pre-existing portal pulmonary hypertension, 2 gastrointestinal hemorrhage due to variceal bleeding and a portal vein thrombosis. Unlike women with portal vein thrombosis or BCS, these hemorrhages occurred despite prophylaxis with beta-blocker therapy [25]. Whether the use of endoscopic band ligation or combining beta-blocker treatment could achieve better results is unknown. In these women at particular risk of thrombosis, a Doppler ultrasound of portal vein at 3 months and 6 months postpartum can be recommended. This study also proposed to investigate porto-pulmonary hypertension prior to conception since pregnancy can worsen it [25].

The prevalence of splenic artery aneurysm in women with porto-sinusoidal vascular disease seems low [26]. Albeit the risk of rupture in these patients is also unknown and the size of aneurysm justifying prophylactic treatment undetermined, the risk of maternal and foetal mortality should be considered [27]. Splenic artery aneurysms should be added to the list of items to be checked prior to pregnancy in women with porto-sinusoidal vascular disease [26].

## Other Vascular Disorders

Hereditary hemorrhagic telangiectasia (HTT) is a rare genetically transmitted vascular disease notably affecting heart and liver circulations, through the development of vascular malformations. Published studies assessing pregnancy outcomes in HTT reported that miscarriages were not more common in those women than in the general population. A recent review article analyzed 5 case series and 31 case reports and described the evolution of 1577 pregnancies in 630 women with HTT [28]. Severe maternal complications were reported in 2.7% to 6.8% of pregnancies, mostly in non-diagnosed and non-screened HTT women. The most frequent complications were related to pulmonary arteriovenous malformations. There were also 8 complications related to hepatic arteriovenous malformations (6 leading to heart failure and 2 leading to hepatobiliary necrosis). The hyperdynamic state of pregnancy likely explains the risk for decompensation of cardiac disease [29].

Regarding peliosis hepatis, pregnancy has not been linked to the development of this liver disease, in contrast to oral contraceptives [9]. There are two cases of hepatic peliosis reported. One patient presenting with massive post-partum hemorrhage and multiorgan failure had a peliotic liver incidentally found at laparotomy [30]. The second patient presenting with signs of portal hypertension in her seventh month of gestation was subsequently diagnosed with hepatic peliosis on liver biopsy; she delivered a baby at full term without any complication but died of portal hypertension related complications 2.5 years later [31].

## Management of Liver Disease and Underlying Prothrombotic Disorders During Pregnancy, Delivery and Puerperium in Women with Vascular Liver Disease

### *Early Counseling*

Managing pregnant women with vascular liver disease remains challenging. To prevent unplanned and potentially high-risk pregnancies in patients with vascular liver disease, counseling and education about potential maternal or fetal risks should be routinely included in the care of these women prior to any pregnancy plan. Women with vascular liver disease should be early informed that pregnancy is not contraindicated. However, women should also be informed that (1) vascular liver disease and underlying prothrombotic disorders need to be well characterized and controlled before conception; and (2) pregnancy needs to be closely monitored, to early detect and prevent unfavorable maternal or fetal outcomes. Higher risk of spontaneous miscarriages or prematurity should be explained.

## Management During Pregnancy

Management of vascular liver disease during pregnancy mainly consists of management of portal hypertension, antithrombotic treatment (anticoagulation and/or aspirin) and management of underlying prothrombotic disorders. For each medication specific information of risks related during pregnancy should be given.

### Management of Portal Hypertension

Gastroesophageal varices should ideally be investigated in the year before conception and otherwise during the second trimester of pregnancy. Non cardioselective beta-blockers can be administered during pregnancy. Beta-blockers have been evaluated in women treated for indications other than portal hypertension. Some studies suggested neonatal adverse effects such as small for gestational age newborns, neonatal hypoglycaemia or bradycardia especially in newborns [32]. Those complications can be easily recognized and managed using specific monitoring at birth. Data on the management of acute variceal bleeding during pregnancy are extremely scarce. The risk and benefits of pharmacologic therapy has not been evaluated. Selected case reports suggest the efficacy of endoscopic band ligation [33, 34]. A total of 9 pregnant women with cirrhosis who underwent TIPS placement to prevent variceal hemorrhage, or to manage ascites, or refractory bleeding varices have been reported [35–39]. These case reports suggest that TIPS can be performed safely during pregnancy, ideally during the second trimester. It is reasonable to recommend that variceal hemorrhage occurring during pregnancy be managed as in the non-pregnant patient [40]. Decisions are probably best guided by current practice guidelines dedicated to non-pregnant subjects.

### Management of Antithrombotic Therapy During Pregnancy

There is no recommendation for anticoagulants before or during pregnancy specific to patients with vascular liver disease. A prophylactic dose of anticoagulants can be proposed at the beginning of pregnancy, and should be proposed after delivery, in patients with vascular liver diseases who are not usually treated with anticoagulants. In patients already treated with anticoagulants, recommendations are extrapolated from those for patients with mechanical heart valves. The American College of Cardiology and American Heart Association guidelines recommend that patients planning a pregnancy can continue warfarin until pregnancy, but with a shift for heparin as soon as pregnancy is identified [41]. Warfarin and all Vitamin K antagonists must be switched to low molecular weight heparin before the sixth weeks of gestation as they cross placenta causing fetal hemorrhage, and fetal vitamin K-antagonist syndrome, especially between 6 and 12 weeks of gestation [42]. New direct oral anticoagulants are contraindicated during whole pregnancy. Low molecular weight heparins are the only anticoagulant to be used for anticoagulation during pregnancy. Their potential advantages include the fact they do not cross the placental barrier which makes them considered safe for the fetus. Unlike other molecules, nadroparin calcium or tinzaparin have the advantage of being administered in a single daily dose for therapeutic treatment. These measures to prevent the risk of thromboembolisms are combined with type-2 venous restraint.

Low-dose aspirin has been largely used and tested during pregnancy for the prevention of preeclampsia and appears to be safe for the fetus [43]. The obstetrical history that could justify this prescription comprises more than three spontaneous miscarriages, pre-eclampsia <32 weeks of gestation and/or intrauterine growth retardation <fifth percentile with a probable vascular origin (professional agreement). Maintenance of aspirin during pregnancy should be discussed on a case-by-case basis, with the lowest possible dosage, i.e. a maximum of 160 mg/day. In these situations, aspirin should be taken in the evening or at least 8 h after waking up (grade B), before 16 gestational weeks, at a dose of 100–160 mg/day (grade A). The use of aspirin at doses ≥500 mg/day beyond the beginning of the sixth month (24 weeks) is formally contraindicated due to an increased risk of fetal heart malformation.

## Management of Underlying Prothrombotic Disorders

If an underlying hematological disease exists, it has to be stabilized before conception. Hydroxycarbamide (hydroxyurea, Hydrea) treatment for myeloproliferative disorder is teratogenic in several animal species. Hydroxycarbamide is also a source of abnormalities in sperm parameters and a 3 month wash-out or a spermatogenesis cycle seems justified before considering conception. Interferon alpha can be prescribed during pregnancy. A recent literature review identified 43 pregnant women with essential thrombocythemia treated with interferon alpha. In this study a decrease platelets count at birth and no adverse events that required the discontinuation of treatment and 93% of healthy babies were observed [44]. There is no data on ruxolitinib in pregnancy.

## *Planning of Labor Phase and Birth*

It has been common wisdom that peak increases in intra-abdominal pressure during the active phase of labor increase the risk of variceal rupture. However, since abdominal pressure during labor increases in parallel with that of chest pressure, it is unlikely that the pushing efforts increase the risk of esophageal or gastric variceal rupture. Furthermore, reported cases of variceal hemorrhage closely linked to delivery are very few [45]. Among recent series of pregnancies in women with vascular disorders of the liver, there were four reported cases of variceal hemorrhage during 135 pregnancies, and only one occurred around delivery [17, 18, 22, 24, 25]. The theoretical risks of vaginal delivery must then be weighed against those associated with cesarean section, which had formerly been proposed to cope with this theoretical risk. Bleedings from specific or nonspecific complications of portal hypertension (injury to porto-systemic collaterals, postoperative ascites and post-partum thromboembolism) have to be considered [46]. Thus, vaginal delivery with adequate analgesia and assistance in the active phase of labor is currently recommended by most authors and caesarian section reserved only for obstetrical indications [9]. Platelet counts generally considered as safe for delivery are over 50,000 G/L for cesarean section, over 20,000 G/L for vaginal delivery, over 75,000 G/L for epidural anesthesia and over 50,000 G/L for spinal anesthesia. Timing and mode of delivery should be based on a consensus between all the disciplines involved and the patient.

## *Puerperium Period*

Postpartum, the use of estrogen-derived oral contraceptives is contra-indicated due to its association with an increased risk of BCS and venous thromboembolism in women with previous thromboembolism [12]. Breastfeeding is possible with beta-blockers therapy and with warfarin but not with other vitamin K antagonists molecules or direct oral anticoagulant [47]. Hydroxycarbamide (hydroxyurea, Hydrea) treatment is contra-indicated during breastfeeding.

In conclusion, although at heightened risk for mother and fetus, pregnancy is still feasible for women with vascular disorders of the liver if the liver disease is well controlled. These patients should be managed by a multidisciplinary medical team with experience in such diseases. Although the risk of miscarriage is heightened, a pregnancy reaching 20 weeks of gestation is very likely to end with the birth of a live baby.

**Conflicts of Interest**  The authors declared no conflicts of interest.

# References

1. Plessier A, Darwish-Murad S, Hernandez-Guerra M, Consigny Y, Fabris F, Trebicka J, et al. Acute portal vein thrombosis unrelated to cirrhosis: a prospective multicenter follow-up study. Hepatology. 2010 Jan;51(1):210–8.
2. Darwish Murad S, Plessier A, Hernandez-Guerra M, Fabris F, Eapen CE, Bahr MJ, et al. Etiology, management, and outcome of the Budd-Chiari syndrome. Ann Intern Med. 2009 Aug 4;151(3):167–75.
3. Valla D-C. Budd-Chiari syndrome and veno-occlusive disease/sinusoidal obstruction syndrome. Gut. 2008 Oct;57(10):1469–78.
4. De Gottardi A, Rautou P-E, Schouten J, Rubbia-Brandt L, Leebeek F, Trebicka J, et al. Porto-sinusoidal vascular disease: proposal and description of a novel entity. Lancet Gastroenterol Hepatol. 2019 May;4(5):399–411.
5. Munnell EW, Taylor HC. Liver blood flow in pregnancy—hepatic vein catheterization 1. J Clin Invest. 1947 Sep 1;26(5):952–6.
6. Mustafa R, Ahmed S, Gupta A, Venuto RC. A comprehensive review of hypertension in Pregnancy. J Pregnancy. 2012;2012:1–19.
7. García-Pagán J-C, Gracia-Sancho J, Bosch J. Functional aspects on the pathophysiology of portal hypertension in cirrhosis. J Hepatol. 2012 Aug;57(2):458–61.
8. Tindall VR, Beazley JM. An assessment of changes in liver function during normal pregnancy--using a modified bromsulphthalein test. J Obstet Gynaecol Br Commonw. 1965 Oct;72(5):717–37.
9. Bissonnette J, Durand F, de Raucourt E, Ceccaldi P-F, Plessier A, Valla D, et al. Pregnancy and vascular liver disease. J Clin Exp Hepatol. 2015 Mar;5(1):41–50.
10. Pabinger I, Grafenhofer H. Thrombosis during pregnancy: risk factors, diagnosis and treatment. Pathophysiol Haemost Thromb. 2002;32(5–6):322–4.
11. Ren W, Li X, Jia J, Xia Y, Hu F, Xu Z. Prevalence of Budd-Chiari syndrome during Pregnancy or puerperium: a systematic review and meta-analysis. Gastroenterol Res Pract. 2015;2015:1–13.
12. Rautou P-E, Plessier A, Bernuau J, Denninger M-H, Moucari R, Valla D. Pregnancy: a risk factor for Budd-Chiari syndrome? Gut. 2009 Apr;58(4):606–8.
13. Randi ML, Bertozzi I, Rumi E, Elena C, Finazzi G, Vianelli N, et al. Pregnancy complications predict thrombotic events in young women with essential thrombocythemia. Am J Hematol. 2014 Mar;89(3):306–9.
14. Denninger M-H, Chaït Y, Casadevall N, Hillaire S, Guillin M-C, Bezeaud A, et al. Cause of portal or hepatic venous thrombosis in adults: the role of multiple concurrent factors. Hepatology. 2000 Mar 1;31(3):587–91.
15. Khuroo MS, Datta DV. Budd-Chiari syndrome following pregnancy. Report of 16 cases, with roentgenologic, hemodynamic and histologic studies of the hepatic outflow tract. Am J Med. 1980 Jan;68(1):113–21.
16. Dilawari JB, Bambery P, Chawla Y, Kaur U, Bhusnurmath SR, Malhotra HS, et al. Hepatic outflow obstruction (Budd-Chiari syndrome). Experience with 177 patients and a review of the literature. Medicine (Baltimore). 1994 Jan;73(1):21–36.
17. Khan F, Rowe I, Martin B, Knox E, Johnston T, Elliot C, et al. Outcomes of pregnancy in patients with known Budd-Chiari syndrome. World J Hepatol. 2017 Jul 28;9(21):945–52.
18. Rautou P-E, Angermayr B, Garcia-Pagan J-C, Moucari R, Peck-Radosavljevic M, Raffa S, et al. Pregnancy in women with known and treated Budd-Chiari syndrome: maternal and fetal outcomes. J Hepatol. 2009 Jul;51(1):47–54.
19. Shukla A, Sadalage A, Gupta D, Gupte A, Mahapatra A, Mazumder D, et al. Pregnancy outcomes in women with Budd Chiari syndrome before onset of symptoms and after treatment. Liver Int Off J Int Assoc Study Liver. 2018;38(4):754–9.
20. Plessier A, Sibert A, Consigny Y, Hakime A, Zappa M, Denninger M-H, et al. Aiming at minimal invasiveness as a therapeutic strategy for Budd-Chiari syndrome. Hepatology. 2006 Nov;44(5):1308–16.

21. Bruckner TA, Mortensen LH, Catalano RA. Spontaneous pregnancy loss in Denmark following economic downturns. Am J Epidemiol. 2016 Apr 15;183(8):701–8.
22. Hoekstra J, Seijo S, Rautou PE, Ducarme G, Boudaoud L, Luton D, et al. Pregnancy in women with portal vein thrombosis: results of a multicentric European study on maternal and fetal management and outcome. J Hepatol. 2012 Dec;57(6):1214–9.
23. Mandal D, Dattaray C, Sarkar R, Mandal S, Choudhary A, Maity TK. Is pregnancy safe with extrahepatic portal vein obstruction? An analysis. Singapore Med J. 2012 Oct;53(10):676–80.
24. Aggarwal N, Chopra S, Raveendran A, Suri V, Dhiman RK, Chawla YK. Extra hepatic portal vein obstruction and pregnancy outcome: largest reported experience. J Obstet Gynaecol Res. 2011 Jun;37(6):575–80.
25. Andrade F, Shukla A, Bureau C, Senzolo M, D'Alteroche L, Heurgué A, et al. Pregnancy in idiopathic non-cirrhotic portal hypertension: a multicentric study on maternal and fetal management and outcome. J Hepatol. 2018 Dec;69(6):1242–9.
26. Andrade F, Shukla A, Bureau C, Senzolo M, D'Alteroche L, Heurgué A, et al. Reply to: "splenic artery aneurysms, portal hypertension and pregnancy". J Hepatol. 2019 May;70(5):1026–7.
27. Hosn MA, Xu J, Sharafuddin M, Corson JD. Visceral artery aneurysms: decision making and treatment options in the new era of minimally invasive and endovascular surgery. Int J Angiol Off Publ Int Coll Angiol Inc. 2019 Mar;28(1):11–6.
28. Dupuis O, Delagrange L, Dupuis-Girod S. Hereditary haemorrhagic telangiectasia and pregnancy: a review of the literature. Orphanet J Rare Dis. 2020 Jan 7;15(1):5.
29. Lai CF, Dennis A, Graham J. High output cardiac failure in a parturient with hereditary haemorrhagic telangiectasia. Anaesth Intensive Care. 2010 Mar;38(2):381–6.
30. Patricot LM, Dumont M, Duvernois JP, Baulieux J, Mercatello A. A case of hepatic and splenic peliosis occurring in the puerperium after normal pregnancy. J Gynecol Obstet Biol Reprod (Paris). 1986;15(3):321–6.
31. Butt MO, Luck NH, Hassan SM, Abbas Z, Mubarak M. Peliosis Hepatis complicating Pregnancy: a rare entity. J Transl Intern Med. 2017 Jun;5(2):132–4.
32. Cissoko H, Jonville-Béra A-P, Swortfiguer D, Giraudeau B, Autret-Leca E. Exposition aux bêtabloquants en fin de grossesse. Arch Pédiatrie. 2005 May;12(5):543–7.
33. Ghidirim G, Mishin I, Dolghii A, Lupashcu A. Prophylactic endoscopic band ligation of esophageal varices during pregnancy. J Gastrointest Liver Dis JGLD. 2008 Jun;17(2):236–7.
34. Starkel P, Horsmans Y, Geubel A. Endoscopic band ligation: a safe technique to control bleeding esophageal varices in pregnancy. Gastrointest Endosc. 1998 Aug;48(2):212–4.
35. Chandramouli S, Lee WM, Lo J, Toomay S, Tujios S. Prophylactic transjugular intrahepatic portosystemic shunt placement for cirrhosis management in pregnancy. Hepatol Baltim Md. 2020 May;71(5):1876–8.
36. Ingraham CR, Padia SA, Johnson GE, Easterling TR, Liou IW, Kanal KM, et al. Transjugular intrahepatic portosystemic shunt placement during Pregnancy: a case series of five patients. Cardiovasc Intervent Radiol. 2015 Oct;38(5):1205–10.
37. Lodato F, Cappelli A, Montagnani M, Colecchia A, Festi D, Azzaroli F, et al. Transjugular intrahepatic portosystemic shunt: a case report of rescue management of unrestrainable variceal bleeding in a pregnant woman. Dig Liver Dis Off J Ital Soc Gastroenterol Ital Assoc Study Liver. 2008 May;40(5):387–90.
38. Savage C, Patel J, Lepe MR, Lazarre CH, Rees CR. Transjugular intrahepatic portosystemic shunt creation for recurrent gastrointestinal bleeding during pregnancy. J Vasc Interv Radiol JVIR. 2007 Jul;18(7):902–4.
39. Wildberger JE, Vorwerk D, Winograd R, Stargardt A, Busch N, Günther RW. New TIPS placement in pregnancy in recurrent esophageal varices hemorrhage--assessment of fetal radiation exposure. ROFO Fortschr Geb Rontgenstr Nuklearmed. 1998 Oct;169(4):429–31.
40. EASL. EASL clinical practice guidelines: vascular diseases of the liver. J Hepatol. 2016 Jan;64(1):179–202.
41. Nishimura RA, Otto CM, Bonow RO, Carabello BA, Erwin JP, Fleisher LA, et al. 2017 AHA/ACC focused update of the 2014 AHA/ACC guideline for the management of patients with

valvar heart disease: a report of the American college of cardiology/American heart association task force on clinical practice guidelines. Circulation. 2017 Jun 20;135(25):e1159–95.
42. Bates SM, Greer IA, Middeldorp S, Veenstra DL, Prabulos A-M, Vandvik PO. VTE, thrombophilia, antithrombotic therapy, and pregnancy: antithrombotic therapy and prevention of thrombosis, 9th ed: American college of chest physicians evidence-based clinical practice guidelines. Chest. 2012 Feb;141(2 Suppl):e691S–736S.
43. Bujold E, Roberge S, Lacasse Y, Bureau M, Audibert F, Marcoux S, et al. Prevention of pre-eclampsia and intrauterine growth restriction with aspirin started in early pregnancy: a meta-analysis. Obstet Gynecol. 2010 Aug;116(2, Part 1):402–14.
44. Sakai K, Ueda A, Hasegawa M, Ueda Y. Efficacy and safety of interferon alpha for essential thrombocythemia during pregnancy: two cases and a literature review. Int J Hematol. 2018 Aug;108(2):203–7.
45. Rosenfeld H, Hochner-Celnikier D, Ackerman Z. Massive bleeding from ectopic varices in the postpartum period: rare but serious complication in women with portal hypertension. Eur J Gastroenterol Hepatol. 2009 Sep;21(9):1086–91.
46. Sultan AA, Tata LJ, West J, Fiaschi L, Fleming KM, Nelson-Piercy C, et al. Risk factors for first venous thromboembolism around pregnancy: a population-based cohort study from the United Kingdom. Blood. 2013 May 9;121(19):3953–61.
47. Qasqas SA, McPherson C, Frishman WH, Elkayam U. Cardiovascular pharmacotherapeutic considerations during pregnancy and lactation. Cardiol Rev. 2004;12(4):201–21.

# Chapter 16
# Antithrombotic Therapy and Liver Disease

**Massimo Primignani and Armando Tripodi**

## Introduction

Vascular diseases of the liver affect the liver and/or the biliary system because of thrombotic or inflammatory disorders of the hepatic vasculature. In their primary form, rare but nowadays increasingly recognized, the liver/biliary damage is caused by the diseased vessels. More frequent is the secondary involvement of the hepatic vasculature by pre-existent liver or biliary diseases, or by vascular invasion/compression by malignant or benign neoplasia or cysts. While several of the primary vascular disorders require anticoagulant treatment, the role of this treatment in parenchymal liver disease with secondary vascular involvement is more controversial.

In this chapter, we will discuss the present knowledge on anticoagulation (or other antithrombotic drugs) in those primary vascular liver diseases in which such treatment is required, as the Budd-Chiari Syndrome (BCS) and acute/recent extrahepatic portal vein obstruction (EHPVO), or could be considered, as in chronic EHPVO, idiopathic non-cirrhotic portal hypertension/porto-sinusoidal vascular disease (INCPH/PSVD) and sinusoidal obstruction syndrome (SOS). In addition, we will discuss the current indications and warnings of anticoagulation in patients with cirrhosis and portal vein thrombosis.

M. Primignani (✉)
Foundation IRCCS Ca' Granda Ospedale Maggiore Policlinico, Division of Gastroenterology and Hepatology, Milan, Italy
e-mail: massimo.primignani@policlinico.mi.it

A. Tripodi
Angelo Bianchi Bonomi Hemophilia and Thrombosis Center, Milan, Italy
e-mail: armando.tripodi@unimi.it

© Springer Nature Switzerland AG 2022
D. Valla et al. (eds.), *Vascular Disorders of the Liver*,
https://doi.org/10.1007/978-3-030-82988-9_16

# Primary Vascular Liver Diseases Requiring Anticoagulant Treatment

## *Budd-Chiari Syndrome/Hepatic Outflow Tract Obstruction (BCS)*

BCS is an eponym for hepatic venous outflow tract obstruction, which can be located from the level of the small hepatic veins to the level of the termination of inferior vena cava into the right atrium. Primary BCS is a rare, life threatening thrombotic disorder. The high rate of thrombophilia (defined as the presence of inherited or acquired prothrombotic hemostasis defects) in BCS motivates the widespread indication for anticoagulant therapy. Although the lack of randomized studies, due to the rarity of the disease, cohort studies clearly show that an early implementation of anticoagulation may prevent thrombosis progression, possibly achieves vein recanalization and improves survival [1–5]. Long-term anticoagulation is mandatory and applies to all patients, although the evidence for BCS patients without identified thrombophilia is inconclusive [6].

Besides long-term anticoagulation, angioplasty/thrombolysis, transjugular intrahepatic portosystemic shunt (TIPS) and liver transplantation are the ensuing recommended steps in the management of BCS. Anticoagulation should be maintained also in patients ultimately undergoing orthotopic liver transplantation (OLT). In fact, BCS recurrence after OLT, common in the past, has dropped since the early implementation and long-term maintenance of anticoagulation after OLT [7].

Low molecular weight heparin (LMWH) and vitamin K antagonists (VKA) are the traditional, commonly used antithrombotic drugs in BCS. A treatment with LMWH followed by VKA targeting at an international normalized ratio (INR) of 2–3 has been shown to achieve a 89% 5-year survival rate [8].

An incidence up to 14% of heparin-induced thrombocytopenia (HIT) has been observed in vascular liver diseases, which is higher than that observed in venous thromboembolism, particularly in BCS patients with underlying myeloproliferative neoplasms [9, 10]. Because unfractioned heparin (UFH) and (to a lesser extent) LMWH can provoke HIT [10] close surveillance of the platelet count during heparin treatment, either with UFH or LMWH, is needed [9–11]. If during treatment, platelet count is reduced >50% and /or other features (i.e., clinical signs or physical examination) suggest the occurrence of HIT, heparin administration must be stopped and replaced by other, non-heparin anticoagulants, such as argatroban or danaparoid. Argatroban is preferred in patients with renal insufficiency [12]. Fondaparinux, that is not associated with HIT, is a good choice, especially in stable, non-critically ill patients [13]. Bleeding is a feared adverse event in BCS patients undergoing anticoagulant therapy. The incidence of major bleeding in BCS patients on anticoagulants has been shown to be as high as 22.8 per 100 patient years, markedly higher than that observed in anticoagulated patients with deep vein thrombosis of the lower limbs [14]. Esophageal varices and invasive therapeutic procedures appear to account for such high bleeding rate [14]. Nonetheless, anticoagulation remains strongly recommended in BCS. Current guidelines recommend treating portal hypertension, which is a major risk factor for bleeding while excess anticoagulation plays a secondary role [6]. Consequently, portal hypertensive bleeding should be prevented (by non-selective beta blocking agents or endoscopic band ligation) or treated as it is done in cirrhosis [6]. Previous history of portal-hypertensive bleeding is not a contra-indication for anticoagulation, if adequate prophylaxis for recurrent bleeding is implemented. Data on thrombolysis are scarce. Major bleedings and limited recanalization rates are reported. Therefore, systemic thrombolysis is not generally recommended in patients with BCS. Transcatheter, local thrombolysis is sometimes used together with angioplasty/stenting of short segment stenosis in the hepatic veins [15, 16]. No recommendation can be presently made on direct oral anticoagulants (DOAC) and anti-platelet drugs due to the limited available data. This issue is discussed in the last section of this chapter.

## Extrahepatic Portal Vein Obstruction (EHPVO)

### *Acute/Recent EHPVO*

Recent formation of thrombi within the portal vein and/or right or left branches defines acute EHPVO. Thrombi may extend into the mesenteric or splenic veins and occlusion may be complete or partial. Therapy is aimed at preventing the extension of thrombosis to mesenteric veins, thus preventing intestinal infarction, and achieving vein recanalization [17, 18]. Both these aims can be achieved by early anticoagulation therapy. In a prospective European study [19], the extension of thrombosis to the superior mesenteric vein was prevented in those patients who had an early start of anticoagulation. Indeed, only 2/95 cases of limited intestinal infarction were observed, although 60% of patients had initial involvement of the superior mesenteric vein. While spontaneous recanalization of symptomatic acute/recent primary EHPVO is quite rare in patients not receiving anticoagulation, and only occurs when associated with self-limiting underlying pathology and/or minimal thrombus extension [20], recanalization of the portal, splenic and superior mesenteric veins was achieved in 39%, 80%, and 73% of anticoagulated patients, respectively [19]. Extension of thrombosis to the splenic vein and ascites, even minimal at baseline, were associated with the absence of recanalization of the portal vein. In addition, it has been observed that delayed initiation of anticoagulation impacts negatively on the recanalization rate [21]. Recanalization of the portal vein does not appear to occur beyond the sixth month of anticoagulation treatment. These findings confirm the results of previous retrospective studies [21–23]. Therefore, expert consensus recommend anticoagulation for at least 6 months in acute EHPVO [6]. Nonetheless, mesenteric vein thrombosis may recanalize even after more than 6 months. Therefore, decision on the optimal duration of anticoagulation should be made on a case-by-case basis, weighting the benefits of a possible improvement of the patency of the porto-mesenteric axis and the risks of prolonged anticoagulation. However, if an underlying persistent prothrombotic defect is recognized, long-term anticoagulation should be considered, and is generally recommended [6]. In most studies, anticoagulation was mainly based on UFH or LMWH given at therapeutic doses and LMWH has been replaced by VKA targeted at an INR from 2 to 3. In the prospective European study, UFH and LMWH were used in 25% and 65% of patients, respectively [19]. As in BCS, HIT has been shown to occur in up to 20% of EHPVO patients treated with UFH, which is a much higher rate compared to HIT in patients without EHPVO [11]. Consequently, UFH should be no longer indicated in the treatment of acute EHPVO. Such an incidence is probably lower, though not negligible in patients treated with LMWH, particularly in those with underlying myeloproliferative neoplasms [9–11].

As far as bleeding is concerned, the prospective European study reported a 9% bleeding rate in patients on anticoagulation, and a 2% mortality rate. The latter was, however, unrelated to bleeding or EHPVO [19]. Current consensus guidelines recommend early treatment with LMWH at therapeutic dose and switching to VKA in stable patients, targeting an INR from 2 to 3 [2, 6, 7]. Data on DOAC are encouraging, though still limited [24–27].

## Thrombolysis in Recent EHPVO

Treatment of acute EHPVO with local thrombolysis, via the transjugular or the transhepatic approach, has been reported in small cohorts or case reports. Recanalization rates vary considerably, ranging from 15 to 60%, not different from those achieved with anticoagulation alone, but with an incidence of bleeding events up to 60% [16, 28, 29], and fatal outcome in some cases [16, 29, 30]. Although the transjugular approach might be associated with fewer complications, data are still limited. Since most patients treated with early anticoagulation have good clinical outcomes, even failure of recanalization does not warrant thrombolysis in most cases [2, 6, 7]. Thrombolysis should be cautiously used, in selected cases, i.e. symptomatic EHPVO with progressive extension of thrombosis and/or signs of mesenteric ischemia, despite anticoagulation. In such cases, local thrombolysis appears to be safer and more effective than systemic thrombolysis [31]. Furthermore, new interventional techniques, combining local thrombolysis and mechanical thrombectomy may add to the effective treatment of patients with acute mesenteric vein thrombosis, particularly in OLT candidates [32, 33].

## Chronic Extrahepatic Portal Vein Obstruction (EHPVO) Non-Cirrhotic, Nonmalignant

Following acute EHPVO, in the absence of portal vein recanalization, porto-portal collaterals veins develop around/inside the thrombus, to bypass the obstructed vessel. Such cavernomatous transformation of the portal vein begins within few days, as a compensatory mechanism to bypass the obstructed vessel, but is unable to normalize blood flow and prevent portal hypertension. Gastroesophageal varices may develop as early as one month after the acute episode and such changes involve a significant risk of severe gastrointestinal bleeding. However, patients with primary chronic EHPVO frequently carry one or more persistent prothrombotic risk factors, leading to an increased risk of recurrent thrombosis [22, 34]. Therefore, the proper management of chronic EHPVO requires careful weighting of the opposite risks of thrombosis and bleeding.

No randomized studies on anticoagulant therapy in patients with chronic EHPVO exist. Evidence for a favorable benefit/risk ratio of anticoagulation in these patients is low and stems from cohort studies, reporting a reduced risk of thrombosis recurrence. At multivariate analysis, long-term anticoagulation was identified as an independent factor of decreased risk of recurrent thrombosis in one study [34] and borderline in another [35]. As for the bleeding risk in patients with chronic EHPVO receiving anticoagulation, it appears to depend more on whether primary prophylaxis for portal hypertensive bleeding was [22, 34] or was not [35] performed, rather than on anticoagulation itself. Moreover, if bleeding occurs, its severity appears to be similar in patients with or without anticoagulation [34]. Overall, multivariate analysis indicated a favorable impact of anticoagulation therapy on survival with a statistically significant decrease in mortality rate in one study [36], and a non-significant decrease in the other [35].

International guidelines recommend long-term anticoagulant therapy in patients with chronic EHPVO and a persistent documented thrombophilia, as well as those with recurrent thrombosis or intestinal infarction, while in patients without underlying prothrombotic conditions there is little information to recommend anticoagulant therapy. In patients with gastroesophageal varices, anticoagulation should be started after adequate portal hypertensive bleeding prophylaxis is implemented [2, 3, 37].

The Baveno VI Consensus Statements [6] on the use of antithrombotic drugs in primary vascular liver disease are listed below [Levels of existing evidence ranked—and recommendations graded—according to the Oxford System*]

**Use of Anticoagulants and Anti-Platelet Drugs in Vascular Liver Diseases: Baveno VI Consensus Statements**

- Low Molecular Weight Heparin (LMWH) and Vitamin K Antagonists (VKA) are widely accepted and used in primary thrombosis of the portal venous system or hepatic venous outflow tract [1b; A].
- No current recommendation can be made on Direct Oral Anticoagulants (DOACs) and anti-platelet drugs due to limited data [5;D].

**Anticoagulation in Budd-Chiari-Syndrome**

- Long-term anticoagulation should be given to all patients, although there is no definitive evidence for patients without identified risk factors (5;D).

                                                  

- Portal hypertension should be treated since it is the major risk factor for bleeding, while excess anticoagulation plays a secondary role (4;C).
- Previous bleeding related to portal hypertension is not considered a major contraindication for anticoagulation, provided appropriate prophylaxis for recurrent bleeding is initiated (4;C).

Anticoagulation in recent EHPVO

- Recent EHPVO rarely resolves spontaneously (3a,A).
- Low molecular weight heparin should be started immediately followed by oral anticoagulant therapy (2b;B). Most patients treated with early anticoagulation have a good clinical outcome. Therefore, even failure of recanalization do not warrant further interventions (e.g. local thrombolysis) in most cases (2b;B).
- Anticoagulation should be given for at least six months. When an underlying persistent prothrombotic state has been documented long-term anticoagulation is recommended (1b;A).

**Anticoagulation in chronic EHPVO**

- In patients without underlying prothrombotic disease, there is scarce information to recommend anticoagulant therapy (5;D).
- In patients with a persistent documented prothrombotic state, recurrent thrombosis or intestinal infarction long-term anticoagulant therapy is recommended (3b;B).
- Anticoagulation should be started after adequate portal hypertensive bleeding prophylaxis has been initiated (5;D).

* http://www.cebm.net/downloads/Oxford_EBM_Levels_5.rtf

## Idiopathic Noncirrhotic Portal Hypertension/Porto-Sinusoidal Vascular Disease

Idiopathic noncirrhotic portal hypertension (INCPH) is characterized by the occurrence of portal hypertension in the absence of liver cirrhosis and other known causes of noncirrhotic portal hypertension [38]. The new proposed term "Porto-Sinusoidal Vascular Disease" (PSVD), that better highlights the assumed pathophysiology of parenchymal vascular obstruction, includes the histopathological features of obliterative venopathy, even in the absence of portal hypertension, as possible different stages or a different expression of the same disease.

The rationale for anticoagulation therapy in INCPH/PSVD, relies on the histologic findings of parenchymal vascular obstruction, the reported frequency of thrombophilia, as high as 40%, in Western countries [39], and the higher incidence of EHPVO as compared to cirrhosis patients, particularly in those with a concomitant HIV infection [40]. Indeed, the occurrence of EHPVO worsens the prognosis of these patients and may jeopardize liver transplantation if extended to the splenic and mesenteric veins. Moreover, after the occurrence of acute EHPVO, the implementation of anticoagulant therapy appears to achieve portal vein recanalization in only half the patients with INCPH/PSVD [41], thus suggesting that prevention of EHPVO by prophylactic anticoagulation might be a better option than its treatment at the time of occurrence. However, although attractive, anticoagulation therapy cannot be generally recommended in INCPH/PSVD, given the lack of controlled studies and the fact that portal hypertensive bleeding is the main complication of the disease. Current expert recommendations consider anticoagulant treatment only in patients with clear underlying prothrombotic defects or in patients who develop EHPVO. Randomized studies of anticoagulant therapy in PSVD patients are warranted. Whether anticoagulant treatment could prevent the progression of disease and the development of portal hypertension in PSVD patients without portal hypertension is also unknown and needs evaluation in prospective studies.

## Sinusoidal Obstruction Syndrome (SOS)

Sinusoidal obstruction syndrome (SOS) (previously known as veno-occlusive disease) is a severe vascular liver disease, characterized by sinusoidal nonthrombotic obstruction [2] (see also the in-depth review in Chap. 11). Toxicity from chemotherapeutic regimens used in the workup for stem cell transplantation is the leading cause of SOS. Other causes include several chemotherapeutic agents used in adjuvant or neo-adjuvant treatments of solid cancer, or immunosuppressors used in the context of organ transplantation or inflammatory bowel diseases. Recognition of risk factors and reduction of the intensity of myeloablative regimens, if possible, may help to prevent SOS, but such adjustments require a careful evaluation of the risk/benefit ratio.

Defibrotide (a mixture of oligodeoxyribonucleotides extracted from porcine intestinal mucosal DNA with antithrombotic, fibrinolytic and angiogenic properties) has demonstrated beneficial effects for SOS prophylaxis in a randomized study of pediatric hematopoietic stem-cell transplantation [42]. Defibrotide was also evaluated in patients with SOS in four studies [43–46] achieving a 32–65% survival at day 100, without bleeding complications, but no firm conclusions can be drawn from the pooled analysis of these studies, due to methodological flaws and heterogeneity. Conversely, a meta-analysis of 12 studies in patients undergoing hematopoietic stem cell transplantation showed that prophylaxis with heparin was unable to decrease the risk of SOS [47].

Overall, the use of defibrotide for preventing SOS in patients undergoing hematopoietic stem cell transplantation is currently recommended. The role of other anticoagulant therapies, in either the prophylaxis or treatment of patients with SOS requires further studies [2].

# Antithrombotic Therapy in Parenchymal Liver Disease with Secondary Vascular Involvement

## *Portal Vein Thrombosis (PVT) in Patients with Cirrhosis*

Recent data [48] indicate that cirrhosis is not an acquired bleeding diathesis, as historically believed because of the frequent finding of prolonged prothrombin time (PT), activated partial thromboplastin time (aPTT), and thrombocytopenia. Indeed, the decreased levels of procoagulant proteins justify the worsening of such classical coagulation tests as the PT and aPTT. However, global tests of hemostasis, as the endogenous thrombin potential, able to take into account also the effect of the anticoagulants (mainly protein C) also synthesized by the liver and decreased in advanced disease, show that the hemostatic system is rebalanced in cirrhosis, although frailer than in healthy individuals. Further developments of research have demonstrated a procoagulant imbalance in cirrhotic patients, likely due to high levels of factor VIII (procoagulant driver) combined with decreased levels of protein C (anticoagulant driver) [48], thus reversing the previous paradigm of cirrhosis as the epitome of spontaneous auto-anticoagulation. Indeed, portal vein thrombosis is a well-known complication of cirrhosis, particularly in the setting of advanced disease. Likewise, venous thromboembolism in the lower limbs and in the lung also occurs in cirrhosis, apparently at an even higher rate than in non-cirrhotic individuals [49, 50]. Based on such clinical and laboratory evidence, anticoagulation treatment is no longer considered as a contraindication in patients with cirrhosis, who present with thrombosis. In addition, animal models of acute or chronic liver failure [51–54], and growing clinical data [55–59] suggest that antithrombotic treatment slows down progression of liver disease and decrease the rate of adverse events related to portal hypertension.

The occurrence of PVT in the course of cirrhosis has been regarded as a determinant of severe prognosis [60, 61] since it is assumed to impair liver perfusion, deteriorate liver function [55, 59–61] and has been shown to worsen the severity of variceal bleeding at the time of occurrence [60]. Further reasons supporting anticoagulation in cirrhosis patients with PVT are the risk of intestinal infarction with the progression of thrombosis into the superior mesenteric vein [62], the increased mortality of patients with occlusive PVT listed for liver transplantation [59] and the increased mortality post liver transplant in patients with occlusive PVT [63]. The favorable effect of anticoagulant treatment, either LMWH or VKA, is suggested by several cohort studies that included 226 patients, most with partial PVT. Repermeation rate ranged from 55% to 75% with the higher rates occurring in patients with partial PVT. Time interval between diagnosis of PVT and start of anticoagulation treatment less than 6 months seems to be the most important predictor of the chance of response to treatment [64].

Another issue refers to the recurrence of PVT after the achievement of repermeation of the portal vein. Recurrence has been reported in up to 38% of cases few months after the discontinuation of anticoagulation, if treatment had been stopped soon after repermeation of the portal vein [65]. This observation suggests that prolonging anticoagulation treatment after repermeation of the portal vein may prevent thrombosis recurrence. Overall, bleeding complications occurred in 17/226 (7.5%) patients and correlated with portal hypertension in eight cases. A multicenter study showed a correlation between platelet counts less than $50 \times 10^9/L$ and bleeding risk [66]. Finally, two meta-analyses confirm that anticoagulant therapy improves the rate of portal vein recanalization and prevents PVT progression in such patients [67, 68].

However, in real-world clinical practice, the implementation of anticoagulation for the management of PVT in cirrhosis is limited by the perceived risk of bleeding and, more importantly, by the still controversial findings on the impact of portal vein recanalization on the clinical outcome. As for the first issue, several reports suggest that anticoagulation with VKA does not increase the risk of portal hypertensive bleeding, compared with patients with cirrhosis non taking these anticoagulants, if patients receive adequate prophylaxis of variceal hemorrhage [6, 56, 69]. Rather, it appears that VKA increase the risk of minor bleeding, compared with patients without cirrhosis [69]. Moreover, at least in patients who achieve complete portal vein recanalization, both transplantation-free survival and portal hypertension-related event-free times appear to be increased [69]. Such benefits of anticoagulation, beyond the resolution of portal vein thrombosis, confirms the data of a randomized trial in which a daily prophylactic administration of LMWH to patients with compensated cirrhosis delayed hepatic decompensation [28], and support the hypothesis of intrahepatic thrombosis as a contributor to the progression of the disease. However, these findings are questioned by a recent study by Nery et al. [70] who found a high rate of spontaneous recanalization and the lack of clinical deterioration associated with PVT in a large cohort of patients with cirrhosis and PVT (mostly partial PVT). Therefore, the role of PVT in the course of liver cirrhosis is still controversial, although most experts agree that occlusive portal vein thrombosis worsens cirrhosis outcome. Randomized clinical trials will assess the benefit/risk ratio of anticoagulation for preventing or treating PVT in cirrhotic patients. At present, anticoagulant treatment in cirrhosis, with LMWH or VKA is recommended for patients with PVT listed for liver transplantation or symptomatic and progressive PVT [6, 7, 71].

The Baveno VI Consensus Statements [6] on the management of portal vein thrombosis in cirrhosis are listed below.

**Anticoagulation and Portal Vein Thrombosis (PVT) in Cirrhosis. Baveno VI Consensus Statements**

---

---

---

(Levels of existing evidence ranked - and recommendations graded - according to the Oxford System* (i.e.: level of evidence from 1 = highest to 5 = lowest; grade of recommendation from A = strongest, to D = weakest)

- Screening for PVT is indicated in patients on the waiting list for liver transplant every 6 months (5;D).
- Anticoagulation should be considered in potential candidates with thrombosis of the main portal vein trunk or progressive PVT (3a;B).

- In this setting, the goal is to permit/facilitate LT and reduce post-transplant mortality/morbidity, and anticoagulation should be maintained until transplantation to prevent re-thrombosis (4;C).
- In untreated potential LT candidates with PVT, an imaging follow-up every 3 months is recommended. Anticoagulation is recommended in case of progression (5;D).
- In non-candidates to LT no recommendation regarding anticoagulation treatment can be made at present. Anticoagulation could be considered in selected cases (extension to superior mesenteric vein, known "strong" prothrombotic conditions) (5;D).
- Patients with low platelet count (e.g. <50 × $10^9$/L) are at higher risk of both PVT and bleeding complications under anticoagulation and require more caution (5;D)
- The benefit/risk ratio of anticoagulation for preventing or treating PVT in cirrhotic patients requires further randomized controlled trials (RCTs) (5;D).
- LMWH and VKA appear to be equally effective in cirrhotic individuals with PVT. Data on DOAC are scarce. There is an urgent need for improved tools for monitoring anticoagulation in cirrhotic patients. Measurement of thrombin generation might be an option (5; D).

---

* http://www.cebm.net/downloads/Oxford_EBM_Levels_5.rtf

## Anticoagulant Drugs: Mechanism of Action and Management

The anticoagulant drugs used to prevent or treat thrombosis (PVT or peripheral thrombosis) in patients affected by liver disease are the same as those used for non-liver disease patients and include UFH, LMWH, fondaparinux, VKA and DOAC. Dosages and management are similar to those used in non-liver disease patients. However, patients with cirrhosis, because of their impaired synthetic capacity, could theoretically represent a challenge both for dosage and management. The following paragraphs describe the most important issues that are related to the use of these drugs in patients with cirrhosis.

**Unfractionated Heparin** UFH is a fast-acting anticoagulant that is administered by intravenous injection and inhibits factor Xa and thrombin upon complexing with endogenous antithrombin. When used to treat acute thrombosis, UFH requires dose-adjustment by the activated partial thromboplastin time (APTT) aimed at a clotting time prolongation from 1.5 to 2.5-fold the baseline value. In cirrhotic patients, antithrombin is reduced and the APTT is often prolonged beyond the upper limit of the normal range. These features together with the associated risk of HIT and osteoporosis make clinicians reluctant to use UFH in cirrhosis.

**Low Molecular Weight Heparin** LMWH is a fast-acting anticoagulant that is administered by subcutaneous injection and inhibits factor Xa and to a lesser extent thrombin. Like UFH, LMWH requires antithrombin, but can be used at fixed body weight adjusted dose without laboratory testing, except for patients with renal failure, pregnancy or obesity. Whenever dose-adjustment is needed, the method of choice should be the anti-factor Xa activity adjusted to correspond from 0.6 to 1.0 IU/mL. LMWH is frequently used in patients with cirrhosis in spite of the fact that there is no firm evidence on the dose required to achieve full protection in this population. When used at prophylactic or therapeutic dose, LMWH proved effective in preventing [57] or treating ongoing PVT [66] even in patients with cirrhosis. LMWH carries less risk of HIT or osteoporosis than UFH.

**Fondaparinux** This is a synthetic penta-saccharide, representing the least monosaccharide sequence able to bind antithrombin. Fondaparinux is administered by subcutaneous injection and inhibits specifically factor Xa. It is used for prophylaxis or treatment at fixed dose without adjustment by laboratory testing and does not carry the risk of HIT.

**Vitamin K Antagonists** VKA (warfarin and congeners) are anticoagulants, which upon oral administration slow down the post ribosomal carboxylation of vitamin K dependent coagulation factors IX, VII, X, II, protein C and protein S. VKA are slow acting anticoagulants (full effect is achieved after approximately one week from the first ingestion) and require dose-adjustment by testing periodically the prothrombin time (PT) with results expressed as international normalized ratio (INR). Dose-adjustment should be aimed to achieve the therapeutic interval from 2.0 to 3.0 INR units (target 2.5). VKA are effective anticoagulants, but are variably affected by the diet and additional drugs that are concomitantly taken by patients. Their effectiveness/safety is dependent on the time for which the patient is maintained within the therapeutic interval. In patients with cirrhosis, the PT-INR as a scale of the degree of anticoagulation represents a challenge that has not yet been entirely resolved. The baseline PT is often abnormal in cirrhosis and therefore it is uncertain whether the VKA dosage required to attain its target prolongation is the same as that used for patients with normal baseline PT. In a recent study, it was however shown that cirrhotic patients on VKA because of PVT have taken the same weekly dosage as the control population of non-cirrhotic patients [72]. An additional unresolved issue is the fact that the INR has been devised as an universal scale to harmonize PT results stemming from different commercial thromboplastins. This system of harmonization requires the determination of the international sensitivity index (ISI) for each thromboplastin, relative to an international thromboplastin standard. The ISI is determined by testing plasma from patient on VKA. The coagulation defect induced by VKA is qualitatively different from that induced by cirrhosis. Therefore, doubts have been cast on the validity of the regular INR when used for patients with cirrhosis [73, 74]. A modified system of INR calibration (tentatively called INRliver) has been proposed, but not implemented yet [75]. It is therefore uncertain whether the regular INR scale, as determined with commercial thromboplastins, is truly representative of the level of anticoagulation achieved by VKA in patients with cirrhosis. Until more information will be available, it is advised that whenever cirrhotic patients need VKA, the dosage should be such to attain a therapeutic interval from to 2.0 to 3.0 INR as for non-cirrhotic patients.

**Direct Oral Anticoagulants** These drugs, at variance with heparins or VKA, target activated coagulation factors without intermediation from antithrombin or carboxylation. Currently there are four DOAC that have been approved by FDA and EMA for treatment/prevention of VTE and prevention of ischemic stroke and systemic embolism in patients with atrial fibrillation. They include dabigatran (a thrombin inhibitor), rivaroxaban, apixaban and edoxaban (factor Xa inhibitors). An additional DOAC, betrixaban is currently under evaluation from FDA and EMA for the prophylaxis of VTE in hospitalized ill patients. Phase III clinical trials showed that DOAC are effective/safe when used at fixed unadjusted dose based on patients' characteristics. Patients with cirrhosis have been deliberately excluded from the DOAC registration trials. Hence, information on their efficacy/safety in this setting is scanty and limited to few observational studies [27, 76–78] or case reports [79–84].

Regarding primary vascular disorders of the liver, as recent EHPVO or portal vein cavernoma and BCS, the experience with DOAC is still limited, though it appears that the adverse events, including major and minor bleeding events and the failure of anticoagulation (thrombosis progression or recurrence), are comparable between DOAC and traditional anticoagulants. Conversely, more experience has been accumulated, though mainly in retrospective studies, on the efficacy/safety of DOAC in patients with cirrhosis (requiring anticoagulation mostly because atrial fibrillation or deep vein thrombosis [27, 76, 85]. A first systematic review and meta-analysis to evaluate the safety of DOAC compared with warfarin or low-molecular weight heparin [86] did not show a significant difference in both all-cause bleeding (risk ratio 0.72; 95% CI, 0.32–1.63) and major bleeding (odd ratio 0.46; 95% CI, 0.10–2.09). A further recent meta-analysis, including a quite large number of patients, suggest that DOAC, as compared to VKA, reduced the incidence of major bleeding by 61%, without any difference in the incidence of gastrointestinal bleeding, and irrespective to Child-Pugh score or the presence of esophageal varices [87]. Overall, these real world data suggest that, compared to VKA, DOAC may be equally effective in cirrhotic patients, with less bleeding events. Focusing particularly on PVT patients with cirrhosis, a recent, relatively small randomized, not blinded trial, including 80 cirrhotic patients with PVT randomly assigned (1:1) to receive rivaroxaban 10 mg/12 h or warfarin showed that such relatively small doses of rivaroxaban achieved higher resolution rates of PVT and improved short-term survival rate, without hemorrhagic effect or other adverse events [88]. A meta-analysis on the use of anticoagulation in PVT patients with cirrhosis demonstrated that anticoagulation was effective and safe as compared to controls and pooled rates of treatment responders and bleeding events were similar between LMWH, VKA, and DOAC [89]. Overall, a small randomized trial, several retrospective studies and meta-analysis nowadays suggest that DOAC can be used in patients with splanchnic vein thrombosis, both cirrhotic and non-cirrhotic. However, high quality, large clinical trials are needed and more data concerning the optimal dose of DOAC and which DOAC could be preferable according to the severity of liver disease are still awaited. DOAC are in principle much more suitable than LMWH or VKA. At variance with heparins, DOAC do not require antithrombin and at variance with VKA, they can be used at fixed dose without dose adjustment by laboratory testing. Hence, circumventing the validity of the INR.

# References


 1. Murad SD, Plessier A, Hernandez-Guerra M, Fabris F, Eapen CE, Bahr MJ, et al. Etiology, management, and outcome of the Budd-Chiari syndrome. Ann Intern Med. 2009;151:167–75.
 2. DeLeve LD, Valla DC, Garcia-Tsao G, American Association for the Study Liver D. Vascular disorders of the liver. Hepatology. 2009;49:1729–64.
 3. Plessier A, Rautou PE, Valla DC. Management of hepatic vascular diseases. J Hepatol. 2012;56(Suppl 1):S25–38.
 4. Zeitoun G, Escolano S, Hadengue A, Azar N, El Younsi M, Mallet A, et al. Outcome of Budd-Chiari syndrome: a multivariate analysis of factors related to survival including surgical Porto-systemic shunting. Hepatology. 1999;30:84–9.
 5. Murad SD, Valla DC, De Groen PC, Zeitoun G, Hopmans JA, Haagsma EB, et al. Determinants of survival and the effect of Porto-systemic shunting in patients with Budd-Chiari syndrome. Hepatology. 2004;39:500–8.
 6. de Franchis R, Baveno VI Faculty. Expanding consensus in portal hypertension: report of the Baveno VI consensus workshop: stratifying risk and individualizing care for portal hypertension. J Hepatol. 2015;63:743–52.
 7. EASL. EASL clinical practice guidelines: vascular diseases of the liver. J Hepatol. 2016;64:179–202.
 8. Langlet P, Escolano S, Valla D, Coste-Zeitoun D, Denie C, Mallet A, et al. Clinicopathological forms and prognostic index in Budd-Chiari syndrome. J Hepatol. 2003;39:496–501.
 9. Plessier ACY, Boudaoud L. Budd-Chiari syndrome (BCS) and heparin induced thrombocytopenia (HIT). J Hepatol. 2006;44:S92.
10. Primignani M. High incidence of heparin induced thrombocytopenia (HIT) in splanchnic vein thrombosis treated with low molecular weight heparin (LMWH). J Hepatol. 2008;48:S113.
11. Randi ML, Tezza F, Scapin M, Duner E, Scarparo P, ScandellariR, et al. Heparin-induced thrombocytopenia in patients with Philadelphia-negative myeloproliferative disorders and unusual splanchnic or cerebral vein thrombosis. Acta Haematol. 2010;123:140–5.
12. Linkins LA, Dans AL, Moores LK, Bona R, Davidson BL, Schulman S, et al. Treatment and prevention of heparin-induced thrombocytopenia: antithrombotic therapy and prevention of thrombosis, 9th ed: American college of chest physicians evidence-based clinical practice guidelines. Chest. 2012 Feb;141(2 Suppl):e495S–530S.
13. Cuker A, Cines DB. How I treat heparin-induced thrombocytopenia. Blood. 2012 Mar 8;119(10):2209–18.
14. Rautou PE, Douarin L, Denninger MH, Escolano S, Lebrec D, Moreau R, et al. Bleeding in patients with Budd Chiari syndrome. J Hepatol. 2011;54:56–63.
15. Sharma S, Texeira A, Texeira P, Elias E, Wilde J, Olliff SP. Pharmacological thrombolysis in Budd Chiari syndrome: a single Centre experience and review of the literature. J Hepatol. 2004;40:172–80.

16. Smalberg JH, Spaander MV, Jie KS, Pattynama PM, van Buuren HR, van den Berg B, et al. Risks and benefits of transcatheter thrombolytic therapy in patients with splanchnic venous thrombosis. Thromb Haemost. 2008;100:1084–8.
17. Plessier A, Ratou PE, Valla DC. Management of hepatic vascular diseases. J Hepatol. 2012;56:S25–38.
18. Senzolo M, Riggio O, Primignani M. Vascular disorders of the liver: recommendations from the Italian Association for the Study of the liver (AISF) ad hoc committee. Dig Liver Dis. 2011;43:503–14.
19. Plessier A, Murad DS, Hernandez-Guerra M, Consigny Y, Fabris F, Trebicka J, et al. European Network for vascular disorders of the liver (EN-vie) l. acute portal vein thrombosis unrelated to cirrhosis: a prospective multicenter follow-up study. Hepatology. 2010;51:210–8.
20. Hall TC, Garcea G, Metcalfe M, Bilku D, Dennison AR. Management of acute non-cirrhotic portal vein thrombosis: a systematic review. World J Surg. 2011;35:2510–20.
21. Turnes J, Garcia-Pagan JC, Gonzalez M, Aracil C, Calleja JL, Ripoll C, et al. Portal hypertension-related complications after acute portal vein thrombosis: impact of early anticoagulation. Clin Gastroenterol Hepatol. 2008;6:1412–7.
22. Amitrano L, Guardascione MA, Scaglione M, Pezzullo L, Sangiuliano N, Armellino MF, et al. Prognostic factors in noncirrhotic patients with splanchnic vein thromboses. Am J Gastroenterol. 2007;102:2464–70.
23. Condat B, Pessione F, Helene DM, Hillaire S, Valla D. Recent portal or mesenteric venous thrombosis: increased recognition and frequent recanalization on anticoagulant therapy. Hepatology. 2000;32:466–70.
24. Priyanka P, Kupec JT, Krafft M, Shah NA, Reynolds GJ. Newer oral anticoagulants in the treatment of acute portal vein thrombosis in patients with and without cirrhosis. Int J Hepatol. 2018;2018:8432781.
25. Scheiner B, Stammet PR, Pokorny S, et al. Anticoagulation in non-malignant portal vein thrombosis is safe and improves hepatic function. Wien Klin Wochenschr. 2018;130(13–14):446–55.
26. Steuber TD, Howard ML, Nisly SA. Direct oral anticoagulants in chronic liver disease. Ann Pharmacother. 2019;53(10):1042–9.
27. De Gottardi A, Trebicka J, Klinger C, et al. Antithrombotic treatment with direct-acting oral anticoagulants in patients with splanchnic vein thrombosis and cirrhosis. Liver Int. 2017;37(5):694–9.
28. Hollingshead M, Burke CT, Mauro MA, Weeks SM, Dixon RG, Jaques PF. Transcatheter thrombolytic therapy for acute mesenteric and portal vein thrombosis. J Vasc Interv Radiol. 2005;16:651–61.
29. Malkowski P, Pawlak J, Michalowicz B, Szczerban J, Wroblewski T, Leowska E, et al. Thrombolytic treatment of portal thrombosis. Hepato-Gastroenterology. 2003;50:2098–100.
30. Ferro C, Rossi UG, Bovio G, Dahamane M, Centanaro M. Transjugular intrahepatic portosystemic shunt, mechanical aspiration thrombectomy, and direct thrombolysis in the treatment of acute portal and superior mesenteric vein thrombosis. Cardiovasc Intervent Radiol. 2007;30:1070–4.
31. Liu K, Li WD, Du XL, Li CL, Li XQ. Comparison of systemic thrombolysis versus indirect thrombolysis via the superior mesenteric artery in patients with acute portal vein thrombosis. Ann Vasc Surg. 2017;39:264–9.
32. Ryu R, Lin TC, Kumpe D, et al. Percutaneous mesenteric venous thrombectomy and thrombolysis: successful treatment followed by liver transplantation. Liver Transpl Surg. 1998;4(3):222–5.
33. Sonavane A, Raut V, Marar S, et al. Preoperative successful thrombectomy and thrombolysis of acute extensive splanchnic venous system and TIPSS thrombosis in a child with Budd-Chiari syndrome—creating a window to enable living donor liver transplantation. Pediatr Transplant. 2020;00:e13857.
34. Condat B, Pessione F, Hillaire S, Denninger MH, Guillin MC, Poliquin M, et al. Current outcome of portal vein thrombosis in adults: risk and benefit of anticoagulant therapy. Gastroenterology. 2001;120:490–7.

35. Spaander MC, Hoekstra J, Hansen BE, van Buuren HR, Leebeek FW, Janssen HL. Anticoagulant therapy in patients with non-cirrhotic portal vein thrombosis: effect on new thrombotic events and gastrointestinal bleeding. J Thromb Haemost. 2013;11:452–9.

36. Orr DW, Harrison PM, Devlin J, Karani JB, Kane PA, Heaton ND, et al. Chronic mesenteric venous thrombosis: evaluation and determinants of survival during long-term follow-up. Clin Gastroenterol Hepatol. 2007;5:80–6.

37. de Franchis R, Baveno V. Revising consensus in portal hypertension: report of the Baveno V consensus workshop on methodology of diagnosis and therapy in portal hypertension. J Hepatol. 2010;53:762–8.

38. Schouten JN, Garcia-Pagan JC, Valla DC, Janssen HL. Idiopathic noncirrhotic portal hypertension. Hepatology. 2011;54:1071–81.

39. Hillaire S, Bonte E, Denninger MH, Casadevall N, Cadranel JF, Lebrec D, et al. Idiopathic noncirrhotic intrahepatic portal hypertension in the west: a re-evaluation in 28 patients. Gut. 2002;51:275–80.

40. Schouten JN, Van der Ende ME, Koeter T, Rossing HH, Komuta M, Verheij J, et al. Risk factors and outcome of HIV-associated idiopathic noncirrhotic portal hypertension. Aliment Pharmacol Ther. 2012;36:875–85.

41. Siramolpiwat S, Seijo S, Miquel R, Berzigotti A, Garcia-Criado A, Darnell A, et al. Idiopathic portal hypertension: natural history and long-term outcome. Hepatology. 2014;59:2276–85.

42. Corbacioglu S, Cesaro S, Faraci M, Valteau-Couanet D, Gruhn B, Rovelli A, et al. Defibrotide for prophylaxis of hepatic veno-occlusive disease in paediatric haemopoietic stem-cell transplantation: an open-label, phase 3, randomised controlled trial. Lancet. 2012;379:1301–9.

43. Chalandon Y, Roosnek E, Mermillod B, Newton A, Ozsahin H, Wacker P, et al. Prevention of veno-occlusive disease with defibrotide after allogeneic stem cell transplantation. Biol Blood Marrow Transpl. 2004;10:347–54.

44. Chopra R, Eaton JD, Grassi A, Potter M, Shaw B, Salat C, et al. Defibrotide for the treatment of hepatic venoocclusive disease: results of the European compassionate-use study. Br J Haematol. 2000;111:1122–9.

45. Richardson PG, Elias AD, Krishnan A, Wheeler C, Nath R, Hoppensteadt D, et al. Treatment of severe venoocclusive disease with defibrotide: compassionate use results in response without significant toxicity in a high-risk population. Blood. 1998;92:737–44.

46. Richardson PG, Murakami C, Jin Z, Warren D, Momtaz P, Hoppensteadt D, et al. Multi-institutional use of defibrotide in 88 patients after stem cell transplantation with severe veno-occlusive disease and multisystem organ failure: response without significant toxicity in a high-risk population and factors predictive of outcome. Blood. 2002;100:4337–43.

47. Imran H, Tleyjeh IM, Zirakzadeh A, Rodriguez V, Khan SP. Use of prophylactic anticoagulation and the risk of hepatic venoocclusive disease in patients undergoing hematopoietic stem cell transplantation: a systematic review and meta-analysis. Bone Marrow Transpl. 2006;37:677–86.

48. Tripodi A, Primignani M, Chantarangkul V, Dell'Era A, Clerici M, de Franchis R, et al. An imbalance of pro-vs. anti-coagulation factors in plasma from patients with cirrhosis. Gastroenterology. 2009;137(6):2105–11.

49. Northup PG, McMahon MM, Ruhl AP, Altschuler SE, Volk-Bednarz A, Caldwell SH, et al. Coagulopathy does not fully protect hospitalized cirrhosis patients from peripheral venous thromboembolism. Am J Gastroenterol. 2006;101:1524–8.

50. Sogaard KK, Horvath-Puho E, Gronbaek H, Jepsen P, Vilstrup H, Sorensen HT. Risk of venous thromboembolism in patients with liver disease: a nationwide population-based case-control study. AmJ Gastroenterol. 2009;104:96–101.

51. Fujita K, Nozaki Y, Wada K, Yoneda M, Endo H, Takahashi H, et al. Effectiveness of antiplatelet drugs against experimental non-alcoholic fatty liver disease. Gut. 2008;57:1583–91.

52. Ganey PE, Luyendyk JP, Newport SW, Eagle TM, Maddox JF, Mackman N, et al. Role of the coagulation system in acetaminophen-induced hepatotoxicity in mice. Hepatology. 2007;46:1177–86.

53. Anstee QM, Goldin RD, Wright M, Martinelli A, Cox R, Thursz MR. Coagulation status modulates murine hepatic fibrogenesis: implications for the development of novel therapies. J Thromb Haemost. 2008;6:1336–43.

54. Anstee QM, Wright M, Goldin R, Thursz MR. Parenchymal extinction: coagulation and hepatic fibrogenesis. Clin Liver Dis. 2009;13:117–26.

55. Wright M, Goldin R, Hellier S, Knapp S, Frodsham A, Hennig B, et al. Factor V Leiden polymorphism and the rate of fibrosis development in chronic hepatitis C virus infection. Gut. 2003;52:1206–10.

56. Assy N, Pettigrew N, Lee SS, Chaudhary RK, Johnston J, Minuk GY. Are chronic hepatitis C viral infections more benign in patients with hemophilia? Am J Gastroenterol. 2007;102:1672–6.

57. Villa E, Camma C, Marietta M, Luongo M, Critelli R, Colopi S. Enoxaparin prevents portal vein thrombosis and liver decompensation in patients with advanced cirrhosis. Gastroenterology. 2012;143:1253–60.

58. La Mura V, Braham S, Tosetti G, Branchi F, Bitto N, Moia M, et al. Harmful and beneficial effects of anticoagulants in patients with cirrhosis and portal vein thrombosis. Clin Gastroenterol Hepatol. 2018;16:1146–52.

59. Englesbe MJ, Kubus J, Muhammad W, Sonnenday CJ, Welling T, Punch JD, et al. Portal vein thrombosis and survival in patients with cirrhosis. Liver Transpl. 2010;16:833–90.

60. Søgaard KK, Darvalics B, Horváth-Puhó E, Sørensen HT. Survival after splanchnic vein thrombosis: a 20-year nationwide cohort study. Thromb Res. 2016;141:1–7.

61. D'Amico G, De Franchis R. Cooperative study group. Upper digestive bleeding in cirrhosis. Post-therapeutic outcome and prognostic indicators. Hepatology. 2003;38:599–612.

62. Francoz C, Belghiti J, Vilgrain V, Sommacale D, Paradis V, Condat B, et al. Splanchnic vein thrombosis in candidates for liver transplantation: usefulness of screening and anticoagulation. Gut. 2005;54:691–7.

63. Amitrano L, Guardascione MA, Brancaccio V, Margaglione M, Manguso F, Iannaccone L, et al. Risk factors and clinical presentation of portal vein thrombosis in patients with liver cirrhosis. J Hepatol. 2004;40:736–41.

64. Rodriguez-Castro KI, Porte RJ, Nadal E, Germani G, Burra P, Senzolo M. Management of nonneoplastic portal vein thrombosis in the setting of liver transplantation: a systematic review. Transplantation. 2012;94:1145–53.

65. Senzolo M, Sartori M, Rossetto V, Burra P, Cillo U, Boccagni P, et al. Prospective evaluation of anticoagulation and transjugular intrahepatic portosystemic shunt for the management of portal vein thrombosis in cirrhosis. Liver Int. 2012;32:919–27.

66. Delgado MG, Seijo S, Yepes I, Achecar L, Catalina MV, Garcia-Criado A, et al. Efficacy and safety of anticoagulation on patients with cirrhosis and portal vein thrombosis. Clin Gastroenterol Hepatol. 2012;10:776–83.

67. Qi X, De Stefano V, Li H, Dai J, Guo X, Fan D. Anticoagulation for the treatment of portal vein thrombosis in liver cirrhosis: a systematic review and meta-analysis of observational studies. Eur J Intern Med. 2015;26:23–9.

68. Loffredo L, Pastori D, Farcomeni A, Violi F. Effects of anticoagulants in patients with cirrhosis and portal vein thrombosis: a systematic review and meta-analysis. Gastroenterology. 2017;153:480–7.

69. Cerini F, Gonzalez JM, Torres F, Puente A, Casas M, Vinaixa C, et al. Impact of anticoagulation on upper-gastrointestinal bleeding in cirrhosis. A retrospective multicenter study. Hepatology. 2015;62:575–83.

70. Nery F, Chevret S, Condat B, de Raucourt E, Boudaoud L, Rautou PE, et al. Causes and consequences of portal vein thrombosis in 1,243 patients with cirrhosis: results of a longitudinal study. Hepatology. 2015;61:660–7.

71. Andriulli A, Tripodi A, Angeli P, Senzolo M, Primignani M, Giannini EG, et al. Hemostatic balance in patients with liver cirrhosis: report of a consensus conference. Dig Liver Dis. 2016;48:455–67.

72. Tripodi A, Primignani M, Braham S, Chantarangkul V, Clerici M, Moia M, et al. Coagulation parameters in patients with cirrhosis and portal vein thrombosis treated sequentially with low molecular weight heparin and vitamin K antagonists. Dig Liv Dis. 2016;48:1208–13.
73. Tripodi A, Chantarangkul V, Primignani M, Fabris F, Dell'Era A, Sei C, et al. The international normalized ratio calibrated for cirrhosis (INR$_{liver}$) normalizes prothrombin time results for model for end-stage liver disease calculation. Hepatology. 2007;46:520–7.
74. Bellest L, Eschwège V, Poupon R, Chazouillères O, Robert A. A modified international normalized ratio as an effective way of prothrombin time standardization in hepatology. Hepatology. 2007;46:528–34.
75. Tripodi A. How to implement the modified international normalized ratio for cirrhosis [INR(liver)] for model for end-stage liver disease calculation. Hepatology. 2008;47:1423–4.
76. Intagliata NM, Henry ZH, Maitland H, Shah NL, Argo CK, Northup PG, et al. Direct oral anticoagulants in cirrhosis patients pose similar risks of bleeding when compared to traditional anticoagulation. Dig Dis Sci. 2016;61(6):1721–7.
77. Hum J, Shatzel JJ, Jou JH, Deloughery TG. The efficacy and safety of direct oral anticoagulants vs traditional anticoagulants in cirrhosis. Eur J Haematol. 2017;98(4):393–7.
78. Janczak DT, Mimier MK, McBane RD, Kamath PS, Simmons BS, Bott-Kitslaar DM, et al. Rivaroxaban and Apixaban for initial treatment of acute venous thromboembolism of atypical location. Mayo Clin Proc. 2018;93(1):40–7.
79. Qi X, Yoshida EM, Mendez-Sanchez N, Guo X. Rivaroxaban recanalized occlusive superior mesenteric vein thrombosis, but increased the risk of bleeding in a cirrhotic patient. Liver Int. 2017;37(10):1574–5.
80. Nery F, Valadares D, Morais S, Gomes MT, De Gottardi A. Efficacy and safety of direct-acting Oral anticoagulants use in acute portal vein thrombosis unrelated to cirrhosis. Gastroenterology Res. 2017;10(2):141–3.
81. Martinez M, Tandra A, Vuppalanchi R. Treatment of acute portal vein thrombosis by nontraditional anticoagulation. Hepatology. 2014;60(1):425–6.
82. Pannach S, Babatz J, Beyer-Westendorf J. Successful treatment of acute portal vein thrombosis with rivaroxaban. Thromb Haemost. 2013;110(4):626–7.
83. Lenz K, Dieplinger B, Buder R, Piringer P, Rauch M, Voglmayr M. Successful treatment of partial portal vein thrombosis (PVT) with low dose rivaroxaban. Z Gastroenterol. 2014;52(10):1175–7.
84. Yang H, Kim SR, Song MJ. Recurrent acute portal vein thrombosis in liver cirrhosis treated by rivaroxaban. Clin Mol Hepatol. 2016;22(4):499–502.
85. Goriacko P, Veltri KT. Safety of direct oral anticoagulants vs warfarin in patients with chronic liver disease and atrial fibrillation. Eur J Haematol. 2018;100(5):488–93.
86. Lapumnuaypol K, DiMaria C, Chiasakul T. Safety of direct oral anticoagulants in patients with cirrhosis: a systematic review and meta-analysis. QJM. 2019 Aug 1;112(8):605–10.
87. Menichelli D, Ronca V, Di Rocco A, Pignatelli P, Marco Podda G. CAR Direct oral anticoagulants and advanced liver disease: a systematic review and meta-analysis. Eur J Clin Invest. 2021;51:e13397.
88. Hanafy AS, Abd-Elsalam S, Dawoud MM. Randomized controlled trial of rivaroxaban versus warfarin in the management of acute non-neoplastic portal vein thrombosis. Vasc Pharmacol. 2019;113:86–91.
89. Mohan BP, Aravamudanb VM, Khan SR, Ponnada S, Asokkumar R, Adler DG. Treatment response and bleeding events associated with anticoagulant therapy of portal vein thrombosis in cirrhotic patients: systematic review and meta-analysis. Ann Gastroenterol. 2020;33:521–7.

**Part II**

# Causes for Vascular Disorders of the Liver

# Chapter 17
# Hemostatic Disorders and the Liver

Ton Lisman

## Liver Diseases and Hemostatic Disorders

### *Hemostatic Changes in Liver Disease*

The liver is a crucial component of the hemostatic system. It is the site of synthesis of the majority of proteins involved in clot formation, regulation of coagulation, and fibrinolysis. In addition, the liver synthesizes thrombopoeitin, a hormone that regulates production of platelets. In patients with advancing liver disease, major changes in the hemostatic system are frequently present [1]. Such changes include thrombocytopenia, decreased plasma levels of pro- and anticoagulant proteins, and decreased plasma levels of fibrinolytic proteins. In addition, elevated plasma levels of a discrete number of hemostatic proteins that are not synthesized by hepatocytes, but by vascular endothelial cells, are frequently present. Such proteins include the platelet adhesive protein von Willebrand factor, and the fibrinolytic components tissue-type plasminogen activator, and plasminogen activator inhibitor type 1.

Hemostatic alterations in patients with liver diseases are likely not only due to defective hepatic synthesis and increased endothelial cell activation. Continuous consumption of hemostatic factors by low-grade activation of hemostasis likely contributes [2]. Such low-grade hemostatic activation may be systemic and induced for example by activated endothelial cells that may activate platelets, and express the natural activator of coagulation, tissue factor (TF) supporting thrombin and fibrin generation. Alternatively, activation of hemostasis may occur within the liver. Intrahepatic activation of hemostasis may occur by activation hepatic TF. In a

T. Lisman (✉)
Surgical Research Laboratory and Section of Hepatobiliary Surgery and Liver Transplantation, Department of Surgery, University of Groningen, University Medical Center Groningen, Groningen, The Netherlands
e-mail: j.a.lisman@umcg.nl

© Springer Nature Switzerland AG 2022
D. Valla et al. (eds.), *Vascular Disorders of the Liver*,
https://doi.org/10.1007/978-3-030-82988-9_17

healthy liver TF is expressed by hepatocytes, but is in a conformation that is not able to support coagulation activation—this non-coagulant form of TF is referred to as 'cryptic' TF. Upon liver injury, hepatic TF can become 'decrypted' and as such support activation of coagulation within the liver [3]. The generation of mice with a liver-specific deletion of TF has unequivocally demonstrated a role for hepatic TF decryption in thrombus formation within the liver and it has been suggested that hepatic TF contributes to the hypercoagulable status of a liver disease patient [4]. In addition, exposure of hepatic collagen may also result in intrahepatic activation and/or deposition of platelets, which in turn can support propagation of coagulation.

## *The Concept of Rebalanced Hemostasis*

Regardless of the exact causes of the profound hemostatic changes of a patient with liver disease, an important question regards the net effect of all these changes for the hemostatic balance. Historically, it has been generally assumed that the hemostatic changes in a patient with liver disease caused a bleeding disorder. Indeed, bleeding in these patients is common, both spontaneously (e.g., variceal bleeding), and procedure-related (notably during liver transplantation). Besides the fact that clinical bleeding is common, routine diagnostic tests of hemostasis in patients with liver disease suggest a hypocoagulable state, with thrombocytopenia and prolongations in clotting tests such as the prothrombin time and activated partial thromboplastin time. The combination of these findings has led to the long-held dogma that liver diseases are associated with a hemostatic defect causing bleeding. However, multiple observations in the clinical setting and various research laboratories have led to a drastic change in this dogma.

From a laboratory perspective, the platelet count and PT/APTT are unsuitable to assess the hemostatic status in patients with complex hemostatic disorders [5]. First, although patients with liver disease frequently are thrombocytopenic, the low platelet count appears to be counteracted, at least in part, by highly elevated levels of the platelet adhesive protein von Willebrand factor (VWF) and decreased levels of the VWF-cleaving protease ADAMTS13 [6, 7]. As such, the thrombocytopenia should not be valued in isolation, but in the context of the functionality of the VWF/ADAMTS13 axis. Second, the PT and APTT are insensitive for plasma levels of natural anticoagulant proteins. Prolongation of the PT and/or APTT therefore only indicate that there are defects or deficiencies in procoagulant proteins. However, in patients with liver disease there is a simultaneous decline in pro- and anticoagulant proteins. When using a laboratory test that is sensitive for the levels of all pro- and anticoagulant proteins, it becomes clear that the coagulation system in patients with liver diseases is as competent of that of healthy individuals [8], or perhaps even hypercoagulable [9–13]. Thrombomodulin-modified thrombin generation testing by calibrated automated thrombinography is currently the test of choice in the research laboratory to assess functionality of the coagulation system in individuals with complex hemostatic changes.

From a clinical perspective, it needs to be acknowledged that although variceal bleeding is a common complication of chronic liver disease, it is unrelated to hemostatic failure but rather a consequence of portal hypertension and the fragility of the varix [14]. In addition, although bleeding during liver transplantation was profound and often massive in the early days of liver transplantation [15], over time there has been a substantial decline in bleeding and blood product transfusion during the procedure. Nowadays, it is possible to perform liver transplantations without the requirement for any blood product transfusion in a proportion of patients [16], which questions the notion that the transplant recipient has an overt bleeding disorder. Finally, in contrast to historic belief, patients with liver diseases are not 'auto-anticoagulated' and therefore protected from thrombotic disease. In contrast, it has now been well established that liver diseases are a risk factor for development of thrombotic disease, most notably venous thrombosis and portal vein thrombosis.

Collectively these and other laboratory and clinical observations have led to the concept of 'rebalanced hemostasis' [17, 18]. This concept states that the 'average' patient with liver disease is in hemostatic balance due to a concomitant decline in pro- and anticoagulant drivers. The new, reset, hemostatic balance of patients with liver disease, however, is less stable that the hemostatic balance in healthy individuals, explaining why both bleeding and thrombotic complications are common. Factors that may tip the balance towards hypo- or hypercoagulability are poorly understood, but may include infection, renal failure and decompensation [19, 20]. A careful inspection of the hemostatic system of both the well compensated as the decompensated patient with liver disease reveals that although the net result of all hemostatic changes is a rebalanced system, there are clear hypo- and hypercoagulable features that within the hemostatic balance may contribute to development of bleeding or thrombosis.

## *Hypercoagulable Features*

Although the concept of rebalanced hemostasis has helped change the dogma of liver diseases as a bleeding disorder, it may be an oversimplification. It will likely be helpful to consider the specific hypo- and hypercoagulable features within the rebalanced system in understanding thrombotic and bleeding complications, and ways to treat or prevent these. Hypercoagulable features that may contribute to thrombotic disease include (1) platelet hyperreactivity, (2) enhanced thrombin generating capacity, (3) a prothrombotic fibrin structure, (4) increased production of intravascular tissue factor, and (5) prothrombotic endothelium. The functionality of platelets in patients with liver disease is debated in literature [21], which in part relates to technical difficulties in assessing platelet functionality, particularly in thrombocytopenic blood. It has been suggested that endotoxemia results in enhanced in vivo platelet activation, which may contribute to thrombosis [22]. Also, the highly elevated plasma levels of von Willebrand factor combined with the low levels of the von Willebrand factor-cleaving protease ADAMTS13 may contribute to thrombotic risk [6, 7]. With respect to thrombin generating capacity: although in a seminal paper published in 2005,

Tripodi and coworkers demonstrated comparable thrombin generating capacity between patients with cirrhosis and healthy controls [8], many subsequent studies by independent laboratories have demonstrated enhanced thrombin generating capacity in patients [9–13]. Enhanced thrombin generating capacity is linked to defects in anticoagulant systems such as antithrombin and the protein C system that are apparently not entirely balanced by defects in procoagulant proteins [23]. In addition to enhanced thrombin generating capacity, it also seems that the thrombogenicity of the fibrin clot eventually formed is enhanced in patients, which may be linked to post-translational modifications of the fibrinogen molecule, notably oxidation [24]. Finally, prothrombotic features in patients with cirrhosis may be linked to cellular systems that are not taken into account in in vitro studies of hemostatic capacity. Notably, tissue factor decryption on hepatocytes and production of tissue factor by white blood cells may lead to activation of coagulation [3, 25]. Furthermore, defective anticoagulant capacity of the endothelial cells may further propagate platelet and coagulation activation. Anticoagulant properties that may be defective in patients with liver disease include the endothelial glycocalix, production of platelet inhibitors such as nitric oxide, and the anticoagulant transmembrane protein thrombomodulin.

## Unbalanced Hemostasis: A Contributor to Vascular Liver Disorders?

Vascular liver disorders comprise of a spectrum of conditions that may occur in patients with preexisting liver disease, but may also occur in previously healthy individuals. A number of vascular liver disorders are characterized by a thrombotic component. In general, the risk of developing thrombotic disease can be linked to Virchov's Triad. i.e., hypercoagulability, stasis, and the vascular wall. This section will outline the contribution of inherited or acquired factors resulting in hypercoagulability to the pathogenesis of vascular liver disorders characterized by a thrombotic component. Both liver-disease associated hypercoagulability, and hypercoagulability in vascular liver disorders unrelated to chronic liver diseases will be considered.

### *Intrahepatic Thrombosis*

Liver injury in animal models of liver disease appear uniformly accompanied by thrombus formation in the liver microcirculation. The first evidence for intrahepatic thrombus formation in experimental liver injury came from studies examining the effects of murine hepatitis virus infection in inbred strains of mice [26]. These studies demonstrated the presence of microthrombi within the hepatic microvasculature in areas of inflammation and subsequent tissue necrosis. Similarly, in mouse models of acute liver failure [27] and in models of cholestatic [4] and non-cholestatic [28] fibrosis, intrahepatic thrombi have been demonstrated. Intrahepatic thrombi appear to drive progression of disease as anticoagulants or antiplatelet agents decrease thrombus formation and disease severity in these animal models [29, 30]. Recent studies have suggested a detrimental role of the platelet adhesive protein von Willebrand factor in progression of acute liver failure in mice and humans [31, 32]. Conversely, hypercoagulable states result in faster progression of disease [33]. It has been proposed that intrahepatic thrombi either drive disease progression by physical obstruction of the microcirculation with subsequent microischemia or that coagulation proteases such as factor Xa or thrombin are key in driving disease progression by their capacity to activate protease activated receptors on cells [34]. Unanswered questions in these experimental settings are the exact composition and location of the thrombi and the exact mechanisms linking thrombus formation or deposition of platelets and fibrin to disease progression. Also, it is unclear whether unbalanced hemostasis lies at the basis of intrahepatic thrombus formation, although a hypercoagulable state likely exacerbates thrombus load. The initiating trigger of intrahepatic activation of coagulation appears to be tissue factor decryption, whereas it is unclear what initiates intrahepatic platelet deposition. Endothelial activation, collagen exposure, alterations in flow, and local thrombin formation could all contribute, but experimental evidence for any of these mechanisms is thus far lacking.

In humans, a role of microvascular thrombus formation in progression of chronic liver injury was first proposed by Wanless and coworkers [35, 36], although in these studies it was never demonstrated that platelets and/or fibrin were present in diseased human livers. Indirect evidence for a role of intrahepatic thrombus formation to disease progression comes from observational studies that suggest inherited hypercoagulability (e.g., carriership of FVleiden) to increase [37] and inherited hypocoagulability (hemophilia) [38] to decrease progression of chronic liver injury. Large epidemiological studies have demonstrated that aspirin use is associated with decreased progression of liver disease [39–41]. Importantly, these results do not necessarily mean that platelets are implicated in disease progression in humans. Aspirin has many platelet-independent effects [42] that could potentially affect progression of chronic liver disease [43]. Finally, a single randomized clinical study has demonstrated anticoagulant therapy with low molecular weight heparin to delay disease progression in patients with cirrhosis [44].

In aggregate, intrahepatic thrombosis has been clearly demonstrated in animals with various forms of liver injury, and thrombus formation appears directly linked to disease progression. It is however unclear whether unbalanced hemostasis is a key component of intrahepatic thrombus formation. In humans, it is unclear whether intrahepatic thrombosis occurs and a causal link with disease progression is yet to be demonstrated.


## *Portal Vein Thrombosis and Budd Chiari Syndrome*

Portal vein thrombosis (PVT) is a common complication of cirrhosis. It is frequently asymptomatic and detected incidentally during imaging studies. It has long been assumed that cirrhotic PVT results in progression of disease and clinical deterioration [45], but recent data have suggested that PVT is merely related to disease severity and not responsible for disease progression [46]. It has been demonstrated by some, but not all studies, that reduced portal flow increases the risk for cirrhotic PVT [46, 47], but it is unclear whether reduced flow is the key initiator of thrombus formation. It has been suggested that unbalanced hemostasis also contributes to development of PVT, but data are inconsistent. Studies have shown inherited thrombophilia, particular the prothrombin G20210A variant to increase the risk for PVT [48], but other studies found no role for inherited thrombophilia in PVT development [46]. Also, it has been demonstrated that patients with NASH-related cirrhosis have an increased incidence of PVT [49]. These data have been interpreted as NASH-associated hypercoagulability to drive PVT development. However, it is still unclear whether NASH is truly associated with an increased hypercoagulable state compared to other etiologies of cirrhosis [50, 51], and other factors (notably obesity) may explain the increased risk of PVT in NASH-cirrhosis. Prospective clinical studies will be required to assess whether hemostatic unbalance is related to risk of PVT development, or whether other factors such as decreased portal flow are key drivers.

Non-cirrhotic portal vein thrombosis is a rare disease, and it is incompletely understood why thrombi occur occasionally in this specific vascular bed. In a large proportion of patients with non-cirrhotic PVT, prothrombotic abnormalities including inherited thrombophilia, oral contraceptive use and myeloproliferative disorders are present, suggesting hemostatic unbalance to drive thrombus development [52]. However, a proportion of patients appears to develop PVT as a consequence of local factors, particularly abdominal inflammatory conditions (which may also cause hypercoagulability), and a proportion of patients has idiopathic disease. Patients with non-cirrhotic portal vein thrombosis are hypercoagulable in terms of thrombin generating capacity, and their hypercoagulability was independent of the etiology, which may indicate that hypercoagulability develops as a consequence of the disease [53]. Similarly, patients with Budd Chiari syndrome (BCS) are characterized by a high incidence of inherited thrombophilia, oral contraceptive use, and myeloproliferative neoplasms [54]. Although the high prevalence of thrombophilia in both non-cirrhotic PVT and BCS suggest a key role for hemostatic unbalance in these diseases, it is unclear why these particular vascular beds are vulnerable for thrombus formation, and why the majority of patients with thrombophilia do not develop these specific thrombotic events. It is likely that the pathogenesis of these rare disease is multifactorial, and a better understanding on the event(s) that initiate thrombus formation is key in obtaining insight in the pathogenesis.

## *Hepatic Artery Thrombosis after Liver Transplantation*

Hepatic artery thrombosis almost exclusively occurs in patients following liver transplantation. Isolated hepatic artery thromboses probably do not occur as the hepatic artery is profoundly protected against atherosclerosis, and thus no trigger for thrombosis develops during life [55]. Hepatic artery thrombosis occurs in approximately 5% of adult liver transplant recipients [56], while the prevalence in children is substantially higher [56, 57]. As the transplanted liver (initially) lacks any collateral circulation, the absence of arterial flow results will invariably lead to ischemia and necrosis of the right hepatic lobe if flow is not restored in time. Furthermore, as the biliary system is fully dependent on arterial flow, rapid biliary ischemic damage occurs in case of a hepatic artery thrombosis. Thrombosis of the hepatic artery is thus associated with morbidity and graft loss [58]. Hepatic artery thrombosis can occur early (within 2–3 months) after transplantation, but may also occur years after the procedure. The clinical outcome of late hepatic artery thrombosis is usually more benign compared to early thrombosis, as collaterals may have developed over time, especially when occlusion of the hepatic artery is preceded by a slowly worsening stenosis [59].

Early hepatic artery thrombosis is envisioned primarily as a surgical complication. Technical imperfections with the anastomosis related for example to aberrant donor or recipient arterial anatomy or complex backtable arterial reconstruction, kinking of the artery, prolonged clamping of the hepatic artery, or the use of an arterial conduit indeed increase the risk for hepatic artery thrombosis substantially [58, 60, 61]. The incidence of early hepatic artery thrombosis has substantially decreased since the first decades of liver transplantation, which also suggests that surgical factors contribute substantially to this complication. Furthermore, low volume transplant centers or less experienced surgeons have a higher rate of hepatic artery thrombosis, which again indicates that the complication has a surgical component. However, additional non-surgical factors also contribute to the risk of early hepatic artery thrombosis. These factors include damage to the graft for example by prolonged cold or warm ischemic times, preoperative transarterial chemoembolisation for HCC, or an otherwise damaged artery for example due to complications during organ procurement [61–63]. Furthermore, retransplantation is also an important risk factor for early hepatic artery thrombosis, with the risk even increasing further in a second retransplantation [63, 64]. Also, insufficient blood flow through the artery, for example in patients with a splenic artery steal syndrome, increases the risk for hepatic artery thrombosis, although in a splenic artery steal syndrome ligation of the splenic artery is sufficient to restore adequate arterial flow [61].

Unbalanced hemostasis, which has been clearly demonstrated early after liver transplantation [65–67], may contribute to development of early HAT. Clinical evidence for a role of the coagulation system in early hepatic artery thrombosis has emerged from a studies in which patients transplanted for familial amyloidotic polyneuropathy (FAP) or acute intermittent porphyria (AIP) were shown to have a substantially increased risk for hepatic artery thrombosis as compared to patients transplanted for end-stage liver disease [68, 69]. In contrast to patients with end-stage liver disease, patients with FAP and AIP have a fully competent hemostatic system, as the synthetic capacity of the liver of these patients is not compromised. Furthermore, the surgical procedure, and the arterial reconstruction is generally much less complicated in a patient with FAP or AIP compared to the end-stage liver disease patient because of the absence of a disturbed liver architecture, portal hypertension, venous collaterals, or perihepatic inflammatory lesions. Although experimental evidence is lacking, it is likely that patients with FAP or AIP have an increased hypercoagulable status posttransplant compared to the end-stage liver disease patients and this notion combined with the substantially reduced technical difficulty of transplantation in these patients suggests that the increased incidence of hepatic artery thrombosis is a result of their increased hypercoagulable status [70].

There is no consensus on risk factors for late hepatic artery thrombosis, but donor age, severe acute rejection, backtable surgery for anatomic variations, blood group-incompatible grafts, active cigarette smoking, usage of a donor iliac artery interposition graft to the aorta, and use of a graft from a donor who died of a cerebrovascular accident have all been suggested as risk factors [59].

Hemostatic unbalance may also contribute to late HAT. One study retrospectively analyzed the effect of aspirin administration to patients with risk factors for late hepatic artery thrombosis (in this study employment of a donor iliac artery interposition graft to the aorta, and use of a graft from a donor who died of a cerebrovascular accident) [71]. Patients who received aspirin indefinitely had a substantially decreased risk of late hepatic artery thrombosis (3.6 vs 0.6%, which is a relative risk reduction of 82%), which suggests that (excessive) platelet activation may be involved in the pathogenesis of this complication [71, 72].

## Effects of Coagulation Disorders on the Liver

It has been well established that liver diseases can lead to profound hemostatic disorders. However, the converse may also be true. Critical illnesses in which profound disseminated activation of coagulation occurs may result in liver failure as a result of thrombus formation within the liver.

## *Disseminated Intravascular Coagulation*

A variety of clinical conditions are associated with clinically silent (systemic) activation of the hemostatic system. However, when activation of hemostasis is more extensive, disseminated intravascular coagulation (DIC) may develop [73]. DIC is characterized by systemic formation of thrombi in the (microvasculature). These clots may jeopardize oxygen delivery to organ systems and therefore can lead to multiple organ failure. Fibrin deposition is found in most organs of patients with DIC. In addition, in experimental animal models of DIC fibrin deposition is also found in various organs, and anticoagulant therapy has been shown to decrease fibrin deposition and to improve organ function in these models [74]. As ongoing clot formation leads to depletion of circulating platelets and coagulation factors, a bleeding tendency frequently accompanies DIC, and bleeding is in fact frequently the presenting symptom [75].

Clinical conditions that may be accompanied by DIC are severe infections and sepsis, trauma, cancer, and obstetrical complications [76]. The diagnosis of DIC is based on clinical findings in combination with laboratory findings. The International Society of Thrombosis and Hemostasis (ISTH) has developed a scoring algorithm for patients with an underlying disorder known to be associated with DIC. In such patients a DIC score consisting of a platelet count, levels of fibrin degradation products (such as D-dimer), the prothrombin time, and the fibrinogen levels can be calculated to determine whether DIC is present [77].

Liver failure may thus complicate DIC as part of the multiple organ failure syndrome that may accompany DIC. An interesting group of patients in this respect are patients with preexisting liver disease. It has been suggested that patients with cirrhosis may have (low-grade) DIC [78], but the fact that all components of the ISTH-DIC score are already abnormal as a consequence of the hemostatic alterations associated with cirrhosis [79], makes a diagnosis of DIC based on these criteria unreliable in patients with cirrhosis. It may be that only those patients with cirrhosis that become critically ill develop 'true' DIC. For example patients with acute-on-chronic liver failure (ACLF) are characterized by an inflammatory state, multiple organ failure, and hemostatic changes on top of the hemostatic changes that are present in the (compensated) cirrhotic [80]. Whether DIC is a cause of ACLF-associated organ failure, or whether organ failure in ACLF is mechanistically distinct from organ failure in patients with DIC without preexisting liver failure remains to be established. Also acute liver failure (ALF) is an inflammatory condition in which multiple organ failure and coagulopathy may develop, and as such may also be a condition in which DIC occurs.

## *Hemostatic Activation in Pregnancy-Associated Liver Diseases*

Pregnancy may occasionally be complicated by severe liver diseases induced by the pregnancy. Severe pregnancy-induced liver diseases are associated with a significant risk of morbidity and mortality for both the mother and the baby. Part of this risk relates to bleeding or thrombotic events, and thrombotic events may drive these specific liver diseases.

Acute fatty liver of pregnancy (AFLP) is a rare complication occurring in ~1:20.000 pregnancies, and is a medical and obstetric emergency [81]. Patients with AFLP have accumulation of microvesicular fat droplets within their hepatocytes, with biochemical evidence of liver injury and liver failure. Hemostatic changes include thrombocytopenia, a prolonged prothrombin time, and reduced fibrinogen levels [82]. It has been debated whether hemostatic changes of AFLP are related to liver failure or that DIC also contributes. It has recently been reported that the vast majority of patients with AFLP have a positive ISTH-DIC score that persists after delivery [83]. Nevertheless, as discussed in the section on DIC it should be noted that the constituents of the ISTH-DIC score (low platelet count, elevated fibrin split products, elevated prothrombin time, and low fibrinogen) are all compatible with synthetic and clearance defects of the liver. Whether DIC is an important component of AFLP and whether DIC-related clot formation within the liver drives the disease thus remains to be established. Importantly, a proportion of patients with AFLP also have preeclampsia (see below).

Preeclampsia, eclampsia, and hemolysis, elevated liver enzymes, low platelets (HELLP) syndrome form a spectrum of diseases that are characterized by pregnancy-induced hypertension combined with proteinuria and organ dysfunction. Eclampsia refers to the onset of seizures in a patient with preeclampsia, while the HELLP syndrome is considered to be a severe form of preeclampsia. Although the etiology of preeclampsia is incompletely understood, abnormal placental development and a generalized inflammatory response resulting in endothelial cell activation are thought to be important contributors. Generalized activation of endothelial cells results in activation of the hemostatic system, resulting in a thrombotic microangiopathy. An increase in plasma levels of highly reactive von Willebrand factor multimers have been suggested to be responsible for the consumptive thrombocytopenia [84]. Histopathologic findings in the liver include intravascular fibrin deposits that are thought to lead to hepatic sinusoidal obstruction, intrahepatic vascular congestion, and increased intrahepatic pressure. This process contributes to liver failure, but also may lead to intraparenchymal and subcapsular hemorrhage, and eventually hepatic rupture [81].

The hemostatic alterations in preeclampsia and HELLP thus are driven by at least 2 mechanisms—an endothelial-driven thrombotic microangiopathy, and a liver disease-induced coagulopathy. The latter, however, may be mild as the prothrombin time may be normal in patients with HELLP syndrome. In those patients that develop coagulation abnormalities, it is generally assumed that DIC has developed, although it cannot be excluded that those patients that have a positive DIC score, the primary factor driving coagulation abnormalities is liver failure as also outlined in the section on AFLP. It has also been argued that the vast majority of women with preeclampsia and HELLP have liver injury, but do not have overt liver failure and no evidence of clinically relevant DIC [85], and that the prime hemostatic abnormality in these patients thus is a profound thrombocytopenia. Whether HELLP-associated liver injury is primarily related to a thrombotic, platelet-mediated microangiopathy or whether DIC with consequent intrahepatic clot formation contributes therefore remains to be established.

## Conclusion

Multiple vascular liver diseases are characterized by a thrombotic component. Whether local or systemic factors drive these thrombotic events in the liver are incompletely understood, and studies on the pathogenesis of these vascular liver diseases have been hampered by the low incidence of these diseases and the absence of suitable animal models. A variety of diseases including infection, sepsis, trauma, cancer, and obstetric diseases may result in systemic generation of thrombi in various organs including the liver. Such thrombi contribute to organ failure. Although anticoagulant strategies may be helpful in preventing or clearing clots and improving organ failure, the use of these drugs is hampered by the fact that a bleeding tendency also accompanies DIC. An interesting area of research regards DIC-like syndromes in patients with underlying liver disease (ALF, ACLF, and pregnancy-associated liver diseases). Although these diseases are characterized by inflammation, coagulopathy, and (multiple) organ failure, it is incompletely understood whether these patients truly have DIC, or whether the positive DIC scores reflect the effects of the underlying liver disease on hemostasis.

# References


 1. Lisman T, Porte RJ. Pathogenesis, prevention, and management of bleeding and thrombosis in patients with liver diseases. Res Pract Thromb Haemost. 2017;1:150–61.
 2. Ferro D, Basili S, Lattuada A, Mantovani B, Bellomo A, Mannucci PM, et al. Systemic clotting activation by low-grade endotoxaemia in liver cirrhosis: a potential role for endothelial procoagulant activation. Ital J Gastroenterol Hepatol. 1997 Oct;29(5):434–40.
 3. Sullivan BP, Kopec AK, Joshi N, Cline H, Brown JA, Bishop SC, et al. Hepatocyte tissue factor activates the coagulation cascade in mice. Blood. 2013 Mar 7;121(10):1868–74.
 4. Rautou PE, Tatsumi K, Antoniak S, Owens AP, Sparkenbaugh E, Holle LA, et al. Hepatocyte tissue factor contributes to the hypercoagulable state in a mouse model of chronic liver injury. J Hepatol. 2016 Jan;64(1):53–9.
 5. Lisman T, Porte RJ. Value of preoperative hemostasis testing in patients with liver disease for perioperative hemostatic management. Anesthesiology. 2017 Dec 2;126(2):338–44.
 6. Lisman T, Bongers TN, Adelmeijer J, Janssen HL, de Maat MP, de Groot PG, et al. Elevated levels of von Willebrand factor in cirrhosis support platelet adhesion despite reduced functional capacity. Hepatology. 2006 Jul;44(1):53–61.
 7. Uemura M, Fujimura Y, Matsumoto M, Ishizashi H, Kato S, Matsuyama T, et al. Comprehensive analysis of ADAMTS13 in patients with liver cirrhosis. Thromb Haemost. 2008 Jun;99(6):1019–29.
 8. Tripodi A, Salerno F, Chantarangkul V, Clerici M, Cazzaniga M, Primignani M, et al. Evidence of normal thrombin generation in cirrhosis despite abnormal conventional coagulation tests. Hepatology. 2005 Mar;41(3):553–8.
 9. Lebreton A, Sinegre T, Pereira B, Lamblin G, Duron C, Abergel A. Plasma hypercoagulability in the presence of thrombomodulin but not of activated protein C in patients with cirrhosis. J Gastroenterol Hepatol. 2017 Apr;32(4):916–24.
10. Gatt A, Riddell A, Calvaruso V, Tuddenham EG, Makris M, Burroughs AK. Enhanced thrombin generation in patients with cirrhosis-induced coagulopathy. J Thromb Haemost. 2010 Sep;8(9):1994–2000.
11. Youngwon N, Kim JE, Lim HS, Han KS, Kim HK. Coagulation proteins influencing global coagulation assays in cirrhosis: hypercoagulability in cirrhosis assessed by thrombomodulin-induced thrombin generation assay. Biomed Res Int. 2013;2013:856754.
12. Kleinegris MC, Habets CA, van de Sande AJ, Henskens YM, Ten Cate-Hoek AJ, van Deursen C, et al. Liver cirrhosis is associated with hypercoagulability, decreased clot strength and normal fibrinolysis. J Thromb Haemost. 2013;11(S2):49–50.
13. Lisman T, Kleiss S, Patel VC, Fisher C, Adelmeijer J, Bos S, et al. In vitro efficacy of pro- and anticoagulant strategies in compensated and acutely ill patients with cirrhosis. Liver Int. 2018;38(11):1988–96.

14. Garcia-Tsao G, Bosch J. Management of varices and variceal hemorrhage in cirrhosis. N Engl J Med. 2010 Mar 4;362(9):823–32.
15. Lewis JH, Bontempo FA, Cornell F, Kiss JE, Larson P, Ragni MV, et al. Blood use in liver transplantation. Transfusion. 1987 May-Jun;27(3):222–5.
16. Massicotte L, Thibeault L, Roy A. Classical notions of coagulation revisited in relation with blood losses, transfusion rate for 700 consecutive liver transplantations. Semin Thromb Hemost. 2015 Jul;41(5):538–46.
17. Lisman T, Porte RJ. Rebalanced hemostasis in patients with liver disease: evidence and clinical consequences. Blood. 2010 Aug 12;116(6):878–85.
18. Lisman T, Stravitz RT. Rebalanced hemostasis in patients with acute liver failure. Semin Thromb Hemost. 2015 Jul;41(5):468–73.
19. Zanetto A, Rinder HM, Campello E, Saggiorato G, Deng Y, Ciarleglio M, Wilson FP, Senzolo M, Gavasso S, Bulato C, Simioni P, Garcia-Tsao G. Acute kidney injury in decompensated cirrhosis is associated with both hypo- and hyper-coagulable features. Hepatology. 2020;72(4):1327–40.
20. Patel VC, Adelmeijer J, Azarian S, Hernandez Tejero M, Calvo A, Fernández J, Bernal W, Lisman T. Mixed fibrinolytic phenotypes in decompensated cirrhosis and acute-on-chronic liver failure with Hypofibrinolysis in those with complications and poor survival. Hepatology. 2020 Apr;71(4):1381–90.
21. Caldwell S, Lisman T. The cirrhotic platelet: shedding light on an enigma. Hepatology. 2017 Feb;65(2):407–10.
22. Raparelli V, Basili S, Carnevale R, Napoleone L, Del Ben M, Nocella C, et al. Low-grade endotoxemia and platelet activation in cirrhosis. Hepatology. 2017 Sep 19;65(2):571–81.
23. Lisman T, Bos S, Intagliata NM. Mechanisms of enhanced thrombin generating capacity in patients with cirrhosis. J Thromb Haemost. 2018 Apr;10:1128–31.
24. Hugenholtz GC, Mccrae FL, Adelmeijer J, Dulfer SE, Porte RJ, Lisman T, et al. Procoagulant changes in fibrin clot structure in patients with cirrhosis are associated with oxidative modifications of fibrinogen. J Thromb Haemost. 2016;15(5):1054–66.
25. Saliola M, Lorenzet R, Ferro D, Basili S, Caroselli C, Santo AD, et al. Enhanced expression of monocyte tissue factor in patients with liver cirrhosis. Gut. 1998 Sep;43(3):428–32.
26. MacPhee PJ, Dindzans VJ, Fung LS, Levy GA. Acute and chronic changes in the microcirculation of the liver in inbred strains of mice following infection with mouse hepatitis virus type 3. Hepatology. 1985 Jul-Aug;5(4):649–60.
27. Ganey PE, Luyendyk JP, Newport SW, Eagle TM, Maddox JF, Mackman N, et al. Role of the coagulation system in acetaminophen-induced hepatotoxicity in mice. Hepatology. 2007 Oct;46(4):1177–86.
28. Hugenholtz GC, Meijers JC, Adelmeijer J, Porte RJ, Lisman T. TAFI deficiency promotes liver damage in murine models of liver failure through defective down-regulation of hepatic inflammation. Thromb Haemost. 2013 May;109(5):948–55.
29. Kopec AK, Joshi N, Luyendyk JP. Role of hemostatic factors in hepatic injury and disease: animal models de-liver. J Thromb Haemost. 2016 Jul;14(7):1337–49.
30. Lisman T, Luyendyk JP. Platelets as modulators of liver diseases. Semin Thromb Hemost. 2018 Mar;44(2):114–25.
31. Cline-Fedewa H, Baker KS, Williams KJ, Roth RA, Mittermeier K, Lisman T, Palumbo JS, Luyendyk JP. Von Willebrand factor delays liver repair after acetaminophen-induced acute liver injury in mice. J Hepatol. 2020 Jan;72(1):146–55.
32. Driever EG, Stravitz RT, Zhang J, Adelmeijer J, Durkalski V, Lee WM, Lisman T. VWF/ADAMTS13 imbalance, but not global coagulation or fibrinolysis, is associated with outcome and bleeding in acute liver failure. Hepatology. 2020;73(5):1882–91.
33. Anstee QM, Goldin RD, Wright M, Martinelli A, Cox R, Thursz MR. Coagulation status modulates murine hepatic fibrogenesis: implications for the development of novel therapies. J Thromb Haemost. 2008 Aug;6(8):1336–43.
34. Anstee QM, Wright M, Goldin R, Thursz MR. Parenchymal extinction: coagulation and hepatic fibrogenesis. Clin Liver Dis. 2009 Feb;13(1):117–26.

35. Wanless IR, Wong F, Blendis LM, Greig P, Heathcote EJ, Levy G. Hepatic and portal vein thrombosis in cirrhosis: possible role in development of parenchymal extinction and portal hypertension. Hepatology. 1995 May;21(5):1238–47.
36. Wanless IR, Liu JJ, Butany J. Role of thrombosis in the pathogenesis of congestive hepatic fibrosis (cardiac cirrhosis). Hepatology. 1995 May;21(5):1232–7.
37. Wright M, Goldin R, Hellier S, Knapp S, Frodsham A, Hennig B, et al. Factor V Leiden polymorphism and the rate of fibrosis development in chronic hepatitis C virus infection. Gut. 2003 Aug;52(8):1206–10.
38. Assy N, Pettigrew N, Lee SS, Chaudhary RK, Johnston J, Minuk GY. Are chronic hepatitis C viral infections more benign in patients with hemophilia? Am J Gastroenterol. 2007 Aug;102(8):1672–6.
39. Jiang ZG, Feldbrugge L, Tapper EB, Popov Y, Ghaziani T, Afdhal N, et al. Aspirin use is associated with lower indices of liver fibrosis among adults in the United States. Aliment Pharmacol Ther. 2016 Mar;43(6):734–43.
40. Poujol-Robert A, Boelle PY, Conti F, Durand F, Duvoux C, Wendum D, et al. Aspirin may reduce liver fibrosis progression: evidence from a multicenter retrospective study of recurrent hepatitis C after liver transplantation. Clin Res Hepatol Gastroenterol. 2014 Oct;38(5):570–6.
41. Shen H, Shahzad G, Jawairia M, Bostick RM, Mustacchia P. Association between aspirin use and the prevalence of nonalcoholic fatty liver disease: a cross-sectional study from the third National Health and nutrition examination survey. Aliment Pharmacol Ther. 2014 Nov;40(9):1066–73.
42. Botting RM. Vane's discovery of the mechanism of action of aspirin changed our understanding of its clinical pharmacology. Pharmacol Rep. 2010 May-Jun;62(3):518–25.
43. Imaeda AB, Watanabe A, Sohail MA, Mahmood S, Mohamadnejad M, Sutterwala FS, et al. Acetaminophen-induced hepatotoxicity in mice is dependent on Tlr9 and the Nalp3 inflammasome. J Clin Invest. 2009 Feb;119(2):305–14.
44. Villa E, Zecchini R, Marietta M, Bernabucci B, Lei B, Vukotic R, et al. Enoxaparin prevents portal vein thrombosis (Pvt) and decompensation in advanced cirrhotic patients: final report of a prospective randomized controlled study. Hepatology. 2011;54:418a–9a.
45. Stine JG, Shah PM, Cornella SL, Rudnick SR, Ghabril MS, Stukenborg GJ, et al. Portal vein thrombosis, mortality and hepatic decompensation in patients with cirrhosis: a meta-analysis. World J Hepatol. 2015 Nov 28;7(27):2774–80.
46. Nery F, Chevret S, Condat B, de Raucourt E, Boudaoud L, Rautou PE, et al. Causes and consequences of portal vein thrombosis in 1,243 patients with cirrhosis: results of a longitudinal study. Hepatology. 2015 Feb;61(2):660–7.
47. Stine JG, Wang J, Shah PM, Argo CK, Intagliata N, Uflacker A, et al. Decreased portal vein velocity is predictive of the development of portal vein thrombosis: a matched case-control study. Liver Int. 2018 Jan;38(1):94–101.
48. Amitrano L, Guardascione MA, Brancaccio V, Margaglione M, Manguso F, Iannaccone L, et al. Risk factors and clinical presentation of portal vein thrombosis in patients with liver cirrhosis. J Hepatol. 2004 May;40(5):736–41.
49. Stine JG, Shah NL, Argo CK, Pelletier SJ, Caldwell SH, Northup PG. Increased risk of portal vein thrombosis in patients with cirrhosis due to nonalcoholic steatohepatitis. Liver Transpl. 2015 Aug;21(8):1016–21.
50. Potze W, Siddiqui MS, Boyett SL, Adelmeijer J, Daita K, Sanyal AJ, et al. Preserved hemostatic status in patients with non-alcoholic fatty liver disease. J Hepatol. 2016 Jun 11;65(5):980–7.
51. Bos S, van den Boom B, Kamphuisen PW, Adelmeijer J, Blokzijl H, Schreuder T, Lisman T. Haemostatic profiles are similar across all Aetiologies of cirrhosis. Thromb Haemost. 2019 Feb;119(2):246–53.
52. Plessier A, Darwish-Murad S, Hernandez-Guerra M, Consigny Y, Fabris F, Trebicka J, et al. Acute portal vein thrombosis unrelated to cirrhosis: a prospective multicenter follow-up study. Hepatology. 2010 Jan;51(1):210–8.
53. Raffa S, Reverter JC, Seijo S, Tassies D, Abraldes JG, Bosch J, et al. Hypercoagulability in patients with chronic noncirrhotic portal vein thrombosis. Clin Gastroenterol Hepatol. 2012 Jan;10(1):72–8.

54. Darwish Murad S, Plessier A, Hernandez-Guerra M, Fabris F, Eapen CE, Bahr MJ, et al. Etiology, management, and outcome of the Budd-Chiari syndrome. Ann Intern Med. 2009 Aug 4;151(3):167–75.

55. Krus S, Turjman MW, Fiejka E. Comparative morphology of the hepatic and coronary artery walls. Part I. differences in the distribution and intensity of non-atherosclerotic intimal thickening and atherosclerosis. Med Sci Monit. 2000 Jan-Feb;6(1):19–23.

56. Duffy JP, Hong JC, Farmer DG, Ghobrial RM, Yersiz H, Hiatt JR, et al. Vascular complications of orthotopic liver transplantation: experience in more than 4,200 patients. J Am Coll Surg. 2009 May;208(5):896–903.

57. Sieders E, Peeters PM, TenVergert EM, de Jong KP, Porte RJ, Zwaveling JH, et al. Early vascular complications after pediatric liver transplantation. Liver Transpl. 2000 May;6(3):326–32.

58. Bekker J, Ploem S, de Jong KP. Early hepatic artery thrombosis after liver transplantation: a systematic review of the incidence, outcome and risk factors. Am J Transplant. 2009 Apr;9(4):746–57.

59. Gunsar F, Rolando N, Pastacaldi S, Patch D, Raimondo ML, Davidson B, et al. Late hepatic artery thrombosis after orthotopic liver transplantation. Liver Transpl. 2003 Jun;9(6):605–11.

60. Stange BJ, Glanemann M, Nuessler NC, Settmacher U, Steinmuller T, Neuhaus P. Hepatic artery thrombosis after adult liver transplantation. Liver Transpl. 2003 Jun;9(6):612–20.

61. Mueller AR, Platz KP, Kremer B. Early postoperative complications following liver transplantation. Best Pract Res Clin Gastroenterol. 2004 Oct;18(5):881–900.

62. Yao FY, Kinkhabwala M, LaBerge JM, Bass NM, Brown R Jr, Kerlan R, et al. The impact of pre-operative loco-regional therapy on outcome after liver transplantation for hepatocellular carcinoma. Am J Transplant. 2005 Apr;5(4 Pt 1):795–804.

63. Silva MA, Jambulingam PS, Gunson BK, Mayer D, Buckels JA, Mirza DF, et al. Hepatic artery thrombosis following orthotopic liver transplantation: a 10-year experience from a single Centre in the United Kingdom. Liver Transpl. 2006 Jan;12(1):146–51.

64. Oh CK, Pelletier SJ, Sawyer RG, Dacus AR, McCullough CS, Pruett TL, et al. Uni- and multivariate analysis of risk factors for early and late hepatic artery thrombosis after liver transplantation. Transplantation. 2001 Mar 27;71(6):767–72.

65. Pereboom IT, Adelmeijer J, van Leeuwen Y, Hendriks HG, Porte RJ, Lisman T. Development of a severe von Willebrand factor/ADAMTS13 dysbalance during orthotopic liver transplantation. Am J Transplant. 2009 May;9(5):1189–96.

66. Lisman T, Bakhtiari K, Pereboom IT, Hendriks HG, Meijers JC, Porte RJ. Normal to increased thrombin generation in patients undergoing liver transplantation despite prolonged conventional coagulation tests. J Hepatol. 2010 Mar;52(3):355–61.

67. Arshad F, Lisman T, Porte RJ. Hypercoagulability as a contributor to thrombotic complications in the liver transplant recipient. Liver Int. 2013 Jul;33(6):820–7.

68. Bispo M, Marcelino P, Freire A, Martins A, Mourao L, Barroso E. High incidence of thrombotic complications early after liver transplantation for familial amyloidotic polyneuropathy. Transpl Int. 2009 Feb;22(2):165–71.

69. Dowman JK, Gunson BK, Mirza DF, Bramhall SR, Badminton MN, Newsome PN, et al. Liver transplantation for acute intermittent porphyria is complicated by a high rate of hepatic artery thrombosis. Liver Transpl. 2012 Feb;18(2):195–200.

70. Lisman T, Porte RJ. Hepatic artery thrombosis after liver transplantation: more than just a surgical complication? Transpl Int. 2009 Feb;22(2):162–4.

71. Vivarelli M, La Barba G, Cucchetti A, Lauro A, Del Gaudio M, Ravaioli M, et al. Can antiplatelet prophylaxis reduce the incidence of hepatic artery thrombosis after liver transplantation? Liver Transpl. 2007 May;13(5):651–4.

72. Lisman T, Porte RJ. Antiplatelet medication after liver transplantation: does it affect outcome? Liver Transpl. 2007 May;13(5):644–6.

73. Levi M, Sivapalaratnam S. Disseminated intravascular coagulation: an update on pathogenesis and diagnosis. Expert Rev Hematol. 2018 Aug;11(8):663–72.

74. Slofstra SH. Van 't veer C, Buurman WA, Reitsma PH, ten Cate H, Spek CA. Low molecular weight heparin attenuates multiple organ failure in a murine model of disseminated intravascular coagulation. Crit Care Med. 2005 Jun;33(6):1365–70.
75. Hunt BJ. Bleeding and coagulopathies in critical care. N Engl J Med. 2014 Feb 27;370(9):847–59.
76. Levi M, Scully M. How I treat disseminated intravascular coagulation. Blood. 2018 Feb 22;131(8):845–54.
77. Toh CH, Hoots WK. SSC on disseminated intravascular coagulation of the ISTH. The scoring system of the scientific and standardisation committee on disseminated intravascular coagulation of the international society on thrombosis and Haemostasis: a 5-year overview. J Thromb Haemost. 2007 Mar;5(3):604–6.
78. Bakker CM, Knot EA, Stibbe J, Wilson JH. Disseminated intravascular coagulation in liver cirrhosis. J Hepatol. 1992 Jul;15(3):330–5.
79. Lisman T, Leebeek FW, de Groot PG. Haemostatic abnormalities in patients with liver disease. J Hepatol. 2002 Aug;37(2):280–7.
80. Fisher C, Patel VC, Stoy SH, Singanayagam A, Adelmeijer J, Wendon J, et al. Balanced haemostasis with both hypo- and hyper-coagulable features in critically ill patients with acute-on-chronic-liver failure. J Crit Care. 2017;43:54–60.
81. Westbrook RH, Dusheiko G, Williamson C. Pregnancy and liver disease. J Hepatol. 2016 Apr;64(4):933–45.
82. Knight M, Nelson-Piercy C, Kurinczuk JJ, Spark P, Brocklehurst P. UK obstetric surveillance system. A prospective national study of acute fatty liver of pregnancy in the UK. Gut. 2008 Jul;57(7):951–6.
83. Nelson DB, Yost NP, Cunningham FG. Hemostatic dysfunction with acute fatty liver of pregnancy. Obstet Gynecol. 2014 Jul;124(1):40–6.
84. Hulstein JJ, van Runnard Heimel PJ, Franx A, Lenting PJ, Bruinse HW, Silence K, et al. Acute activation of the endothelium results in increased levels of active von Willebrand factor in hemolysis, elevated liver enzymes and low platelets (HELLP) syndrome. J Thromb Haemost. 2006 Dec;4(12):2569–75.
85. Cunningham FG, Nelson DB. Disseminated intravascular coagulation syndromes in obstetrics. Obstet Gynecol. 2015 Nov;126(5):999–1011.

# Chapter 18
# Primary Hepatic Vascular Neoplasms and Hematologic Neoplasms Affecting Liver Vessels

**Maxime Ronot and Dominique Cazals-Hatem**

Apart from hepatocytes, cholangiocytes, Kupffer cells and stellate cells, the liver contains endothelial cells within the arterial, portal, sinusoids, and hepatic venous systems. These cells may give rise to various benign and malignant lesions of vascular origin. The spectrum of tumors stretches from very common ones such as hemangiomas to very rare neoplasms such as angiosarcomas. Despite a common vascular origin, clinical course, pathologic features, imaging appearance and prognosis of these neoplasms are highly variable and heterogeneous.

All haematopoietic and lymphoid neoplasms described in the 2017-WHO classification may infiltrate the liver during their course. Beside lymphomas and leukemias, some disorders like amyloidosis or systemic mastocytosis affect predominantly sinusoids or the venous beds and generate secondary vascular disorders.

The purpose of this chapter is to provide an overview of primary vascular tumors most frequently observed in adult-livers. Pediatric tumors, especially infantile hemangioma will not be discussed herein. In the second part, hematologic neoplasms known for their propensity to affect liver vessels are detailed, focusing on pathological features in order to improve diagnosis when hepatic involvement by the hemopathy is the first manifestation of the disease. The chapter will focus on clinical presentation, imaging and pathology while the complex issues of treatment and prognosis will not be considered.


M. Ronot (✉)
Department of Radiology, APHP. Nord, Beaujon, Clichy, France

Université de Paris, Paris, France
e-mail: maxime.ronot@aphp.fr

D. Cazals-Hatem
Department of Pathology, APHP. Nord, Beaujon, Clichy, France
e-mail: dominique.cazals-hatem@aphp.fr



© Springer Nature Switzerland AG 2022
D. Valla et al. (eds.), *Vascular Disorders of the Liver*,
https://doi.org/10.1007/978-3-030-82988-9_18

# Primary Hepatic Vascular Neoplasms

## *Cavernous Haemangioma*

Cavernous haemangioma is probably the most frequent benign liver lesion. Its prevalence is evaluated between 1.2 and 20% [1] in the general population. It affects all ages. The female-to-male ratio varies from 2.1 to 5 between surveys [2–4].

### Pathology

Macroscopic examination shows well-delineated, flat spongy lesions of red-blue color. Microscopically, haemangiomas are easy to recognize. They are made of cavernous vascular spaces lined by flattened regular endothelium underlying fibrous septa of various widths (Fig. 18.1, Table 18.1). Small haemangiomas may become entirely fibrous, appearing as "a solitary fibrous nodule" corresponding microscopically to sclerosed haemangioma [5]. Differential diagnoses are mentioned in

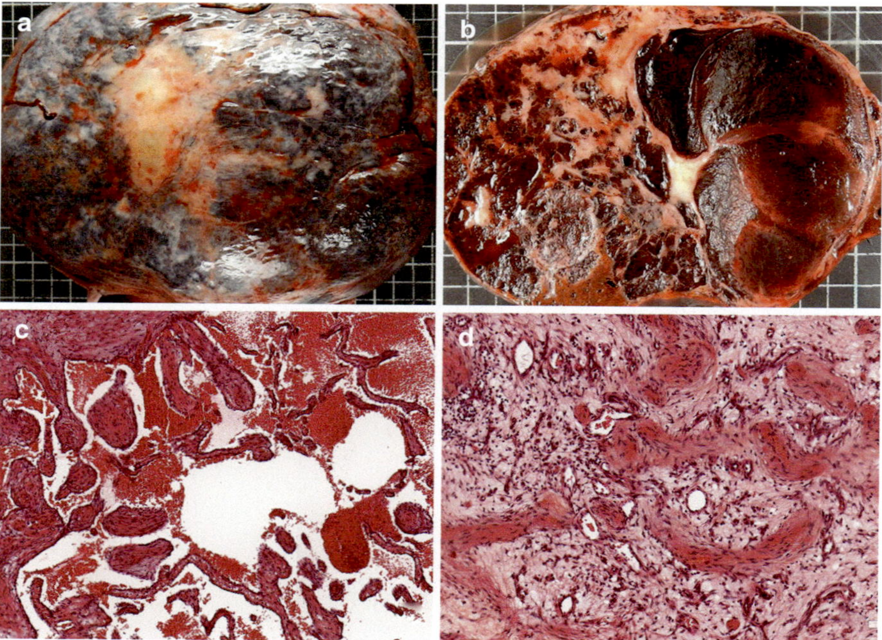

**Fig. 18.1** Giant cavernous hemangioma. (**a**) External aspect of a 21 cm large giant hemangioma resected by lobectomy. (**b**) Cut section shows a well-demarcated spongy dark red tumor with fibrous septa and scars corresponding to internal thrombi. (**c**) Histology shows a cavernous architecture with vascular spaces lined by regular endothelial cells and filled with hematies. (**d**) Sclerosing zones exhibit abundant fibrous stroma and tiny vascular lumen

**Table 18.1**  Histopathological characteristics of the main hepatic vascular neoplasms

| Vascular tumors | Macroscopy | Microscopy | Phenotype | Differential diagnosis |
|---|---|---|---|---|
| Cavernous hemangioma<br>*Benign* | Solitary/multiple/Giant<br>Well-circumscribed<br>Dark red and spongy<br>Cavernous pattern<br>Filled with red blood cells | Uniform vascular pattern<br>Bland flat endothelial cells<br>No nuclear pleomorphism<br>No mitosis, no necrosis<br>*Sclerosed/hyalinized/calcified variant*<br>*Capillary variant* | CD31, CD34, ERG, factor VIII | Infantile hemangioma<br>Hepatic small vessel neoplasm<br>Lymphangioma<br>Hereditary hemorrhagic telangiectasia |
| Epithelioid hemangioendothelioma<br>*Low grade malignant* | Solitary/multiple<br>Fuzzy borders<br>White and firm<br>Fibrous pattern | Gradual and centrifugal cellularity<br>Sinusoidal infiltration by single cells<br>Dendritic/epithelioid/vacuolar cells<br>Intra-cytoplasmic red blood cells<br>Sclerotic fibrous center ± calcification<br>Nuclear pleomorphism<br>No mitosis | CD31, CD34, ERG, factor VIII<br>D2-40<br>± EMA<br>± cytokeratin | Cholangiocarcinoma<br>Signet-ring cells carcinoma |
| Angiosarcoma<br>*High grade malignant* | Multiple/diffuse infiltration<br>Poorly circumscribed<br>Dark red heterogeneous<br>Spongious pattern<br>Filled with red blood cells<br>Necrosis, infarction | Heterogeneous cavernous/solid pattern<br>Irregular and atypical endothelial cells<br>Nuclear pleomorphism<br>Mitosis, necrosis<br>Extramedullary hematopoiesis | CD31, CD34, ERG, factor VIII<br>Ki67 > 10%<br>± GLUT-1<br>± P53<br>± c-MYC | Hepatic small vessel neoplasm<br>Kaposi sarcoma |

Table 18.1. Strong expression of GLUT-1 characterizes infantile haemangioma in children. Lymphangioma has no red blood cells and reacts with D2-40. Hepatic small vessel neoplasms, recently recognized as a distinct entity, may mimic capillary infiltrative haemangioma [6].

## Manifestations and Course

Most of the time, the lesion is asymptomatic and incidentally found during examinations of the abdomen for unrelated reasons. Most lesions remain stable in size [7] or demonstrate minimal increase in diameter over time [8]. Liver tests are normal. The evolution is fully benign and haemangioma never transform into a malignant form.

Complications are rare and mostly observed with large haemangiomas. They can be divided into (a) alterations of internal architecture such as inflammation; (b) coagulation abnormalities and (c) compression of adjacent structures.

- Some cases of inflammatory processes complicating giant haemangioma have been initially reported by Bornman et al. [9]. Signs and symptoms of an inflammatory process include low-grade fever, weight loss, abdominal pain, accelerated erythrocyte sedimentation rate, normal white blood cell count, anemia, thrombocytosis, and increased fibrinogen level. In imaging, visualization of a spontaneously hyperattenuating structure corresponding to a thrombosis comforts the diagnosis. Abnormalities disappear after surgical resection of the haemangioma [9–11].
- Kasabach-Merritt syndrome is an exceptional complication of hepatic haemangioma in adults Characterized by an intravascular coagulaction activation. The syndrome is reversible after removal of the hemangioma. Intratumoral hemorrhage is rarely encountered in hepatic haemangioma.

## Imaging Appearance

Typical Aspect

Haemangioma is typically a homogenous hyperechoic lesion less than 3 cm in diameter, with sharp margins and acoustic enhancement. No vascular pattern is identified on color Doppler [12]. A hypoechoic center but no peripheral hypoechoic rim can be observed. The larger the haemangiomas is, more heterogeneous it can appear [13]. Contrast-enhanced ultrasound reveals peripheral globular enhancement in the portal phase. Isoechoic pattern on late phase is seen in most atypical haemangiomas [14]. Therefore, this technique, which has a sensitivity of 84 to 89% and a specificity of 92 to 100%, should be performed in equivocal lesions [14–16].

On computed tomography (CT), the three major criteria for the diagnosis of haemangioma are the following: (a) spontaneous low attenuation on pre-contrast images in comparison with surrounding liver; (b) peripheral and globular enhancement of the lesion followed by a central enhancement on contrast-enhanced images; and (c) contrast enhancement of the lesion on delayed scans [17]. Among these criteria, the most important is the second one as the presence of peripheral puddles at arterial phase has a sensitivity of 67%, a specificity of 99%, and a positive predictive value of 86% for haemangioma [18]. One of the most precious features for diagnosis is the parallel evolution of lesion and aorta enhancement after contrast injection [18].

Magnetic Resonance imaging (MRI) is the key imaging modality in the characterization of liver haemangiomas [19, 20]. The classical appearance of liver haemangiomas is that of a homogeneous well delineated hypointenselesion on T1-weightened sequences and strongly hyperintenselesion on heavily T2-weighted sequences with a "light bulb" pattern. Dynamic multiphasic T1-weightened sequences, after gadolinium chelate administration show findings similar to that on contrast-enhanced CT phases (Fig. 18.2) [21]. The diagnostic value is very high with a sensitivity of 90%, a specificity of 92% and a global accuracy of 90% [21]. Diffusion-weighted sequences (DW-MRI) show a spontaneous hyperintensity on low-b-value acquisitions and persistent high signal intensity on high b value corresponding to a «shrine-through» and related to the T2 effect. ADC maps that are automatically generated by the system are therefore very important to confirm the diffusion restriction [22]. Hepatospecific contrast agents may show a paradoxical pseudo-wash out on the transitional of hepatobiliary phase in case of rapidly filling haemangioma [23].

## Variants

Two variants commonly cause atypical presentation at imaging, the giant haemangioma and the rapidly filling haemangioma:

- Giant haemangiomas are defined by a large size exceeding 6 (or 12) cm in diameter. They are often heterogeneous [24, 25] with marked central areas corresponding to thrombosis, extensive hyalinization and fibrosis. However, usually the typical early, peripheral, globular enhancement is observed as well as strong hyperintensity on T2-weightened images at the periphery. The progressive centripetal enhancement of the lesion, although present, does not lead to complete filling (Fig. 18.2) [24, 26, 27].
- Rapidly filling haemangiomas are not uncommon and appear to occur significantly more often in small lesions (42% of haemangiomas <2 cm in diameter) [28]. CT and MR imaging show an immediate homogeneous enhancement at arterial-phase which makes differentiation from other hypervascular tumors difficult. Their diagnosis is based on strong hyperintensity on T2-weighted images, the parallel enhancement with arterial structures, and the persistent enhancement on delayed-phase imaging. Interestingly, shunts are observed in 20 to 25% of liver haemangiomas [28, 29]. They seem very much related to the rapidly filling type rather than to the size [29, 30].

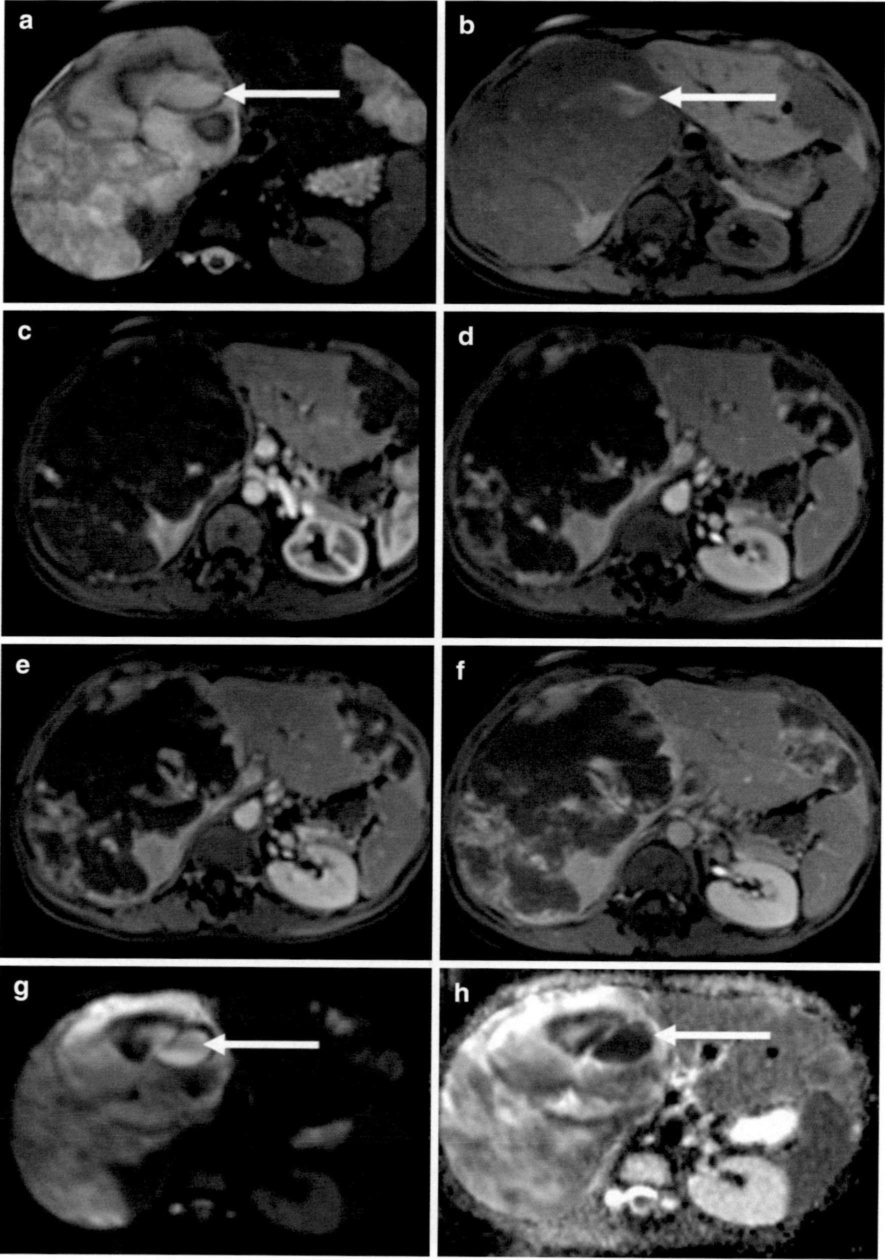

Other haemangiomas may uncommonly have an atypical presentation, including very slow filling haemangiomas (represent 8 to 16% of all haemangiomas [31]), sclerosed or hyalinized/calcified haemangiomas, cystic haemangiomas, pedunculated haemangiomas, haemangiomas with fluid-fluid level, and haemangiomas with capsular retraction [32–35]. Hyalinization, which corresponds to an end-stage involution secondary to thrombosis or internal infarction is histologically characterized by abundant hyalinized tissue, obliterated vascular channels and small residual vessels. On imaging, it shows atypical features such as hypointensity on T2-weighted MR images and lack of enhancement. For this reason, sclerosed hemangioma may be misdiagnosed with malignancy.

## Epithelioid Hemangioendothelioma

Hepatic epithelioid hemangioendothelioma (HEH) is a rare low-grade malignant tumor that arises from liver endothelial cells [36–40]. HEH is seen in adults with a 2:1 female: malesex ratio. It is rarely solitary, and most patients show multifocal disease at diagnosis. Most tumors are incidentally discovered.

### *Pathology*

Grossly, nodules are round, white or grey and firm. They are non-encapsulated and ill-circumscribed with fuzzy infiltrative borders around central hyalinized scar. Microscopically, no vascular space is noticed. Endothelial differentiation is unobvious: neoplastic cells are ovoid, spindle or round singly sited in an abundant fibrous stroma. The pathognomonic vacuolated cell centered by red blood cell may be inconspicuous. At the periphery, cells display an epithelioid pattern forming endovascular cords or tufts. Nuclei are irregular and pleomorphic without mitosis (Fig. 18.3—Table 18.1). Aberrant focal expression of cytokeratin or EMA may mislead the diagnosis with poorly differentiated carcinoma, cholangiocarcinoma or metastasis.

---

**Fig. 18.2** Giant cavernous hemangioma. MR imaging performed in the same patient as Fig. 18.1 shows that lesions are bilobar. They show high signal intensity on T2-weighted images (**a**), and hypointensity on T1-weighted images (**b**). After extracellular contrast medium injection, lesions present with a peripheral nodular and discontinuous enhancement and progressive centripetal filling (from **c** to **f**). On high b value diffusion weighted imaging (**g**) lesions show a high signal intensity, with high ADC values (**h**) consistent with a typical 'T2 shine thought effect'. Note the presence of inner focal areas of signal hyperintensity on T1-w and hypointensity on T2-w images, that appear heterogeneous and hypointense on diffusion-w images, and are associated with low ADC values (arrows). These areas correspond to intratumoral thrombosis

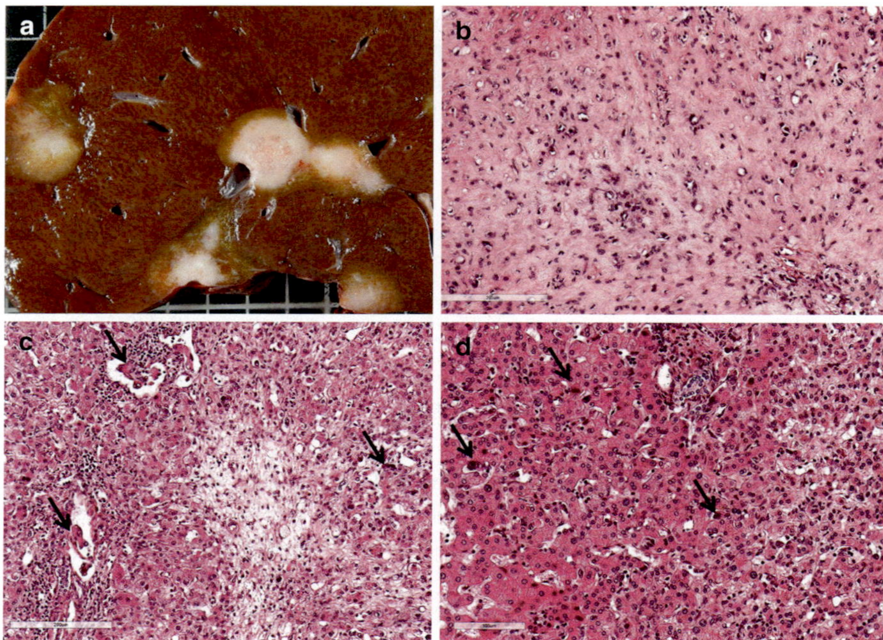

**Fig. 18.3** Epithelioid hemangioendothelioma. (**a**) Cut section of a liver explant presenting multiples well-circumcribed tumors with white centers and fuzzy outlines. (**b**) The center of epithelioid hemangioendothelioma is sclerotic with scattered vacuolar small cells containing red blood cells. (**c**) The periphery of epithelioid hemangioendothelioma shows tuffs of tumoral cells in portal veins and sinusoids (→) between well-preserved hepatic plates. (**d**) Tumoral outlines are indistinct with tumoral cells still present at the interface with normal liver (→)

## *Manifestations and Course*

The natural course of evolution of HEH significantly varies between patients, some remaining completely asymptomatic over a long period of time, while others may rapidly progress to extensive liver parenchymal replacement, metastasis and death.

## *Imaging Appearance*

It is classically considered that HEH can be divided into three distinct imaging patterns: a solitary nodule, multiple nodules, and diffuse and confluent nodules. Single nodules are believed to progress to multiple nodules and eventually to confluent diffuse disease.

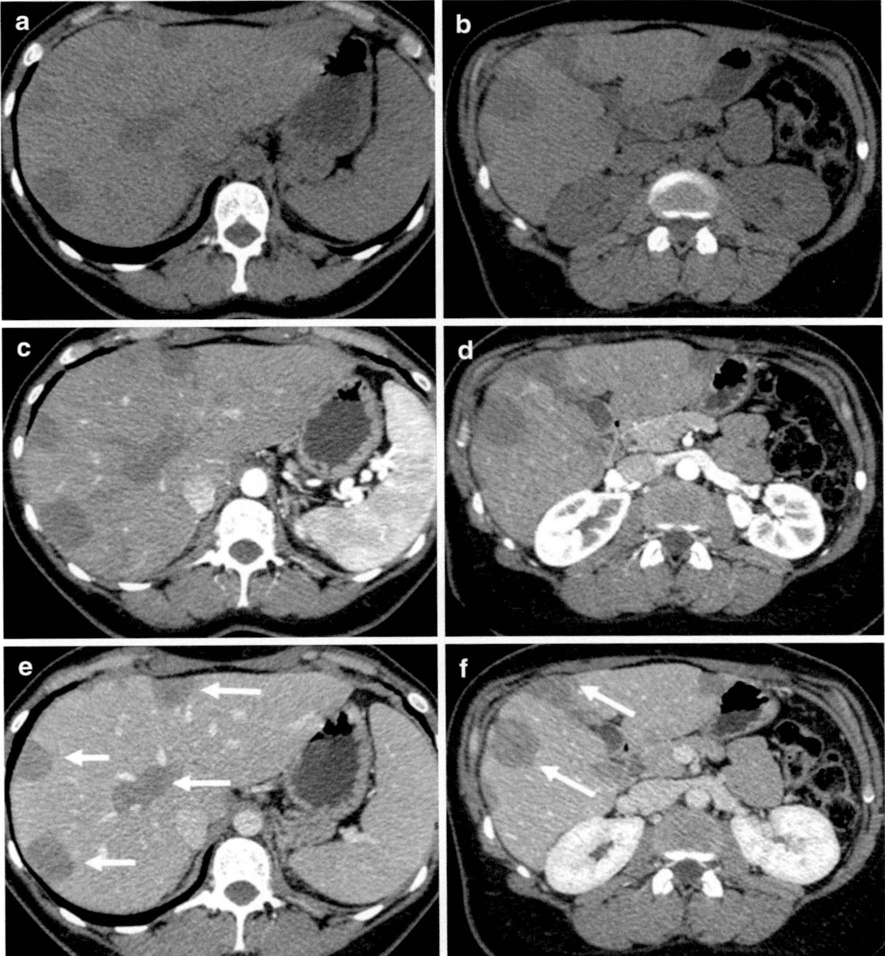

**Fig. 18.4** Epithelioid hemangioendothelioma. CT performed in the same patient as Fig. 18.3 shows that lesions are bilobar (arrows). They show hypoattenuation on precontrast images (**a** and **b**), and remain hypoattenuating relative to the liver on contrast-enhanced arterial phase (**c** and **d**) and portal venous phase (**e** and **f**). Lesions are predominantly subcapsular

Solitary nodules usually measure up to 5 centimeters and are typically located in the subcapsular area of the right liver lobe [41]. Multifocal disease is more variable, with lesions of different size, located at the periphery or more deeply in the liver [42]. Lesions frequently demonstrate focal capsular retraction, while capsular bulge is not observed (Figs. 18.4 and 18.5).

M. Ronot and D. Cazals-Hatem

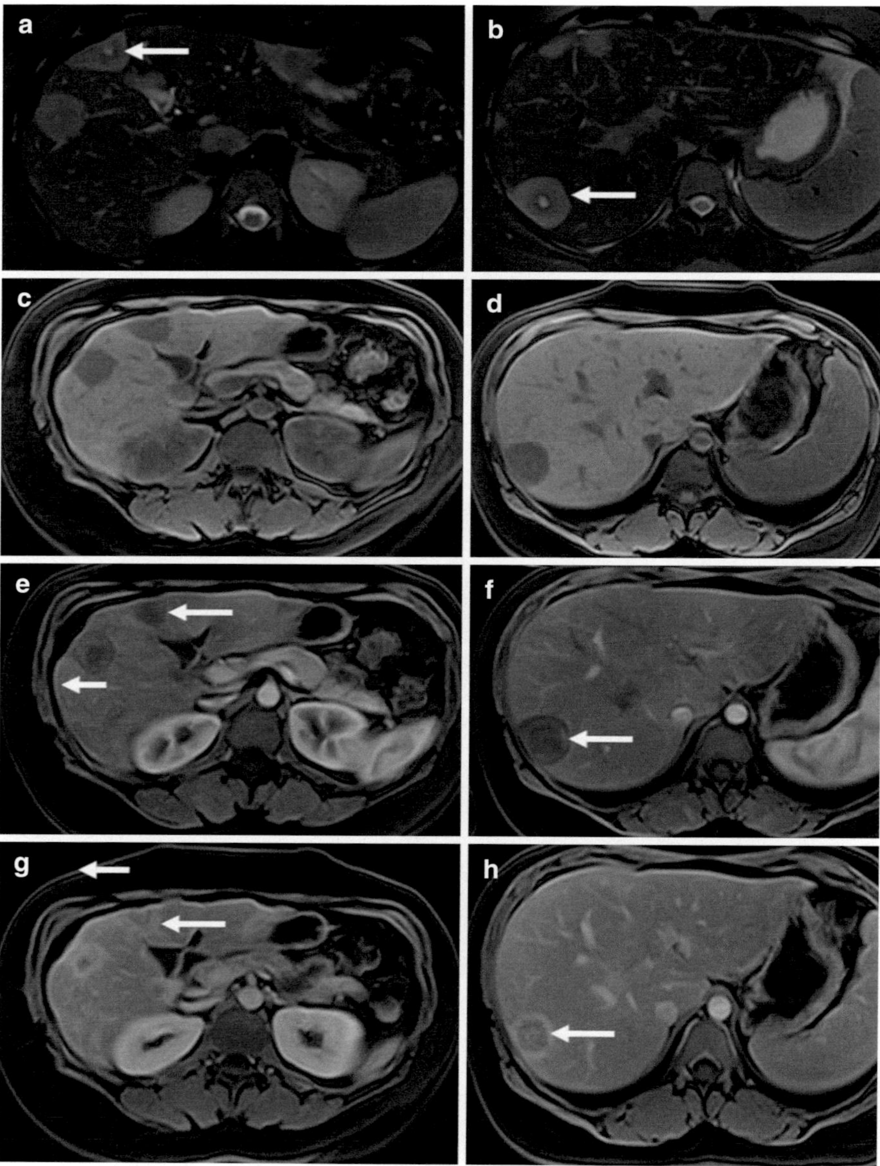

**Fig. 18.5** Epithelioid hemangioendothelioma. MR imaging performed in the same patient as Figs. 18.3 and 18.4. Lesions show high signal intensity on T2-weighted images (**a** and **b**), and hypointensity on T1-weighted images (**c** and **d**). After extracellular contrast medium injection, lesions remain hypoattenuating to the liver on arterial phase (**e** and **f**) and show delayed contrast enhancement (**g** and **h**). Note that some lesion present with a target appearance (arrows) with central hyperintensity on T2-w images, followed centrifugally by a layer of hypointensity, and by an external hyperintensity. This layered appearance is also visible on contrast-enhanced images, with core and peripheral delayed enhancement

On ultrasound examination, tumors are typically hypoechoic to adjacent liver. However, a small proportion may show hyperechogenicity. On CT, lesions are typically hypoattenuating on pre-contrast and contrast-enhanced images when compared to the liver, and may contain calcifications (Fig. 18.4). At MRI, lesions are hypointense on T1-weighted images and may present with a typical concentric target appearance with central hypointensity, a thin rim of hyperintensity, and a peripheral rim of hypointensity. This is referred to as the "dark-bright-dark ring sign" [43]. On T2-weighted images, lesion show variable signal intensity: no rim, and sometimes double- or triple-layered target pattern with a hyperintense center followed by alternating layers of T2-weighted intermediate or hypointensity, the majority of tumors presenting a T2-weighted hyperintense central core corresponding to fibrous stroma (Fig. 18.5). The same layered aspect is visible on diffusion-weighted imaging that often shows a rim of diffusion restriction in the periphery of the lesion but more variable signal in the core. On contrast-enhanced images, most HEH initially shownone to mild central enhancement, some showing an early rim enhancement. On delayed phase, the lesions appear more homogeneous. Globular peripheral enhancement and early arterial enhancement followed by washout are not frequently seen. After injection ofliver-specific MR contrast agents, some degree of "trapping" of the contrast agent can be depicted, with a hypointense rim and central hyperintensity on hepatobiliary phase [42]. Extrahepatic involvement, when present, is most commonly seen in the lung, lymph nodes, peritoneum, spleen, and bone marrow.

## Angiosarcoma

Angiosarcoma is a rare high-grade malignant endothelial neoplasm representing the commonest sarcoma arising in the liver. There is a male predominance.

### *Pathology*

Tumors are multifocal with involvementof both hepatic lobes in nearly all patients have lesions ranging from 3 to 20 cm large size. Metastatic disease at presentation is seen in 45–60% of patients, the spleen, peritoneum, lung and bone marrow being the most common locations [44]. Grossly, angiosarcoma appears as an ill-defined heterogeneous spongy mass, with solid and cavernous areas admixed with infarcted zones [44]. Microscopically, endothelial differentiation is patent and cells exhibit obvious malignant features (bizarre hyperchromatic nuclei, mitosis) (Fig. 18.6—Table 18.1). If a solid sarcomatous or epithelioid pattern predominates, an immunohistochemistry is required for

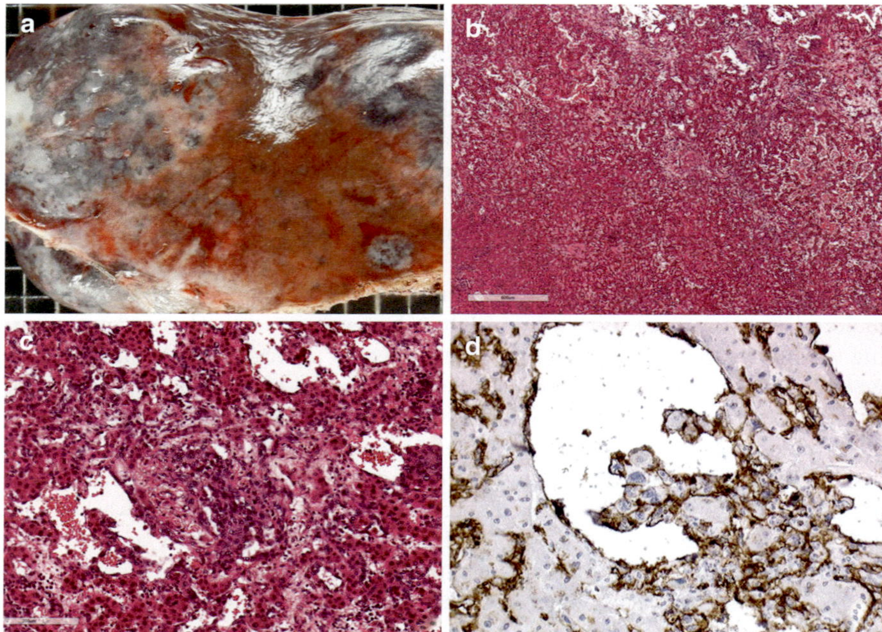

**Fig. 18.6** Angiosarcoma. (**a**) Liver resection shows multifocal dark red lesions corresponding to an extensive angiosarcoma. (**b**) Histology shows diffuse infiltration by a cavernous and hemorrhagic tumor. (**c**) Vascular spaces are lined by atypical irregular endothelial cells and filled with hematies. (**d**) Endothelial cells express endothelial cell marker CD34 and CD31

confirmation (endothelial markers CD31, CD34, ERG, Factor VIII). A sinusoidal growth pattern admixed with prominent peliotic changes may pose diagnostic difficulty on biopsy sample and require additional immunostaining for mutant p53expression and high Ki-67 proliferative index. Indeed, well-differentiated angiosarcomas with subtle atypia must be distinguished from hepatic small vessel neoplasm recently described as a rare vascular neoplasm with uncertain malignant potential (see below) [6].

## *Etiology*

Angiosarcoma had been linked to exposure to thorium dioxide (Thorotrast), inorganic arsenic, or vinyl chloride, but most cases are currently diagnosed in patients without such a past exposure [45].

## *Manifestations and Course*

Patients typically present with non-specific symptoms and advanced stage disease in the fifth to seventh decade of life. Rapid fatal outcome year of diagnosis is the rule [46]. Liver lesions on initial imaging often progress to multifocal or even fulminant disease during the course of workup.

## *Imaging Appearance*

Typically, when seen at CT, tumors follow blood pool attenuation and are therefore hypoattenuating to the surrounding liver on pre-contrast images. Inner areas of internal hemorrhage can be seen. On the late hepatic arterial phase, focal enhancement is seen in up to 90% of tumors [47] but several patterns of enhancement have been described, including nodular, rim, branching, or more diffuse. The smallest lesions may show no arterial enhancement. On portal venous and delayed phases, tumors show progressive enhancement, and a minority of tumors may remain poorly- or non-enhanced. Typical haemangioma-like pattern (peripheral nodular enhancement followed by central in-fill), and 'reverse haemangioma pattern'(early central enhancement withperipheral progressive enhancement on delayed phases) have been described [47, 48]. On MRI, tumors are usually hyperintense and heterogeneous on T2-weighted images, hypointense to the liver on T1-weighted images, with possible areas of high signal intensity indicating intralesions bleeding. Diffusion-weighted images frequently show heterogeneous signal. Enhancement patterns using extracellular contrast agents are the same as seen at CT. Washout is not seen in angiosarcomas, nor is hepatic or portal venous invasion (Fig. 18.7).

## Hepatic Small Vessel Neoplasm

Hepatic small vessel neoplasm (HSVN), recently described, is a very rare infiltrative vascular neoplasm of the liver. Lesions present as an incidental encapsulated nodule (size from 0.2 to 16 cm in diameter). Histologically, well-differentiate small vessels predominate with typical sinusoidal growth pattern and infiltrative borders. Endothelial cells are flat and regular without nuclear atypia, mitosis or metastasis; low Ki67 staining and negative stains with p53 and c-MYC help to exclude angiosarcoma [6]. Recurrent mutations recently found in these neoplasms (GNAQ or GNA14 affecting the G proteins) are suggestive of benign or congenital lesions and this signature looks consistent with the indolent course of HSVN [49].

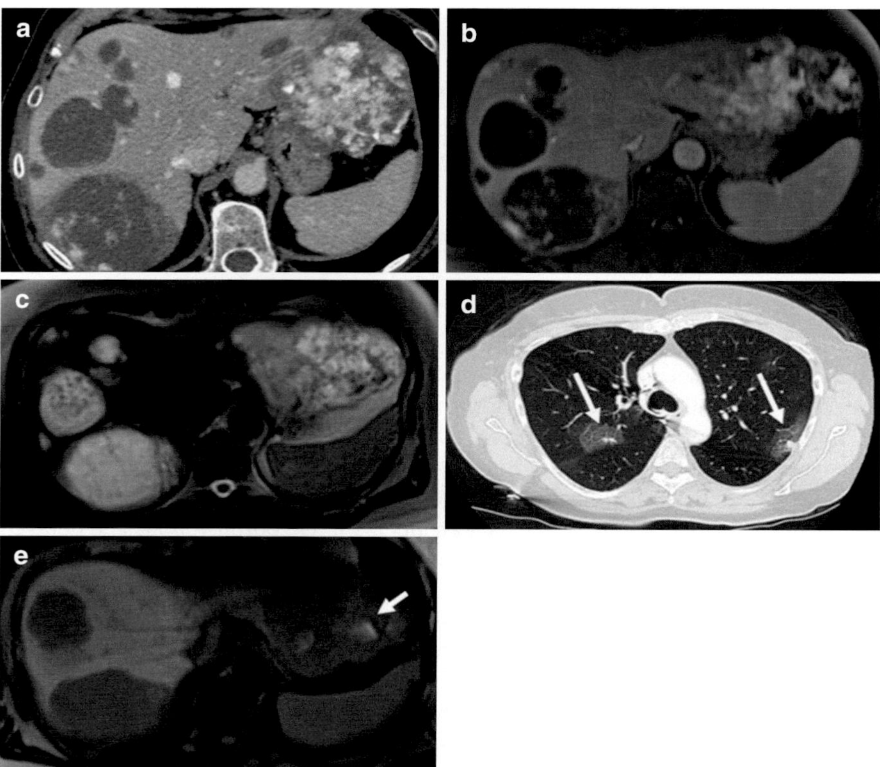

**Fig. 18.7** Angiosarcoma. Abdominal CT (**a**), liver MR imaging (**b-d**) and chest CT (**e**) performed in the same patient as Fig. 18.6. CT shows bilobar lesions with different sizes, showing multiple focal enhancement in the largest ones. The smallest lesions may show no arterial enhancement. On MR imaging, tumors are hyperintense and heterogeneous on T2-weighted images (**b**), hypointense to the liver on T1-wighted images (**c**), and areas of high signal intensity indicating intra-lesions bleeding (arrows). Enhancement patterns using extracellular contrast agents is the same as seen on CT (**d**). Chest CT shows bilateral subcentimetric nodules surrounded by ground glass, consistent with intra-alveolar hemorrhage, and corresponding to lung metastases

Imaging features of HSVN have been poorly described. While angiosarcoma is the main differential on pathology, hemangioma is the main one on imaging. Paisant et al. recently reported four cases in which tumors consistently show continuous irregular thick, rim arterial enhancement with a "flower petal shape" due to early septa enhancement on contrast-enhanced CT, MRI or ultrasound [50].

# Hematologic Neoplasms Affecting Liver Vessels

## *Malignant Lymphoproliferative Disorders*

### Clinical Presentations

Hepatic infiltration by lymphoproliferative diseases may be observed in all non-Hodgkin's B-cell or T-cell lymphomas, Hodgkin's disease and leukemia or myeloma classified according to the WHO classification [51]. Liver is the main organ secondarily affected by lymphoproliferative diseases after lymph nodes, bone marrow and spleen. Involvement of the liver is common in late or advanced stages of the disease and generally associated with splenic infiltration. It remains rare at initial stages. In a German retrospective series of 668 consecutive patients treated for malignant blood disorders, the prevalence of hepatic infiltration diagnosed on the initial radiological examination for staging was 3.3% in non-Hodgkin's lymphoma, 12% in Hodgkin's disease, 1.8% in myeloma and 0% in leukemia [52]. Clinical manifestations of hepatic involvement are diverse, ranging from liver enlargement and abdominal pain to a hemophagocytic syndrome related to systemic activation of macrophages especially in lymphoma associated to Epstein-Barr virus (EBV). Most patients are asymptomatic so that hepatic involvement may be recognized only on imaging for staging, or on needle biopsy done for the evaluation of abnormal liver tests (raised transaminases or cholestasis). Severe hepatic dysfunction including ascites related to a massive hepatic infiltration is extremely rare. A definite diagnosis is reached at trans-jugular liver biopsy performed to investigate for acute liver failure [53]. Jaundice is rare and carries a poor prognosis.

### Imaging Appearance

Lymphomatous involvement of the liver may present as a focal liver mass or masses, or as a diffuse infiltrating disease. Rarely, it corresponds to an ill-defined mass in the porta hepatis [54]. The most frequent imaging presentation of primary lymphoma is that of a solitary lesion, reported in about 60% of cases. Multiple lesions are seen in the remaining patients. Multifocal lesions or diffuse infiltration is the most common aspect of secondary hepatic lymphoma (90%). Innumerable small focal nodules distributed throughout the liver are observed in about 10% of cases of secondary non-Hodgkin lymphoma or Hodgkin disease. At CT, nodules are iso or hypoattenuating to the liver, and enhance less than the surroundingliver parenchyma on arterial, portal venous, or delayed phase images. The lesions may contain hemorrhage, or necrosis, but calcification are rare before treatment. At

MRI, the nodules are hypo- or isointense on T1-weighted images and mildly hyperintense on T2-weighted images. On contrast-enhanced images the enhancement pattern is similar to that above described at CT. Diffusion-weighted images is important component because the highly cellular content of lymphoma translates into a markedlyrestricted diffusion. Whole-body diffusion-weighted imaging has been suggested to be as sensitive as FDG PET/CT for tumor staging [55–57]. FDGPET/CT demonstrates avid hypermetabolism in primary and secondary liver lymphoma, and it is usually an imaging modality of choice for staging and for assessing treatment response.


**Histopathological Features**

The hepatic involvement varies according to the type of disorder. Three main patterns of infiltration can be described: the prominent portal infiltration, the nodular growth pattern, and the sinusoidal infiltration [58]. Most hepatic lymphomas correspond to secondary dissemination, although elevated liver tests may be the first manifestation. Primary hepatic lymphoma is exceptional and corresponds to a diffuse large B-cell lymphoma with a typical nodular pattern, mainly associated with HCV infection.

Curently, the vast majority of hepatic lymphoma are non-Hodgkin lymphomas (90% of all lymphomas). Hepatic infiltration by Hodgkin's lymphoma (10% of all lymphomas) is therefore rare. When present, it is classically restricted to portal tracts without sinusoidal infiltration. Among non-Hodgkin lymphomas, B-cell lymphomas dominate (>80%). Most of the B-cell lymphomas present initially with minimal systemic diffusion, so that a liver infiltration is observed mainly in advanced stages or in relapses. Aggressive diffuse large B-cell lymphomas (including Burkitt lymphoma)– representing half of the patients— display a typical nodular pattern with macroscopic nodulation in the liver visible and easily identified at imaging. Mature B-cell indolent lymphomas (lymphocytic, follicular, marginal zone or mantle B-cell lymphomas…) infiltrate liver parenchyma preferentially in portal tracts without nodulation (Fig. 18.8). Only hairy B-cell leukemia, lymphoblastic B-cell lymphoma/leukemia and plasmoblastic leukemia predominantly infiltrate sinusoids [58, 59]. Sinusoidal infiltration by plasma cells is observed in 32-48% of multiple myeloma and clinical manifestation of liver failure is generally present in terminal phase of the disease; it may exceptionally be the initial manifestation [60]. Intravascular large B-cell lymphoma is exceptional and characterized by predominant growth of centroblastes in blood vessels of brain, spleen, liver and bone-marrow, associated with hemophagocytic syndrome in Asian patients [61].

Peripheral T-cell lymphoma differs from B-cell lymphoma in clinical presentation by a frequent systemic diffusion in spleen, liver and bone marrow without lymphadenopathy or bulky mass. Histologically, diffuse sinusoidal infiltrate without nodulation dominate in most of T-cell lymphomas. According to the WHO

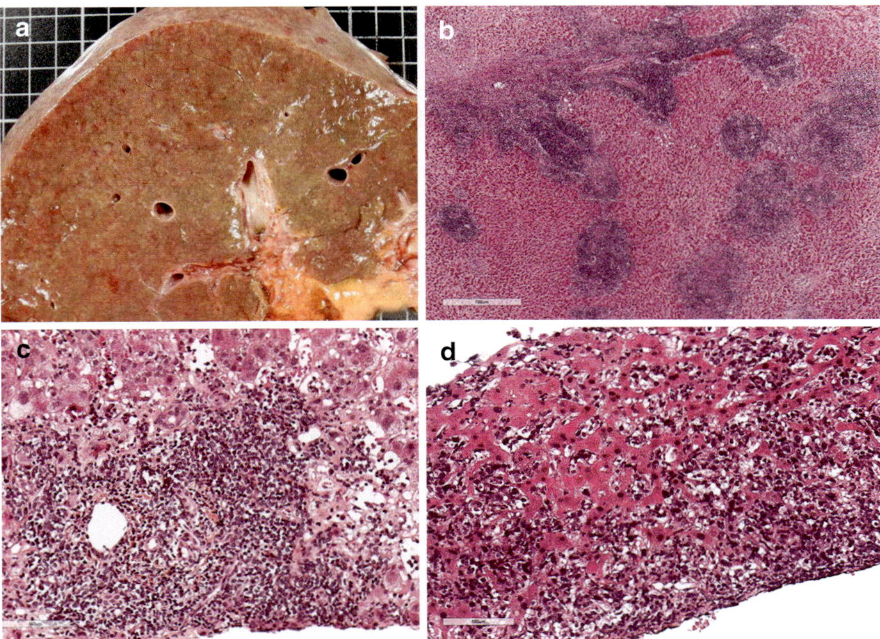

**Fig. 18.8** Liver infiltration by B-cell lymphoma/leukemia. (**a/b**) Chronic lymphocytic leukemia (CLL) at terminal stage (autopsy). (**a**) Hepatic enlargement with on cut section an homogeneous and pale parenchyma without nodule. (**b**) Histological section shows massive infiltration of all portal tracts by CLL. (**c**) B-lymphoblastic leukemia infiltration initially presenting as an acute liver failure (transjugular biopsy): medium and monomorphic lymphoblasts engorge all portal tracts with peri-portal necrosis. (**d**) Diffuse large B-cell lymphoma at a relapse stage forming nodulation at imaging: lymphomatous infiltration generate a diffuse parenchymal destruction

classification, two variants of T-cell lymphomas (representing less than 2% of non-Hodgkin lymphomas and rapidly lethal) may present with primary (or early) hepatic infiltration. First, the extranodal natural killer (NK)/T-cell lymphoma associated to EBV observed preferentially in Asia because of a high EBV prevalence that area: it expresses activated cytotoxic markers (TiA1/Granzyme B), while inducing extensive tissue necrosis, angiodestruction and cytokinemia with macrophage stimulation and hemophagocytosis [62]. Second, the hepatosplenic $\gamma\delta$ T-cell lymphoma occurs *de novo* (80%) in young male (median age 35 year-old), or during immunosuppressive therapy inducing clonal expansion of $\gamma\delta$ T-cells (20%): it presents with hepatosplenomegaly, deep thrombocytopenia and severe B-symptoms. Microscopically, the infiltrate consists of small size monomorphic T-cells in hepatic sinusoids (CD3 +, CD5-, CD4¬, CD8-, CD56+, Granzyme-B-, EBV-), in bone marrow sinuses and red splenic pulp [63] (Fig. 18.9). Specific cytogenetic abnormalities (isochromosome 7q, trisomy 8), and more recently mutations in STAT3, STAT5B genes (in 10 and 30% of cases respectively) have been involved in the pathogenesis through inducing activation of JAK/STAT pathway [63]. Progress in genetic studies could rapidly lead to novel targeted therapy. T-cell large granular lymphocytic

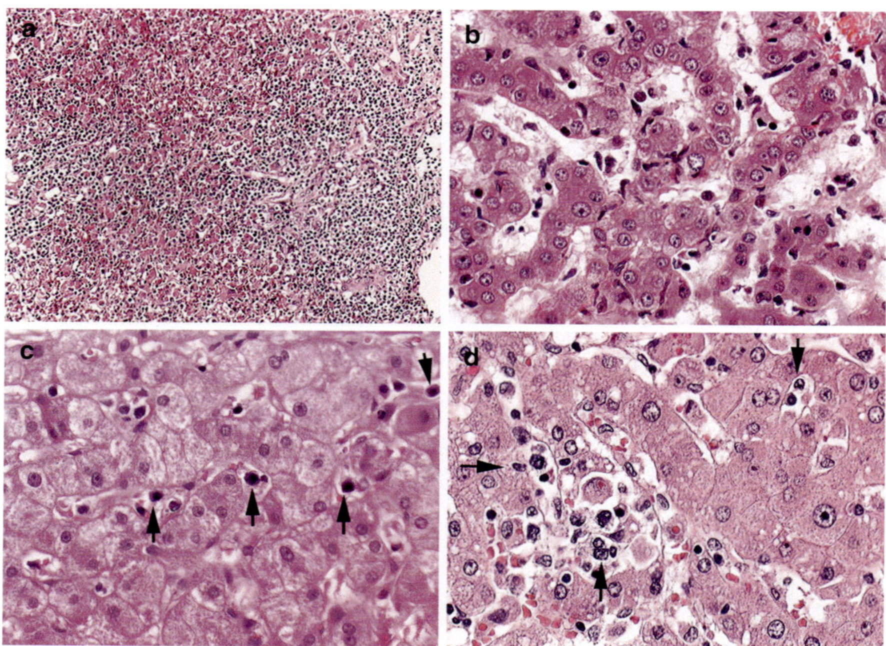

**Fig. 18.9** Liver infiltration by T-cell lymphoma/leukemia. (**a**) T/NK lymphoblastic leukemia presenting as an acute liver failure with a rapid fatal course (post-mortem biopsy): parenchyma is hemorrhagic and necrotic and diffusely infiltrate by medium lymphoblasts. (**b**) Peripheral T-cell lymphoma with liver involvement characterized by atypical small T-cell in dilated sinusoids admixed with Kupffer hyperplasia. (**c**) Hepatosplenic T-cell lymphoma presenting with hepatosplenomegaly: small size atypical lymphocytes with irregular nuclei (arrow) are sited in sinusoids without heptocellular damage. (**d**) NK/T-cell EBV+ lymphoma presenting initially with hepatic infiltration and an hemophagocytic syndrome: pleomorphic large T-cell (arrow) are seen in dilated sinusoids with hemophagocytosis in Kupffer cells

leukemia with azurophilic cytoplasmic granules in cytology is the main differential diagnosis. Liver infiltration of acute leukemia/lymphoma (myeloid, T, B or NK-cell type) may generate massive portal and sinusoidal infiltration producing acute liver failure.

The reactive hemophagocytic syndrome is a hyperinflammatory syndrome potentially fatal caused by dysregulated immune response to a trigger. Malignant lymphoproliferations (mainly EBV-related lymphoma) and infections (viral, fungic, bacterial) are the major triggers inducing cytokinemia and macrophage activation (INF-g, TNF-a, IL-1/6/18) [64]. Clinically it is characterized by fever, jaundice, hepatosplenomegaly, cytopenia, hypertriglyceridemia, hyperferritinemia. Bone marrow or liver biopsy is necessary to detect hemophagocytosis. In the liver, hemophagocytosis is seen inKupffer cells locatedin dilated sinusoids [65].

# Mastocytosis

Systemic mastocytosis is a clonal neoplastic mast-cell proliferation characterized by atypical mast-cells in organs other than the skin, including the liver, the spleen, the gastrointestinal tract and lymph nodes. New WHO classification encompasses indolent systemic mastocytosis, aggressive systemic mastocytosis, systemic mastocytosis associated with another neoplastic hematopoietic disease, and mast cell leukemia [66]. The symptoms of systemic mastocytosis are non-specific, linked to histamine-releasing, including flush, pruritus, diarrhea, abdominal pain, bronchospasm or headache. Hepatic involvement during systemicmastocytosis is frequent [67] presenting with liver enlargement, ascites, portal hypertension, jaundice or isolated abnormalities of liver tests. In the absence of suggestive skin involvement, the diagnosis of systemic mastocytosis is based on histologic features including sinusoid and portal infiltration by atypical mast-cells forming clusters of at least 15 atypical mast-cells (Fig. 18.10). Identification of mast-cells needs immunohistochemistry (expression of CD117, Tryptase, CD25) since neoplastic mast cells characteristic of systemic mastocytosis are degranulated on conventional Toluidine or Giemsa

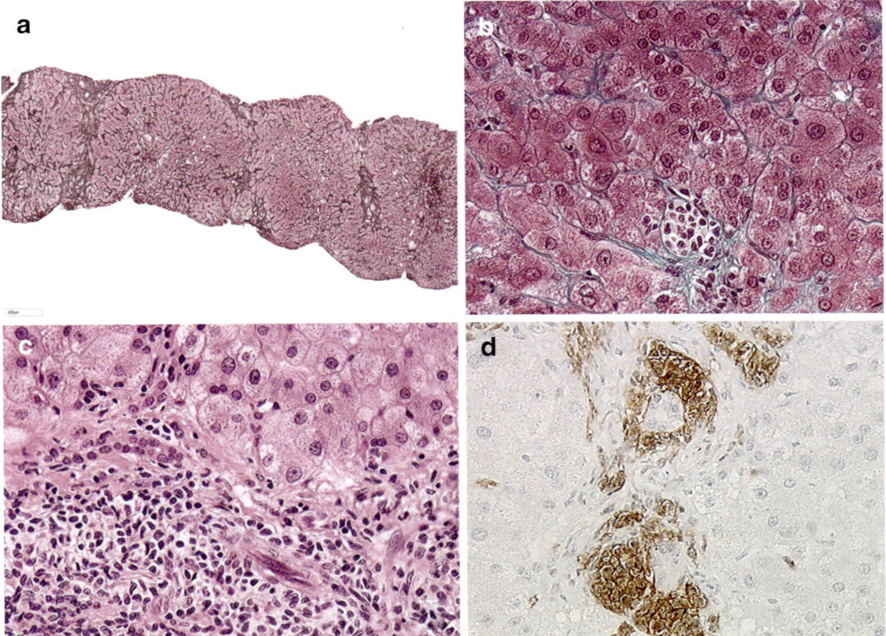

**Fig. 18.10** Liver infiltration by systemic mastocytosis (patients presenting with portal hypertension and ascites). (**a**) Liver parenchyma exhibits on argentic stain regenerative changes without cirrhosis and a diffuse sinusoidal fibrosis. (**b**) Nests of atypical mast-cell are seen in sinusoids. (**c**) A portal tract is infiltrate by spindle degranulated mast-cells. (**d**) Mast-cells express c-KIT in immunohistochemistry

staining. Affected portal spaces and sinusoids present with fibrosis deposit correlated with the amount of neoplastic mast-cells. Secondarily, a nodular regenerative hyperplasia with obliterative portal venopathy mimicking vascular portal-sinusoidal disease with clinically non-cirrhotic portal hypertension may develop [68, 69].

## Myeloid Metaplasia

Portal hypertension is a well-known complication of myeloproliferative neoplasms arising in around 10% of patients with polycythemia vera, thrombocytemia or primary myelofibrosis. Portal hypertension results from various causes: thrombosis of portal veins (extrahepatic and intrahepatic), thrombosis of hepatic veins, sinusoidal fibrosis with or without myeloid metaplasia and nodular regenerative hyperplasia [70]. Wanless et al. described these lesions in details in a large series of patients with myelofibrosis and polycythemia vera collected on autopsy before 1990 [71]: thrombotic processes in large, medium and small portal veins associated with sinusoidal fibrosis/dilation and nodular regenerative hyperplasia play a major role in causing non-cirrhotic portal hypertension. Microvascular portal alteration characterized by obliterative portal venopathy is highly correlated withmacrovascular portal thrombosis and may reflect thromboembolic extension to terminal portal venules.

Myeloid infiltration of sinusoids is classically observed in advanced fibrotic stage of myelofibrosis representing extramedullary hematopoiesis in spleen and liver; it is isolated or associated with perisinusoidal fibrosis and hepatocellular regenerative changes (Fig. 18.11). Extra-medullary hematopoiesis observed in all patients of Wanless's series was severe in a minority of patients and displays no correlation with portal hypertension. Long-term improvement after anticoagulation of portal hypertension in myeloproliferative neoplasmsis in agreement with the major role of thrombosis in the genesis of vascular portal–sinusoidal disease [72]. Radiological features (hepatosplenomegaly and lymphadenopathies) are the result of extramedullary haematopoiesis, causing global hepatomegaly without nodulation.

## Amyloidosis

Hepatic amyloidosis is observed in systemic amyloidosis and classically associated with cardiac and renal involvement which are highly related to the outcome [73]. Hepatic amyloidosis is rarely symptomatic but can be a presenting feature: less than 30% of patients show clinical symptoms but palpable hepatomegaly is present in 80% of patients directly related to parenchymal infiltration [74]. Portal hypertension is rare and ascites may be secondary to liver infiltration, hypoproteinemia and heart failure. Jaundice is exceptional and lately associated with renal failure and apoor short-term outcome [75]. Liver tests abnormalities (elevations of gamma-GT and alkaline phosphatase) are unrelated with the degree of amyloid infiltration.

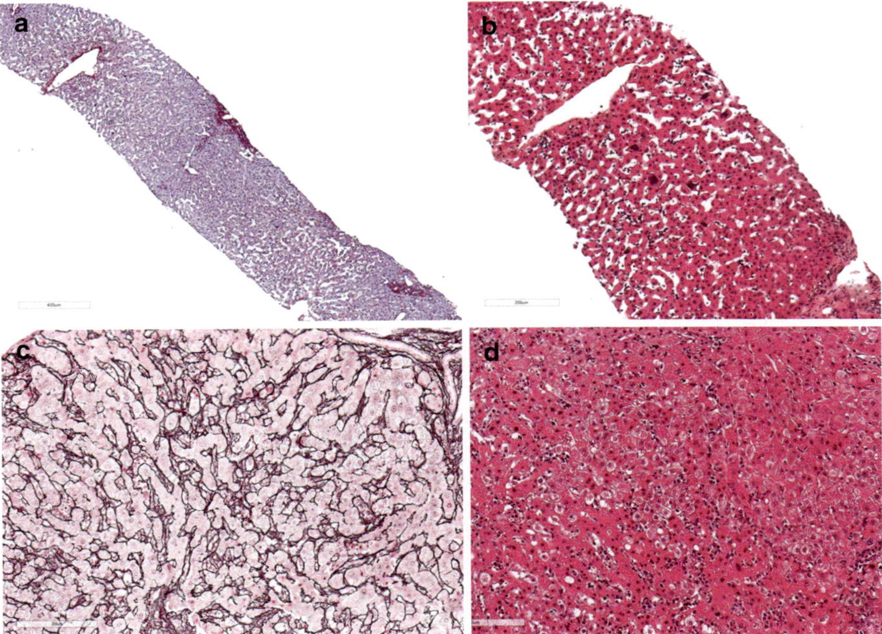

**Fig. 18.11** Myeloid metaplasia in liver. (**a**/**b**) Myeloid metaplasia associated with JAK2 mutated polycythemia vera (biopsy done for portal hypertension). (**a**) Parenchyma shows isolated sinusoidal dilation. (**b**) Neoplastic hematopoiesis (megakaryocytes and erythroblasts) is noticed in dilated sinusoids. (**c**/**d**) Myeloid metaplasia associated with myelofibrosis at a fibrotic stage (biopsy done for refractory ascites). (**c**) Argentic stain shows diffuse sinusoid fibrosis. (**d**) The myeloid infiltration in sinusoids generates focal hepatocellular atrophy

Rare cases of spontaneous intrahepatic hematomas have been reported in patients with AL type amyloidosis [76]. Diagnosis of amyloidosis requires a liver biopsy. However, amyloidosis is deemed to expose to an increased risk of biopsy related bleeding [74]. The transjugular transvenous routemay therefore prove particularly helpful. Histological examination shows amorphous eosinophilic deposits in artery walls and Disse's spaces causing atrophy of hepatocyte trabeculae when abundant (Fig. 18.12). Pathologists must be informed of amyloidosis suspicion in order to use specific stains for diagnostic confirmation: Congo red stains extra-cellular deposits and gives a characteristic yellow-green birefringence in polarized light. Amyloid deposits are classified into type AA or AL depending on clinical context. SAA parafin-immunostain is performed to characterize AA type amyloidosis; direct immunofluorescence technics on frozen sections are necessary for AL amyloidosis. AL type amyloidosis is associated with hemopathies producing B-clones, wether initially known or diagnosed using electrophoresis of serum and urinary proteins, myelogram and/or osteomedullary biopsy and cytogenetics for myeloma. Imaging features of liver amyloidosis are non-specific, including hepatomegaly due to massive amyloid deposition. Occasionally, focal areas of low attenuation within

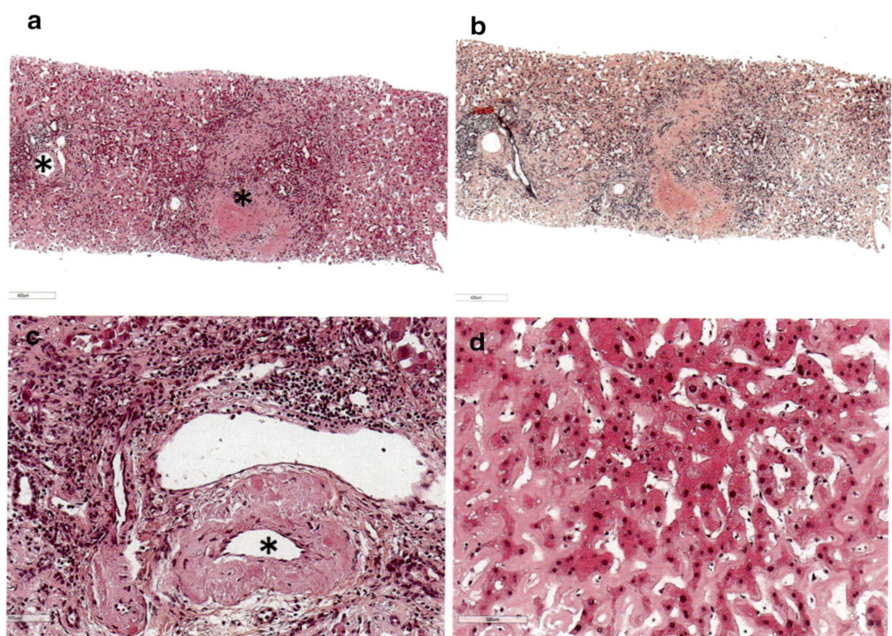

**Fig. 18.12** Hepatic amyloidosis in a multivisceral AL amyloidosis (a-d). (**a**) Hepatic infiltration by amyloidosis involving all sinusoids and some portal tracts (*). (**b**) Amyloid deposit is stained in red with Red Congo. (**c**) Portal veins look normal whereas hepatic arteries have thickened infiltrated walls. (**d**) Disse spaces are filled with amorphous pale acellular deposit leading to hepatocellular atrophy

the liver and spleen can be seen at CT, corresponding to sites of amyloid deposition named "amyloid pseudotumor appearance". Delayed enhancement has also been reported.

# Conclusion

Hepatic tumors of vascular origin include both very common and very rare lesions. On one hand, hemangioma is, by far, the most frequent solid hepatic tumor. It follows an indolent course of evolution, and rarely exposes patients to complications. The diagnosis can be reached non-invasively by imaging in the vast majority of the patients. On the other end of the spectrum, a heterogeneous group of very rare neoplasms present with different clinical course, pathologic features, imaging appearance and prognosis. While epithelioid hemangioendothelioma may present with a wide range of clinical presentations, angiosarcomas are very aggressive and rapidly progressive tumors with a dismal prognosis. In both cases, imaging can approach the diagnosis but pathology is always mandatory.

Hepatic vessels may also be infiltrated by various haematopoietic and lymphoid neoplasms. In most cases of leukemia and lymphoma, the liver may secondarily be involved. Imaging may suggest the diagnosis but definite diagnosis relies on liver biopsy for extensive pathological analysis. Other disorders, e.g. amyloidosis or systemic mastocytosis, affect predominantly sinusoids or the venous beds and therefore induce secondary vascular disorders.

# References


1. Semelka RC, Sokka CM. Hepatic hemangiomas. Magn Reson Imaging Clin N Am. 1997;5:241–53.
2. Mergo PJ, Ros PR. Benign lesions of the liver. Radiol Clin N Am. 1998;36:319–31.
3. Trotter JF, Everson GT. Benign focal lesions of the liver. Clin Liver Dis. 2001;5:17–42.
4. Biecker E, Fischer HP, Strunk H, et al. Benign hepatic tumours. Z Gastroenterol. 2003;41:191–200.
5. Craig JR, Peters RL, Edmondson HA. Tumors of the liver and intrahepatic bile ducts. AFIP 1988, Washington p. 64–75.
6. Gill RM, Buelow B, Mather C, Joseph NM, Alves V, Brunt EM, Liu TC, Makhlouf H, Marginean C, Nalbantoglu I, Sempoux C, Snover DC, Thung SN, Yeh MM, Ferrell LD. Hepatic small vessel neoplasm, a rare infiltrative vascular neoplasm of uncertainmalignant potential. Hum Pathol. 2016 Aug;54:143–51.
7. Takayasu K, Makuuchi M, Takayama T. Computed tomography of a rapidly growing hepatic hemangioma. J Comput Assist Tomogr. 1990;14:143–5.
8. Nghiem HV, Bogost GA, Ryan JA, et al. Cavernous hemangiomas of the liver: enlargement over time. AJR. 1997;169:137–40.
9. Bornman PC, Terblanche J, Blumgart RL, et al. Giant hepatic hemangiomas: diagnostic and therapeutic dilemmas. Surgery. 1987;101:445–9.
10. Pateron D, Babany G, Belghiti J, et al. Giant hemangioma of the liver with pain, fever, and abnormal liver tests: report of two cases. Dig Dis Sci. 1991;36:524–7.
11. Pol B, Disdier P, Le Treut YP, et al. Inflammatory process complicating giant hemangioma of the liver: a report of three cases. Liver Transplant Surg. 1998;4:204–7.
12. Bree RL, Schwab RE, Glazer GM, Fink-Bennett D. The varied appearances of hepatic cavernous hemangiomas with sonography, computed tomography, magnetic resonance imaging and scintigraphy. Radiographics. 1987;7:1153–75.
13. Tano S, Veno N, Tomiyama T, Kimura K. Possibility of differentiating small hyperechoic liver tumors using contrast enhanced colour Doppler ultrasonography: a preliminary study. Clin Radiol. 1997;52:41–5.
14. Quaia E, Bertolotto M, Dalla PL. Characterization of liver hemangiomas with pulse inversion harmonic imaging. Eur Radiol. 2002;12:537–44.
15. Youk JH, Kim CS, Lee JM. Contrast-enhanced agent detection imaging: value in the characterization of focal hepatic lesions. J Ultrasound Med. 2003;22:897–910.
16. Leen E, Ceccotti P, Kalogeropoulos C, et al. Prospective multicenter trial evaluating a novel method of characterizing focal liver lesions using contrast-enhanced sonography. AJR Am J Roentegenol. 2006;186:1551–9.
17. Freeny PC, Marks WM. Hepatic hemangioma: dynamic bolus CT. AJR. 1986;147:711–9.
18. Nino-Murcia M, Olcott EW, Brooke Jeffrey R, et al. Focal liver lesions: pattern-based classification scheme for enhancement at arterial phase CT. Radiology. 2000;215:746–51.
19. Itai Y, Ohtomo K, Furui S, et al. Noninvasive diagnosis of small cavernous hemangioma of the liver: advantage of MRI. AJR Am J Roentgenol. 1985;145:1195–9.

20. Starck DD, Felder RC, Wittenberg J, et al. Magnetic resonance imaging of cavernous hemangioma of the liver: tissue-specific characterization. AJR. 1985;145:213–22.
21. Semelka RC, Brown ED, Ascher SM, et al. Hepatic hemangiomas: a multi-institutional study of appearance on T2-weighted and serial gadolinium-enhanced gradient-echo MR images. Radiology. 1994;192:401–6.
22. Taouli B, Koh DM. Diffusion-weighted MR imaging of the liver. Radiology. 2010;254:47–66.
23. Doo KW, Lee CH, Choi JW, et al. "Pseudo washout" sign in high-flow hepatic hemangioma on gadoxetic acid contrast-enhanced MRI mimicking hypervascular tumor. AJR Am J Roentgenol. 2009;193:490–6.
24. Danet IM, Semelka RC, Braga L, et al. Giant hemangioma of the liver: MR imaging characteristics in 24 patients. Magn Reson Imaging. 2003;21:95–101.
25. Coumbaras M, Wendum D, Monnier-Cholley L, et al. CT and MR imaging features of pathologically proven atypical giant hemangioma of the liver. AJR. 2002;179:1457–63.
26. Valls C, Rene M, Gil M, et al. Giant cavernous hemangioma of the liver: atypical CT and MR findings. Eur Radiol. 1996;6:448–50.
27. Choi BI, Han MC, Park JH, et al. Giant cavernous hemangioma of the liver: CT and MR imaging in 10 cases. AJR Am J Roentgenol. 1989;152:12221–1226.
28. Hanafusa K, Ohashi I, Himeno Y, et al. Hepatic hemangioma: findings with two-phase CT. Radiology. 1995;196:465–9.
29. Kim KW, Kim TK, Han JK, et al. Hepatic hemangiomas with arterio-portal shunt: findings at two-phase CT. Radiology. 2001;219:707–11.
30. Byun JH, Kim TK, Lee CW, et al. Arterioportal shunt: prevalence in small hemangiomas versus that in hepatocellular carcinomas 3 cm or smaller at two-phase helical CT. Radiology. 2004;232:354–60.
31. Jang HJ, Kim TK, Lim HK, et al. Hepatic hemangioma: atypical appearances on CT, MR imaging, and sonography. AJR Am J Roentgenol. 2003;180:135–41.
32. Hihara T, Araki T, Katou K, et al. Cystic cavernous hemangioma of the liver. Gastrointest Radiol. 1990;15:112–4.
33. Soyer P, Bluemke DA, Fishman EK, et al. Fluid-fluid levels within focal hepatic lesions: imaging appearance and etiology. Abdom Imaging. 1998;23:161–5.
34. Yang DM, Yoon MH, Kim HS, et al. Capsular retraction in hepatic giant hemangioma: CT and MR features. Abdom Imaging. 2001;26:36–8.
35. Matsuhita M, Takehara Y, Nasu H, et al. Atypically enhanced cavernous hemangiomas of the liver: centrifugal enhancement does not preclude the diagnosis of hepatic hemangioma. J Gastroenterol. 2006;41:1227–30.
36. Weiss SW, Enzinger F. Epithelioid hemangioendothelioma a vascular tumor often mistaken for a carcinoma. Cancer. 1982;50(5):970–81.
37. Makhlouf HR, Ishak KG, Goodman ZD. Epithelioid hemangioendothelioma of the liver. Cancer. 1999;85(3):562–82.
38. Uchimura K, Nakamuta M, Osoegawa M, et al. Hepatic epithelioid hemangioendothelioma. J Clin Gastroenterol. 2001;32(5):431–4.
39. Mehrabi A, Kashfi A, Fonouni H, et al. Primary malignant hepatic epithelioid hemangioendothelioma. Cancer. 2006;107(9):2108–21.
40. Amin S, Chung H, Jha R. Hepatic epithelioid hemangioendothelioma: MR imaging findings. Abdom Imaging. 2011;36(4):407–14.
41. Miller W, Dodd G 3rd, Federle M, Baron R. Epithelioid hemangioendothelioma of the liver: imaging findings with pathologic correlation. AJR Am J Roentgenol. 1992;159(1):53–7.
42. Paolantonio P, Laghi A, Vanzulli A, et al. MRI of hepatic epithelioid hemangioendothelioma (HEH). J Magn Reson Imaging. 2014;40(3):552–8.
43. Kim HR, Rha SY, Cheon SH, et al. Clinical features and treatment outcomes of advanced stage primary hepatic angiosarcoma. Ann Oncol. 2009;20(4):780–7. https://doi.org/10.1093/annonc/mdn702.

44. Yasir S, Torbenson MS. Angiosarcoma of the liver: Clinicopathologic Featuresand morphologic patterns. Am J Surg Pathol. 2019 May;43(5):581–90.
45. Falk H, Herbert J, Crowley S, et al. Epidemiology of hepatic angiosarcoma in the United States: 1964-1974. Environ Health Perspect. 1981;41:107–13.
46. Locker GY, Doroshow JH, Zwelling LA, Chabner BA. The clinical features of hepatic angiosarcoma: a report of four cases and a review of the English literature. Medicine. 1979;58(1):48–64.
47. Pickhardt PJ, Kitchin D, Lubner MG, et al. Primary hepatic angiosarcoma: multi-institutional comprehensive cancer Centre review of multiphasic CT and MR imaging in 35 patients. Eur Radiol. 2015;25(2):315–22. https://doi.org/10.1007/s00330-014-3442-0.
48. Koyama T, Fletcher JG, Johnson CD, et al. Primary hepatic angiosarcoma: findings at CT and MR imaging. Radiology. 2002;222(3):667–73.
49. Joseph NM, Brunt EM, Marginean C, Nalbantoglu I, Snover DC, Thung SN, Yeh MM, Umetsu SE, Ferrell LD, Gill RM. Frequent GNAQ and GNA14 mutations in hepatic small vessel neoplasm. Am J Surg Pathol. 2018 Sep;42(9):1201–120.
50. Paisant A, Bellal B, Lebigot J, Canivet CM, Michalak S, Aubé C imaging features of hepatic small vessel neoplasm: case series. Hepatology. 2021 Jun 15. https://doi.org/10.1002/hep.31779. Online ahead of print.
51. Swerdlow SH, Campo E, Pileri SA, Harris NL, Stein H, Siebert R, et al. The 2016 revision of the World Health Organization classification of lymphoid neoplasms. Blood. 2016;127(20):2375–90.
52. Bach AG, Behrmann C, Holzhausen HJ, Spielmann RP, Surov A. Prevalence and imaging of hepatic involvement in malignant lymphoproliferative disease. Clin Imaging. 2012 Oct;36(5):539–46.
53. Rich NE, Sanders C, Hughes RS, Fontana RJ, Stravitz RT, Fix O, et al. Malignant infiltration of the liver presenting as acute liver failure. Clin Gastroenterol Hepatol Off Clin Pract J Am Gastroenterol Assoc. 2015 May;13(5):1025–8.
54. Tomasian A, Sandrasegaran K, Elsayes KM, Shanbhogue A, Shaaban A, Menias CO. Hematologic malignancies of the liver: spectrum of disease. Radiographics. 2015 Jan-Feb;35(1):71–86.
55. Foschi FG, Dall'Aglio AC, Marano G, et al. Role of contrastenhanced ultrasonography in primary hepatic lymphoma. J Ultrasound Med. 2010;29(9):1353–6.
56. Kwee TC, Takahara T, Vermoolen MA, Bierings MB, Mali WP, Nievelstein RA. Whole-body diffusion-weighted imaging for staging malignant lymphoma in children. Pediatr Radiol. 2010;40(10):1592–602. quiz 1720–1721
57. Lin C, Itti E, Luciani A, Haioun C, Meignan M, Rahmouni A. Whole-body diffusion-weighted imaging in lymphoma. Cancer Imaging. 2010;10(A):S172–8.
58. Loddenkemper C, Longerich T, Hummel M, Ernestus K, Anagnostopoulos I, Dienes H-P, et al. Frequency and diagnostic patterns of lymphomas in liver biopsies with respect to the WHO classification. Virchows Arch Int J Pathol. 2007 May;450(5):493–502.
59. Kim M-J, Park H-S, Yhim H-Y. Intravascular large b-cell lymphoma diagnosed via transjugular liver biopsy in a patient with liver dysfunction and thrombocytopenia: a case report. Medicine (Baltimore). 2017 May;96(19):e6925.
60. Coffey D, Fain B, Thompson C, Chan ED, Nawaz S. Liver failure as the only clinical manifestation of multiple myeloma. Ann Hematol. 2012 Apr;91(4):625–7.
61. Ponzoni M, Campo E, Nakamura S. Intravascular large B-cell lymphoma: a chameleon with multiple faces and many masks. Blood. 2018 Oct 11;132(15):1561–7.
62. Zing NPC, Fischer T, Zain J, Federico M, Rosen ST. Peripheral T-cell lymphomas: incorporating new developments in diagnostics, prognostication, and treatment into clinical practice-PART 2: ENKTL, EATL, indolent T-cell LDP of the GI tract, ATLL, and Hepatosplenic T-cell lymphoma. Oncol Williston Park N. 2018;32(8):e83–9.
63. Yabe M, Miranda RN, Medeiros LJ. Hepatosplenic T-cell lymphoma: a review of clinicopathologic features, pathogenesis, and prognostic factors. Hum Pathol. 2018 Apr;74:5–16.

64. Wang H, Xiong L, Tang W, Zhou Y, Li F. A systematic review of malignancy-associated hemophagocytic lymphohistiocytosis that needs more attentions. Oncotarget. 2017 Aug 29;8(35):59977–85.
65. De Gottardi J, Montani M, Angelillo-Scherrer A, Rovo A, Berzigotti A. Hepatic sinusoidal hemophagocytosis with and without hemophagocytic lymphohistiocytosis. PLoS One. 2019 Dec 30;14(12):e0226899.
66. Valent P, Akin C, Metcalfe DD. Mastocytosis: 2016 updated WHO classification and novel emerging treatment concepts. Blood. 2017;129(11):1420–7.
67. Mican JM, Di Bisceglie AM, Fong TL, Travis WD, Kleiner DE, Baker B, et al. Hepatic involvement in mastocytosis: clinicopathologic correlations in 41 cases. Hepatol Baltim Md. 1995 Oct;22(4 Pt 1):1163–70.
68. Martins C, Teixeira C, Ribeiro S, Trabulo D, Cardoso C, Mangualde J, et al. Systemic mastocytosis: a rare cause of non-cirrhotic portal hypertension. World J Gastroenterol. 2016 Jul 28;22(28):6559–64.
69. Yoshida M, Nishikawa Y, Yamamoto Y, Doi Y, Tokairin T, Yoshioka T, et al. Mast cell leukemia with rapidly progressing portal hypertension. Pathol Int. 2009 Nov;59(11):817–22.
70. Degott C, Capron JP, Bettan L, Molas G, Bernuau D, Potet F, et al. Myeloid metaplasia, perisinusoidal fibrosis, and nodular regenerative hyperplasia of the liver. Liver. 1985 Oct;5(5):276–81.
71. Wanless IR, Peterson P, Das A, Boitnott JK, Moore GW, Bernier V. Hepatic vascular disease and portal hypertension in polycythemia vera and agnogenic myeloid metaplasia: a clinicopathological study of 145 patients examined at autopsy. Hepatol Baltim Md. 1990 Nov;12(5):1166–74.
72. Cazals-Hatem D, Hillaire S, Rudler M, Plessier A, Paradis V, Condat B, et al. Obliterative portal venopathy: portal hypertension is not always present at diagnosis. J Hepatol. 2011 Mar;54(3):455–61.
73. Gertz MA, Kyle RA. Hepatic amyloidosis: clinical appraisal in 77 patients. Hepatology. 1997 Jan;25(1):118–21.
74. Park MA, Mueller PS, Kyle RA, Larson DR, Plevak MF, Gertz MA. Primary (AL) hepatic amyloidosis: clinical features and natural history in 98 patients. Medicine (Baltimore). 2003 Sep;82(5):291–8.
75. Peters RA, Koukoulis G, Gimson A, Portmann B, Westaby D, Williams R. Primary amyloidosis and severe intrahepatic cholestatic jaundice. Gut. 1994 Sep;35(9):1322–5.
76. Tam M, Seldin DC, Forbes BM, Connors LH, Skinner M, Oran B, et al. Spontaneous rupture of the liver in a patient with systemic AL amyloidosis undergoing treatment with high-dose melphalan and autologous stem cell transplantation: a case report with literature review. Amyloid Int J Exp Clin Investig Off J Int Soc Amyloidosis. 2009;16(2):103–7.

# Chapter 19
# Primary Immunodeficiencies and Non Malignant Hematologic Disease Associated with Disorders of Hepatic Vessels

Marion Malphettes

## Primary Immunodeficiencies Associated with Disorders of Hepatic Vessels

Primary immunodeficiency diseases (PIDs) encompass more than 400 distinct disorders usually characterized by increased susceptibility to infection, and sometimes associated to auto-immunity, inflammation, lymphoproliferation or malignancy [1]. PIDs are often inherited and may be caused by defects affecting any component of the adaptative or the innate immune system. Some patients with PIDs may develop disorders of hepatic vessels. These PIDs will be reviewed in the next sections, where they will be categorized according to the classification from the International Union of Immunological Societies [1]. As hepatic vessel disorders may occasionally be the first manifestation of these PIDs, liver specialists should be aware of the main clinical and biological characteristics of each disorder, in order to ensure rapid accurate PID diagnosis (Table 19.1).

### *Predominantly Antibody Deficiencies*

#### Common Variable Immunodeficiency Disorders

Common variable immunodeficiency disorders (CVIDs) are a group of late onset primary antibody failures characterized by hypogammaglobulinemia of at least 2 immunoglobulin (Ig) isotypes and inability to generate effective antibody responses [1]. CVID is categorized as a B-cell disorder, but T-cell defects are frequently

M. Malphettes (✉)
Department of Clinical Immuno-Pathology, Hospital Saint-Louis Paris, Paris, France
e-mail: marion.malphettes@aphp.fr

© Springer Nature Switzerland AG 2022
D. Valla et al. (eds.), *Vascular Disorders of the Liver*,
https://doi.org/10.1007/978-3-030-82988-9_19

**Table 19.1** Main clinical and biological characteristics of immuno-hematological disorders likely revealed by hepatic vessel disorders

|  | Clinical clues | Biological tools |
|---|---|---|
| **PAD** | Consanguinity, personal or family history of infection, auto-immunity or lymphoproliferation | IgG, IgA, IgM trough level Immunophenotype: T and B cell naïve and memory subsets |
| **CGD** | Consanguinity, personal or family history of typical infection (*Serratia marcescens, Burkholderia cepacia, aspergillus, liver abscess)* or inflammatory diseases (IBD) | Nitroblue tetrazolium test (NBT) or flow cytometry with dihydrorhodamine (DHR) |
| **TBD** | Personal or family history of unexplained cytopenias, pulmonary fibrosis, abnormal skin pigmentation, nail dystrophy, oral leukoplakia or premature greying of hair | Telomere length measurement |
| **PNH** | Personal history of cytopenia, hemolysis or thrombosis | Flow *cytometric* analysis of GPI-anchored proteins |

*PAD* predominantly antibody deficiencies; *CGD* chronic granulomatous disease; *TBD* telomere biology disorders; *PNH* paroxysmal nocturnal hemoglobinuria. *IBD* inflammatory bowel diseases

associated [2]. It is the most frequent form of clinically significant primary immune deficiency, affecting between 1/25000 to 1/500000 of the population. CVID patients are highly susceptible to respiratory infections due to encapsulated bacteria and are also prone to intestinal infections due, among others, to *Giardia, Campylobacter, Salmonella* or *Norovirus* [3–5]. CVID patients have a tendency to develop a range of associated non-infectious complications. These complications are believed to result from the underlying immune dysregulation rather than from infection, even though infection may sometimes act as a trigger. Within the group of CVID, there appear to be distinct clinical phenotypes. Patients can be divided by complication, with some patients experiencing autoimmunity, enteropathy, granuloma, polyclonal lymphoproliferative infiltration or lymphoid malignancies, these belonging to the «Disease-related complications» group; others have no disease-related complications, and belong to the «Infections only» group [6, 7]. The «Infections only» group accounts for two thirds of the CVID patients and the «Disease-related complications» group for the remaining third. The phenotype can be defined early in the follow-up of the patients and the prognosis is markedly different as «Infections only» patients have an almost normal life expectancy while the overall survival of «Disease-related complications» patients is around 50% at 30 years from diagnosis [8]. Liver involvement is present in at least 10% of CVID patients and is associated with increased mortality [8, 9]. Notably, liver damage is a late complication in the natural history of CVID, occurring with a median delay of 8.3 years, IQR (4–16.6) after CVID diagnosis (personal unpublished data from the French DEFI cohort). Overall, infection, lymphoproliferation, granuloma and mostly hepatic vessel disorders, contributes to liver damage in the setting of CVID. Four large studies report on liver disease in CVID, highlighting the high prevalence of hepatic vessel disorders, found in 5 to 12% of patients [10–13]. Of note, hepatitis C virus was occasionally transmitted through contaminated intravenous immunoglobulin preparation before 1991. About 40% of these HCV-infected patients had a rapid progression of HCV infection to end-stage liver disease while ten percent of patients spontaneously cleared the virus [14, 15].

## Pathology

The French study by Malamut et al., published in 2007, reported on 51 primary antibody deficiency patients, including 40 CVID, with liver abnormalities [10]. Among the 23 patients with liver biopsy, 20 had nodular regenerative hyperplasia of the liver (NRH). Eighteen patients had intra-sinusoidal infiltrate associated to NRH, composed of CD8 + T lymphocytes (Fig. 19.1). In seven patients, marked intra-sinusoidal lymphocytic infiltrates were co-localized with sinusoidal dilatation. Eight NRH patients had repeated liver biopsies showing steady or progressive sinusoidal infiltrate over time in respectively 6 and 2 patients. Ten patients had epithelioid granuloma associated to NRH. The presence of granuloma was not associated with the grade of liver cell plate abnormalities, nor with the amount of

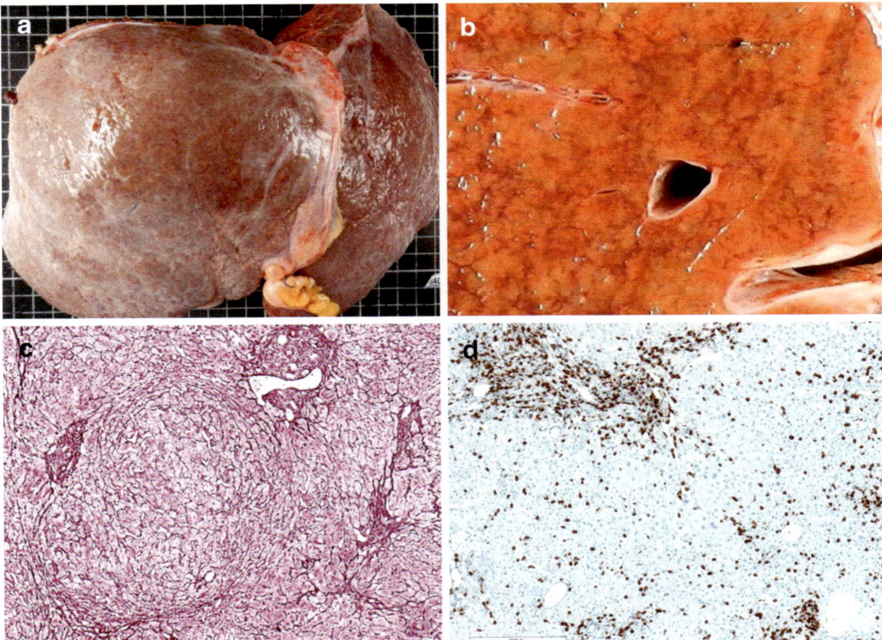

**Fig. 19.1** Common variable immunodeficiency disorder associated with portal-sinusoidal disease (observed in a patient transplanted for non-cirrhotic portal hypertension). (**a**) The liver explant has a rough surface. (**b**) Cut section shows micronodules in non-cirrhotic parenchyma suggestive of nodular regenerative hyperplasia (NRH). (**c**) Histologically, argentation stain emphasizes NRH; portal tracts are round, with small or invisible portal veinules. (**d**) Numerous CD8 T lymphocytes infiltrate portal tracts and sinusoids (Courtesy of Dr. Cazals-Hatem)

intra-sinusoidal infiltrate. Ward et al., reported in 2008 a study focusing on liver disease in 108 CVID patients from their local database [12]. NRH was found in 13 out of 16 reviewed biopsies. NRH was associated with moderate fibrosis in 5 patients, three of whom had granuloma. In the American study from Fuss et al., [11] published in 2013, 14 out of 216 CVID patients were identified as having NRH. NRH was accompanied by peri-sinusoidal fibrosis in 3 patients as well as spotty lobular inflammatory foci, made of lymphocytes and rare microgranuloma in two patients. In six patients, mild to moderate focal portal inflammatory infiltrates were observed. The cells in the infiltrates were CD8+ T lymphocytes, found in both the parenchyma and the portal areas. Activated Kupfer cells were also present, predominantly in the parenchyma areas. Quantitation of cytokine production was conducted in liver samples obtained from 6 patients. IncreasedIFN-γ mRNA was demonstrated in 5 patients, and was most prominent in those with the most severe NRH.

Last, in 2014, Pulvirenti et al. reported an observational single-center study on 111 CVID patients from a single Italian center [13]. Abnormalities of spleno-portal axis were found in 28 CVID patients. Only 5 patients had liver biopsy, each showing NRH, sinusoidal dilatation and mild portal lympho-histiocytic infiltrate.

Of note, an association of NRH and lymphocytic intra-sinusoidal infiltrate was found in up to 87% of liver biopsies in the French study. The issue of a possible relationship between intra-sinusoidal CD8+ T cells and endothelial cell damage has been addressed in the study from Ziol et al. [16]. In this study, an intra-sinusoidal infiltrate was described in 14 of 44 patients with NRH associated with diverse diseases, including a few CVID patients. Some patients had complete resolution of lymphocyte infiltrate on repeated biopsies, suggesting that it could be either transient or patchy. On biopsy samples, intra-sinusoidal lymphocytes were not randomly distributed, but were preferentially located next to atrophic liver cell plates, in close contact with apoptotic endothelial cells. Comparison of T-cell repertoires from liver lymphoid infiltrate and from blood lymphocytes showed marked differences, indicating that the liver T-cell expansions were liver-specific. Among other, endothelial sinusoidal cells can act as antigen presenting cells, leading to CD8+ cytotoxic T cells activation at high antigen concentration [17]. In CVID patients, the activated cytotoxic T cells infiltrating the liver sinusoids might arise from a local antigen driven process targeting the endothelium and being responsible for the chronic sinusoidal cell injury and NRH. The hypothetic antigen presented by the liver endothelial cells and driving this immune activation is not known. Of note, liver damage is strongly associated with enteropathy in CVID patients [12], suggesting a pathogenic role of the gut-liver axis [18]. The association ofhepatic vessel disorders with hepatic granulomas, reported in a few CVID patients, has already been described in the setting of sarcoidosis, with a report of 100 liver biopsy showing 20% of patients having vascular changes, consisting of sinusoïdal dilatation (14 patients) or NRH (9 patients) [19]. In addition, this association is also described in chronic granulomatous disease (see below).

## Evolution and Outcome

In the study by Fuss et al., most NRH patients presented initially with increased alkaline phosphatase (ALP) level, first observed at a mean of 7.8 +/− 2.8 years (range 2 to 19 years) after the time of CVID diagnosis [11]. Regarding liver disease course, there seems to be several patterns, and the authors suggest that NRH could evolve through three distinct courses: in a minority of patients (3/14), the liver disease remained non-progressive, while in a larger proportion (6/14) the disease developed slowly towards portal hypertension and hypersplenism. Finally, a small group of patients, presenting with an associated auto-immune hepatitis like liver disease, had a more severe course, developing severe liver dysfunction within a short period of time (1–2 years), leading in most case to death.

In the British study from Ward et al., 12 out of 13 NRH patients had raised ALP. Three different types of ALP course were identified: the most common pattern of ALP derangement was a progressive elevation, observed in 6 of 13 patients; 2 patients had fluctuating ALP; and four had only a transient increase [12]. In this study, NRH was a common complication, but had an overall benign clinical course, rarely complicated by portal hypertension. This is in contrast with the former study by Fuss et al., but it is possible that these patients were not followed for a sufficient length of time to identify more severe liver disease. Conversely, the French study by Malamut et al. reported a high prevalence of portal hypertension (affecting as much as 75% of CVID patients with NRH, and 50% of all tested CVID patients), which may reflect a selection bias of the study population [10]. Hepato-pulmonary syndrome (HPS), an uncommon complication of hepatic vessel disorders, has been occasionally reported in CVID [20]. Interestingly, HPS was reported in two monozygotic twin brothers with CVID [21].

Malamut et al. showed a significant association of NRH with autoimmune diseases; this, combined to the observation of intra-sinusoidal T-cell infiltration and general lymphocytic abnormalities prompted the authors to propose an auto-immune mechanism [10]. At variance with the French study by Malamut et al., there was no associationbetween NRH and autoimmune condition in the study by Ward et al. [12]. Interestingly, in this study, enteropathy was reported in 6 out of 13 NRH patients and in 5 out of the 95 patients without proven NRH, ($P < 0.0001$). NRH was also associated with granuloma elsewhere in the body: 38% of patients with NRH had granuloma anywhere compared with only 10% of those without NRH. There was a strong association of NRH with lymphoproliferation ($p = 0.0002$), but no associations between NRH and age at CVID onset ($P = 0.84$), age at CVID diagnosis ($p = 0.43$), delay in diagnosis ($p = 0.15$) or length of Ig therapy ($p = 0.17$). In the Italian study by Pulvirenti et al., spleno-portal axis abnormalities were more frequent in the CVID group with profound T cell impairment, referred to as LOCID, for Late Onset Combined Immune Deficiency (7 of 17, 2 patients with NRH) [13, 22]. In this study, CVID patients with NRH had a higher prevalence of gastroenteritis ($p = 0.0002$), lymphoid nodular hyperplasia ($p = 0.009$) and auto-immune manifestations ($p = 0.03$). Overall, CVID patients with NRH are more likely to have « Disease-related complications » than those without NRH.

Unlike other « Disease-related complications » usually diagnosed close to CVID diagnosis, NRH is a late event in the course of the disease, occurring several years after CVID diagnosis.

## Primary Predominantly Antibody Deficiencies (PAD) Due to Monogenic Defects

Interestingly, prior studies have demonstrated disorders of hepatic vessels in a constellation of inherited primary antibody deficiencies resulting from disease-causing genes, and thus excluded from CVID by definition. For example, NRH was occasionally reported in the setting of X-linked agammaglobulinemia and in hyper IgM syndrome [10, 13], in ADA2 deficiency [23], in leaky severe combined immune deficiency due to mutation in *interleukin-2 receptor gamma chain* gene [24]. In our center, NRH was also identified in two siblings with X-linked lymphoproliferative disease; in one patient with gain-of-function mutation of *STAT1*; in one patient with Immunodeficiency, Centromeric Instability and Facial Anomalies (ICF) type 2 syndrome due to mutation in *ZBTB24*; in one patient with mutation in *LRBA;* and in one patient with mutation in *CTLA4* (unpublished personal observations).

In summary, hepatic vessel disorders are scarcely reported in several different monogenic defects having in common an impaired antibody immune response, which is in favor of disorders of hepatic vessels being a consequence of hypogammaglobulinemia. Few cases of hepatic vessel disorders have been reported prior to any Ig perfusion, making unlikely the hypothesis that these disorders would be the consequence of regular infusion of plasma derived products.

## Treatment and Liver Transplantation

Correction of serum immunoglobulin G trough level by IgG perfusion is not sufficient to prevent hepatic vessel injury, as the majority of hepatic vessel disorders cases develop after several years of Ig replacement therapy. It is worth noting that IgA are the main Ig found in mucous secretion of the gastro-intestinal tract, playing a crucial role in its defense, yet, Ig preparations contain only trace amounts of IgA. At present, there is no way to correct IgA deficiency. Finally, genetic alterations identified in some PADs may open the way to targeted biotherapy, such as recombinant CTLA4 in *CTLA4* and *LRBA* mutants or anti-TNF in ADA2 deficiency [23, 25–27]. It is still unclear whether these therapies are effective in inhibiting the progression of liver disease.

The literature on orthotopic liver transplantation for CVID related liver disease is limited, with only 12 adult patients reported in a study using meta-analized data [28]. Histological examination of liver explants shows portal-sinusoidal disease with prominent NRH lesions and CD8 T lymphocytes infiltrate in sinusoids without cirrhosis (Fig. 19.1). HPS was the indication for transplantation in four patients, while ascites and liver failure was the main reason for liver transplantation in the other patients. The average age at liver transplantation was 45 years, with a MELD score of 15. Only 52% of patients were alive after 3 years. Post-transplant course was challenging, due to severe immunodeficiency, leading to opportunistic infections, including cytomegalovirus, toxoplasmosis and invasive fungal infections, and malignancy in one case. Early disease recurrence was another issue, affecting 50% of patients with a more rapid course of graft NRH compared to pretransplant NRH. Recurrence of NRH after transplant has already been described in non CVID patients [28]. Furthermore, NRH is not infrequent post-transplant, even when the original indication for transplantation is not NRH [29]. It has been postulated that post-transplant NRH may be due to azathioprine toxicity or immune-mediated damages. The reason for the very short timescale to graft NRH recurrence in CVID remains unknown. Finally, liver transplantation in CVID remains a challenge, prompting a need for discussion to reduce post-transplant risk, with immunosuppression reduction and with a better control of infections.

**Conclusion**

Predominantly antibody deficiency should be suspected in patients with unexplained hepatic vessel disorders. In this respect, personal or family history of infection, auto-immunity or lymphoproliferation, should be looked for. Serum immunoglobulin classes and sub-classes quantitative analysis and extensive immunophenotype should be performed (Table 19.1).

## *Chronic Granulomatous Disease*

Chronic granulomatous disease (CGD) is an inherited deficiency of phagocyte function caused by defects in any of the five subunits of the NADPH oxidase complex responsible for the respiratory burst. CGD diagnosis can be made by measurement of NADPH oxidase activity through the dihydrorhodamine (DHR) flow cytometry assayor the nitroblue tetrazolium test (NBT). Patients with CGD are at increased risk of life-threatening infections with catalase-positive bacteria and fungi and they are prone to inflammatory complications such as colitis mimicking inflammatory bowel diseases. CGD usually manifests within the first years of life, however, it may be first diagnosed in adulthood. Effective management of CGD relies on prophylactic antibiotics and antifungals along with management of acute infections as they occur. In addition, allogenic bone marrow transplantation, best performed early in life, can lead to stable remission of CGD [30]. CGD patients are highly susceptible to respiratory infections, but other sites are also commonly affected. Liver abscess are occurring in as much as 27% of a 368-patient registry [31]. Staphylococcal species are the most common organisms responsible for liver abscesses, accounting for over 50% of infections. Gram-negative rods (*Serratia marcescens*, *Burkholderia cepacia*) and fungi (*Aspergillus* species) are also commonly reported. The marked improvement in prophylaxis and management of infectious complications has resulted in a dramatic reduction in mortality of CGD patients. Because patients are living longer, noninfectious complications are emerging. Among these complications, liver disease is common. Hepatic involvement was studied in a cohort of 194 patients with CGD followed as part of a natural history protocol [32, 33]. Liver specimens from 38 patients were reviewed. Granuloma was found in 75% and portal or lobular hepatitis in 95% of specimen. A portal venopathy, consisting of a narrowing or an obliteration of portal veins was present in 24 patients, associated in some cases with hypertrophy of the vein wall. Similar changes were found in the central vein in 20 patients. Portal and central venopathy were both present in 19 patients. By multivariate analysis, only the total episodes of liver abscess was significantly associated with central venopathy (OR 9.35, 95% CI 1.04–83.3; $p$ = 0.046). Nodular regenerative hyperplasia was seen in 9 patients, including 6 of 12 autopsy specimens. In contrast, only 2 of 19 (10.5%) biopsy specimens from patients alive at the end of the follow-up period showed established NRH ($P = .044$). Twenty-four patients died during the study (12%), all from infection. Regression analysis identifies progressive thrombocytopenia, ALP increases and a history of liver abscess as independent predictors of mortality. Autopsy data and prospective evaluation of sinusoidal portal pressure as well as portal vein diameter, support the connection between progressive thrombocytopenia and portal hypertension, suggesting that portal hypertension may herald a poor prognosis in CGD and that mortality in CGD is associated with the development of non-cirrhotic portal hypertension.

## Combined Immune-Deficiencies with Associated or Syndromic Features

### Telomere Biology Disorders

Telomeres are non-coding repetitive DNA sequences, located on linear chromosome ends that are essential in maintaining chromosomal integrity and stability. They are coated by a protein protecting complex, named shelterin, which recruits and modulates the telomerase complex, the enzyme responsible for telomere elongation. Telomerase consist of a 4-protein scaffold (dyskerin, NOP10, NHP2, and GAR), an RNA template (TERC) and a reverse transcriptase (TERT) [34, 35]. Telomerase is active in cells with high replicative demands. Telomere maintenance is essential to slow the shortening that occurs with each cell division. When critical telomere shortening happens, the cell becomes either senescent or undergoes apoptosis. Telomere biology disorders (TBDs) are accelerated ageing syndromes caused by inherited gene mutations resulting in shortened telomeres. They are also referred to as telomeropathies, or syndromes of telomere shortening. Assessment of telomere length by flow-fluorescence *in situ* hybridization (flow-FISH) on white blood cells is used for laboratory diagnosis. At least 14 genes have been found mutated in the TBDs to date [36]. Mutations in genes encoding components of the telomerase or the shelterin protection complex are the most frequent causative aberrations. TBDs encompass a large spectrum of conditions. Dyskeratosis congenita, a disorder at the severe end of the spectrum, presents in childhood with the triad of abnormal skin pigmentation, nail dystrophy and oral leukoplakia, associated with a high risk of bone marrow failure, pulmonary fibrosis and liver disease. The less severe end of the spectrum consists of adults with just one of these features. They may show other premature aging features like early hair graying and osteoporosis. Liver disease can be a first adult-onset presentation of TBDs and is estimated to complicate around 10% of TBDs. Liver disease pathology is heterogeneous among telomerase-mutation carriers, including cryptogenic cirrhosis and NRH [37–39]. Though, some pathologic findings are recurrent, and most patients have both inflammatory and fibrotic components. Histological examination of liver explants shows extensive portal fibrosis or incomplete septal cirrhosis with obliterative portal venopathy and NRH-changes in non-fibrotic areas (Fig. 19.2).

Liver disease is also heterogeneous in severity. Notably, the presence of a telomerase gene mutation and very short telomeres does not necessarily translate into liver disease in each mutation carrier from the same family, and some other genetic

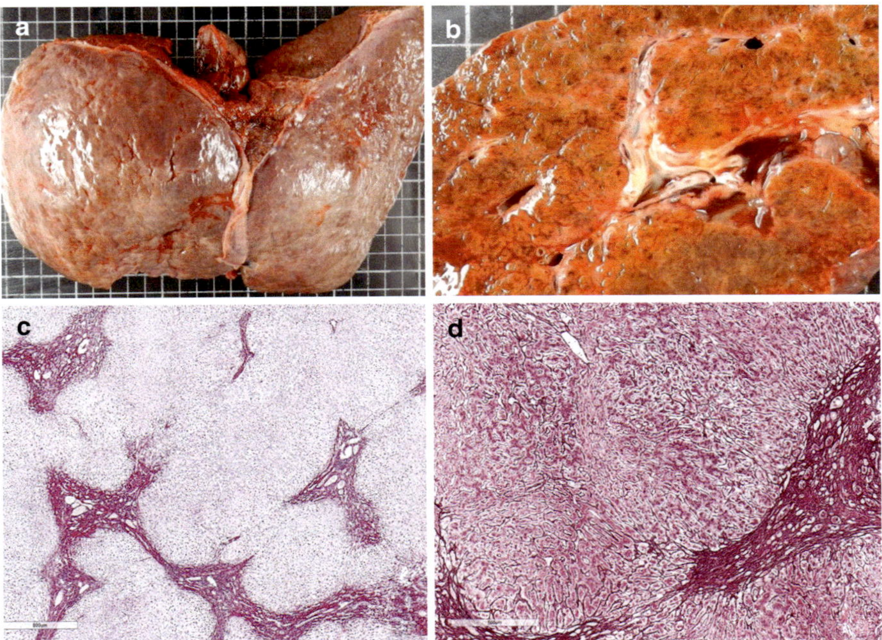

**Fig. 19.2** Telomeropathy associated with hepatopathy (observed in a patient affected with h-TERT gene mutation and transplanted for a severe portal hypertension with hepatopulmonary syndrome). (**a**) The liver explant looks dysmorphic and fibrous. (**b**) Cut section shows a macronodular parenchyma with fine septa. (**c**) Histologically, portal tracts are enlarged by fibrosis creating incomplete septa without cirrhosis. (**d**) Argentation stain reveals nodular regenerative hyperplasia (NRH) (Courtesy of Dr. Cazals-Hatem)

and environmental factors may be involved to result in the diverse phenotypes. Hepato-pulmonary syndrome (HPS) has been described in several cases of TBD. HPS was reported in 9 of 42 patients presenting with dyspnea as an initial presentation, out of 150 TBD subjects included in the Johns Hopkins Telomere syndrome registry [40]. In this series of HPS, median time to death or liver transplantation was 6 years (range, 4–10 years; n = 6). The 9 patients with HPS were significantly younger compared to the 33 patients whose dyspnea was related to pulmonary fibrosis (median, 25 years versus 55 years; P < .001). NRH was the most frequent histopathologic abnormality (67%), and it was seen in the absence of cirrhosis. Perivascular and intrahepatocyte iron deposits were also noted, even in the absence of prior red blood cell transfusion. The frequent reports of HPS with NRH in the genetically homogenous group of patients TBD is remarkable and suggests a specific association of HPS with telomere dysfunction. The physiopathology of NRH in TBD is unknown. The finding of perivascular iron deposits supports the hypothesis that vascular fragility may be a driving event. Environmental factors may be involved. One patient developed fatal liver disease after azathioprine administration [39]. Some patients with dyskeratosis congenital have fatal hepatic complications after bone marrow transplant [41]. Notably, in the general population, prevalence of NRH increases with age as demonstrated in a large autopsy study, occurring in 5.6% of individuals over age 80, suggesting an age-dependent mechanism [42].

Liver transplantation (LT) outcomes in patients with TBD are variable. Only four cases of LT in adult patients have been reported so far. One patient presented with progressive HPS post bone marrow transplantationand showed significant symptomatic improvement at 12 months and was alive and well 22 months after LT [43]. Another patient underwent successful liver transplantation at age twenty for a non-A, non-B hepatitis that rapidly evolved to sub-massive hepatic necrosis with early fibrosis. The patient was alive and well 18 years after transplantation [39]. Finally, two other patients underwent LT for HPS [40]. Hypoxia resolved within 3 months but both patients subsequently developed idiopathic pulmonary fibrosis, 18 months and 12 years post-transplant respectively.

In conclusion, because of their wide-range of possible clinical presentations, TBDs are often difficult to identify and diagnose. TBDs should be suspected in every patient with idiopathic portal hypertension. In this respect, personal or family history of unexplained cytopenias, premature greying of hair or pulmonary fibrosis should be looked for. If TBDs were suspected, patient telomere length should be assessed (Table 19.1).

## Hepatic Veno-Occlusive Disease with Immunodeficiency Syndrome (VODI)

Hepatic veno-occlusive disease with immunodeficiency syndrome (VODI, OMIM235550) is an autosomal recessive primary immunodeficiency associated with terminal hepatic lobular vascular occlusion and hepatic lobule zone 3 fibrosis [44]. Onset is usually before the age of 6 months. Hepatic veno-occlusive disease in

VODI is indistinguishable clinically and pathologically from the sinusoidal obstruction syndromedescribed after hematopoietic cell transplantation. Immunodeficiency in VODI is combined, associating severe hypogammaglobulinemia, absence of memory B cells, of lymph node germinal centers, and of tissue plasma cells to clinical evidence of T-cell immunodeficiency (defined by occurrence of opportunistic infections including *Pneumocystis jirovecii* infection, mucocutaneous candidiasis, and enteroviral or cytomegalovirus infections) with normal numbers of circulating T cellsbut absence of CD4$^+$ memory T cells [45]. VODI is caused by mutations in the *SP110* gene [46]. *SP110* is expressed in T and B lymphocytes, lymph nodes, spleen and liver, its structure is consistent with a role in transcriptional regulation. The mechanism by which mutations in SP110 leads to decreased T cell and B cell function and to sinusoidal injury have yet to be elucidated. VODI has been almost only described in patients of Lebanese descent. Patients with VODI often die in the first year of life due to either hepatic failure or fulminant infections, if unrecognized and untreated with intravenous immunoglobulin and *Pneumocystis jiroveci* prophylaxis. Hematopoietic stem cell transplantation may cure the disease, but high transplant-related mortality has been reported, partly because chemotherapy conditioning may exacerbate hepatic veno-occlusion.

In the case of VODI, the very early onset of the liver disease and its invariable association with the immune deficiency suggests that it is a primary feature in this syndrome. Conversely, in the other PIDs described above, the liver injury is occasional and occurs late in the natural history of the PID, suggesting that it is a secondary event.

## Non Malignant Hematologic Disorders Associated with Hepatic Vessel Disorders

### *Paroxysmal Nocturnal Hemoglobinuria*

Paroxysmal nocturnal hemoglobinuria (PNH) is a clonal hematopoietic stem cell disorder that manifests with hemolytic anemia, bone marrow failure, and thrombosis. The disease is caused by a somatic mutation in the phosphatidylinositol glycan A (*PIGA*) gene. The *PIGA* gene product is essential for the correct assembly of glycosylphosphatidylinositol (GPI) anchors, used to link several proteins to the cell membrane. The acquired mutation in bone marrow stem cells results in a clone of blood cells deficient in GPI anchored proteins. Flow cytometric analysis of GPI-anchored proteins on blood cells is the gold standard for diagnosis of PNH. Lack of GPI anchored complement inhibitory proteins CD55 and CD59 accounts for most of the clinical manifestations. CD55 inhibits C3 convertase and CD59 prevents the assembly of the complement membrane attack complex at the cell surface. Their lack results in increased sensibility to complement-mediated intravascular hemolysis and free hemoglobin release in the plasma leading to nitric oxide (NO) scavenging. NO depletion inhibits smooth muscle relaxation, causing symptoms like abdominal pain and pulmonary hypertension. Apart from hemolysis, another prominent feature is a highly increased risk of thrombosis [47] only partially alleviated by anticoagulation [48]. The development of thrombosis is one of the most important factors negatively influencing survival. According to the data from the international PNH registry, the incidence of thrombosis is 15.5% [49]. Thrombosis may occur at any site, although venous thrombosis is more common than arterial, affecting unusual location such as splanchnic veins. Hepatic vein thrombosis (Budd-Chiari syndrome) accounts for approximately 40% of thrombotic events with an associated high mortality [50]. Histological analysis of liver explants for chronic Budd Chiari syndrome in this context shows typical inverted cirrhosis with veno-venous fibrosis and ancient thrombosis in hepatic veins (Fig. 19.3).

Thrombosis pathogenesis is not fully understood but likely multifactorial [51]. Among the many different mechanisms suspected to account for the thrombophilic state in PNH are the following factors. First, the absence of GPI-anchored complement regulatory proteins on PNH platelets results in the formation of prothrombotic

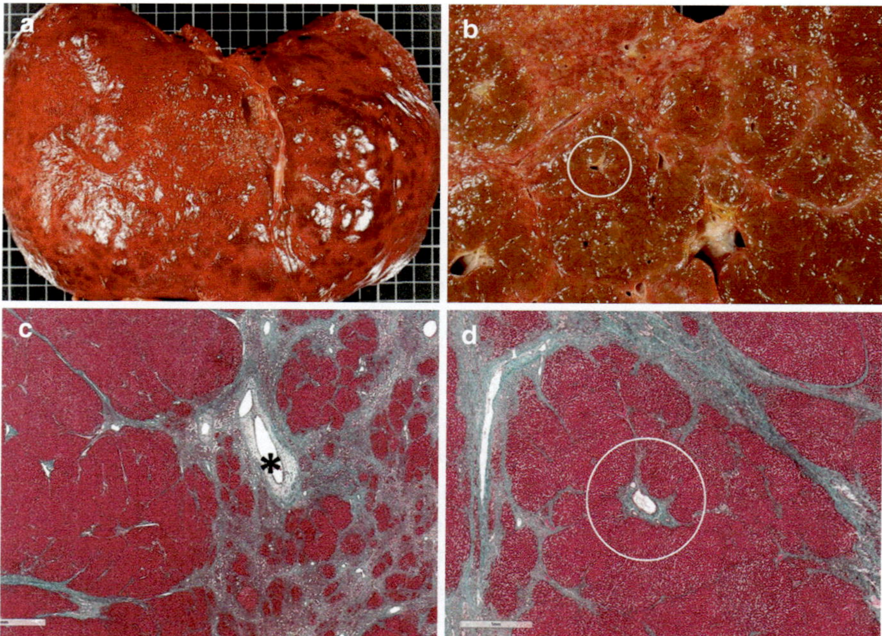

**Fig. 19.3** Paroxysmal nocturnal hemoglobinuria associated with hepatic veins thrombosis (observed in a patient transplanted for chronic Budd Chiari syndrome). (**a**) The liver explant has a congestive and macronodular aspect. (**b**) Liver cut section shows macronodular cirrhosis with congestive parenchymal extinction (top) and well-preserved portal spaces (circle). (**c**) Histologically, fibrosis predominates around obstructed hepatic veins (*) forming veno-venous bridges. (**d**) Regenerative nodules are centered by normal portal tract (circle) indicative of veno-centric cirrhosis (Courtesy of Dr. Cazals-Hatem)

microparticles [52]. Second, NO depletion subsequent to hemolysis contributes to platelet activation and aggregation [53]. Third, plasma free hemoglobin can directly activate endothelial cells [54]. Finally, C5a release may result in the generation of inflammatory cytokines such as IL-6, which promotes thrombin formation. It is unclear which of these mechanisms contributes most to thrombosis in PNH. Notably, thrombosis risk correlates with PNH clone size [55, 56]. Furthermore, complement inhibition is the most effective strategy to reduce thrombosis in PNH [57]. HPN management has been dramatically improved by the development of eculizumab, approved by the FDA in 2007. This humanized monoclonal antibody blocks the activation of terminal complement C5. Eculizimab has been shown to improve anemia [58] and to reduce the incidence rate of thromboembolic events [57]. Thrombosis is the most urgent indication to start eculizumab, and many patients will be able to discontinue anticoagulation if their PNH is controlled with eculizumab. However, thrombosis remains a risk in patients on eculizumab, in particular at times of break-through haemolysis, triggered for example by infection [50]. Bone marrow transplantation is an alternative curative option in patients with aplastic anemia in countries where eculizimab is not available. However it has historically been associated with a high treatment related mortality of 40–50% [50].

Prior to eculizimab, thrombosis recurrence risk was high despite anticoagulation and patients often required procedure such as transjugular intrahepatic portosystemic shunt [59]. In the eculizimab era, patients with Budd Chiari syndrome have successfully undergone liver transplantation supported by long term eculizimab treatment [60].

## Sickle Cell Disease

Sickle cell disease (SCD) is an autosomal recessive disorder caused by mutations in the gene encoding the β-globin chain of hemoglobin. Its incidence is estimated to be between 300,000 and 400,000 neonates each year, mostly in individuals of sub-Saharan Africa descent [61]. SCD encompasses a group of disorders characterized by the presence of at least one mutated hemoglobin S allele (HbS; p.Glu6Val) and a second pathogenic variant, resulting in abnormal hemoglobin polymerization. Homozygous Hb S/Saccounts for 60%–70% of SCD in the United States. Other forms of SCD, usually result from coinheritance of HbS with other abnormal β-globin chain variants, the most common being sickle-hemoglobin C disease (Hb S/C), a less severe form [62]. In SCD, the mutated β-globin chain causes red blood cells to havea sickle shape, especially when under low oxygen tension. The sickled erythrocytes are poorly deformable and prone to hemolysis, resulting in acute complications such as severe anemia and ischemic vaso-occlusive accidents related to vessel obstruction by red blood cells. Liver acute vaso-occlusive crisis has been noted in nearly 10% of patients. It occurs predominantly in patients with homozygous S/S sickle cell anemia, and to a lesser extent in patients with HbS/C disease [63]. Liver biopsy performed during hepatic crises shows sinusoidal distension and obstruction by sickle cell aggregates, mild centrilobular necrosis and Kupfer cell hypertrophy (Fig. 19.2). The syndrome is self-limited, usually resolving within 3 to 14 days with intravenous hydration and analgesia. If acute liver failure develops, the only potentially effective therapeutic option is liver transplantation, which is challenging but feasible [64].

Repeated vaso-occlusive crisis and ongoing haemolytic anaemia, even when subclinical, lead to parenchymal injury and chronic organ damage, causing progressive multiorgan failure and early mortality. Irreversible chronic organ damages involve mainly the brain and kidney; still, chronic liver disease accounts for up to 11% of death in SCD [65]. Two pathologic studies suggest that chronic hepatic lesions are mainly vascular [66, 67]. Altogether, sinusoidal dilatation is observed in 71 to 88%, ischemic necrosis in up to 35% of liver biopsies, perisinuoidal fibrosis in 82% and regenerative changes in 20% as illustrated in Fig. 19.4. Chronic hepatic vessel injuries could either result from recurrent microvascular occlusions, subsequent necrosis and repair or from an endothelial activation mediated by plasma free hemoglobin. Still, iron deposition and accumulation are also important determinants of liver damage in these chronically transfused patients [68]. In SCD, currently available disease modifying treatments are limited to transfusions and

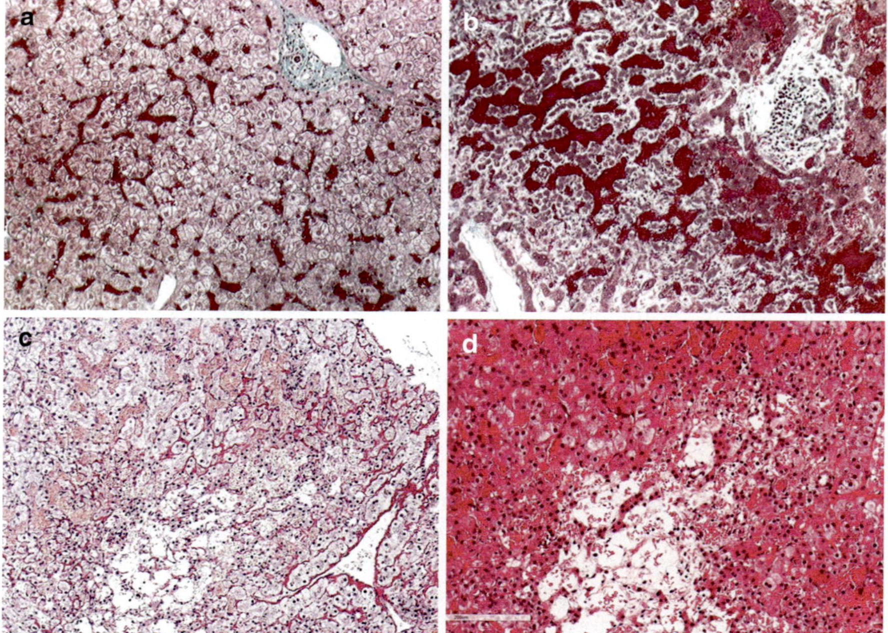

**Fig. 19.4** Hepatic and sinusoidal lesions in Sickle-cell disease (liver biopsies done for abnormal liver tests). (**a**) Sickled-red cells are fortuitously found in dilated sinusoids. (**b**) In vaso-occlusive crisis, extensive centrilobular necrosis is observed admixed with massive congestive sinusoidal dilatation. (**c**- **d**) Sickle-cell disease can generate sinusoidal disruption with slight perisinusoidal fibrosis (**c**) and peliosis (**d**) (Courtesy of Dr. Cazals-Hatem)

hydroxycarbamide. Deeper insights into the pathophysiology of SCD have led to the development of novel agents targeting cellular adhesion, inflammation or oxidant injury, aimed at preventing acute vaso-occlusive pain events. For example, crizanlizumab, a monoclonal antibody directed at P-selectin, an adhesion molecule that facilitates cell-to-cell interactions of red blood cells, endothelial cells, white blood cells, and platelets, was shown to significantly lower the rate of vaso-occlusive crisis in a recent trial [69].

Hematopoetic stem cell transplant is the only curative therapeutic approach, but barriers to treatment are substantial and include a lack of suitable donors, immunologic transplant rejection and long-term adverse effects. Pre-transplant poor end-organ function can be an issue for older patients. Gene therapy to correct the HbS β chain point mutation is under investigation as another curative modality [70].

# References


1. Picard C, Bobby Gaspar H, Al-Herz W, Bousfiha A, Casanova J-L, Chatila T, et al. International Union of Immunological Societies: 2017 primary immunodeficiency diseases committee report on inborn errors of immunity. J Clin Immunol. 2018 Jan;38(1):96–128.
2. Mouillot G, Carmagnat M, Gérard L, Garnier J-L, Fieschi C, Vince N, et al. B-cell and T-cell phenotypes in CVID patients correlate with the clinical phenotype of the disease. J Clin Immunol. 2010 Sep;30(5):746–55.
3. Oksenhendler E, Gérard L, Fieschi C, Malphettes M, Mouillot G, Jaussaud R, et al. Infections in 252 patients with common variable immunodeficiency. Clin Infect Dis Off Publ Infect Dis Soc Am. 2008 May 15;46(10):1547–54.
4. Rolfes MC, Sriaroon P, Dávila Saldaña BJ, Dvorak CC, Chapdelaine H, Ferdman RM, et al. Chronic norovirus infection in primary immune deficiency disorders: an international case series. Diagn Microbiol Infect Dis. 2018 Aug;12:69–73.
5. Dion J, Malphettes M, Bénéjat L, Mégraud F, Wargnier A, Boutboul D, et al. Campylobacter infection in adult patients with primary antibody deficiency. J Allergy Clin Immunol Pract. 2018 Jul;6:1038–1041.e4.
6. Chapel H, Lucas M, Lee M, Bjorkander J, Webster D, Grimbacher B, et al. Common variable immunodeficiency disorders: division into distinct clinical phenotypes. Blood. 2008 Jul 15;112(2):277–86.
7. Chapel H, Lucas M, Patel S, Lee M, Cunningham-Rundles C, Resnick E, et al. Confirmation and improvement of criteria for clinical phenotyping in common variable immunodeficiency disorders in replicate cohorts. J Allergy Clin Immunol. 2012 Nov;130(5):1197–1198.e9.
8. Resnick ES, Moshier EL, Godbold JH, Cunningham-Rundles C. Morbidity and mortality in common variable immune deficiency over 4 decades. Blood. 2012 Feb 16;119(7):1650–7.
9. Song J, Lleo A, Yang GX, Zhang W, Bowlus CL, Gershwin ME, et al. Common variable immunodeficiency and liver involvement. Clin Rev Allergy Immunol. 2017 Aug 7;55(3):340–51.
10. Malamut G, Ziol M, Suarez F, Beaugrand M, Viallard JF, Lascaux AS, et al. Nodular regenerative hyperplasia: the main liver disease in patients with primary hypogammaglobulinemia and hepatic abnormalities. J Hepatol. 2008 Jan;48(1):74–82.
11. Fuss IJ, Friend J, Yang Z, He JP, Hooda L, Boyer J, et al. Nodular regenerative hyperplasia in common variable immunodeficiency. J Clin Immunol. 2013 May;33(4):748–58.
12. Ward C, Lucas M, Piris J, Collier J, Chapel H. Abnormal liver function in common variable immunodeficiency disorders due to nodular regenerative hyperplasia. Clin Exp Immunol. 2008 Sep;153(3):331–7.

13. Pulvirenti F, Pentassuglio I, Milito C, Valente M, De Santis A, Conti V, et al. Idiopathic non cirrhotic portal hypertension and spleno-portal axis abnormalities in patients with severe primary antibody deficiencies. J Immunol Res. 2014;2014:672458.
14. Webster AD, Brown D, Franz A, Dusheiko G. Prevalence of hepatitis C in patients with primary antibody deficiency. Clin Exp Immunol. 1996 Jan;103(1):5–7.
15. Quinti I, Pierdominici M, Marziali M, Giovannetti A, Donnanno S, Chapel H, et al. European surveillance of immunoglobulin safety--results of initial survey of 1243 patients with primary immunodeficiencies in 16 countries. Clin Immunol Orlando Fla. 2002 Sep;104(3):231–6.
16. Ziol M, Poirel H, Kountchou GN, Boyer O, Mohand D, Mouthon L, et al. Intrasinusoidal cytotoxic CD8+ T cells in nodular regenerative hyperplasia of the liver. Hum Pathol. 2004 Oct;35(10):1241–51.
17. Shetty S, Lalor PF, Adams DH. Liver sinusoidal endothelial cells–gatekeepers of hepatic immunity. Nat Rev Gastroenterol Hepatol. 2018 Sep;15(9):555–67.
18. Daniels JA, Torbenson M, Vivekanandan P, Anders RA, Boitnott JK. Hepatitis in common variable immunodeficiency. Hum Pathol. 2009 Apr;40(4):484–8.
19. Devaney K, Goodman ZD, Epstein MS, Zimmerman HJ, Ishak KG. Hepatic sarcoidosis. Clinicopathologic features in 100 patients. Am J Surg Pathol. 1993 Dec;17(12):1272–80.
20. Azzu V, Elias JE, Duckworth A, Davies S, Brais R, Kumararatne DS, et al. Liver transplantation in adults with liver disease due to common variable immunodeficiency leads to early recurrent disease and poor outcome. Liver Transplant Off Publ Am Assoc Study Liver Dis Int Liver Transplant Soc. 2018;24(2):171–81.
21. Holmes SN, Condliffe A, Griffiths W, Baxendale H, Kumararatne DS. Familial hepatopulmonary syndrome in common variable immunodeficiency. J Clin Immunol. 2015 Apr;35(3):302–4.
22. Bertinchamp R, Gérard L, Boutboul D, Malphettes M, Fieschi C, Oksenhendler E, et al. Exclusion of patients with a severe T-cell defect improves the definition of common variable immunodeficiency. J Allergy Clin Immunol Pract. 2016 Dec;4(6):1147–57.
23. Springer JM, Gierer SA, Jiang H, Kleiner D, Deuitch N, Ombrello AK, et al. Deficiency of adenosine deaminase 2 in adult siblings: many years of a misdiagnosed disease with severe consequences. Front Immunol. 2018;9:1361.
24. Neves JF, Martins C, Cordeiro AI, Neves C, Plagnol V, Curtis J, et al. Novel IL2RG mutation causes leaky TLOWB+NK+ SCID with nodular regenerative hyperplasia and Normal IL-15 STAT5 phosphorylation. J Pediatr Hematol Oncol. 2018 Jun;22:328–33.
25. Kostel Bal S, Haskologlu S, Serwas NK, Islamoglu C, Aytekin C, Kendirli T, et al. Multiple presentations of LRBA deficiency: a single-center experience. J Clin Immunol. 2017 Nov;37(8):790–800.
26. Lee S, Moon JS, Lee C-R, Kim H-E, Baek S-M, Hwang S, et al. Abatacept alleviates severe autoimmune symptoms in a patient carrying a de novo variant in CTLA-4. J Allergy Clin Immunol. 2016 Jan;137(1):327–30.
27. Lo B, Zhang K, Lu W, Zheng L, Zhang Q, Kanellopoulou C, et al. AUTOIMMUNE DISEASE. Patients with LRBA deficiency show CTLA4 loss and immune dysregulation responsive to abatacept therapy. Science. 2015 Jul 24;349(6246):436–40.
28. Loinaz C, Colina F, Musella M, Lopez-Rios F, Gomez R, Jimenez C, et al. Orthotopic liver transplantation in 4 patients with portal hypertension and non-cirrhotic nodular liver. Hepato-Gastroenterology. 1998 Oct;45(23):1787–94.
29. Hübscher SG. What is the long-term outcome of the liver allograft? J Hepatol. 2011 Sep;55(3):702–17.
30. Holland SM. Chronic granulomatous disease. Hematol Oncol Clin North Am. 2013;27(1):89–99. viii
31. Winkelstein JA, Marino MC, Johnston RB, Boyle J, Curnutte J, Gallin JI, et al. Chronic granulomatous disease. Report on a national registry of 368 patients. Medicine (Baltimore). 2000 May;79(3):155–69.
32. Feld JJ, Hussain N, Wright EC, Kleiner DE, Hoofnagle JH, Ahlawat S, et al. Hepatic involvement and portal hypertension predict mortality in chronic granulomatous disease. Gastroenterology. 2008 Jun;134(7):1917–26.

33. Hussain N, Feld JJ, Kleiner DE, Hoofnagle JH, Garcia-Eulate R, Ahlawat S, et al. Hepatic abnormalities in patients with chronic granulomatous disease. Hepatology. 2007 Mar;45(3):675–83.

34. Armanios M, Blackburn EH. The telomere syndromes. Nat Rev Genet. 2012 Oct;13(10):693–704.

35. Bertuch AA. The molecular genetics of the telomere biology disorders. RNA Biol. 2016;13(8):696–706.

36. Savage SA. Beginning at the ends: telomeres and human disease. F1000Research. 2018;7.

37. Patnaik MM, Kamath PS, Simonetto DA. Hepatic manifestations of telomere biology disorders. J Hepatol. 2018 Sep;69(3):736–43.

38. Dokal I. Dyskeratosis congenita in all its forms. Br J Haematol. 2000 Sep 1;110(4):768–79.

39. Calado RT, Regal JA, Kleiner DE, Schrump DS, Peterson NR, Pons V, et al. A spectrum of severe familial liver disorders associate with telomerase mutations. PLoS One. 2009 Nov 20;4(11):e7926.

40. Gorgy AI, Jonassaint NL, Stanley SE, Koteish A, DeZern AE, Walter JE, et al. Hepatopulmonary syndrome is a frequent cause of dyspnea in the short telomere disorders. Chest. 2015 Oct;148(4):1019–26.

41. Rocha V, Devergie A, Socié G, Ribaud P, Espérou H, Parquet N, et al. Unusual complications after bone marrow transplantation for dyskeratosis congenita. Br J Haematol. 1998 Oct;103(1):243–8.

42. Wanless IR. Micronodular transformation (nodular regenerative hyperplasia) of the liver: a report of 64 cases among 2,500 autopsies and a new classification of benign hepatocellular nodules. Hepatology. 1990 May;11(5):787–97.

43. Mahansaria SS, Kumar S, Bharathy KGS, Kumar S, Pamecha V. Liver transplantation after bone marrow transplantation for end stage liver disease with severe Hepatopulmonary syndrome in Dyskeratosis Congenita: a literature first. J Clin Exp Hepatol. 2015 Dec 1;5(4):344–7.

44. Mellis C, Bale PM. Familial hepatic venoocclusive disease with probable immune deficiency. J Pediatr. 1976 Feb;88(2):236–42.

45. Cliffe ST, Bloch DB, Suryani S, Kamsteeg E-J, Avery DT, Palendira U, et al. Clinical, molecular, and cellular immunologic findings in patients with SP110-associated veno-occlusive disease with immunodeficiency syndrome. J Allergy Clin Immunol. 2012 Sep;130(3):735–742.e6.

46. Roscioli T, Cliffe ST, Bloch DB, Bell CG, Mullan G, Taylor PJ, et al. Mutations in the gene encoding the PML nuclear body protein Sp110 are associated with immunodeficiency and hepatic veno-occlusive disease. Nat Genet. 2006 Jun;38(6):620–2.

47. Van Bijnen STA, Van Heerde WL, Muus P. Mechanisms and clinical implications of thrombosis in paroxysmal nocturnal hemoglobinuria. J Thromb Haemost JTH. 2012 Jan;10(1):1–10.

48. Hall C, Richards S, Hillmen P. Primary prophylaxis with warfarin prevents thrombosis in paroxysmal nocturnal hemoglobinuria (PNH). Blood. 2003 Nov 15;102(10):3587–91.

49. Schrezenmeier H, Muus P, Socié G, Szer J, Urbano-Ispizua A, Maciejewski JP, et al. Baseline characteristics and disease burden in patients in the international paroxysmal nocturnal hemoglobinuria registry. Haematologica. 2014 May;99(5):922–9.

50. Griffin M, Munir T. Management of thrombosis in paroxysmal nocturnal hemoglobinuria: a clinician's guide. Ther Adv Hematol. 2017 Mar;8(3):119–26.

51. Hill A, Kelly RJ, Hillmen P. Thrombosis in paroxysmal nocturnal hemoglobinuria. Blood. 2013 Jun 20;121(25):4985–96.

52. Wiedmer T, Hall SE, Ortel TL, Kane WH, Rosse WF, Sims PJ. Complement-induced vesiculation and exposure of membrane prothrombinase sites in platelets of paroxysmal nocturnal hemoglobinuria. Blood. 1993 Aug 15;82(4):1192–6.

53. Rother RP, Bell L, Hillmen P, Gladwin MT. The clinical sequelae of intravascular hemolysis and extracellular plasma hemoglobin: a novel mechanism of human disease. JAMA. 2005 Apr 6;293(13):1653–62.

54. Helley D, de Latour RP, Porcher R, Rodrigues CA, Galy-Fauroux I, Matheron J, et al. Evaluation of hemostasis and endothelial function in patients with paroxysmal nocturnal hemoglobinuria receiving eculizumab. Haematologica. 2010 Apr;95(4):574–81.

55. Nishimura J-I, Kanakura Y, Ware RE, Shichishima T, Nakakuma H, Ninomiya H, et al. Clinical course and flow cytometric analysis of paroxysmal nocturnal hemoglobinuria in the United States and Japan. Medicine (Baltimore). 2004 May;83(3):193–207.

56. Moyo VM, Mukhina GL, Garrett ES, Brodsky RA. Natural history of paroxysmal nocturnal haemoglobinuria using modern diagnostic assays. Br J Haematol. 2004 Jul;126(1):133–8.

57. Hillmen P, Muus P, Dührsen U, Risitano AM, Schubert J, Luzzatto L, et al. Effect of the complement inhibitor eculizumab on thromboembolism in patients with paroxysmal nocturnal hemoglobinuria. Blood. 2007 Dec 1;110(12):4123–8.

58. Schubert J, Hillmen P, Röth A, Young NS, Elebute MO, Szer J, et al. Eculizumab, a terminal complement inhibitor, improves anaemia in patients with paroxysmal nocturnal haemoglobinuria. Br J Haematol. 2008 Jun;142(2):263–72.

59. Hoekstra J, Leebeek FWG, Plessier A, Raffa S, Darwish Murad S, Heller J, et al. Paroxysmal nocturnal hemoglobinuria in Budd-Chiari syndrome: findings from a cohort study. J Hepatol. 2009 Oct;51(4):696–706.

60. Singer AL, Locke JE, Stewart ZA, Lonze BE, Hamilton JP, Scudiere JR, et al. Successful liver transplantation for Budd-Chiari syndrome in a patient with paroxysmal nocturnal hemoglobinuria treated with the anti-complement antibody eculizumab. Liver Transplant Off Publ Am Assoc Study Liver Dis Int Liver Transplant Soc. 2009 May;15(5):540–3.

61. Kato GJ, Piel FB, Reid CD, Gaston MH, Ohene-Frempong K, Krishnamurti L, et al. Sickle cell disease. Nat Rev Dis Primer. 2018 Mar 15;4:18010.

62. Bender MA. Sickle cell disease. In: Adam MP, Ardinger HH, Pagon RA, Wallace SE, Bean LJ, Stephens K, et al., editors. GeneReviews® [Internet]. Seattle (WA): University of Washington; 1993. [cited 2018 Oct 11]. Available from: http://www.ncbi.nlm.nih.gov/books/NBK1377/.

63. Banerjee S, Owen C, Chopra S. Sickle cell hepatopathy. Hepatology. 2001 May;33(5):1021–8.

64. Hurtova M, Bachir D, Lee K, Calderaro J, Decaens T, Kluger MD, et al. Transplantation for liver failure in patients with sickle cell disease: challenging but feasible. Liver Transplant Off Publ Am Assoc Study Liver Dis Int Liver Transplant Soc. 2011 Apr;17(4):381–92.

65. Darbari DS, Kple-Faget P, Kwagyan J, Rana S, Gordeuk VR, Castro O. Circumstances of death in adult sickle cell disease patients. Am J Hematol. 2006 Nov;81(11):858–63.

66. Bauer TW, Moore GW, Hutchins GM. The liver in sickle cell disease. A clinicopathologic study of 70 patients. Am J Med. 1980 Dec;69(6):833–7.

67. Charlotte F, Bachir D, Nénert M, Mavier P, Galactéros F, Dhumeaux D, et al. Vascular lesions of the liver in sickle cell disease. A clinicopathological study in 26 living patients. Arch Pathol Lab Med. 1995 Jan;119(1):46–52.

68. Hankins JS, Smeltzer MP, McCarville MB, Aygun B, Hillenbrand CM, Ware RE, et al. Patterns of liver iron accumulation in patients with sickle cell disease and thalassemia with iron overload. Eur J Haematol. 2010 Jul;85(1):51–7.

69. Kutlar A, Kanter J, Liles DK, Alvarez OA, Cançado RD, Friedrisch JR, et al. Effect of crizanlizumab on pain crises in subgroups of patients with sickle cell disease: a SUSTAIN study analysis. Am J Hematol. 2018 Oct;8:55–61.

70. Kapoor S, Little JA. Pecker LH. Mayo Clin Proc: Advances in the Treatment of Sickle Cell Disease; 2018 Nov 7.

# Chapter 20
# Systemic Diseases Affecting Liver Vessels

A. Le Joncour and D. Saadoun

## Introduction

The liver may be injured during the course of many systemic diseases. A systemic etiology of vascular liver disease is found in more than 50% of cases. Systemic diseases such as connective tissue diseases or vasculitis are rare, but they may induce hepatic vessel damage and require specific therapeutic management. Therefore, systemic diseases need to be ascertained in every patient with vascular liver disease. The mechanisms of injury can be broadly divided into three pathways: vascular, toxic, and immune. Vascular obstruction may be an early event but is also the late common pathway from all mechanisms. The exact prevalence of these diseases is often unknown because of their rarity. We describe here the vascular liver complications of the main systemic diseases affecting liver vessels (Tables 20.1 and 20.2).

A. Le Joncour · D. Saadoun (✉)
Sorbonne Universités, UPMC University Paris, 06, INSERM, UMR S 959, Immunology-Immunopathology-Immunotherapy (I3), Paris, France

Biotherapy (CIC-BTi), Hôpital Pitié-Salpêtrière, AP-HP, Paris, France

Department of Internal Medicine and Clinical Immunology, AP-HP, Groupe Hospitalier Pitié-Salpêtrière, Centre national de références Maladies Autoimmunes et systémiques rares, Centre national de références Maladies Autoinflammatoires rares et Amylose inflammatoire, Paris, France
e-mail: alexandre.lejoncour@aphp.fr; david.saadoun@aphp.fr

© Springer Nature Switzerland AG 2022
D. Valla et al. (eds.), *Vascular Disorders of the Liver*,
https://doi.org/10.1007/978-3-030-82988-9_20

**Table 20.1** Type of vascular liver disease according to systemic disease[a]

| Systemic Disease | Vascular liver Disease |
|---|---|
| **Vasculitis** | |
| Behcet's disease | BCS 1–3% (8–26% among angio-Behçet) |
| | Portal vein thrombosis <1% |
| | Arterial aneurysm <1% |
| | NRH < 1% |
| PAN | Cholecystis 2–17% |
| | Hepatic aneurysm <0–20%, spontaneuous rupture: Rare |
| **Connective tissue disease** | |
| Anti-phospholipid syndrome | BCS <1% |
| | Portal vein thrombosis <<1% |
| | PSVD <<1% |
| | HVOD <<1% |
| | Hepatic infarction << 1% (except in catastrophic APS: 3%) |
| Lupus | PSVD (NRH) 0.3–5% |
| | Hepatic arteritis (autopsy): 20% |
| Systemic sclerosis | NRH 1–4% |
| Sarcoidosis | Portal hypertension: 3% |
| | PSVD (NRH) 0–9% |
| | HVOD (sinusoidal dilatation) 0–14% |
| | BCS <<1% |

*BCS* Budd-Chiari Syndrome; *PAN* Periarteritis nodosa; *PSVD* porto-sinusoidal vascular disease; *HVOD* hepatic-veno-occlusive disease; *NRH* nodular regenerative hyperplasia
[a]from [1–23]

**Table 20.2** Type of systemic disease according to vascular liver disease[a]

| Vascular liver disease | Systemic disease |
|---|---|
| BCS | Behcet's disease 2–10% |
| | APS: |
| | Positive aPL: 17–25% |
| | Definite APS: Estimate 10–15% |
| Portal vein thrombosis | Behcet's disease <<1% |
| | APS: |
| | Positive aPL: 11% |
| | Definite APS: Estimate 5% |
| PSVD | RA 9–16% |
| | APS: |
| | Positive aPL: 4–8% |
| | Definite APS: Unknown |
| | Lupus: 1–4% |
| | SSc: 1–2% |
| HVOD | APS: |
| | Positive aPL: Unknown |
| | Lupus: Unknown |
| | SSc: Unknown |
| Hepatic aneurysm | PAN: 5% |
| | Takayasu: Unknown |

*BCS* Budd-Chiari Syndrome; *APS* Antiphospholipid syndrome; *aPL* antiphospholipid antibodies; *RA* rheumatoid arthritis; *SSc* Systemic sclerosis; *PAN* Periarteritis nodosa; *PSVD* porto-sinusoidal vascular disease; *HVOD* hepatic-veno-occlusive disease.
[a]from [1–23]

## Proposed General Pathophysiology

As chronic inflammatory/auto immune diseases are known to increase cardiovascular risk, mechanisms underlying vascular dysfunction have been widely studied and thus help us to understand the pathophysiology of systemic diseases associated liver vascular lesions.

Various key players may be involved in vascular damage:

(a) Inflammatory cytokines such as TNF alpha, IL-6 and IL-1beta interact with specific receptors and activate endothelial cells (through JAK-STAT, NF-kappaB, and Smad signaling pathways) leading to an inflammatory response involving cell adhesion, permeability and apoptosis [24].

(b) Growing evidences show that innate immunity play a major role in vascular homeostasis and dysfunction. Activated neutrophils and macrophages (through ROS generation, matrix metalloproteinase, extracellular Traps release) increase endothelial expression of adhesion molecules and widens cell–cell junctions, which facilitate the migration of leukocytes into inflamed tissue. Proteases secreted from leukocytes can damage the glycocalyx layer [25].

(c) Dysregulation of the adaptive immunity, especially the increase of TH-1/Th-17 lymphocytes have been show to participate to endothelial cell dysfunction [26, 27]. Moreover, in some circumstances, autoantibodies have been shown to activate endothelial cells directly or through activation of the complement system [28, 29].

Activated endothelial cells can in turn enhance immune cells chemotactism and adhesion thus creating a deleterious loop.

More specifically, liver vessel dysfunction has been studied in inflammatory conditions [30]: during inflammation, expression of ICAM-1 increases and expression of vascular cell adhesion molecule-1 (VCAM-1) and CD31 are induced, leading to the transendothelial migration of leucocytes. This hepatic endothotelial activation and leucocytes recruitment can lead to local microthrombi [31]. The hemodynamic disturbances at the level of the hepatic microvasculature lead to apoptosis and hepatocyte atrophy, coexisting with maintained or increased blood supply to adjacent acini cells. The local hyperperfusion leads, in turn, to elevated levels of cell growth activators which act as autocrine or paracrine peptides. All together these phenomena create an "atrophy-hypertrophy complex" characteristic of nodular regenerative hyperplasia (NRH) [32].

## Vasculitis

### *Behçet's Disease*

Behçet's disease (BD) is a chronic systemic vasculitis characterized by mucocutaneous, ocular, gastrointestinal and cerebral recurrent lesions. Diagnosis of BD is primarily based on clinical manifestations and new criteria of the International

Team for the revision of the international criteria for Behçet's disease are now used in numerous studies [33] (Table 20.3). This auto-inflammatory disorder involves different vessel types and sizes of the vascular tree and is often complicated by recurrent thrombosis, particularly in the venous compartment (found in that almost 30%). The physiopathology of thrombosis is unknown but may related to innate immunity activation. Neutrophils in BD exhibit increased superoxide production which potentially contributes to clot formation by fibrinogen oxidation [34]. Neutrophils are also prone to undergo NEtosis leading to endothelial activation and thrombosis (Le Joncour A et al., submitted).

Budd-Chiari syndrome (BCS) is the most common hepatic manifestation. In large series including more than 800 patients, Budd-Chiari syndrome occurs in 1 to 3% of patients and accounts for 8–26% of patients with vein thrombosis [1–6]. Patients with BCS are usually male and younger than those without BCS. The prevalence of BD in series of BCS ranges from 2% to more than 10%. Prevalence varies depending on the area where from reports originates [7, 35–38]. BD has ranked third among causes in countries where BD is prevalent [37]. BD related BCS affects young males mainly originating from North Africa and Middle East but may also occur in Caucasians. BCS usually presents with fever as part of a systemic inflammatory reaction syndrome [3]. Concomitant vena cava thrombosis is more frequent in BD-related BCS than in BCS of other aetiology, occurring in 70% of patients. An intracardiac thrombus is found in almost 30% of patients [3, 5, 8]. Thus, hepatic vein thrombosis could represent an extension of the vena cava thrombus [8] although cases of pure hepatic vein involvement are not rare. Approximately two third of the BD patients with BCS had liver-related symptoms and signs (ascites, oesophageal varices, etc.). They were at high risk of death, as 58% of them died at 5 years compared to 10% of those without liver-related

**Table 20.3** Classification criteria for Behçet's disease

| Signs/Symptoms | Points |
|---|---|
| Ocular lesions | 2 |
| Genitial aphthosis | 2 |
| Oral aphthosis | 2 |
| Skin lesions | 1 |
| Neurological manifestations | 1 |
| Vascular manifestations | 1 |
| Positive pathergy test | 1 |
| **Score** | **Plausibility of BD** |
| 4 | Probable BD |
| 5 | BD highly likely |
| ≥ 6 | Almost certainly BD |

*BD* Behçet's disease
Adapted from the International Criteria for Behçet's Disease (ICBD)[1]

symptoms, $p = 0.01$ [5]. The remaining patients, who lacked liver related manifestations, had a better prognosis probably due to (a) intensive immunosuppressive treatment started before the full-blown disease onset, (b) mild obstruction of the hepatic venous outflow, and (c) slowly progressing disease with more chance for extensive collateral formation [3, 4]. It is noteworthy that oesophageal varices can be a sign of superior vena cava obstruction without hepatic vein obstruction [39]. Such oesophageal varices constitute cavocaval collaterals running through the portal venous territory. Management of BD-related BCS has not been studied in randomized studies. Retrospective data support the idea that immunosuppressive treatments are more efficient than anticoagulant alone in BD thrombosis [40], and that anti-TNF alpha might be more effective than conventional immunosuppressive therapy [41]. Endovascular angioplasty is often not feasible because of long-length of vena cava obstruction. However, in the selected cases where it appears feasible, angioplasty should be considered after immunosuppressive treatment has been initiated in order to avoid stent thrombosis (Table 20.4).

Portal vein thrombosis is less prevalent than BCS among BD patients, having been reported in a few cases reports [1, 42]. In a series of 844 BD patients, 6 had cavernous transformation of the portal vein of whom 5 also had BCS [9].

In BD patients, arterial disorders are less common than venous thrombosis but constitute a major cause of death. Aortic aneurysms are the most frequent arterial lesions. Aneurysm of the hepatic artery is exceptional as spontaneous rupture has been described in only three cases [43–45].

**Table 20.4** Differences between Behcet's disease and antiphospholipid syndrome related BCS[a]

|  | **Behçet's disease** | **Antiphospholipid syndrome** |
| --- | --- | --- |
| Epidemiology | Young men, African- middle east | Women>men |
| Medical history | Oral and/or genital aphtosis, arthralgia, thrombo phlebitis, uveitis | Repeated miscarriage, obstetrical complication Idiopathic venous and/or arterial thrombosis |
| Clinical | Fever IVC thrombosis, Intra cardiac thrombosis | Livedo, mitral valvulopathy, stroke, lupus signs |
| Laboratory findings | Inflammatory syndrome | Repeatedly detectable: - Lupus anticoagulant - Anticardiolipid antibodies - Antibeta2 gp1 antibodies |
| Treatment | High dose steroids Plus immunosuppressive drugs or monoclonal anti-anti-TNF and anticoagulation | Anticoagulation |

*IVC* inferior vena cava
[a]from [1–9, 13–16]

## *Periarteritis Nodosa*

Polyarteritis nodosa (PAN) is a systemic vasculitis that commonly involves the skin, kidneys, nerves, and gastrointestinal tract. When the gallbladder is involved as part of a systemic vasculitis, PAN is, by far, the most likely cause. Cholecystitis was reported in 2% to 17% of patients with PAN and in up to 40% of autopsied patients [46–48].

In an autopsy series of 11 patients with PAN, all patients had hepatic arteritis [10]. In a series of 36 patients with hepatic aneurysms, 2 had PAN [11]. PAN is a vasculitis involving small-sized and medium-sized arteries, leading to occurrence of microaneurysms in mesenteric vessels. Medium-sized arteries involvement is present in about 40% of cases [12, 48]. Aneurysms of hepatic arteries are observed in 0–20% of cases [12, 48]. Rare cases report have described spontaneous rupture of hepatic aneurysm [49–52]. Besides hepatic aneurysms, artermal occlusions can account for 80% of vasculitis lesions [12].

## *Other Vasculitis*

1. Giant Cell Arteritis

Giant cell arteritis is a large vessel granulomatous vasculitis. Abnormal liver test results—mostly increased serum alkaline phosphatase and gamma-glutamyl transpeptidase levels are found in in 50–70% of cases. The mechanisms for abnormal liver tests remain uncertain. It has been hypothesized that cholestasis result from ischaemic injury and cytokine release. Some cases report demonstrated non-caseating epithelioid cell granulomatous inflammation of medium-sized arterioles within the portal tracts and disruption of the elastic laminae [53, 54]. Liver involvement does not seem to impact the prognosis of giant cell arteritis. Hepatic lesions, such as arteritis, are segmental and focal and are thus difficult to highlight in histologic samples. Thus, it is not mandatory to perform systematic liver biopsy in patients with giant cell arteritis.

2. Takayasu arteritis

Takayasu arteritis is a chronic inflammatory vasculitis that affects aorta and its major branches. Hepatic artery involvement has not been described in Takayasu arteritis.

However, two cases of sinusoidal dilatation in patients with Takayasu arteritis have been published. They responded to steroids therapy [55].

3. ANCA-associated vasculitis

Abnormal liver test results are found in half of the patient with ANCA-associated vasculitis and are correlated with disease activity [56]. Similar to giant cell arteritis, one explanation could be a gallbladder or bile duct vasculitis. Indeed, charts review of 61 cases of gallbladder vasculitis found that ANCA-associated vasculitis was the present in 13% of cases [57]. The other possible explanation for abnormal liver test results is granulomatous hepatitis [58].

## Connective Tissue Disease

### *Anti-Phospholipid Syndrome*

The antiphospholipid syndrome (APS) is an acquired thrombophilic disorder in which autoantibodies to a variety of phospholipids determinants of cell membranes or phospholipid binding proteins are produced. Clinical features for definite APS include vascular thrombosis (arterial and/or venous or small-vessels) that must be diagnosed on the basis of objective criteria; and pregnancy morbidity. APS is characterized by a hypercoagulable state potentially resulting in thrombosis of all segments of the vascular bed. APS is considered "primary" when not associated with other underlying disease; or "secondary" when it appears in association with other autoimmune disorders, mainly systemic lupus erythematosus (SLE). It is suggested that thrombosis in APS is the consequence of complement system activation by aPL antibodies that in turn lead to endothelial cell activation and thrombosis [59].

In series of BCS patients, anti-phospholipids antibodies tested positive in 17–25% [7, 13]. Thus APS might be regarded as the third most common prothrombotic factor in BCS patients. However, APS diagnosis is challenging due to the poor specificity of antiphospholipid antibodies, especially in patients with chronic liver disease. Indeed, in a systematic review and meta-analysis, Qi et al. suggested that there is insufficient evidence regarding the association between anti-phospholipid antibodies and BCS [60]. In BCS patients, the estimated prevalence of definite APS is about 10–15% of BCS. Presence of lupus anticoagulant provides stronger evidence for antiphospholipid syndrome than anti beta2 glycoprotein-1 antibodies, while anticardiolipin antibodies appear to be the least specific feature unless repeatedly detected at high titers [61] (Table 20.4).

BCS seems to be an uncommon thrombotic manifestation of APS. In a cohort of 1000 European patients 0.7% had a BCS [14], while among 450 Asian patients, none had a BCS [62]. Espinosa et al. reviewed 43 cases of APS related BCS reported in the literature. In 65% of the patients, BCS was inaugural. The acute, chronic and fulminant variants of BCS were found in 70%, 23 and 7% of cases respectively [63].

In series of patients with portal vein thrombosis, anti-phospholipid antibodies are found in 10% of cases [64, 65] but the estimated prevalence of definite APS is probably around 5% [66]. Rare case reports describe definite APS with portal vein thrombosis.

APS associated venous thrombosis requires prolonged anticoagulation therapy with vitamin K antagonist (VKA). Direct oral anticoagulants (DOAC) are currently not recommended in this situation [67]. Indeed, a recent randomised study comparing efficacy and safety of VKA and DOAC in primary APS patients was prematurely stopped because of a high number of thrombotic events in the DOAC arm [67]. However, this study only included patients with so-called triple positivity of aPL antibodies, i.e. APS patients that are at highest risk of recurrent thrombosis [68]. Furthermore, another randomised open label controlled study enrolling 116 patients with APS did not find statistical differences between VKA and DOAC (but thrombotic event did not occur in any group) [69]. Hydroxychloroquine and specific immunosuppressive agent can be needed in secondary APS.

The term porto-sinusoidal vascular disease (PSVD) has been recently proposed to group together with idiopathic non-cirrhotic portal hypertension, nodular regenerative hyperplasia (NRH) and/or obliterative portal venopathy. Several reports have documented a relationship between NRH and APS [15, 70–72]. Perez-Ruiz et al. first suggested a role for aPL in the pathogenesis of NRH, four out of seven patients with rheumatic disorders and NRH, had positive lupus anticoagulant test [15]. Sera from 13 patients with histologically defined NRH were tested for aPL, 77% of the NRH patients had aPL compared with 14% of the patients with autoimmune liver diseases and healthy controls ($P < 0.05$) [73]. NRH may be more prevalent among secondary APL. Indeed, NRH can also be a complication of other connective diseases such as rheumatoid arthritis and SLE (see below).

The association between hepatic-veno-occlusive disease (HVOD) and APS was first described by Pappas et al. [74] in a patient with systemic lupus erythematosus (SLE) and false positive VDRL. Still, in SLE, only rare cases with aPL in association with HVOD have been documented [75, 76]. Saadoun et al. described 11 cases of sinusoidal dilatation in patient positive for antiphospholipid antibodies [16].

Several cases of hepatic infarction have been reported in association with APS, especially in pregnant or post-term women [77, 78]. Most of these cases were present in catastrophic APS, which is characterized by thrombosis occurring in at least three organs within 1 week. It is an extremely rare variant of APS carrying a mortality rate of 46% to 50%. Gomez-Puerta et al. analysed 15 patients with catastrophic APS during pregnancy and found manifestations resembling HELLP syndrome in half of the cases, including three cases of hepatic infarction [79]. In a retrospective review of the abdominal computed tomographic scans in 215 APS patients, out of 42 patients with abdominal thrombosis, only one patient with hepatic infarction was reported [80].

In a review of 250 patients with catastrophic APS, there was liver involvement in 34% of patients, while at autopsies 84.5% had hepatic microthrombi and 3.1% hepatic infarction [81, 82].

## Systemic Lupus

Systemic lupus erythematosus (SLE) is an autoimmune disease known to affect a variety of organ systems.

The association NRH, a component of PSVD, and SLE was described in several cases reports. It has been found in 0.3–6% of autopsy cases [17], and 5% of 35 patients who systematically underwent Doppler ultrasonography [18]. The exact prevalence in SLE as well as the relationship with antiphospholipid antibodies are difficult to assess and both may be underestimated in population-based studies.

An autopsy series found hepatic arteritis in 21% and peliosis in 12% of cases [17] but the clinical significance of these findings remain unclear.

## *Systemic Sclerosis*

Systemic sclerosis is a connective tissue disease characterized by vasculopathy, fibrosis, and immune dysfunction.

In a series, 278 patients with established systemic sclerosis 4 patients were diagnosed with biopsy-proven NRH resulting in a prevalence of 1.4% [19]. Graf et al. also collected 22 other cases in the literature [19]. It is important to note that none of the reported patients were under treatment with azathioprine, a drug associated with the development of NRH (see Chap. 21). Most of the patients had portal hypertension symptoms and increased serum alkaline phosphate land gamma glutamyl transpeptidase levels. Therefore, patients with systemic sclerosis and features of persistent cholestasis of unknown origin should be considered for Doppler ultrasound and liver biopsy to check for PVSD.

## *Rheumatoid Arthritis*

The association of NRH and rheumatoid arthritis (RA) (i.e. especially in Felty's syndrome) is generally accepted although its exact prevalence among RA patients is unknown. Blendis et al. did not observe any instance of NRH at autopsy in 51 RA patients [83]. On the other hand, the prevalence of RA among patients with NRH has been well studied. Wanless et al. reviewed 2500 autopsies, and found 64 having NRH. Among the latter, 6 had RA (9%) and among them, two third presented with Felty's syndrome. In a review of the literature, 180 cases of NRH were analyzed, 30 of whom had RA (16.7%). Among the 30 patients with RA and NRH, 25 (83%) had Felty's syndrome. They estimated that patient with RA had five-fold increased risk having NRH compare to controls [15, 84–86]. It is difficult to assess the exact role of medication in these autopsy cases.

Sinusoidal dilatation is a rare condition. A survey of 100 consecutive patients with adult RA without clinical evidence of liver disease identified 32 cases with - mostly minor - abnormalities of liver test results. Liver biopsies were obtained in eight of these patients. The most striking finding was the presence of sinusoidal dilation in all samples, with a normal central vein and preservation of hepatic architecture [87]. Such findings results were not found in other studies [20, 83].

# Sarcoidosis

Sarcoidosis is a systemic granulomatous disease of unknown aetiology and involves many organs. The liver is frequently involved but rarely does this involvement give rise to symptoms. The most common histopathological manifestation consist in non-caseating hepatic granulomas found in approximately 24–85% of patients with sarcoidosis.

Sarcoidosis and portal hypertension is not uncommon, having mostly been reported as single cases or small series. Portal hypertension was described in only 3% of 180 patients with hepatic sarcoidosis [20]. Portal hypertension is associated with, and likely secondary to cirrhosis in 25% of cases of portal hypertension. In the remaining cases the aetiology is not completely understood. NRH is found in 9% [20, 21]. Maddrey et al. suggested that small arterial-venous shunts may be formed in the region of the granulomas in the liver, resulting in elevated portal blood flow that leads to a compensatory increase in intrahepatic resistance [22]. Another proposed mechanism is that presinusoidal obstruction by granulomas in the portal vein causes an increase in pressure and restrict flow [21].

Management of symptomatic liver involvement in sarcoidosis requires systemic steroids and occasionally immune suppressants. Bilal et al. have reported encouraging long term results of liver transplantation in a single center experience [23].

Budd Chiari syndrome has been described in rare patients with sarcoidosis. It can be speculated that hepatic vein obstruction resulted from extrinsic compression by inflammation and oedema related to sarcoid granulomas.

# Drug Toxicity

As all clinical or biological manifestations that occur during the clinical course of systemic diseases, hepatic disorders (including vascular liver disorders) may be secondary to drug toxicity. Indeed, azathioprine, a drug commonly used to treat vasculitis and connective tissue diseases has been associated with vascular liver disease. This aspect is discussed in Chap. 21.

# References


1. Bayraktar Y, Balkanci F, Bayraktar M, Calguneri M. Budd-Chiari syndrome: a common complication of Behçet's disease. Am J Gastroenterol. 1997 May;92(5):858–62.
2. Cansu DU, Temel T, Erturk A, Kasifoglu T, Acu B, Korkmaz C. The long-term outcomes for patients with Budd-Chiari syndrome caused by Behcet's disease: a case series on the results, from cirrhosis to death. Hepat Mon. 2016 Oct;16(10):e32457.
3. Desbois AP. How might we increase success in marine-based drug discovery? Expert Opin Drug Discov. 2014 Sep;9:985–90.

4. Seyahi E, Caglar E, Ugurlu S, Kantarci F, Hamuryudan V, Sonsuz A, et al. An outcome survey of 43 patients with Budd-Chiari syndrome due to Behçet's syndrome followed up at a single, dedicated center. Semin Arthritis Rheum. 2015 Apr;44(5):602–9.

5. Tascilar K, Melikoglu M, Ugurlu S, Sut N, Caglar E, Yazici H. Vascular involvement in Behçet's syndrome: a retrospective analysis of associations and the time course. Rheumatol Oxf Engl. 2014 Nov;53(11):2018–22.

6. Wu X, Li G, Huang X, Wang L, Liu W, Zhao Y, et al. Behçet's disease complicated with thrombosis: a report of 93 Chinese cases. Medicine (Baltimore). 2014 Dec;93(28):e263.

7. Darwish Murad S, Plessier A, Hernandez-Guerra M, Fabris F, Eapen CE, Bahr MJ, et al. Etiology, management, and outcome of the Budd-Chiari syndrome. Ann Intern Med. 2009 Aug 4;151(3):167–75.

8. Bismuth E, Hadengue A, Hammel P, Benhamou JP. Hepatic vein thrombosis in Behçet's disease. Hepatol Baltim Md. 1990 Jun;11(6):969–74.

9. Bayraktar Y, Balkanci F, Kansu E, Dundar S, Uzunalimoglu B, Kayhan B, et al. Cavernous transformation of the portal vein: a common manifestation of Behçet's disease. Am J Gastroenterol. 1995 Sep;90(9):1476–9.

10. Matsumoto T, Kobayashi S, Shimizu H, Nakajima M, Watanabe S, Kitami N, et al. The liver in collagen diseases: pathologic study of 160 cases with particular reference to hepatic arteritis, primary biliary cirrhosis, autoimmune hepatitis and nodular regenerative hyperplasia of the liver. Liver. 2000 Oct;20(5):366–73.

11. Abbas MA, Fowl RJ, Stone WM, Panneton JM, Oldenburg WA, Bower TC, et al. Hepatic artery aneurysm: factors that predict complications. J Vasc Surg. 2003 Jul 1;38(1):41–5.

12. Stanson AW, Friese JL, Johnson CM, McKusick MA, Breen JF, Sabater EA, et al. Polyarteritis Nodosa: Spectrum of angiographic findings. Radiographics. 2001 Jan 1;21(1):151–9.

13. Cheng D, Xu H, Lu Z, Hua R, Qiu H, Du H, et al. Clinical features and etiology of Budd–Chiari syndrome in Chinese patients: a single-center study. J Gastroenterol Hepatol. 2013 Jun 1;28(6):1061–7.

14. Cervera R, Piette J-C, Font J, Khamashta MA, Shoenfeld Y, Camps MT, et al. Antiphospholipid syndrome: clinical and immunologic manifestations and patterns of disease expression in a cohort of 1,000 patients. Arthritis Rheum. 2002 Apr;46(4):1019–27.

15. Perez Ruiz F, Orte Martinez FJ, Zea Mendoza AC. Ruiz del Arbol L, Moreno Caparros a. nodular regenerative hyperplasia of the liver in rheumatic diseases: report of seven cases and review of the literature. Semin Arthritis Rheum. 1991 Aug;21(1):47–54.

16. Saadoun D, Cazals-Hatem D, Denninger M, Boudaoud L, Pham B, Mallet V, et al. Association of idiopathic hepatic sinusoidal dilatation with the immunological features of the antiphospholipid syndrome. Gut. 2004;53(10):1516–9.

17. Matsumoto T, Yoshimine T, Shimouchi K, Shiotu H, Kuwabara N, Fukuda Y, et al. The liver in systemic lupus erythematosus: pathologic analysis of 52 cases and review of Japanese autopsy registry data. Hum Pathol. 1992 Oct;23(10):1151–8.

18. Berzigotti A, Frigato M, Manfredini E, Pierpaoli L, Mulè R, Tiani C, et al. Liver hemangioma and vascular liver diseases in patients with systemic lupus erythematosus. World J Gastroenterol. 2011 Oct 28;17(40):4503–8.

19. Graf L, Dobrota R, Jordan S, Wildi LM, Distler O, Maurer B. Nodular regenerative hyperplasia of the liver: a rare vascular complication in systemic sclerosis. J Rheumatol. 2017 Nov 1;jrheum.170292.

20. Devaney K, Goodman ZD, Epstein MS, Zimmerman HJ, Ishak KG. Hepatic sarcoidosis: clinicopathologic features in 100 patients. Am J Surg Pathol. 1993;17(12):1272–80.

21. Blich M, Edoute Y. Clinical manifestations of sarcoid liver disease. J Gastroenterol Hepatol. 2004 Jul;19(7):732–7.

22. Maddrey WC, Johns CJ, Boitnott JK, Iber FL. Sarcoidosis and chronic hepatic disease: a clinical and pathologic study of 20 patients. Medicine (Baltimore). 1970 Sep;49(5):375–95.

23. Seksik P, Mary J-Y, Beaugerie L, Lémann M, Colombel J-F, Vernier-Massouille G, et al. Incidence of nodular regenerative hyperplasia in inflammatory bowel disease patients treated with azathioprine. Inflamm Bowel Dis. 2011 Feb;17(2):565–72.

24. Sprague AH, Khalil RA. Inflammatory cytokines in vascular dysfunction and vascular disease. Biochem Pharmacol. 2009 Sep 15;78(6):539–52.
25. Huber-Lang M, Lambris JD, Ward PA. Innate immune responses to trauma. Nat Immunol. 2018 Apr;19(4):327.
26. Hata T, Takahashi M, Hida S, Kawaguchi M, Kashima Y, Usui F, et al. Critical role of Th17 cells in inflammation and neovascularization after ischaemia. Cardiovasc Res. 2011 May 1;90(2):364–72.
27. Razakandrainibe R, Pelleau S, Grau GE, Jambou R. Antigen presentation by endothelial cells: what role in the pathophysiology of malaria? Trends Parasitol. 2012 Apr 1;28(4):151–60.
28. Meier LA, Binstadt BA. The contribution of autoantibodies to inflammatory cardiovascular pathology. Front Immunol [Internet]. 2018 Apr 27;9. Available from: https://www.ncbi.nlm.nih.gov/pmc/articles/PMC5934424/
29. Savage COS, Williams JM. Anti–endothelial cell antibodies in Vasculitis. J Am Soc Nephrol. 2007 Sep 1;18(9):2424–6.
30. Poisson J, Lemoinne S, Boulanger C, Durand F, Moreau R, Valla D, et al. Liver sinusoidal endothelial cells: physiology and role in liver diseases. J Hepatol. 2017 Jan 1;66(1):212–27.
31. Lalor PF, Shields P, Grant AJ, Adams DH. Recruitment of lymphocytes to the human liver. Immunol Cell Biol. 2002 Feb 1;80(1):52–64.
32. Hartleb M, Gutkowski K, Milkiewicz P. Nodular regenerative hyperplasia: evolving concepts on underdiagnosed cause of portal hypertension. World J Gastroenterol WJG. 2011 Mar 21;17(11):1400–9.
33. International Team for the Revision of the International Criteria for Behçet's Disease (ITR-ICBD). The international criteria for Behçet's disease (ICBD): a collaborative study of 27 countries on the sensitivity and specificity of the new criteria. J Eur Acad Dermatol Venereol JEADV. 2014 Mar;28(3):338–47.
34. Becatti M, Emmi G, Silvestri E, Bruschi G, Ciucciarelli L, Squatrito D, et al. Neutrophil activation promotes fibrinogen oxidation and thrombus formation in Behcet disease. Circulation. 2016 Jan 19;133:302–11.
35. Afredj N, Guessab N, Nani A, Faraoun SA, Ouled Cheikh I, Kerbouche R, et al. Aetiological factors of Budd-Chiari syndrome in Algeria. World J Hepatol. 2015 Apr 28;7(6):903–9.
36. Ollivier-Hourmand I, Allaire M, Goutte N, Morello R, Chagneau-Derrode C, Goria O, et al. The epidemiology of Budd–Chiari syndrome in France. Dig Liver Dis [Internet]. 2018 Apr 12 [cited 2018 Aug 6];0(0). Available from: https://www.dldjournalonline.com/article/S1590-8658(18)30701-1/fulltext
37. Uskudar O, Akdogan M, Sasmaz N, Yilmaz S, Tola M, Sahin B. Etiology and portal vein thrombosis in Budd-Chiari syndrome. World J Gastroenterol. 2008 May 14;14(18):2858–62.
38. Valla D-C. Primary Budd-Chiari syndrome. J Hepatol. 2009 Jan 1;50(1):195–203.
39. Ennaifer R, Bacha D, Romdhane H, Cheikh M, Nejma HB, BelHadj N. Budd-Chiari syndrome: an unusual presentation of multisystemic sarcoidosis. Clin Pract [Internet]. 2015 Dec 21;5(3). Available from: https://www.ncbi.nlm.nih.gov/pmc/articles/PMC4736049/
40. Desbois AC, Wechsler B, Resche-Rigon M, Piette JC, Huong DLT, Amoura Z, et al. Immunosuppressants reduce venous thrombosis relapse in Behçet's disease. Arthritis Rheum. 2012 Aug;64(8):2753–60.
41. Desbois AC, Biard L, Addimanda O, Lambert M, Hachulla E, Launay D, et al. Efficacy of anti-TNF alpha in severe and refractory major vessel involvement of Behcet's disease: a multicenter observational study of 18 patients. Clin Immunol Orlando Fla. 2018 Aug 18;197:54–9.
42. Benjilali L, Essaadouni L. Splanchnic venous thrombosis: a monocentric study of 31 cases. J Mal Vasc. 2016 Feb;41(1):26–35.
43. Ahmed I, Fotiadis NI, Dilks P, Kocher HM, Fotheringham T, Matson M. Multiple intrahepatic artery aneurysms in a patient with Behçet's disease: use of transcatheter embolization for rupture. Cardiovasc Intervent Radiol. 2010 Apr;33(2):398–401.
44. Hatzidakis A, Petrakis J, Krokidis M, Tsetis D, Gourtsoyiannis N. Hepatic artery aneurysm presenting with hemobilia in a patient with Behçet's disease: treatment with percutaneous transcatheteral embolization. Diagn Interv Radiol Ank Turk. 2006 Mar;12(1):53–5.

45. Jung NY, Kim SK, Chung EC, Park H, Cho YK. Endovascular treatment for rupture of intrahepatic artery aneurysm in a patient with Behçet's syndrome. AJR Am J Roentgenol. 2007 May;188(5):W400–2.
46. Pagnoux C, Mahr A, Cohen P, Guillevin L. Presentation and outcome of gastrointestinal involvement in systemic necrotizing vasculitides: analysis of 62 patients with polyarteritis nodosa, microscopic polyangiitis, Wegener granulomatosis, Churg-Strauss syndrome, or rheumatoid arthritis-associated vasculitis. Medicine (Baltimore). 2005 Mar;84(2):115–28.
47. Le Thi HD, Wechsler B, Guillevin L, Bletry O, Langlois P, Baumer R, et al. Digestive manifestations of periarteritis nodosa in a series of 120 cases. Gastroenterol Clin Biol. 1985;9(10):697–703.
48. Guillevin L, Mahr A, Callard P, Godmer P, Pagnoux C, Leray E, et al. Hepatitis B virus-associated polyarteritis nodosa: clinical characteristics, outcome, and impact of treatment in 115 patients. Medicine (Baltimore). 2005;84(5):313–22.
49. Battula N, Tsapralis D, Morgan M, Mirza D. Spontaneous liver haemorrhage and haemobilia as initial presentation of undiagnosed polyarteritis nodosa. Ann R Coll Surg Engl. 2012 May;94(4):e163–5.
50. Parent BA, Cho SW, Buck DG, Nalesnik MA, Gamblin TC. Spontaneous rupture of hepatic artery aneurysm associated with polyarteritis nodosa. Am Surg. 2010 Dec;76(12):1416–9.
51. Stambo GW, Guiney MJ, Cannella XF, Germain BF. Coil embolization of multiple hepatic artery aneurysms in a patient with undiagnosed polyarteritis nodosa. J Vasc Surg. 2004 May;39(5):1122–4.
52. Wicherts DA, Bruntink MM, Demirkiran A, van Santvoort HC, van Lienden KP, Ambarus CA, et al. Ruptured hepatic artery aneurysm: an unusual presentation of polyarteritis nodosa. BMJ Case Rep [Internet]. 2015 Apr 1;2015. Available from: https://www.ncbi.nlm.nih.gov/pmc/articles/PMC4401939/
53. Lee T, Ra HD, Park YJ, Park HS, Kim SJ. New routing alternative for proximal anterior tibial artery bypass in patients with Buerger disease. J Vasc Surg. 2011 Dec;54(6):1839–41.
54. Rousselet MC, Kettani S, Rohmer V, Saint-Andre JP. A case of temporal arteritis with intrahepatic arterial involvement. Pathol Res Pract. 1989 Sep;185(3):329–31.
55. Durant C, Martin J, Hervier B, Gournay J, Hamidou M. Takayasu arteritis associated with hepatic sinusoidal dilatation. Ann Hepatol. 2011 Dec;10(4):559–61.
56. Willeke P, Schlüter B, Limani A, Becker H, Schotte H. Liver involvement in ANCA-associated vasculitis. Clin Rheumatol. 2015 Jan 30;35(2):387–94.
57. Hernández-Rodríguez J, Tan CD, Rodríguez ER, Hoffman GS. Single-organ gallbladder vasculitis: characterization and distinction from systemic vasculitis involving the gallbladder. An analysis of 61 patients. Medicine (Baltimore). 2014 Nov;93(24):405–13.
58. Sironen RK, Seppä A, Kosma VM, Kuopio T. Churg-Strauss syndrome manifested by appendicitis, cholecystitis and superficial micronodular liver lesions--an unusual clinicopathological presentation. J Clin Pathol. 2010 Sep;63(9):848–50.
59. Keragala CB, Draxler DF, McQuilten ZK, Medcalf RL. Haemostasis and innate immunity–a complementary relationship: A review of the intricate relationship between coagulation and complement pathways. Br J Haematol. 2018 Mar;180(6):782–98.
60. Qi X, De Stefano V, Su C, Bai M, Guo X, Fan D. Associations of antiphospholipid antibodies with splanchnic vein thrombosis: a systematic review with meta-analysis. Medicine (Baltimore). 2015 Jan;94(4):e496.
61. Valla D-C. Budd-Chiari syndrome/hepatic venous outflow tract obstruction. Hepatol Int. 2018 Feb;12(Suppl 1):168–80.
62. Jatuworapruk K, Bhoopat L, Hanvivadhanakul P. Clinical and immunological characteristics of antiphospholipid syndrome in an Asian population: a retrospective study. Asian Pac J Allergy Immunol. 2018 Jul;8:1006–10.
63. Espinosa G, Font J, Garcia-Pagan JC, Tassies D, Reverter JC, Gaig C, et al. Budd-Chiari syndrome secondary to antiphospholipid syndrome: clinical and immunologic characteristics of 43 patients. Medicine (Baltimore). 2001;80(6):345–54.

64. Denninger M, Chaït Y, Casadevall N, Hillaire S, Guillin M, Bezeaud A, et al. Cause of portal or hepatic venous thrombosis in adults: the role of multiple concurrent factors. Hepatology. 2000;31(3):587–91.
65. Amarapurkar P, Bhatt N, Patel N, Amarapurkar D. Primary extrahepatic portal vein obstruction in adults: a single center experience. Indian J Gastroenterol. 2014 Jan 1;33(1):19–22.
66. Valla DC, Condat B. Portal vein thrombosis in adults: pathophysiology, pathogenesis and management. J Hepatol. 2000 May;32(5):865–71.
67. Pengo V, Denas G, Zoppellaro G, Padayattil Jose S, Hoxha A, Ruffatti A, et al. Rivaroxaban vs warfarin in high-risk patients with antiphospholipid syndrome. Blood. 2018 Jul 12;132(13):1365–71.
68. Dufrost V, Risse J, Reshetnyak T, Satybaldyeva M, Du Y, Yan X-X, et al. Increased risk of thrombosis in antiphospholipid syndrome patients treated with direct oral anticoagulants. Results from an international patient-level data meta-analysis. Autoimmun Rev. 2018 Aug 11;17(10):1011–21.
69. Cohen H, Hunt BJ, Efthymiou M, Arachchillage DRJ, Mackie IJ, Clawson S, et al. Rivaroxaban versus warfarin to treat patients with thrombotic antiphospholipid syndrome, with or without systemic lupus erythematosus (RAPS): a randomised, controlled, open-label, phase 2/3, non-inferiority trial. Lancet Haematol. 2016 Sep;3(9):e426–36.
70. Keegan AD, Brooks LT, Painter DM. Hepatic infarction and nodular regenerative hyperplasia of the liver with associated anticardiolipin antibodies in a young woman. J Clin Gastroenterol. 1994 Jun;18(4):309–13.
71. Cadranel JF, Demontis R, Guettier C, Bouraya D, Dautreaux M, Ghazali A, et al. Nodular regenerative hyperplasia associated with primary antiphospholipid syndrome. Gastroenterol Clin Biol. 1996;20(10):901–4.
72. Morlà RM, Ramos-Casals M, García-Carrasco M, Cervera R, Font J, Bruguera M, et al. Nodular regenerative hyperplasia of the liver and antiphospholipid antibodies: report of two cases and review of the literature. Lupus. 1999;8(2):160–3.
73. Klein R, Goller S, Bianchi L. Nodular regenerative hyperplasia (NRH) of the liver--a manifestation of "organ-specific antiphospholipid syndrome"? Immunobiology. 2003;207(1):51–7.
74. Pappas SC, Malone DG, Rabin L, Hoofnagle JH, Jones EA. Hepatic veno-occlusive disease in a patient with systemic lupus erythematosus. Arthritis Rheum. 1984 Jan 1;27(1):104–8.
75. Nakamura H, Uehara H, Okada T, Kambe H, Kimura Y, Ito H, et al. Occlusion of small hepatic veins associated with systemic lupus erythematosus with the lupus anticoagulant and anticardiolipin antibody. Hepato-Gastroenterology. 1989 Oct;36(5):393–7.
76. Greisman SG, Thayaparan RS, Godwin TA, Lockshin MD. Occlusive vasculopathy in systemic lupus erythematosus. Association with anticardiolipin antibody. Arch Intern Med. 1991 Feb;151(2):389–92.
77. Mor F, Beigel Y, Inbal A, Goren M, Wysenbeek AJ. Hepatic infarction in a patient with the lupus anticoagulant. Arthritis Rheum. 1989 Apr;32(4):491–5.
78. Young N, Wong KP. Antibody to cardiolipin causing hepatic infarction in a post partum patient with systemic lupus erythematosus. Australas Radiol. 1991 Feb;35(1):83–5.
79. Gómez-Puerta JA, Cervera R, Espinosa G, Asherson RA, García-Carrasco M, da Costa IP, et al. Catastrophic antiphospholipid syndrome during pregnancy and puerperium: maternal and fetal characteristics of 15 cases. Ann Rheum Dis. 2007 Jun;66(6):740–6.
80. Kaushik S, Federle MP, Schur PH, Krishnan M, Silverman SG, Ros PR. Abdominal thrombotic and ischemic manifestations of the antiphospholipid antibody syndrome: CT findings in 42 patients 1. Radiology. 2001;218(3):768–71.
81. Asherson RA. Multiorgan failure and antiphospholipid antibodies: the catastrophic antiphospholipid (Asherson's) syndrome. Immunobiology. 2005;210(10):727–33.
82. Bucciarelli S, Espinosa G, Cervera R, Erkan D, Gómez-Puerta JA, Ramos-Casals M, et al. Mortality in the catastrophic antiphospholipid syndrome: causes of death and prognostic factors in a series of 250 patients. Arthritis Rheum. 2006 Aug;54(8):2568–76.

83. Blendis LM, Parkinson MC, Shilkin KB, Williams R. Nodular regenerative hyperplasia of the liver in Felty's syndrome. Q J Med. 1974 Jan;43(169):25–32.
84. Wanless IR. Micronodular transformation (nodular regenerative hyperplasia) of the liver: a report of 64 cases among 2,500 autopsies and a new classification of benign hepatocellular nodules. Hepatology. 1990 May;11(5):787–97.
85. Bissonnette J, Généreux A, Côté J, Nguyen B, Perreault P, Bouchard L, et al. Hepatic hemodynamics in 24 patients with nodular regenerative hyperplasia and symptomatic portal hypertension. J Gastroenterol Hepatol. 2012 Aug;27(8):1336–40.
86. Morris JM, Oien KA, McMahon M, Forrest EH, Morris J, Stanley AJ, et al. Nodular regenerative hyperplasia of the liver: survival and associated features in a UK case series. Eur J Gastroenterol Hepatol. 2010 Aug;22(8):1001–5.
87. Laffón A, Moreno A, Gutierrez-Bucero A, Ossorio C, Sabando P, Moreno-Otero R. Hepatic sinusoidal dilatation in rheumatoid arthritis. J Clin Gastroenterol. 1989 Dec;11(6):653–7.

# Chapter 21
# Drugs and Toxins Affecting Liver Vessels

**Laure Elkrief and Laura Rubbia-Brandt**

## Abbreviations

DILI    drug induced liver injury
HIV     human immunodeficiency virus
NRH     nodular regenerative hyperplasia
SOS     sinusoidal obstruction syndrome

## Introduction

Drug-induced hepatotoxicity includes toxicity related to conventional medications, as well as herbal medicine and dietary supplements [1]. Drugs can affect all liver structures, including hepatic vessels. Drugs have thus been associated with a wide spectrum of vascular liver diseases, including thromboses of the large veins (i.e Budd-Chiari syndrome and portal vein thrombosis) as well as microvascular injury - including porto-sinusoidal vascular disease (PSVD) - and sinusoidal lesions, including sinusoidal obstruction syndrome (SOS) also named veno-occlusive disease,

L. Elkrief
Services de Transplantation et Hépato-gastroentérologie, Hôpitaux Universitaires de Genève, Geneva, Switzerland

Service d'hépato-gastroentérologie, Hôpital Trousseau, CHRU de Tours, Chambray-lès-Tours, France
e-mail: l.elkrief@chu-tours.fr

L. Rubbia-Brandt (✉)
Service de Pathologie clinique, Hôpitaux Universitaires et Faculté de Médecine de Genève, Geneva, Switzerland
e-mail: laura.rubbia-brandt@hcuge.ch

© Springer Nature Switzerland AG 2022
D. Valla et al. (eds.), *Vascular Disorders of the Liver*,
https://doi.org/10.1007/978-3-030-82988-9_21

peliosis, and isolated sinusoidal distension. The most frequently reported drugs associated with vascular liver injury are as follows, in decreasing order of frequency: (i) hormones, (ii) thiopurines, (iii) didanosine, (iv) oxaliplatin, and (vi) toxins. This chapter provides an overview of the spectrum of vascular liver lesions related to these agents, and discusses the responsibility of individual agents in the development of vascular liver lesions. For a discussion of vascular disorder occurring in the context of hematopoietic stem cell transplantation the reader is referred to Chap. 10.

## Epidemiology and Diagnosis of Drug-Induced Vascular Liver Diseases

The incidence of drug induced liver injury (DILI) in general is largely unknown because of the paucity of prospective studies and the relatively low frequency of liver injury attributable to drugs. Reported incidence in recent studies ranges from 14 to 19 per 100,000 inhabitants per year [2, 3]. There is marked geographic variability in the agents responsible for drug-induced liver diseases. In Western countries, the majority of cases are associated with conventional medications, whereas in Asian countries, herbal and dietary supplements rather than conventional medications constitute the most common causes [4]. Of note, the proportion of DILI related to herbals and dietary supplements appears to be increasing in Western countries [5]. Diagnosing DILI is challenging; especially since alternative causes for liver injury and/or concomitant medications are frequent [6]. DILI mainly represents a clinical diagnosis that relies on several parameters in the medical history, presentation, laboratory results, and subsequent course. The elements for the diagnosis of DILI are summarized in Table 21.1 [7], relying particularly on the exclusion of

**Table 21.1** Key elements for the diagnosis of drug-induced liver injury (adapted from Roussel Uclaf Causality Assessment Method (RUCAM) in Drug Induced Liver Injury [7])

| |
|---|
| 1. **Time to damage onset**<br>From the beginning of the drug<br>From the discontinuation of the drug |
| 2. **Course after drug discontinuation** |
| 3. **Presence of risk factors**<br>Alcohol<br>Pregnancy<br>Age > 55 years |
| 4. **Concomitant medications** |
| 5. **Known hepatotoxicity of the implicated drug**<br>Labeled on the product characteristics<br>Previously published |
| 6. **Exclusion of other causes of liver diseases** |
| 7. **Response to re-challenge** |
| 8. **Pattern of injury at histology ("drug morphological signature")** |

other cause of liver diseases. Liver histology, although dispensable, is most helpful for the diagnosis. The pattern of histologic lesions can contribute to identifying the causative drug and is particularly helpful when interpreted together with clinical presentation.

Vascular liver injury has been reported for more than 1300 conventional medications, herbal teas, as well as recreative agents. The possible mechanisms of toxicity to liver vessels include metabolite-mediated endothelial lesions and activation of hepatic stellate cells [8]. The resulting vascular changes consist in sinusoidal cell alterations, as well as fibrosis (Table 21.2). The incidence of drug induced vascular liver disease, although unknown, is considered to be much less frequent than the "classical" DILI encompassing mainly hepatocellular, cholestatic, or mixed pattern of injury. Indeed, several specific aspects of drug-induced vascular liver diseases, likely hamper the diagnosis, including the following: (i) the clinical presentation of drug-induced vascular liver diseases is highly variable, ranging from asymptomatic forms with or without mild abnormal liver blood tests, to a clinical syndrome of portal hypertension; (ii) the duration between drug therapy initiation and the first symptoms varies from days to years, contrasting with the usual timeframe criteria accepted for a diagnosis of classical DILI; (iii) liver biopsy is usually indispensable for the diagnosis; and (iv) alternative causes for vascular liver disease are frequently present.

**Table 21.2**  Summary of drug-induced vascular changes

| Mechanism involved | Lesions | Drug examples | Toxin example |
|---|---|---|---|
| **Hypercoagulability** | Venous thrombosis | Oral contraceptive | |
| **Drug-metabolite mediated sinusoidal damage** | Sinusoidal dilatation | Oral contraceptive Azathioprine Oxaliplatin Didanosin | Pyrrozilidine alcaloids Arsenic Vinyl chloride monomer |
| | Peliosis | Anabolic steroids Azathioprine Oxaliplatin Didanosin Arsenical | Pyrrozilidine alcaloids Arsenic |
| | Sinusoidal obstruction syndrome | Azathioprine Oxaliplatin | Pyrrozilidine alcaloids |
| | Porto-sinusoidal vascular disease | Azathioprine Oxaliplatin Didanosin | |
| | Perisinusoidal fibrosis | Azathioprine Oxaliplatin Didanosin | Arsenic Vinyl chloryd monomer |
| **Hepatic stellate cells activation** | Perisinusoidal fibrosis | | Vitamin A |

# Hormones-Associated Vascular Liver Lesions

## *Oral Contraceptive Agents*

The vascular toxicity of oral contraceptive agents has been attributed to the combination of ethynylestradiol and a progestogen. Vascular liver changes associated with oral contraceptive agents include thrombosis of the large veins (i.e Budd-Chiari syndrome and portal vein thrombosis), and sinusoidal dilatation.

### Budd-Chiari Syndrome and Portal Vein Thrombosis

Since the early 1960s, it has been well documented that combined estroprogestative oral contraceptives are associated with a two- to six-fold increase in the risk of venous thrombosis [9]. The risk of venous thrombosis has been related to the dose of ethynilestradiol and the type of progestogen [10]. Up to 74% of western women with Budd-Chiari syndrome had been using oral contraceptive agents [11, 12]. This might explain the female predominance observed in patients with Budd-Chiari syndrome [12]. The risk of Budd-Chiari syndrome was significantly increased in recent first-generation oral contraceptive users (i.e containing 150 µg of ethynilestradiol) than in non-users [13]. However, when an extensive workup is performed, an additional factor was found in 80% of women with Budd-Chiari syndrome using oral contraceptive agents; moreover, oral contraceptive use was the only causal factor in only 10% of Budd-Chiari women [14]. The manifestations of Budd-Chiari syndrome were similar between oral contraceptive users and non-users [13].

Oral contraceptive use has also been frequently found (up to 48%) in women with portal vein thrombosis [15, 16]. However, the mere exposure to oral contraceptive agents does not appear to cause portal vein thrombosis. Indeed, a female predominance has not been reported among patients with portal vein thrombosis, which contrasts with what has been observed in patients with Budd Chiari syndrome [15, 17–19]. Furthermore, in an Italian case-control study, oral contraceptive use was associated with deep vein thrombosis, but not with portal vein thrombosis [17]. Oral contraceptive use was associated with portal vein thrombosis only when local or other general prothrombotic factors were present [14, 16].

Altogether, these data suggest that combined first generation oral contraceptive agents are a causal factor for Budd-Chiari syndrome; this association is less clear for second or third generation contraceptive agents. The association between oral contraceptive agents and portal vein thrombosis has not been well-established. Oral combined contraception discontinuation is recommended both in women with Budd-Chiari syndrome and in those with portal vein thrombosis [20]. Progestin-only contraception does not increase the risk of venous thromboembolism [21] and therefore can be considered in women with a history of Budd-Chiari syndrome or portal vein thrombosis. Data on safety of hormonal substitution in these patients are not available.

## Sinusoidal Dilatation

Isolated sinusoidal dilatation (i.e. in the absence of more specific histologic lesions, namely SOS, atrophy or regenerative changes of hepatocytes, or perisinusoidal fibrosis) has been reported in oral contraceptive users. Most cases were reported in the 1970s when the estrogen content of oral contraceptives was high [22–25]. Reported clinical manifestations included abdominal pain, hepatomegaly, and elevated serum alkaline phosphatases [22, 23, 25]. Time to resolution after oral contraceptives discontinuation ranged from days to years [26].

The direct role of oral contraceptives as a cause for sinusoidal dilatation is far from clear, because in most reported cases the criteria for causality assessment were not fulfilled [26]. (Table 21.1).

## *Anabolic Steroids*

Anabolic androgen steroids may be used for treatment of aplastic anemia or hypogonadism as well as for enhancing performance and muscles development in body building. Anabolic androgen steroids have been mainly associated with peliosis. Peliosis is characterized by different-sized lobular cystic blood lakes, randomly distributed throughout the lobule [27]. Peliosis harbors a total rupture of the reticulin fibers of the perisinusoidal space. The mechanism by which peliosis affects steroids users is not known. Clinical manifestations have varied from right upper quadrant discomfort and hepatomegaly to sudden abdominal pain and hemorrhagic shock due to hepatic rupture and hemoperitoneum. Peliosis may also be a purely incidental finding. Importantly, another cause for liver disease was not present in the reported cases. Peliosis associated with anabolic androgen steroids usually reverses, at least in part, after discontinuation [26, 28].

Altogether, these data are in favor or a direct role of anabolic steroids as a causal factor for peliosis, although the mechanism is not known.

## Thiopurines

Thiopurines include azathioprine, mercaptopurine and thioguanine, all of which are sulphur substituted purine bases. The prototype of this class is mercaptopurine which was introduced into clinical medicine in the 1950's, largely as an antineoplastic agent. Azathioprine was developed and introduced into clinical medicine in the mid-1960's.

## *Azathioprine*

Azathioprine is used as an immunosuppressive agent in organ transplantation to prevent rejection and in autoimmune diseases as a corticosteroid sparing agent. Azathioprine has been long regarded as a leading cause of vascular liver lesions. Nodular regenerative hyperplasia (NRH) has been the most frequently reported entity [29, 30]. Other reported lesions include SOS [31, 32], peliosis [33–35], and sinusoidal dilatation [36].

Azathioprine has mostly been associated with NRH in patients with ulcerative colitis and Crohn's disease [37–39]. It has also been associated with vascular liver injury (including sinusoidal lesions and NRH) after liver [40], or renal transplantation [29, 30, 34, 41, 42] (Fig. 21.1). NRH has also been reported in patients with other inflammatory disorders, treated with azathioprine [43–45]. Vascular lesions have not been reported in patients with autoimmune hepatitis treated with azathioprine.

In patients with Crohn's disease treated with azathioprine, the cumulative incidence of NRH was 0.6% and 1.3% at 5 and 10 years, respectively [37]. Male gender, older age, and stricturing disease/small bowel resection have been associated with NRH [37, 39]. Of note, NRH has been reported in 6% of the patients with inflammatory bowel disease naïve of thiopurines [46]. NRH has also been reported in liver transplant recipients not treated with azathioprine [47].

Azathioprine has been postulated to directly damage hepatic sinusoidal endothelial cells and/or small hepatic and portal veins [29]. DeLeve et al. demonstrated in vitro that azathioprine was selectively toxic to murine sinusoidal endothelial cells (but not hepatocytes), by depleting cellular glutathione stores [48]. However, the link between azathioprine and vascular liver lesions remain unclear, for the

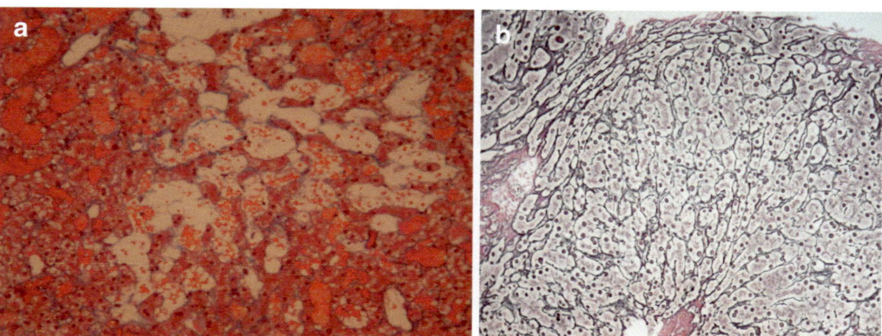

**Fig. 21.1** Liver biopsy performed in a patient with abnormal liver blood tests, treated with azathioprine after renal transplantation (**a**) Low-power examination on hematoxyllin & Eosin stain shows severe sinusoidal dilatation and peliosis. (**b**) A new liver biopsy was performed 2 years later (and azathioprine discontinuation): high-power field examination on reticulin stain shows a regenerative nodule made of enlarged hepatocytic cells centred by portal tracts and delineated at the periphery by atrophic hepatocytes corresponding to nodular regenerative hyperplasia

following reasons: (i) there is no animal model of azathioprine induced vascular liver injury; (ii) dose relationship is not obvious; and (iii) underlying conditions for which azathioprine was administered have been reported to be associated with sinusoidal changes. Regression after azathioprine discontinuation has been reported [49].

Altogether, these data indicate that azathioprine has been mostly associated with the occurrence of NRH. However, the imputability is low (Table 21.3). Despite the low level of evidence for a direct role of azathioprine on vascular liver lesions, drug discontinuation has to be considered, especially if an alternative therapy is available.

## Thioguanine

Thioguanine has been commonly used in the therapy of hematologic neoplasms, as well as a steroid sparing agent in the treatment of autoimmune diseases, especially in patients with inflammatory bowel diseases.

SOS [50, 51] and peliosis [52] have been reported in patients with hematological neoplasm, treated with high-dose chemotherapy including thioguanine. NRH and/ or SOS have also been reported in patients with inflammatory bowel diseases treated with thioguanine. The incidence is highly variables among studies, ranging from

**Table 21.3** Summary of the criteria for the imputability of azathioprine and oxaliplatin related vascular liver disease

|  | Thiopurines | Oxaliplatin |
| --- | --- | --- |
| **Time to damage onset and dose relationship** | **Variable** <br> No dose relationship for azathioprine therapy <br> Dose relationship in patients treated with thioguanine | **Yes** <br> More frequent in patients who received more than 6 chemotherapy cycles <br> Vascular lesions not described in patients treated with surgery alone |
| **Course after drug discontinuation** | **Variable** <br> (improvement, stability or aggravation) | **Regression after discontinuation** |
| **Presence of risk factors** | In patients with IBD, NRH is associated with <br> History of intestinal resection <br> Age |  |
| **Concomitant medications** | **Not reported** | **Not reported** |
| **Pathophysiological rationale** | No animal model | Animal model developed <br> Bevacizumab has a protective affect |
| **Exclusion of other causes of liver diseases** | **No** <br> Underlying conditions are known to be associated with vascular liver lesions | **Yes** |

*IBD* inflammatory bowel disease; *NRH* nodular regenerative hyperplasia

0% to 62% [39, 53]. The incidence of SOS and/or NRH may be related to thioguanine dosing, since it was more frequently observed in patients receiving high-dose thioguanine or with high circulating thioguanine nucleotides levels [39]. In a recent study of 111 patients with inflammatory bowel disease who were treated with low-dose thioguanine (daily dose of 0.3 mg/kg for a median duration of 20 (4–64) months), and who had liver biopsy as part of the toxicity screening, nodular regenerative hyperplasia was detected in only 6% of the patients. No patient had manifestations of portal hypertension [54]. Thioguanine discontinuation has been associated with a decrease in hepatic venous pressure gradient [55]. Ability of thioguanine to induce SOS has recently been validated in an animal model [56]. In this model, SOS occurrence is dependent on thioguanine dose, and mediated by thioguanine nucleotides. These data suggest that split dosing regimen of thioguanine can prevent SOS, by reducing the concentration of thioguanine nucleotides in the hepatic circulation. Cotherapy of thioguanine and allopurinol, to optimize therapeutic thioguanine nucleotides levels, may also be an effective preventive strategy [57].

Altogether these data suggest that the incidence of SOS and/or NRH is low in patients treated with current low-dose thioguanine regimens.


## Oxaliplatin


The liver toxicity of oxaliplatin has been described in the context of neoadjuvant chemotherapy regimen used for downstaging colorectal liver metastasis before surgical hepatic resection. Vascular liver lesions have been described in up to 60% of patients receiving oxaliplatin-based chemotherapy for colon cancer [58–62]. By contrast, they have not been described in patients with colorectal metastasis treated with surgery alone or with other chemotherapy regimens [58, 59]. The anti-VEGF bevacizumab appears to decrease the risk of vascular liver injury following oxaliplatin administration [59, 63]. Oxalipatin has been associated with various types of microvascular hepatic lesions, which may all occur in various combinations. Sinusoidal alterations, including SOS, sinusoidal dilatation and peliosis, are the most frequent, [58–62] (Fig. 21.2). Occlusion of the centrilobular veins, which is considered to be a criterion for increased SOS severity, is found in 50% of oxaliplatin related-SOS [58, 59, 61]. In addition to sinusoidal lesions, NRH occurs in up to 25% of the patients treated with oxaliplatin [59, 62, 64].

Clinical data supporting the link between oxaliplatin and vascular lesions mostly relies on (i) the absence of vascular lesions in patients who had surgery alone; and (ii) the protective effect of bevacizumab, an antiangiogenic monoclonal antibody, on the development of vascular liver lesions. In addition, human and animal studies identified shared key processes associated with oxaliplatin-related SOS. These pathways include the activation of the IL-6/STAT3 pathway, the activation of the coagulation system, as well as an overexpression of genes involved in cellular hypoxia and oxidative stress [65–67].

Before surgery, oxaliplatin-related vascular liver lesions are either asymptomatic or only associated with mildly abnormal liver blood tests. AST-to-platelet-ratio-index

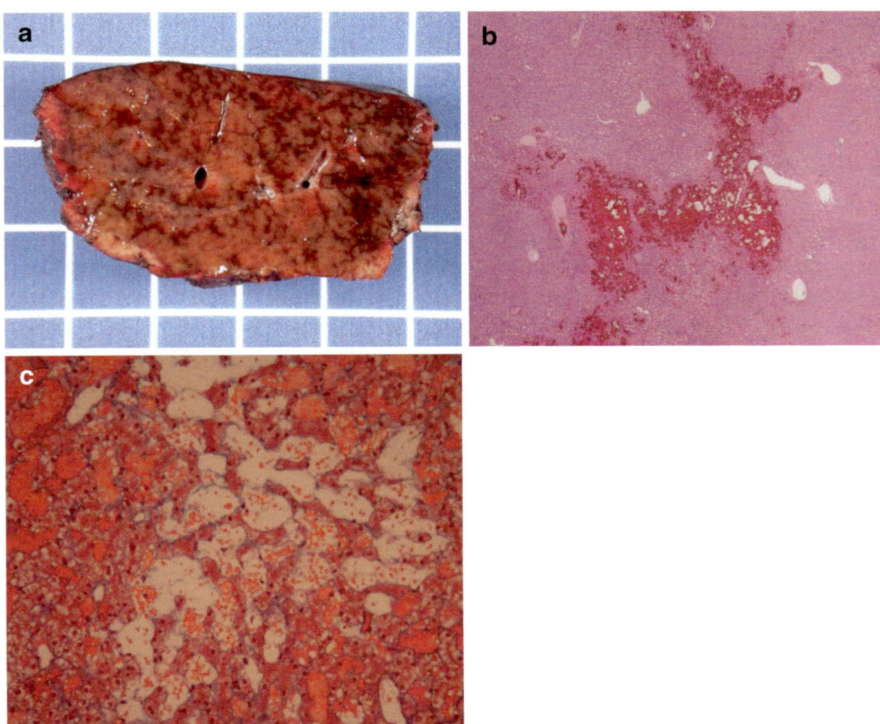

**Fig. 21.2** SOS in a patient treated with oxaliplatin before hepatic resection for colorectal liver metastasis. (**a**) Macroscopically, on the cut surface, the liver has congested areas. (**b**) Low-power examination on hematoxyllin & Eosin stain shows large areas of sinusoidal congestion involving centrilobular and mediolobular lobular surface. (**c**) At high-power examination on Trichrome stain, severe sinusoidal dilatation outlined by atrophic or interrupted hepatocyte trabeculae. The perisinusoidal space of Disse contains several erythrocytes in close contact with hepatocytes

(APRI) may be helpful for a non-invasive estimation of SOS [60] or NRH [64]. Oxaliplatin-based chemotherapy has been associated with non-specific signs of portal hypertension, including thrombocytopenia [60, 64], spleen enlargement [68, 69]. Portal-hypertension related complications, including variceal bleeding or ascites unrelated to surgery have been rarely reported [70]. Oxaliplatin-related vascular liver lesions, especially NRH, negatively impact peri- and post-operative outcomes. Oxaliplatin-related vascular liver lesions have been associated with increased red blood cell transfusion [61], hepatic complications [60, 71], and postoperative liver failure [60, 62], especially after major hepatectomy [64, 72], and more than 6–12 cycles of oxaliplatin-based chemotherapy [61, 72], but not with an increased post-operative mortality [62]. Vascular liver changes can regress after nine months without chemotherapy [62].

Altogether, these data bring strong support for an association between oxaliplatin and vascular liver lesions, especially SOS and NRH. These lesions have been associated with an increased incidence of post-operative complications, but not with increased mortality. There are no clear recommendation for the practical management of patients with oxaliplatin-related vascular liver injury.

## Didanosine

Vascular liver lesions in patients with human immunodeficiency virus (HIV) have been mostly associated with didanosine. This purine nucleoside analogue and first-generation reverse transcriptase inhibitor was widely used in combination with other agents in the therapy HIV infection. More than 100 cases of noncirrhotic portal hypertension related to HIV infections have been reported worldwide [73]. The reported histological lesions include hepatoportal sclerosis, obliterative portal venopathy, sinusoidal lesions and fibrosis (centrilobular, perisinusoidal or portal) [73–80]. NRH is the most frequent of these lesions, since it accounts for three quarters of the cases. In a recent study of 29 HIV patients with vascular liver alterations (of which 90% had been exposed to didanosine), NRH was found in 72% of the biopsies, sinusoidal dilatation in 55% and peliosis in 8% [80].

The association between NRH and antiretroviral therapy has been identified mostly through case reports and small case-control studies [73, 74, 77, 78]. In these studies, 100% of the patients had been exposed to didanosine. However, the evidence for a direct role of didanosine in HIV-related vascular liver diseases remains unclear. First, the association between vascular liver diseases and didanosine may be related to confounding factors. In particular, the long duration of HIV infection may explain that the majority of the patients received didanosine. Furthermore, in patients with HIV, vascular liver diseases may be related to other conditions, such as increased levels of anti–protein S antibodies [80, 81], or infections. In addition, the regression of vascular liver lesions after didanosine discontinuation has not been described. Finally, the underlying mechanisms of vascular liver injury is unclear. Nucleoside reverse transcriptase inhibitors are known to cause mitochondrial toxicity. The link between the association of steatosis and lactic acidosis and mitochondrial toxicity is clear. By contrast, the relationship between vascular liver lesions and mitochondrial toxicity is unclear. Nucleoside reverse transcriptase inhibitors can cause endothelial dysfunction [82]; in all reports however, the causative agent was azathioprine but not didanosine. Lastly, no animal model of vascular liver disease related to nucleoside reverse transcriptase inhibitors exists.

## Medicinal Plants and Toxins

### *Pyrrolizidine Alcaloids*

Pyrrozilidine alcaloids are found in more than 6000 plants worldwide [83]. The main implicated species are: Heliotroprium, Senecio, Crotalaria, and Symphytum (Comfrey) as well as Gynura segetum [84].

Pyrrozilidine alcaloids have been related to SOS in different contexts. This entity was first described in South Africa in 1920 as cirrhosis resulting from Senecio poisoning in humans [85]. Epidemics of SOS were described in the 1970's in India and Afghanistan, caused by consumption of wheat contaminated with seeds of Crotalaria sp. [86, 87]. Pyrrolizidine poisoning is endemic in areas such as Africa and Jamaica, where toxic alkaloids are ingested as infusions, herbal teas, decoctions, or used as an enema [84]. In China, SOS is usually caused by herbal medicine containing pyrrolizidine alkaloids. The most frequent herbal medicine reported is Tusanqi (i.e., Gynura segetum), which is used to relieve pain, improve blood circulation, and dissipate blood stasis. Hepatotoxicity has occurred because of the misuse of G. segetum instead of non-toxic plants in the preparation [88].

The typical histopathological feature of pyrrozilidine alcaloids hepatic toxicity is SOS [89], which may lead to complication such as parenchymal necrosis and in some cases, fibrosis and even cirrhosis. Different clinical subtypes have been described [90]. (i) Acute presentation with marked elevated transaminases, massive abdominal swelling and pain; when lesions are extensive, hepatic failure may occur, leading to death. This presentation has been associated with hemorrhagic centrilobular necrosis. (ii) A subacute presentation with recurrent ascites, splenomegaly and hepatomegaly. This presentation has been associated with extensive fibrosis in centrilobular areas. And (iii), a chronic variant indistinguishable at bedside from cirrhosis of other origin, but showing a venocentric type of cirrhosis at histological examination. In a recent systematic review of Tusanqi-related SOS, reported after 1999, ascites was present in all patients [88]. Other symptoms included hepatomegaly (85%), jaundice (58%), pleural effusion (37%), lower limb edema (37%), and splenomegaly (31%). Gastro-esophageal varices and upper gastrointestinal bleeding are rarely observed. Contrast enhanced computed tomography may be helpful for non-invasive diagnosis of pyrrozilidine-associated related SOS: patchy enhancement and heterogeneous hypoattenuation of the liver parenchyma are features. Other findings include ascites (100%), hepatomegaly (80%), gallbladder wall thickening (87%), pleural effusion (70%), hepatic vein narrowing (87%) [91]. One-year cumulative survival was 80% in patients with Tusanqi-related SOS and after Tusanqi discontinuation, complete recovery occurred in around 40% of the patients, [88]. The detection of pyrrole–protein adducts is specific of pyrrozilidine alkaloids-related toxicity, and thus could be used as diagnostic biomarker of pyrrozilidine alkaloids related SOS [92].

The direct responsibility of pyrrolizidine alkaloids in inducing liver sinusoidal lesions has been demonstrated using animal models [93]. A reproducible rat model was eventually developed consisting of gavage with monocrotaline, a pyrrolizidine alkaloid, for 1 to 10 days before sacrifice [48]. This model showed early injury to sinusoidal and central vein endothelium, preceding the development of veno-occlusive lesions. Coagulative necrosis of hepatocytes occurs later than endothelial injury [48]. Pyrrozilidine alcaloids toxicity is the consequence of the biotransformation of unsaturated alkaloids into toxic metabolites by cytochrome P450 leading mainly to lesions of endothelial cells. In Europe, dietary exposure to pyrrozilidine alkaloids is common, especially in honey, tea, herbal infusions and food supplements users. An exposure to 2 mg/kg of body weight per day of pyrrozilidine alkaloids is considered the lowest dose associated with toxicity. Chronic and acute dietary exposure to pyrrolizidine alkaloids was estimated in the European population via the consumption of plant-derived foods. This resulted in highest estimates of mean chronic dietary exposure which were 10 thousand times lower than the toxic dose, even in the highly exposed population [94].

## *Vitamin A*

The generic term "vitamin A" is used for compounds having the biological activity of retinol or its metabolic products. Dietary sources of vitamin A are carotenoids, such as β-carotene (rich plant sources are sweet potatoes, carrots, and dark green leafy vegetables like spinach) and retinyl esters (rich animal sources are liver, eggs, and fish). Vitamin A is an essential fat-soluble vitamin. Adequate daily intake (~700–900 µg for humans) and hepatic storage (~80% in a healthy individual) are required to maintain plasma adequate retinol levels. Vitamin A plays important physiological roles in vision, reproduction, growth, development, immunity, and metabolic programs [95]. Hypervitaminosis A results from excessive intake of exogenous vitamin A. By contrast, pro-vitamin carotenoids - such as beta-carotene – do not cause toxicity, as their conversion to retinol is highly regulated [96]. The major causes of hypervitaminosis A are medications, especially synthetic retinoids derived from vitamin A – for example psoriasis treatments acitretin or bexarotene used to treat the skin effects of T-cell lymphoma; and dietary supplements taken above recommended dosage, such as cod liver oil, which contains high concentrations of vitamin A. Hypervitaminosis A related to topics has also been reported.

Liver toxicity may occur after prolonged exposure, i.e. at least 3 months and usually several years. Manifestations include mild liver blood tests abnormalities, hepatomegaly, splenomegaly, and manifestations of portal hypertension, such as splenomegaly, ascites or gastro-esophageal varices [97]. Extra-hepatic manifestations include dry skin, cheilosis, gingivitis, muscle and joint pains, fatigue, mental dullness or depression [98]. Improvement after vitamin A withdrawal is inconstant [97, 98].

Histological features include the direct visualization of hypertrophied hepatic stellate cells (which cannot be seen at light microscopy in normal condition) that contain abundant lipid droplets, located in the space of Disse between the sinusoidal endothelial lining cells and the hepatocytes. Hypertrophic stellate cells are often accompanied by sinusoidal dilatation, and less frequently peliosis. The most typical feature is prominent perisinusoidal fibrosis. Immunohistochemistry is helpful, showing the expression of α-smooth muscle actin by hepatic stellate cells [99]. Cirrhosis may develop after prolonged exposition [97, 99, 100]. Perisinusoidal fibrosis is the consequence of direct, dose-dependent, vitamin A toxicity. The excess vitamin A is stored in hepatic stellate cells. In consequence, activation of hepatic stellated cells leads to excess collagen production. The amount of fibrosis is correlated to the dose of vitamin A, namely the dose and the duration of exposition [99].

## *Vinyl Chloride Monomer Toxicity*

Vinyl chloride is a colourless gas at room temperature. Polyvinyl chloride (PVC) is a polymerized form of vinyl chloride that is extensively used in the plastics industry. Vinyl chloride does not occur naturally, and thus is found almost exclusively in factories making PVC. Vinyl chloride has not been identified in food, pharmaceuticals or cosmetic products in recent years. Vinyl chloride-related liver toxicity has exclusively been reported among exposed workers in PVC factories.

Vinyl chloride has been implicated in the development of noncirrhotic portal hypertension, and angiosarcoma of the liver. Vinyl chloride has also been related to hepatocellular carcinoma [101]; however, the direct relationship between vinyl chloride toxicity and hepatocellular carcinoma is poorly demonstrated [102].

The pathology of vinyl chloride-related liver disease is related to endothelial sinusoidal injury. Histological features include sinusoidal dilatation, with or without hypertrophy of the sinusoids [103]. Various degrees of fibrosis have been reported, including perisinusoidal, portal and subcapsular fibrosis, the latter being a typical feature of vinyl chloride-related toxicity [103–105]. Ultimately, cirrhosis may occur. Importantly, these changes were described in an era before hepatitis C was identified, and one cannot exclude that fibrosis was related to hepatitis C. Clinical features include manifestation of portal hypertension, including splenomegaly, varices, gastrointestinal bleeding, and ascites, even in the absence of cirrhosis [102].

Animal models have validated the responsibility of vinyl chloride in liver injury: similar lesions develop in animals after exposure to vinyl chloride [102, 105]. In humans, most reported cases of vascular lesions related vinyl chloride were describe in patients with concomitant angiosarcoma of the liver, which is a rapidly lethal disease. Thus, the course of vascular liver lesions after vinyl chloride exposure discontinuation is unknown.

## Conclusion

Endothelial injury appears to account for the vast majority of drug- and toxin-related vascular liver injury. A large spectrum of different vascular lesions can be observed, either isolated or concomitant one with the other. The diagnosis of drug- and toxin-related vascular liver injury is based on the suggestive context, the exclusion of alternative cause of liver disease, and histological findings. There is a strong level of imputability for oxaliplatin and pyrrolizidine alcaloids-related liver injury. By contrast, the data for a direct relationship between oral contraceptives, didanosine, and thiopurin derivatives are still not fully conclusive. Pyrrozilidine-alcaloids-related sinusoidal injury is still a major concern in terms of public health, especially in Asia and Africa.

# References


1. European Association for the Study of the Liver. Electronic address: easloffice@easloffice.eu, Clinical Practice guideline panel: chair:, panel members, EASL governing board representative: EASL Clinical Practice Guidelines: drug-induced liver injury. J Hepatol. 2019;70:1222–1261.
2. Sgro C, Clinard F, Ouazir K, Chanay H, Allard C, Guilleminet C, et al. Incidence of drug-induced hepatic injuries: a French population-based study. Hepatol Baltim Md. 2002;36:451–5.
3. Björnsson ES, Bergmann OM, Björnsson HK, Kvaran RB, Olafsson S. Incidence, presentation, and outcomes in patients with drug-induced liver injury in the general population of Iceland. Gastroenterology. 2013;144:1419–25. 1425.e1–3; quiz e19-20
4. Wai C-T, Tan B-H, Chan C-L, Sutedja DS, Lee Y-M, Khor C, et al. Drug-induced liver injury at an Asian center: a prospective study. Liver Int Off J Int Assoc Study Liver. 2007;27:465–74.
5. Chalasani N, Fontana RJ, Bonkovsky HL, Watkins PB, Davern T, Serrano J, et al. Causes, clinical features, and outcomes from a prospective study of drug-induced liver injury in the United States. Gastroenterology. 2008;135:1924–34. 1934.e1–4
6. Teschke R, Danan G. Drug induced liver injury with analysis of alternative causes as confounding variables. Br J Clin Pharmacol. 2018;84:1467–77.
7. Danan G, Benichou C. Causality assessment of adverse reactions to drugs—I. a novel method based on the conclusions of international consensus meetings: application to drug-induced liver injuries. J Clin Epidemiol. 1993;46:1323–30.
8. Larrey D. Drug-induced liver diseases. J Hepatol. 2000;32:77–88.
9. Stegeman BH, de Bastos M, Rosendaal FR, van Hylckama VA, Helmerhorst FM, Stijnen T, et al. Different combined oral contraceptives and the risk of venous thrombosis: systematic review and network meta-analysis. BMJ. 2013;347:f5298.
10. van Hylckama VA, Helmerhorst FM, Vandenbroucke JP, Doggen CJM, Rosendaal FR. The venous thrombotic risk of oral contraceptives, effects of oestrogen dose and progestogen type: results of the MEGA case-control study. BMJ. 2009;339:b2921.
11. Chait Y, Condat B, Cazals-Hatem D, Rufat P, Atmani S, Chaoui D, et al. Relevance of the criteria commonly used to diagnose myeloproliferative disorder in patients with splanchnic vein thrombosis. Br J Haematol. 2005;129:553–60.
12. Darwish Murad S, Plessier A, Hernandez-Guerra M, Fabris F, Eapen CE, Bahr MJ, et al. Etiology, management, and outcome of the Budd-Chiari syndrome. Ann Intern Med. 2009;151:167–75.
13. Valla D, Le MG, Poynard T, Zucman N, Rueff B, Benhamou JP. Risk of hepatic vein thrombosis in relation to recent use of oral contraceptives. A case-control study. Gastroenterology. 1986;90:807–11.
14. Denninger MH, Chaït Y, Casadevall N, Hillaire S, Guillin MC, Bezeaud A, et al. Cause of portal or hepatic venous thrombosis in adults: the role of multiple concurrent factors. Hepatology. 2000;31:587–91.
15. Plessier A, Darwish-Murad S, Hernandez-Guerra M, Consigny Y, Fabris F, Trebicka J, et al. Acute portal vein thrombosis unrelated to cirrhosis: a prospective multicenter follow-up study. Hepatology. 2010;51:210–8.
16. Janssen HL, Meinardi JR, Vleggaar FP, van Uum SH, Haagsma EB, van Der Meer FJ, et al. Factor V Leiden mutation, prothrombin gene mutation, and deficiencies in coagulation inhibitors associated with Budd-Chiari syndrome and portal vein thrombosis: results of a case-control study. Blood. 2000;96:2364–8.
17. Amitrano L, Guardascione MA, Scaglione M, Pezzullo L, Sangiuliano N, Armellino MF, et al. Prognostic factors in noncirrhotic patients with splanchnic vein thromboses. Am J Gastroenterol. 2007;102:2464–70.
18. Rajani R, Björnsson E, Bergquist A, Danielsson A, Gustavsson A, Grip O, et al. The epidemiology and clinical features of portal vein thrombosis: a multicentre study. Aliment Pharmacol Ther. 2010;32:1154–62.

19. Janssen HL, Wijnhoud A, Haagsma EB, van Uum SH, van Nieuwkerk CM, Adang RP, et al. Extrahepatic portal vein thrombosis: aetiology and determinants of survival. Gut. 2001;49:720–4.
20. Clinical Practice Guidelines EASL. Vascular diseases of the liver. J Hepatol. 2016;64:179–202.
21. Mantha S, Karp R, Raghavan V, Terrin N, Bauer KA, Zwicker JI. Assessing the risk of venous thromboembolic events in women taking progestin-only contraception: a meta-analysis. BMJ. 2012;345:e4944.
22. Case records of the Massachusetts General Hospital. Weekly clinicopathological exercises. Case 40-1982. Tender hepatomegaly in a 29-year-old woman. N Engl J Med. 1982;307:934–42.
23. Fischer D, Kémény F, Rauturseau J, Marty M, Karsenti P. Massive, painful hepatomegaly, sinusoidal dilatation and prolonged use of estroprogestational agents. Gastroenterol Clin Biol. 1982;6:302–4.
24. Ishak KG. Hepatic lesions caused by anabolic and contraceptive steroids. Semin Liver Dis. 1981;1:116–28.
25. Spellberg MA, Mirro J, Chowdhury L. Hepatic sinusoidal dilatation related to oral contraceptives. A study of two patients showing ultrastructural changes. Am J Gastroenterol. 1979;72:248–52.
26. Marzano C, Cazals-Hatem D, Rautou P-E, Valla D-C. The significance of nonobstructive sinusoidal dilatation of the liver: impaired portal perfusion or inflammatory reaction syndrome. Hepatology. 2015;62:956–63.
27. Zafrani ES, Cazier A, Baudelot AM, Feldmann G. Ultrastructural lesions of the liver in human peliosis. A report of 12 cases. Am J Pathol. 1984;114:349–59.
28. AndrogenicSteroids [Internet]. [cited 2018 Sep 3]; Available from: https://livertox.nlm.nih.gov/AndrogenicSteroids.htm
29. Haboubi NY, Ali HH, Whitwell HL, Ackrill P. Role of endothelial cell injury in the spectrum of azathioprine-induced liver disease after renal transplant: light microscopy and ultrastructural observations. Am J Gastroenterol. 1988;83:256–61.
30. Jones MC, Best PV, Catto GR. Is nodular regenerative hyperplasia of the liver associated with azathioprine therapy after renal transplantation? Nephrol Dial Transplant Off Publ Eur Dial Transpl Assoc - Eur Ren Assoc. 1988;3:331–3.
31. Read AE, Wiesner RH, LaBrecque DR, Tifft JG, Mullen KD, Sheer RL, et al. Hepatic veno-occlusive disease associated with renal transplantation and azathioprine therapy. Ann Intern Med. 1986;104:651–5.
32. Katzka DA, Saul SH, Jorkasky D, Sigal H, Reynolds JC, Soloway RD. Azathioprine and hepatic venocclusive disease in renal transplant patients. Gastroenterology. 1986;90:446–54.
33. Degott C, Rueff B, Kreis H, Duboust A, Potet F, Benhamou JP. Peliosis hepatis in recipients of renal transplants. Gut. 1978;19:748–53.
34. Buffet C, Cantarovitch M, Pelletier G, Fabre M, Martin E, Charpentier B, et al. Three cases of nodular regenerative hyperplasia of the liver following renal transplantation. Nephrol Dial Transplant Off Publ Eur Dial Transpl Assoc - Eur Ren Assoc. 1988;3:327–30.
35. Bouhnik Y, Lémann M, Mary JY, Scemama G, Taï R, Matuchansky C, et al. Long-term follow-up of patients with Crohn's disease treated with azathioprine or 6-mercaptopurine. Lancet. 1996;347:215–9.
36. Gerlag PG, van Hooff JP. Hepatic sinusoidal dilatation with portal hypertension during azathioprine treatment: a cause of chronic liver disease after kidney transplantation. Transplant Proc. 1987;19:3699–703.
37. Seksik P, Mary J-Y, Beaugerie L, Lémann M, Colombel J-F, Vernier-Massouille G, et al. Incidence of nodular regenerative hyperplasia in inflammatory bowel disease patients treated with azathioprine. Inflamm Bowel Dis. 2011;17:565–72.
38. Vernier-Massouille G, Cosnes J, Lemann M, Marteau P, Reinisch W, Laharie D, et al. Nodular regenerative hyperplasia in patients with inflammatory bowel disease treated with azathioprine. Gut. 2007;56:1404–9.

39. Musumba CO. Review article: the association between nodular regenerative hyperplasia, inflammatory bowel disease and thiopurine therapy. Aliment Pharmacol Ther. 2013;38:1025–37.
40. Sterneck M, Wiesner R, Ascher N, Roberts J, Ferrell L, Ludwig J, et al. Azathioprine hepatotoxicity after liver transplantation. Hepatology. 1991;14:806–10.
41. Nataf C, Feldmann G, Lebrec D, Degott C, Descamps JM, Rueff B, et al. Idiopathic portal hypertension (perisinusoidal fibrosis) after renal transplantation. Gut. 1979;20:531–7.
42. Degos F, Degott C, Bedrossian J, Camilieri JP, Barbanel C, Duboust A, et al. Is renal transplantation involved in post-transplantation liver disease? A prospective study. Transplantation. 1980;29:100–2.
43. Barge S, Grando V, Nault J-C, Broudin C, Beaugrand M, Ganne-Carrié N, et al. Prevalence and clinical significance of nodular regenerative hyperplasia in liver biopsies. Liver Int. off. J. Int. Assoc. Study Liver. 2016;36:1059–66.
44. Lemley DE, DeLacy LM, Seeff LB, Ishak KG, Nashel DJ. Azathioprine induced hepatic veno-occlusive disease in rheumatoid arthritis. Ann Rheum Dis. 1989;48:342–6.
45. Mion F, Napoleon B, Berger F, Chevallier M, Bonvoisin S, Descos L. Azathioprine induced liver disease: nodular regenerative hyperplasia of the liver and perivenous fibrosis in a patient treated for multiple sclerosis. Gut. 1991;32:715–7.
46. De Boer NKH, Tuynman H, Bloemena E, Westerga J, Van Der Peet DL, Mulder CJJ, et al. Histopathology of liver biopsies from a thiopurine-naïve inflammatory bowel disease cohort: prevalence of nodular regenerative hyperplasia. Scand J Gastroenterol. 2008;43:604–8.
47. Sebagh M, Azoulay D, Roche B, Hoti E, Karam V, Teicher E, et al. Significance of isolated hepatic veno-occlusive disease/sinusoidal obstruction syndrome after liver transplantation. Liver Transplant Off Publ Am Assoc Study Liver Dis Int Liver Transplant Soc. 2011;17:798–808.
48. DeLeve LD, Wang X, Kuhlenkamp JF, Kaplowitz N. Toxicity of azathioprine and monocrotaline in murine sinusoidal endothelial cells and hepatocytes: the role of glutathione and relevance to hepatic venoocclusive disease. Hepatology. 1996;23:589–99.
49. Seiderer J, Zech CJ, Diebold J, Schoenberg SO, Brand S, Tillack C, et al. Nodular regenerative hyperplasia: a reversible entity associated with azathioprine therapy. Eur J Gastroenterol Hepatol. 2006;18:553–5.
50. Gill RA, Onstad GR, Cardamone JM, Maneval DC, Sumner HW. Hepatic veno-occlusive disease caused by 6-thioguanine. Ann Intern Med. 1982;96:58–60.
51. Krivoy N, Raz R, Carter A, Alroy G. Reversible hepatic veno-occlusive disease and 6-thioguanine. Ann Intern Med. 1982;96:788.
52. Larrey D, Fréneaux E, Berson A, Babany G, Degott C, Valla D, et al. Peliosis hepatis induced by 6-thioguanine administration. Gut. 1988;29:1265–9.
53. Dubinsky MC, Vasiliauskas EA, Singh H, Abreu MT, Papadakis KA, Tran T, et al. 6-thioguanine can cause serious liver injury in inflammatory bowel disease patients. Gastroenterology. 2003;125:298–303.
54. van Asseldonk DP, Jharap B, Verheij J, den Hartog G, Westerveld DB, Becx MC, et al. The prevalence of nodular regenerative hyperplasia in inflammatory bowel disease patients treated with Thioguanine is not associated with clinically significant liver disease. Inflamm Bowel Dis. 2016;22:2112–20.
55. Ferlitsch A, Teml A, Reinisch W, Ulbrich G, Wrba F, Homoncik M, et al. 6-thioguanine associated nodular regenerative hyperplasia in patients with inflammatory bowel disease may induce portal hypertension. Am J Gastroenterol. 2007;102:2495–503.
56. Oancea I, Png CW, Das I, Lourie R, Winkler IG, Eri R, et al. A novel mouse model of veno-occlusive disease provides strategies to prevent thioguanine-induced hepatic toxicity. Gut. 2013;62:594–605.
57. Simsek M, Seinen ML, de Boer NKH. Nodular regenerative hyperplasia in inflammatory bowel disease patients with allopurinol-thiopurine cotherapy. Eur J Gastroenterol Hepatol. 2018;30:1254–5.

58. Rubbia-Brandt L, Audard V, Sartoretti P, Roth AD, Brezault C, Le Charpentier M, et al. Severe hepatic sinusoidal obstruction associated with oxaliplatin-based chemotherapy in patients with metastatic colorectal cancer. Ann Oncol Off J Eur Soc Med Oncol. 2004;15:460–6.
59. Rubbia-Brandt L, Lauwers GY, Wang H, Majno PE, Tanabe K, Zhu AX, et al. Sinusoidal obstruction syndrome and nodular regenerative hyperplasia are frequent oxaliplatin-associated liver lesions and partially prevented by bevacizumab in patients with hepatic colorectal metastasis. Histopathology. 2010;56:430–9.
60. Soubrane O, Brouquet A, Zalinski S, Terris B, Brézault C, Mallet V, et al. Predicting high grade lesions of sinusoidal obstruction syndrome related to oxaliplatin-based chemotherapy for colorectal liver metastases: correlation with post-hepatectomy outcome. Ann Surg. 2010;251:454–60.
61. Aloia T, Sebagh M, Plasse M, Karam V, Lévi F, Giacchetti S, et al. Liver histology and surgical outcomes after preoperative chemotherapy with fluorouracil plus oxaliplatin in colorectal cancer liver metastases. J Clin Oncol Off J Am Soc Clin Oncol. 2006;24:4983–90.
62. Vigano L, De Rosa G, Toso C, Andres A, Ferrero A, Roth A, et al. Reversibility of chemotherapy-related liver injury. J Hepatol. 2017;67:84–91.
63. van der Pool AEM, Marsman HA, Verheij J, Ten Kate FJ, Eggermont AMM, Ijzermans JNM, et al. Effect of bevacizumab added preoperatively to oxaliplatin on liver injury and complications after resection of colorectal liver metastases. J Surg Oncol. 2012;106:892–7.
64. Viganò L, Rubbia-Brandt L, De Rosa G, Majno P, Langella S, Toso C, et al. Nodular regenerative hyperplasia in patients undergoing liver resection for colorectal metastases after chemotherapy: risk factors, preoperative assessment and Clinical impact. Ann Surg Oncol. 2015;22:4149–57.
65. Rubbia-Brandt L, Tauzin S, Brezault C, Delucinge-Vivier C, Descombes P, Dousset B, et al. Gene expression profiling provides insights into pathways of oxaliplatin-related sinusoidal obstruction syndrome in humans. Mol Cancer Ther. 2011;10:687–96.
66. Agostini J, Benoist S, Seman M, Julié C, Imbeaud S, Letourneur F, et al. Identification of molecular pathways involved in oxaliplatin-associated sinusoidal dilatation. J Hepatol. 2012;56:869–76.
67. Robinson SM, Mann J, Vasilaki A, Mathers J, Burt AD, Oakley F, et al. Pathogenesis of FOLFOX induced sinusoidal obstruction syndrome in a murine chemotherapy model. J Hepatol. 2013;59:318–26.
68. Miura K, Nakano H, Sakurai J, Kobayashi S, Koizumi S, Arai T, et al. Splenomegaly in FOLFOX-naïve stage IV or recurrent colorectal cancer patients due to chemotherapy-associated hepatotoxicity can be predicted by the aspartate aminotransferase to platelet ratio before chemotherapy. Int J Clin Oncol. 2011;16:257–63.
69. Angitapalli R, Litwin AM, Kumar PRG, Nasser E, Lombardo J, Mashtare T, et al. Adjuvant FOLFOX chemotherapy and splenomegaly in patients with stages II-III colorectal cancer. Oncology. 2009;76:363–8.
70. Slade JH, Alattar ML, Fogelman DR, Overman MJ, Agarwal A, Maru DM, et al. Portal hypertension associated with Oxaliplatin administration: Clinical manifestations of hepatic sinusoidal injury. Clin Colorectal Cancer. 2009;8:225–30.
71. Wicherts DA, de Haas RJ, Sebagh M, Ciacio O, Lévi F, Paule B, et al. Regenerative nodular hyperplasia of the liver related to chemotherapy: impact on outcome of liver surgery for colorectal metastases. Ann Surg Oncol. 2011;18:659–69.
72. Nakano H, Oussoultzoglou E, Rosso E, Casnedi S, Chenard-Neu M-P, Dufour P, et al. Sinusoidal injury increases morbidity after major hepatectomy in patients with colorectal liver metastases receiving preoperative chemotherapy. Ann Surg. 2008;247:118.
73. Sood A, Castrejón M, Saab S. Human immunodeficiency virus and nodular regenerative hyperplasia of liver: a systematic review. World J Hepatol. 2014;6:55–63.
74. Maida I, Núñez M, Ríos MJ, Martín-Carbonero L, Sotgiu G, Toro C, et al. Severe liver disease associated with prolonged exposure to antiretroviral drugs. J Acquir Immune Defic Syndr. 1999. 2006;42:177–82.

75. Mallet V, Blanchard P, Verkarre V, Vallet-Pichard A, Fontaine H, Lascoux-Combe C, et al. Nodular regenerative hyperplasia is a new cause of chronic liver disease in HIV-infected patients. AIDS. 2007;21:187–92.

76. Saifee S, Joelson D, Braude J, Shrestha R, Johnson M, Sellers M, et al. Noncirrhotic portal hypertension in patients with human immunodeficiency virus-1 infection. Clin Gastroenterol Hepatol Off Clin Pract J Am Gastroenterol Assoc. 2008;6:1167–9.

77. Kovari H, Ledergerber B, Peter U, Flepp M, Jost J, Schmid P, et al. Association of noncirrhotic portal hypertension in HIV-infected persons and antiretroviral therapy with didanosine: a nested case-control study. Clin Infect Dis Off Publ Infect Dis Soc Am. 2009;49:626–35.

78. Cotte L, Bénet T, Billioud C, Miailhes P, Scoazec J-Y, Ferry T, et al. The role of nucleoside and nucleotide analogues in nodular regenerative hyperplasia in HIV-infected patients: a case control study. J Hepatol. 2011;54:489–96.

79. Vispo E, Moreno A, Maida I, Barreiro P, Cuevas A, Albertos S, et al. Noncirrhotic portal hypertension in HIV-infected patients: unique clinical and pathological findings. AIDS. 2010;24:1171–6.

80. Hollande C, Mallet V, Darbeda S, Vallet-Pichard A, Fontaine H, Verkarre V, et al. Impact of Obliterative portal Venopathy associated with human immunodeficiency virus. Medicine (Baltimore). 2016;95:e3081.

81. Mallet VO, Varthaman A, Lasne D, Viard J-P, Gouya H, Borgel D, et al. Acquired protein S deficiency leads to obliterative portal venopathy and to compensatory nodular regenerative hyperplasia in HIV-infected patients. AIDS. 2009;23:1511–8.

82. Kline ER, Sutliff RL. The roles of HIV-1 proteins and antiretroviral drug therapy in HIV-1-associated endothelial dysfunction. J Investig Med Off Publ Am Fed Clin Res. 2008;56:752–69.

83. Fu PP, Xia Q, Lin G, Chou MW. Pyrrolizidine alkaloids--genotoxicity, metabolism enzymes, metabolic activation, and mechanisms. Drug Metab Rev. 2004;36:1–55.

84. Larrey D, Faure S. Herbal medicine hepatotoxicity: a new step with development of specific biomarkers. J Hepatol. 2011;54:599–601.

85. Willmot F, Robertson G. SENECIO disease, or cirrhosis of the liver due to SENECIO poisoning. Lancet. 1920;196:848–9.

86. Tandon BN, Tandon HD, Tandon RK, Narndranathan M, Joshi YK. An epidemic of veno-occlusive disease of liver in Central India. Lancet. 1976;2:271–2.

87. Mohabbat O, Younos MS, Merzad AA, Srivastava RN, Sediq GG, Aram GN. An outbreak of hepatic veno-occlusive disease in North-Western Afghanistan. Lancet. 1976;2:269–71.

88. Wang X, Qi X, Guo X. Tusanqi-related sinusoidal obstruction syndrome in China: a systematic review of the literatures. Medicine (Baltimore). 2015;94:e942.

89. Tandon HD, Tandon BN, Mattocks AR. An epidemic of veno-occlusive disease of the liver in Afghanistan. Pathologic features. Am J Gastroenterol. 1978;70:607–13.

90. Stuart KL, Bras G. Veno-occlusive disease of the liver. Q J Med. 1957;26:291–315.

91. Kan X, Ye J, Rong X, Lu Z, Li X, Wang Y, et al. Diagnostic performance of contrast-enhanced CT in pyrrolizidine alkaloids-induced hepatic sinusoidal obstructive syndrome. Sci Rep. 2016;6:37998.

92. Lin G, Wang JY, Li N, Li M, Gao H, Ji Y, et al. Hepatic sinusoidal obstruction syndrome associated with consumption of Gynura segetum. J Hepatol. 2011;54:666–73.

93. Helmy A. Review article: updates in the pathogenesis and therapy of hepatic sinusoidal obstruction syndrome. Aliment Pharmacol Ther. 2006;23:11–25.

94. Dietary exposure assessment to pyrrolizidine alkaloids in the European population. EFSA J. 2016;14:e04572.

95. Saeed A, Dullaart RPF, Schreuder TCMA, Blokzijl H, Faber KN. Disturbed vitamin a metabolism in non-alcoholic fatty liver disease (NAFLD). Nutrients [Internet]. 2017 [cited 2018 Sep 18]; 10. Available from: https://www.ncbi.nlm.nih.gov/pmc/articles/PMC5793257/

96. Penniston KL, Tanumihardjo SA. The acute and chronic toxic effects of vitamin a. Am J Clin Nutr. 2006;83:191–201.

97. Geubel AP, De Galocsy C, Alves N, Rahier J, Dive C. Liver damage caused by therapeutic vitamin a administration: estimate of dose-related toxicity in 41 cases. Gastroenterology. 1991;100:1701–9.
98. VitaminARetinoids [Internet]. [cited 2018 Sep 17]; Available from: https://livertox.nih.gov/VitaminARetinoids.htm
99. Nollevaux M-C, Guiot Y, Horsmans Y, Leclercq I, Rahier J, Geubel AP, et al. Hypervitaminosis A-induced liver fibrosis: stellate cell activation and daily dose consumption. Liver Int Off J Int Assoc Study Liver. 2006;26:182–6.
100. Bioulac-sage P, Balabaud C. Chapter 40 - Toxic and drug-induced disorders of the liver [internet]. In: Odze RD, Goldblum JR, editors. Surgical pathology of the GI tract, liver, biliary tract, and pancreas (2nd Edition). Philadelphia: W.B. Saunders; 2009 [cited 2018 Sep 17]. p. 1059–1086. Available from: http://www.sciencedirect.com/science/article/pii/B9781416040590500436
101. Mastrangelo G, Fedeli U, Fadda E, Valentini F, Agnesi R, Magarotto G, et al. Increased risk of hepatocellular carcinoma and liver cirrhosis in vinyl chloride workers: synergistic effect of occupational exposure with alcohol intake. Environ Health Perspect. 2004;112:1188–92.
102. Sherman M. Vinyl chloride and the liver. J Hepatol. 2009;51:1074–81.
103. Tamburro CH, Makk L, Popper H. Early hepatic histologic alterations among chemical (vinyl monomer) workers. Hepatology. 1984;4:413–8.
104. Thomas LB, Popper H, Berk PD, Selikoff I, Falk H. Vinyl-chloride-induced liver disease. From idiopathic portal hypertension (Banti's syndrome) to Angiosarcomas. N Engl J Med. 1975;292:17–22.
105. Popper H, Maltoni C, Selikoff IJ. Vinyl chloride-induced hepatic lesions in man and rodents. A comparison Liver. 1981;1:7–20.

# Chapter 22
# Liver Transplantation and Hepatic Vessels

Darwish Murad Sarwa

## Introduction

The liver has a dual blood supply consisting of the portal vein and the hepatic artery. In a native liver, a complete occlusion of either the portal vein or the hepatic artery may not immediately lead to total liver necrosis, because some hepatic inflow will continue from the other, non-occluded vessel, and in time, collaterals will develop. In liver transplantation (LT), however, this compensation mechanism does not exist, as all attachments that might have served for the development of collaterals, have been surgically divided. Therefore, an acute impairment of the hepatic inflow, being either portal or arterial can be detrimental for the newly transplanted graft. This may result in allograft loss or long-term allograft dysfunction and often necessitates salvage re-transplantation. The same holds true for acute hepatic outflow obstruction in the setting of LT. Considering the ongoing scarcity of organ donors, such vascular complications also have a profound impact on the application of liver transplantation as a whole. Therefore, strategies to detect or prevent vascular complications are vital for the existence of liver transplantation as definite treatment for end-stage liver disease.

## Standard Vascular Anastomoses during Liver Transplantation

In order to understand the various types of vascular complications that may occur, it is crucial to understand the operative procedure with regards to the vascular anastomoses. In a standard liver transplantation, with normal donor and recipient

D. M. Sarwa (✉)
Department of Gastroenterology and Hepatology, Erasmus MC University Medical Center Rotterdam, 3015 GD, Rotterdam, The Netherlands
e-mail: s.darwishmurad@erasmusmc.nl



D. Valla et al. (eds.), *Vascular Disorders of the Liver*,
https://doi.org/10.1007/978-3-030-82988-9_22

vascular anatomy, the most common vascular anastomoses include an end-to-end portal anastomosis, end-to-end arterial anastomosis and a cavo-cavostomy (Fig. 22.1). However, many alternative techniques exist in case of non-standard anatomy. For example, when the portal vein is unsuitable for direct anastomosis (e.g. due to longstanding portal vein thrombosis prior to LT) a portal conduit is created, using the donor iliac vein brought along after donor hepatectomy. The donor

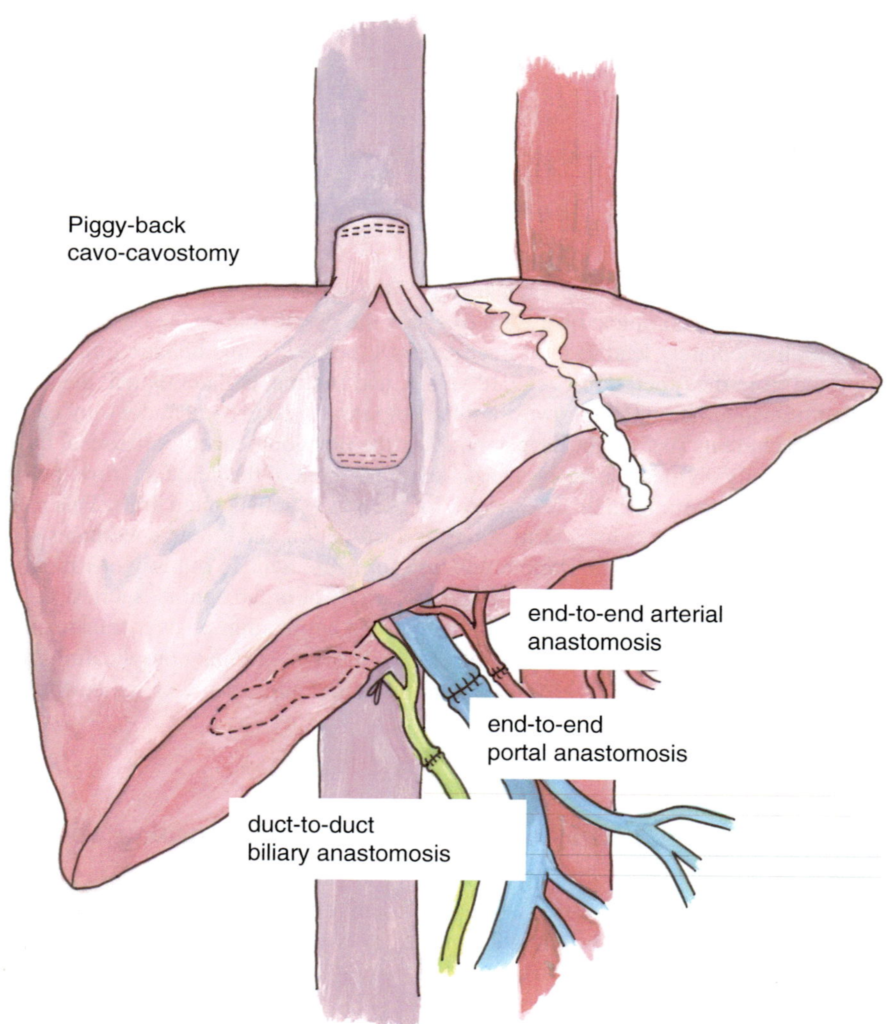


*Original artwork, courtesy of Elsbeth Leeffers and Hermien Hartog*

**Fig. 22.1** Ilustration of an implanted liver graft using the standard vascular and biliary anastomoses. Original artwork, courtesy of Elsbeth Leeffers and Hermien Hartog, the Netherlands

iliac vein is then interposed between the donor portal vein and the recipient superior mesenteric vein. Rarely, a large nearby portal collateral (e.g. in the subhepatic area) is used for inflow instead.

In addition, the use of an arterial conduit is an alternative technique to reconstruct a hepatic artery anastomosis in case of inadequate length of donor or recipient hepatic artery or when the recipient hepatic artery is of poor quality and hence unsuitable for primary anastomosis. Such can be the case in arterial dissection, endovascular damage after trans-arterial chemoembolization (TACE) in hepatocellular carcinoma or a revascularised hepatic artery in case of retransplantation for hepatic artery thrombosis. Although many venous, arterial and synthetic grafts are used to this end, most use the donor iliac artery for grafting. In some cases, the arterial conduit will be directly anastomosed on the celiac trunk or the aorta.

Finally, the cavo-cavostomy technique used in most recent decades is according to the so-called piggy-back technique. The piggy-back technique was first described by Calne et al. in 1968 [1] as a caval anastomosis with preservation of the recipient caval vein, hence avoiding cross clamping of the caval vein and allowing venous blood return from the inferior vena cava during the anhepatic phase. The three (or two) hepatic vein orifices of the recipient are joined to create a common cloaca (cuff), which is eventually anastomosed to the donor suprahepatic caval vein in an end-to-side fashion. The shift from the classical end-to-end caval anastomosis to the piggy-back technique signified an improvement as it resulted in less haemodynamic instability, shorter cold ischaemia times and less renal damage and eliminated the need for a veno-venous bypass [2].

## Types of Complications and Risk Factors

In general, vascular complications can be divided in three large categories: thrombosis, stenosis and endovascular damage (i.e. pseudoaneurysms). In addition, a haemorrhagic leakage at the site of the anastomosis may occur as a rare event, which results directly from a technical malfunction and requires immediate surgical correction. As such, this type of complication is beyond the scope of this chapter.

Thrombotic complications may partly result from an imbalance in coagulation factors. Indeed, the event of liver transplantation is generally considered to represent a hypercoagulable state. A very elegant study showed that all procoagulant factors (except for factor VIII) reach normal levels by day 3 after liver transplantation, which is reflected in the normalisation of the prothrombin time (PT) and activated partial thromboplastin time (aPTT) [3]. However, the anticoagulant protein (protein C, S and antithrombin) levels show delayed recovery and most patients remain deficient for these proteins in the first 10 days. At the same time active thrombin/anti-thrombin complexes are being generated, further predisposing to a prothrombotic state in the early days after LT [3]. Other reported prothrombotic risk factors are related to the allograft (such as ABO incompatibility, viral mismatch, rejection), donor (e.g. age) and recipient smoking history (Table 22.1).

**Table 22.1** Risk factors for vascular complications

| Category | Risk factor |
| --- | --- |
| **General risk factors for vascular complications** | |
| Coagulation system | Low protein C [3, 4]<br>Low protein S [3]<br>Low anti-thrombin [3]<br>High fibrinogen [4] |
| Allograft factors | ABO incompatibility [5]<br>Gender incompatibility [6]<br>Split grafts [7]<br>Allograft rejection [6]<br>Cytomegalovirus (CMV) mismatch [6] |
| Donor factors | Advanced donor age [7–9]<br>Death from intracerebral haemorrhage [7] |
| Life style | Cigarette smoking [10] |
| **Specific risk factors for arterial complications** | |
| Surgical factors | Graft number [6, 7, 11–13]<br>Variant donor anatomy [8, 12, 14, 15]<br>Small donor artery [7]<br>Arterial reconstruction [5, 12, 14]<br>Arterial conduit [8, 12]<br>Multiple anastomoses [12]<br>Delay in arterial reperfusion [12]<br>Intraoperative blood transfusions [5, 12, 13]<br>Duration of arterial anastomosis [5]<br>Prolonged total surgery time [5, 13]<br>Transarterial chemoembolization pre-LT [9, 14]<br>Low recipient weight [6]<br>Roux-en-Y biliary anastomosis [13] |
| **Specific risk factors for portal complications** | |
| Recipient factors | Pre-LT portal vein thrombosis [14] |
| Surgical factors | Portal conduit or portal reconstruction [14, 16–18]<br>Size mismatch donor and recipient portal vein [16–18]<br>Excessive portal vein length [16–18]<br>Concomitant splenectomy [16–18]<br>Prior shunt surgery or splenorenal shunt [16–18] |

Stenosis is generally thought to result from suboptimal circumstances for surgery including, but not restricted to vascular size mismatch, need for vascular reconstruction, use of conduits or prolonged duration of surgery (Table 22.1). Pseudoaneursyms, exclusively of arterial origin, are either iatrogenic or related to the local presence of bile, pancreatic or infectious fluids or fluid collections, which directly damage the vascular wall.

It is very important to recognize, however, that all three types of vascular complications may occur in isolation or in conjunction. For example, thrombosis may result in fibrin deposition, fibrosis and hence stenosis; a stenotic trajectory may give rise to vascular stasis, clot formation and subsequently thrombosis; and pseudoaneurysms can occur in stenotic area's while turbulence of flow within the pseudoaneurysm may lead to clot formation.

## Post-operative Imaging

Doppler ultrasonography (US) is the established first-line imaging modality for the surveillance of vascular integrity after LT, while angiography (CT, MRI or conventional angiography) is often used for confirmation. Doppler US has the advantage of being inexpensive, widely available, reproducible and easily accessible at the patient bedside. Ultrasonography can directly visualize the vessel and detect any interruption, kinking, narrowing or compression of the vessel. The Doppler signals give additional information on vessel patency and blood flow direction, pattern and velocity. Flow velocity is measured by pulse wave mode, correcting for the directional angle. For the hepatic artery, a resistive index (RI) is additionally calculated which reflects the difference between systolic and diastolic flow velocity divided by the systolic flow velocity. A RI of 0.5–0.7 is considered normal, although in arterially reconstructed vessels this may exceed 0.8 in the early post-operative phase (Fig. 22.2). Normal portal flow is continuous, hepatopetal and shows mild respiratory variation, although not infrequently, flow is turbulent and of high velocity in the immediate post-operative period. When the discrepancy in diameter of the donor and recipient portal vein (i.e. size-mismatch) exceeds 50% a helical flow can be seen distally from the anastomosis. Patency of the cavo-cavostomy is picked up by direct visualisation of flow by Doppler and hepatic vein flow is considered normal when it is triphasic or biphasic.

Whenever Doppler US is inconclusive or challenging, contrast enhanced US (CEUS) can provide additional information on vessel patency by the intravenous administration of, preferably, second-generation perfluorocarbon-based contrast agents [19]. The presence of a vascular complication can be confirmed by the use of cross-sectional or conventional angiography, although this should be used sparingly as the use of intravenous iodine-based contrast agents and radiation impose additional risks to the recipient. Computed Tomographic Angiography (CTA) has the added advantage of being fast, accurate and non-invasive with a sensitivity of 100% and a specificity of 89% [20].

Given the profound impact of vascular complications on the allograft most transplant centres have adopted protocols to monitor the patency of the vascular anastomoses in the early post-operative period, although the frequency and timing of imaging vary considerably between centres. As one example, our institution employs a strict schedule of Doppler ultrasonography performed intraoperatively (before abdominal closure), in the ICU immediately after abdominal closure and post-transplantation at day 1 and 7, as well as at any time thereafter as part of the work up of abnormal liver function tests. The introduction of systematic postoperative screening has resulted in many centres in significantly decreased requirements for retransplantation [21].

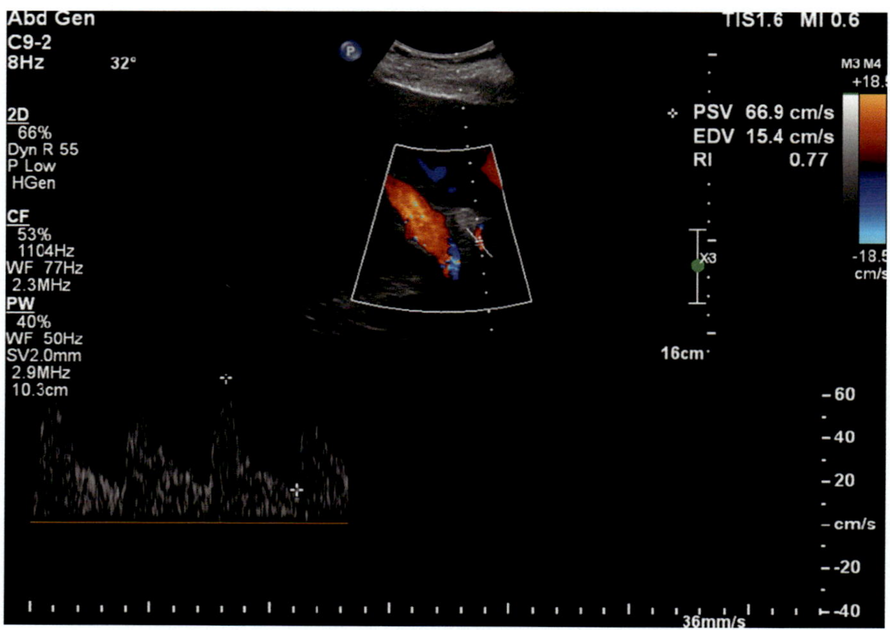

Fig. 22.2 Routine Doppler ultrasound 7 days after liver transplantation. Here the hepatic artery is depicted with a peak systolic velocity (PSV) of 66.9 cm/sec and end diastolic velocity (EDV) 15.4 cm/sec. The resistive index shown here is 0.77, indicating satisfactory arterial flow. (courtesy of the author)

## Post-transplantation Arterial Complications

### *Hepatic Artery Thrombosis (HAT)*

During the early years of liver transplantation, the reported incidence of hepatic artery thrombosis (HAT) was high, 12% in adults and 42% in paediatric recipients [22]. With improvement in surgical techniques and rigorous peri- and postoperative screening, HAT rates have decreased to 1.7 to 9% in more recent series (Table 22.2).

Time of onset of HAT has been correlated with the severity of the subsequent complications. Therefore, HAT is divided in two categories, early HAT (defined as HAT occurring within the first 2 months after LT) and late HAT (occurring any time thereafter) [37]. A pooled analysis of 71 case series including 21,822 recipients showed that the overall median prevalence of early HAT was 4.4% [37]. Late HAT is presumed to occur more infrequent, with a reported prevalence of 0.8%–3.8% [28, 29, 38] (Fig. 22.3).

Clinical presentation of early HAT ranges from fulminant hepatic failure, through recurrent biliary sepsis and delayed biliary leaks, to an asymptomatic presentation in which HAT is detected either during routine postoperative ultrasonography

**Table 22.2**  Prevalence of arterial complications in published case series

| Study (first author, year, [ref]) | Transplant centre | Total number of patients | Prevalence HAT (%) | Prevalence HAS (%) | Prevalence HA pseudo-aneurysm (%) |
|---|---|---|---|---|---|
| Wozney 1986[b] [22] | Pittsburgh, PA, USA | 86 | 12 | 11 | 3 |
| Langnas, 1991[b] [23] | Omaha, NE, USA | 430 | 6 | – | – |
| Abbasoglu, 1997 [11] | Baylor, Tx, USA | 857 | – | 5 | |
| Cavallari, 2000 [21] | Bologna, Italy | 384 | 4 | 2 | 0.5 |
| Settmacher, 2000 [24] | Berlin, Germany | 837 | 2.7 | 3.2 | 0.7 |
| Oh, 2001 [6] | Charlottesville, VA, USA | 424 | 6.8 | – | – |
| Marshall, 2001 [25] | King's college, London, UK | 1327 | – | – | 1.0 |
| Pungpapong, 2002 [10] | Philadelphia, PA, USA | 288 | 5.9 | 3.8 | – |
| Leelaudomlipi, 2003 [26] | Birmingham, UK | 1575 | – | – | 0.5 |
| Stange, 2003 [27] | Berlin, Germany | 1192 | 2.5 | – | – |
| Gunsar, 2003 [28] | Royal Free, London, UK | 634 | 1.7[a] | – | – |
| Leonardi, 2004 [29] | Sao Paolo, Brazil | 178 | 3.8[a] | – | – |
| Silva, 2006 [13] | Birmingham, UK | 1257 | 4.9 | – | – |
| Fistouris, 2006 [30] | Gothenburg, Sweden | 825 | – | – | 2.6 |
| Horrow, 2007 [31] | Philadelphia, PA, USA | 522 | 4.8 | – | – |
| Duffy, 2009 [14] | UCLA, CA, USA | 4234 | 5 | – | – |
| Stewart, 2009 [7] | UNOS data, USA | 54,992 | 2.3 | – | – |
| Pareja, 2010 [32] | Valencia, Spain | 1560 | 2.8 | – | – |
| Ayala, 2011[c] [4] | Madrid, Spain | 441 | 9 | – | – |
| Warner, 2011 [12] | Royal Free, London, UK | 915 | 7.1 | – | – |
| Frongillo, 2013 [33] | Rome, Italy | 258 | – | 9.3 | – |
| Volpin, 2014 [34] | Reims, France | 787 | – | – | 1.5 |
| Yi Yang, 2014 [5] | Chengdu, China | 744 | 2.7 | – | – |
| Pulitano, 2015 [35] | Sydney, Australia | 662 | – | 8.2 | |
| Fujiki, 2017 [36] | Cleveland, OH, USA | 1783 | 2.6 | – | – |

– not reported

[a] late HAT

[b] included adult and paediatric transplantations

[c] included living donor liver transplantation

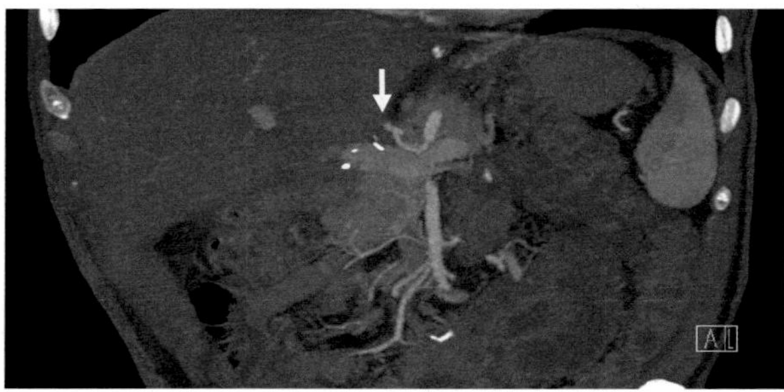

**Fig. 22.3** Computed Tomogram (CT) showing complete hepatic artery occlusion, caused by late hepatic artery thrombosis in a patient after liver transplantation

screening or in the work-up of abnormal liver function tests. Since the peribiliary plexus is dependent predominantly on arterial blood supply, non-fulminant HAT inevitably still results in ischaemic damage to the biliary tree (i.e. ischaemic cholangiopathy). Hence, late HAT is generally diagnosed when patients present with relapsing fever, jaundice, pruritus, hepatic abscess, cholangitis, non-anastomotic biliary strictures, hepatic necrosis or during the work-up for abnormal liver tests in asymptomatic patients [28, 29]. Risk factors for the development of arterial complications are listed in Table 22.1.

HAT is diagnosed by radiological imaging, with Doppler Ultrasonography being the best initial test. Although in the immediate postoperative period the acoustic window of Doppler US may be limited by interference from excessive bowel gas, mechanical ventilation or surgical dressing materials, the reported sensitivity and specificity rates for the detection of hepatic artery thrombosis (HAT) range from 54%–92% and 64%–88%, respectively [31, 39, 40]. HAT is diagnosed when the arterial signal is absent on Doppler US and is imminent when the RI is increased. False positive results have been observed in hypovolemia and low cardiac output state, arterial spasms or severe parenchymal or periportal (lymph)oedema, while false negative results have been found when flow is accidentally measured in arterial collaterals in the setting of subacute or late HAT.

There is a lack of consensus on the management of HAT, largely due to a paucity of comparative studies. Treatment options include urgent retransplantation, arterial revascularisation or wait and see. Revascularisation options include surgical or radiological interventions to restore arterial blood supply through thrombectomy, thrombolysis, balloon angioplasty with/without stenting or surgical revision of the arterial anastomosis. The success rate of revascularisation attempts seems to depend on the early diagnosis of HAT [38]. Indeed, in centres in which daily US was performed, the success rate was as high as 61% vs. 45% in those without daily screening [37]. The choice of intervention depends on the patient condition and the centre's expertise. The potential of revascularisation using endovascular procedures needs to be weighed against the risk of bleeding from thrombolysis or risk of intima dissection or stent occlusion after angioplasty. Even after initial successful revascularisation of the arterial flow, ischaemic cholangiopathy, however, may still be a problem in the long-term. Retransplantation is eventually needed in over half of the cases of HAT, more often in early than late HAT [27, 37].

In contrast to early HAT, long-term survival following late HAT has been reported, with the majority of such cases having developed arterial collaterals at initial presentation. These collaterals can develop as early as 2 months after the HAT event and are more prevalent in paediatric recipients [31, 39]. The results of revascularisation in late HAT are often disappointing and biliary complications occur frequently, compromising long-term graft outcome and quality of life. Therefore, in late HAT, treatment is generally aimed at treating the complications (drainage of abscess or bile leak, antibiotics and biliary drainage, stenting and dilation) and an expectant management is usually followed, allowing time for neovascularisation to occur which may obviate the need for retransplantation.

Low dose aspirin has been used as prophylaxis for (late) HAT in some centres, however its efficacy is still debated. Some reports show no benefit [41] while others show favourable results, especially in high-risk settings [42, 43]. One example thereof is the use of arterial conduits, since these are known to have lower patency rates than end-to-end arterial anastomoses [44].

## *Hepatic Artery Stenosis (HAS)*

Stenosis of the hepatic artery occurs most commonly at the level of the anastomosis or the donor artery [11]. Prevalence ranges from 2–11% (Table 22.2). Ultrasonographic features suggesting hepatic artery stenosis (HAS) include increased peak systolic flow velocity > 200 cm/s, poststenotic turbulent flow and parvus-tardus waveform (prolonged acceleration time > 0.08 s and RI < 0.5) [45], which combined carry a sensitivity of 81% and specificity of 60% [46]. Risk factors for HAS include poor surgical techniques, clamp injury, preservation injury and allograft rejection (Table 22.1). Clinical presentation mimics that of HAT and HAS in fact carries an increased risk for development of HAT. Therefore, it is imperative to diagnose and treat HAS as early as possible. Treatment classically consists of surgical revision of the anastomosis, however lately many reports of successful balloon angioplasty, with or without stenting, have shown to restore long-term patency in 68–78% [11, 47]. If the HAS is however longstanding and untreated, biliary complications are likely to occur, similarly to HAT. Indeed, non-anastomotic and anastomotic biliary strictures occur in 60% of patients with HAS compared to 9.7% in those with normal arterial patency [48]. The need for endovascular/surgical treatment needs to be balanced against the potential risks (bleeding, restenosis) in each individual case. For example, a conservative approach is justified in a patient with HAS who has formed collaterals and shows no signs of biliopathy. Requirement for re-intervention due to restenosis is thought to occur in up to 25% and retransplantation is still needed in 20–24%.

## *Hepatic Artery Pseudoaneurysms (HAP)*

Hepatic artery pseudoaneurysms (HAP) are amongst the most fearsome and life-threatening complications after liver transplantation. These can occur in the intrahepatic or extrahepatic part of the hepatic artery. Reported prevalence ranges from 0.5 to 3% (Table 22.2). A study reviewing 81 published cases reported a pooled prevalence of 0.9%, in which HAP was diagnosed after a median of 58.8 days post LT [49]. The clinical presentation of HAP is non-specific and includes haemobilia, unexplained fever, graft dysfunction, dropping haemoglobin level, gastrointestinal bleeding, hemodynamic instability and haemorrhagic shock. Therefore, a high index of suspicion is required to make the diagnosis before rupture occurs. Major risk factors for the development of intrahepatic HAP are related to direct iatrogenic injury of the hepatic artery in the setting of transhepatic invasive procedures, such as liver biopsy, percutaneous transhepatic cholangiography and transhepatic drainage procedures (Table 22.1) [25]. On the other hand, extrahepatic HAP is mostly related to local infection (mostly mycotic infections), bile leak, pancreatitis, small bowel perforation and presence of a Roux-en-Y hepaticojejunostomy (presumably due to colonization of the subhepatic space with enteric micro-organisms) [49]. While most of the intrahepatic HAP are asymptomatic and detected incidentally, extrahepatic HAP can rupture without warning into the bile duct (arteriobiliary fistula), peritoneal or retroperitoneal cavity (massive haemo(retro)peritoneum) or gastrointestinal tract (arterio-enteric fistula), causing a life-threatening event with a very high mortality rate of up to 69% [25].

Colour Doppler Ultrasound is the most useful initial examination. Intrahepatic HAP may present as an-echogenic area with swirling colour flow, and a high velocity jet flow at the site of the feeding arterial leak or fistula [50]. CT findings are less specific as local inflammation may obscure the image and sensitivity is also lower, reportedly between 25–78% [25, 26]. Angiography remains the gold standard, allowing confirmation and localization of the HAP, assessment of presence of a fistula or active bleeding and direct access to immediate coil embolization.

Various management strategies have been reported, including acute surgical excision, ligation or super-selective radiological embolization and/or stenting. Embolization is mostly effective as primary treatment in intrahepatic HAP, if done super selectively to spare the non-affected area of the graft. For ruptured extrahepatic HAP however, embolization, excision or ligation is only used as a bridging procedure while awaiting retransplantation. In the setting of an active infection results from retransplantation are compromised and long-term antibiotics are often needed. Treating the HAP before rupture occurs is associated with better outcome [51] but has to be weighed against potential induction of graft ischemia and the imminent availability of a rescue retransplantation in that scenario [25].

# Post-transplantation Portal Complications

## *Portal Vein Thrombosis (PVT)*

In contrast to the pre-transplant period, where portal vein thrombosis (PVT) is a common complication of liver cirrhosis, after liver transplantation PVT occurs rather infrequently. The reported prevalence is 0.5–7% (Table 22.3). PVT is generally detected by the absence of Doppler flow in the portal vein, with or without delineation of intraluminal echogenic thrombus material. Risk factors for the development of PVT include pre-existing PVT requiring thrombectomy during transplant surgery, size mismatch between donor and recipient portal vein, excessive portal vein length, use of venous conduits or alternative portal anastomosis, concomitant splenectomy and prior shunt surgery or splenorenal shunt (causing a portal steal-phenomenon) [16–18]. Also, paediatric split liver and living donor liver transplantations carry a higher risk for development of PVT [17]. Patients developing PVT often present with recurrent signs of portal hypertension (ascites, varices, variceal bleeding). Over two third of the patients present with abnormal liver enzymes [14]. However over half of the patients are asymptomatic and PVT is found incidentally during routine ultrasound [16]. Acute, early PVT, however, may lead to imminent graft failure due to the lack of time to develop compensatory, portal-portal or portal-venous collaterals. Salvage retransplantation may be needed in such cases. Finally, contrasting the common belief that the peribiliary plexus exclusively depends on the arterial inflow, one report described 3 cases in which ischaemic biliopathy occurred in the setting of PVT, suggesting the possibility of a biliary consequence to portal compromise [53].

**Table 22.3** Prevalence of portal complications in published case series

| Study (first author, year, [ref]) | Centre | Total number of transplants | Prevalence PVT (%) | Prevalence PVS (%) |
|---|---|---|---|---|
| Wozney, 1986[a] [22] | Pittsburgh, PA, USA | 86 | 6 | 7 |
| Langnas, 1991[a] [23] | Omaha, NE, USA | 430 | 2 | – |
| Cavallari, 2000 [21] | Bologna, Italy | 384 | 0.5 | 0.5 |
| Settmacher, 2000 [16] | Berlin, Germany | 966 | 1.3 | 1.3 |
| Pungpapong, 2002 [10] | Philadelphia, PA, USA | 288 | 1.7 | – |
| Kishi, 2008[b] [17] | Tokyo, Japan | 287 | 7 | – |
| Duffy, 2009[a] [14] | UCLA, CA, USA | 4234 | 2 | – |
| Mullan, 2010[ab] [52] | Harvard, Boston, MA, USA | 181 | – | 7.2 |
| Ayala, 2011[b] [4] | Madrid, Spain | 441 | 1.8 | – |

– not reported
[a]included adult and paediatric transplantations
[b]included living donor liver transplantation

Management options for PVT post transplantation are diverse, varying from systemic anticoagulation, local thrombolysis, surgical revision of the portal anastomosis and retransplantation. Some patients, however, do well with conservative management alone, aimed at treating the portal hypertensive symptoms. Anticoagulation may salvage the graft in almost half of patients [14] and is probably the treatment of choice when the graft is not endangered. In addition, prophylactic use of anticoagulation or antiplatelet therapy is often employed in high-risk patients, such as those after portal reconstruction or conduits, and is usually continued for 1–3 months after liver transplantation to prevent PVT. Although PVT is reported to compromise patient and graft survival [14] as well as limit re-grafting options, especially when PVT is extensive with involvement of the mesenteric and/or splenic vein, cases in which death is directly attributed to PVT are rare.

## *Portal Vein Stenosis (PVS)*

Stenosis of the portal vein anastomosis (PVS) is considered haemodynamically significant when the lumen of the smallest portal vein (either donor or recipient) is reduced by >50% [52] and considered clinically significant when >80% of the lumen is obliterated [16]. The reported prevalence of PVS ranges from 0.5% to 7.2% (Table 22.3). Clinical symptoms consist of recurrence of portal hypertension but are generally milder than with portal vein thrombosis. Of note, the presence of a PVS may predispose to PVT through Virchow's triad of venous stasis, endothelial injury and a hypercoagulable setting (such as is the case post-transplant). Diagnosis can be made through Doppler US, showing relative narrowing at the site of the portal anastomosis. Furthermore, an angle-corrected peak systolic velocity of the portal vein of 80 cm/s or greater is associated with a 100% sensitivity and 84% specificity to detect haemodynamically significant PVS [52]. Likewise, a change in peak systolic velocity across the anastomosis from donor to recipient portal vein of 60 cm/s or greater yields similar sensitivity and specificity. However, the presence of varices or portal collaterals may confound this observation, as portal flow velocity across the stenosis may be lower due to redistribution of blood flow. Other signs include a velocity gradient pre- and post anastomosis of >3:1, persistence of helical/turbulent flow, post-anastomotic portal vein dilatation and signs of portal hypertension. After the suspicion is raised on Doppler US, portal venography remains the gold standard to confirm the diagnosis and assess feasibility for percutaneous interventional therapy including balloon angioplasty with or without stenting.

In the decision making whether or not to proceed with endoluminal therapy one should take into consideration the degree of stenosis. Low-grade stenosis (<80% of the lumen) is not likely to benefit from therapy. Indeed, in one study measuring pre- and post-stenting peak velocities, no difference was found in patients with low grade stenosis, while in high grade stenosis, the peak velocity dropped significantly below the threshold for effect [52]. In some cases, a mild stenosis that does not cause graft dysfunction may even resolve spontaneously over time [54].

# Post Transplantation Hepatic Venous Outflow Obstruction

An outflow obstruction following liver transplantation can occur at two levels, either at the cavo-cavostomy or at the level of the hepatic veins. The hepatic venous outflow obstruction (HVOO) can be due to stenosis and/or a venous thrombosis at these sites. Hepatic vein stenosis is seen almost exclusively in the setting of living donor or split donor liver transplantation, where the donor hepatic vein is directly anastomosed on the recipient inferior vena cava or on the common trunk of two hepatic veins [55]. Diagnosis of HVOO is usually made by Doppler ultrasound. Findings include absence or reversal of venous flow, accelerated turbulent flow with colour aliasing beyond the stenosis, a velocity gradient pre- and post-anastomosis of >3:1 or direct visualisation of the stenosis [19, 56, 57]. Although biphasic or triphasic flow generally excludes stenosis, monophasic flow has high sensitivity but very low specificity for the detection of venous stenosis [19]. Finally, thrombosis can be detected as echogenic intravascular material in the absence of venous flow. The gold standard for confirmation of the diagnosis and measurement of pressure gradient across the anastomosis is invasive venography. There is debate about what exactly defines an abnormal pressure gradient, as gradients anywhere from 2–20 mm Hg have been used as thresholds, but generally a gradient above 10 mm Hg is accepted as clinically relevant.

For deceased liver transplantation, HVOO due to stenosis at the caval anastomosis is the most common venous complication, and it is thought to occur more frequently when employing the piggy-back technique (i.e. preservation of the recipient vena cava and end-to-side cavo-cavostomy) as compared to the classical end-to-end cavo-cavostomy. Prevalence in various series ranges from 0.8–5.4% (Table 22.4). Technical problems, compression, inadequate graft size, kinking, malrotation or caval size mismatch account for the majority of the HVOO due to early stenosis, whereas thrombosis of the caval anastomosis or of the hepatic veins occurs mostly in the setting of recurrence of Budd-Chiari Syndrome [56]. Late stenosis can be caused by intimal hyperplasia and perivascular fibrosis and, in case of partial liver grafts, due to rapid growth leading to twisting. The classic presentation of HVOO consists of abdominal pain, new ascites, rapidly deteriorating liver function and hepatomegaly in case of suprahepatic caval stenosis and lower limb oedema and renal insufficiency in case of infrahepatic caval stenosis [16]. Graft congestion can lead to rapid graft loss and is associated with mortality as high as 17–24% if left untreated [59, 60].

Management is aimed at restoring the venous outflow. The first step is endovascular balloon angioplasty, preferably with prolonged inflation (1–2 minutes) of a high-pressure, oversized balloon to induce overstretching of the stenotic tissue and prevent immediate elastic recoil. When a thrombosis is present, endovascular thrombolysis has been recommended but this carries an inherent risk of bleeding, especially in the early post-transplant period, and hence should be reserved only in highly selected cases. Because of high risk of restenosis, the next step is often deployment of a vascular stent that bridges the stenosis. The choice of stent

**Table 22.4** Prevalence of venous complications in published case series

| Study (first author, year, [ref]) | Centre | Total number of transplants | Prevalence venous thrombosis (%) | Prevalence stenosis cavo-cavostomy (%) |
|---|---|---|---|---|
| Brouwers, 1994 [58] | Groningen, the Netherlands | 245 | – | 2.5 |
| Navarro, 1999 [59] | Nimes, France | 1361 | 0.07 | 1.5 |
| Cavallari, 2000[a] [21] | Bologna, Italy | 384 | 0.2 | 2.6 |
| Settmacher, 2000 [16] | Berlin, Germany | 911 | 0.6 | 1.1 |
| Akun, 2012 [60] | Istanbul, Turkey | 744 | 0.3 | 0.8 |
| Ferro, 2014 [61] | Genoa, Italy | 316 | – | 1.9 |
| Viteri-Ramirez, 2015 [62] | Pamplona, Spain | 295 | – | 5.4 |
| Chu, 2016 [63] | Seoul, South Korea | 449 | – | 1.1 |

– not reported

[a]included adult and paediatric transplantations

appears important also, as too small interstices (such as in Wall stents) may theoretically lead to occlusion of small venous branches in the area [61]. Stent migration, albeit rare, is a much-feared complication. With most types of stents however, excellent long-term patency has been shown in the vast majority of patients [62, 64].

After restoration of the venous outflow, clinical symptoms usually dissipate quite quickly. Failure to do so should raise suspicion for restenosis, in-stent thrombosis or graft dysfunction due to other causes. Rarely, the prolonged hepatic venous congestion causes irreversible damage and graft necrosis, necessitating retransplantation.

# References


1. Calne RY, Williams R. Liver transplantation in man. I. Observations on technique and organization in five cases. Br Med J. 1968;4(5630):535–40.
2. Jovine E, Mazziotti A, Grazi GL, Ercolani G, Masetti M, Morganti M, et al. Piggy-back versus conventional technique in liver transplantation: report of a randomized trial. Transpl Int. 1997;10(2):109–12.
3. Stahl RL, Duncan A, Hooks MA, Henderson JM, Millikan WJ, Warren WD. A hypercoagulable state follows orthotopic liver transplantation. Hepatology. 1990;12(3 Pt 1):553–8.
4. Ayala R, Martinez-Lopez J, Cedena T, Bustelos R, Jimenez C, Moreno E, et al. Recipient and donor thrombophilia and the risk of portal venous thrombosis and hepatic artery thrombosis in liver recipients. BMC Gastroenterol. 2011;11:130.
5. Yang Y, Zhao JC, Yan LN, Ma YK, Huang B, Yuan D, et al. Risk factors associated with early and late HAT after adult liver transplantation. World J Gastroenterol. 2014;20(30):10545–52.
6. Oh CK, Pelletier SJ, Sawyer RG, Dacus AR, McCullough CS, Pruett TL, et al. Uni- and multivariate analysis of risk factors for early and late hepatic artery thrombosis after liver transplantation. Transplantation. 2001;71(6):767–72.

 7. Stewart ZA, Locke JE, Segev DL, Dagher NN, Singer AL, Montgomery RA, et al. Increased risk of graft loss from hepatic artery thrombosis after liver transplantation with older donors. Liver Transpl. 2009;15(12):1688–95.
 8. Cescon M, Zanello M, Grazi GL, Cucchetti A, Ravaioli M, Ercolani G, et al. Impact of very advanced donor age on hepatic artery thrombosis after liver transplantation. Transplantation. 2011;92(4):439–45.
 9. Goel A, Mehta N, Guy J, Fidelman N, Yao F, Roberts J, et al. Hepatic artery and biliary complications in liver transplant recipients undergoing pretransplant transarterial chemoembolization. Liver Transpl. 2014;20(10):1221–8.
10. Pungpapong S, Manzarbeitia C, Ortiz J, Reich DJ, Araya V, Rothstein KD, et al. Cigarette smoking is associated with an increased incidence of vascular complications after liver transplantation. Liver Transpl. 2002;8(7):582–7.
11. Abbasoglu O, Levy MF, Vodapally MS, Goldstein RM, Husberg BS, Gonwa TA, et al. Hepatic artery stenosis after liver transplantation–incidence, presentation, treatment, and long term outcome. Transplantation. 1997;63(2):250–5.
12. Warner P, Fusai G, Glantzounis GK, Sabin CA, Rolando N, Patch D, et al. Risk factors associated with early hepatic artery thrombosis after orthotopic liver transplantation - univariable and multivariable analysis. Transpl Int. 2011;24(4):401–8.
13. Silva MA, Jambulingam PS, Gunson BK, Mayer D, Buckels JA, Mirza DF, et al. Hepatic artery thrombosis following orthotopic liver transplantation: a 10-year experience from a single centre in the United Kingdom. Liver Transpl. 2006;12(1):146–51.
14. Duffy JP, Hong JC, Farmer DG, Ghobrial RM, Yersiz H, Hiatt JR, et al. Vascular complications of orthotopic liver transplantation: experience in more than 4,200 patients. J Am Coll Surg. 2009;208(5):896–903. Discussion 903–5
15. Ishigami K, Zhang Y, Rayhill S, Katz D, Stolpen A. Does variant hepatic artery anatomy in a liver transplant recipient increase the risk of hepatic artery complications after transplantation? AJR Am J Roentgenol. 2004;183(6):1577–84.
16. Settmacher U, Nussler NC, Glanemann M, Haase R, Heise M, Bechstein WO, et al. Venous complications after orthotopic liver transplantation. Clin Transpl. 2000;14(3):235–41.
17. Kishi Y, Sugawara Y, Matsui Y, Akamatsu N, Makuuchi M. Late onset portal vein thrombosis and its risk factors. Hepato-Gastroenterology. 2008;55(84):1008–9.
18. Nikitin D, Jennings LW, Khan T, Vasani S, Ruiz R, Sanchez EQ, et al. Twenty years' follow-up of portal vein conduits in liver transplantation. Liver Transpl. 2009;15(4):400–6.
19. Girometti R, Como G, Bazzocchi M, Zuiani C. Post-operative imaging in liver transplantation: state-of-the-art and future perspectives. World J Gastroenterol. 2014;20(20):6180–200.
20. Brancatelli G, Katyal S, Federle MP, Fontes P. Three-dimensional multislice helical computed tomography with the volume rendering technique in the detection of vascular complications after liver transplantation. Transplantation. 2002;73(2):237–42.
21. Cavallari A, Vivarelli M, Bellusci R, Jovine E, Mazziotti A, Rossi C. Treatment of vascular complications following liver transplantation: multidisciplinary approach. Hepato-Gastroenterology. 2001;48(37):179–83.
22. Wozney P, Zajko AB, Bron KM, Point S, Starzl TE. Vascular complications after liver transplantation: a 5-year experience. AJR Am J Roentgenol. 1986;147(4):657–63.
23. Langnas AN, Marujo W, Stratta RJ, Wood RP, Shaw BW Jr. Vascular complications after orthotopic liver transplantation. Am J Surg. 1991;161(1):76–82. Discussion 82–3
24. Settmacher U, Stange B, Haase R, Heise M, Steinmuller T, Bechstein WO, et al. Arterial complications after liver transplantation. Transpl Int. 2000;13(5):372–8.
25. Marshall MM, Muiesan P, Srinivasan P, Kane PA, Rela M, Heaton ND, et al. Hepatic artery pseudoaneurysms following liver transplantation: incidence, presenting features and management. Clin Radiol. 2001;56(7):579–87.
26. Leelaudomlipi S, Bramhall SR, Gunson BK, Candinas D, Buckels JA, McMaster P, et al. Hepatic-artery aneurysm in adult liver transplantation. Transpl Int. 2003;16(4):257–61.
27. Stange BJ, Glanemann M, Nuessler NC, Settmacher U, Steinmuller T, Neuhaus P. Hepatic artery thrombosis after adult liver transplantation. Liver Transpl. 2003;9(6):612–20.

28. Gunsar F, Rolando N, Pastacaldi S, Patch D, Raimondo ML, Davidson B, et al. Late hepatic artery thrombosis after orthotopic liver transplantation. Liver Transpl. 2003;9(6):605–11.
29. Leonardi MI, Boin I, Leonardi LS. Late hepatic artery thrombosis after liver transplantation: clinical setting and risk factors. Transplant Proc. 2004;36(4):967–9.
30. Fistouris J, Herlenius G, Backman L, Olausson M, Rizell M, Mjornstedt L, et al. Pseudoaneurysm of the hepatic artery following liver transplantation. Transplant Proc. 2006;38(8):2679–82.
31. Horrow MM, Blumenthal BM, Reich DJ, Manzarbeitia C. Sonographic diagnosis and outcome of hepatic artery thrombosis after orthotopic liver transplantation in adults. AJR Am J Roentgenol. 2007;189(2):346–51.
32. Pareja E, Cortes M, Navarro R, Sanjuan F, Lopez R, Mir J. Vascular complications after orthotopic liver transplantation: hepatic artery thrombosis. Transplant Proc. 2010;42(8):2970–2.
33. Frongillo F, Grossi U, Lirosi MC, Nure E, Sganga G, Avolio AW, et al. Incidence, management, and results of hepatic artery stenosis after liver transplantation in the era of donor to recipient match. Transplant Proc. 2013;45(7):2722–5.
34. Volpin E, Pessaux P, Sauvanet A, Sibert A, Kianmanesh R, Durand F, et al. Preservation of the arterial vascularisation after hepatic artery pseudoaneurysm following orthotopic liver transplantation: long-term results. Ann Transplant. 2014;19:346–52.
35. Pulitano C, Joseph D, Sandroussi C, Verran D, Strasser SI, Shackel NA, et al. Hepatic artery stenosis after liver transplantation: is endovascular treatment always necessary? Liver Transpl. 2015;21(2):162–8.
36. Fujiki M, Hashimoto K, Palaios E, Quintini C, Aucejo FN, Uso TD, et al. Probability, management, and long-term outcomes of biliary complications after hepatic artery thrombosis in liver transplant recipients. Surgery. 2017;162(5):1101–11.
37. Bekker J, Ploem S, de Jong KP. Early hepatic artery thrombosis after liver transplantation: a systematic review of the incidence, outcome and risk factors. Am J Transplant. 2009;9(4):746–57.
38. Scarinci A, Sainz-Barriga M, Berrevoet F, van den Bossche B, Colle I, Geerts A, et al. Early arterial revascularization after hepatic artery thrombosis may avoid graft loss and improve outcomes in adult liver transplantation. Transplant Proc. 2010;42(10):4403–8.
39. Flint EW, Sumkin JH, Zajko AB, Bowen A. Duplex sonography of hepatic artery thrombosis after liver transplantation. AJR Am J Roentgenol. 1988;151(3):481–3.
40. Crossin JD, Muradali D, Wilson SR. US of liver transplants: normal and abnormal. Radiographics. 2003;23(5):1093–114.
41. Wolf DC, Freni MA, Boccagni P, Mor E, Chodoff L, Birnbaum A, et al. Low-dose aspirin therapy is associated with few side effects but does not prevent hepatic artery thrombosis in liver transplant recipients. Liver Transpl Surg. 1997;3(6):598–603.
42. Vivarelli M, La Barba G, Cucchetti A, Lauro A, Del Gaudio M, Ravaioli M, et al. Can antiplatelet prophylaxis reduce the incidence of hepatic artery thrombosis after liver transplantation? Liver Transpl. 2007;13(5):651–4.
43. Shay R, Taber D, Pilch N, Meadows H, Tischer S, McGillicuddy J, et al. Early aspirin therapy may reduce hepatic artery thrombosis in liver transplantation. Transplant Proc. 2013;45(1):330–4.
44. Muralidharan V, Imber C, Leelaudomlipi S, Gunson BK, Buckels JA, Mirza DF, et al. Arterial conduits for hepatic artery revascularisation in adult liver transplantation. Transpl Int. 2004;17(4):163–8.
45. Dodd GD 3rd, Memel DS, Zajko AB, Baron RL, Santaguida LA. Hepatic artery stenosis and thrombosis in transplant recipients: doppler diagnosis with resistive index and systolic acceleration time. Radiology. 1994;192(3):657–61.
46. Platt JF, Yutzy GG, Bude RO, Ellis JH, Rubin JM. Use of Doppler sonography for revealing hepatic artery stenosis in liver transplant recipients. AJR Am J Roentgenol. 1997;168(2):473–6.
47. Rostambeigi N, Hunter D, Duval S, Chinnakotla S, Golzarian J. Stent placement versus angioplasty for hepatic artery stenosis after liver transplant: a meta-analysis of case series. Eur Radiol. 2013;23(5):1323–34.
48. Dacha S, Barad A, Martin J, Levitsky J. Association of hepatic artery stenosis and biliary strictures in liver transplant recipients. Liver Transpl. 2011;17(7):849–54.

49. Harrison J, Harrison M, Doria C. Hepatic artery pseudoaneurysm following orthotopic liver transplantation: increasing clinical suspicion for a rare but lethal pathology. Ann Transplant. 2017;22:417–24.
50. Worthy SA, Olliff JF, Olliff SP, Buckels JA. Color flow Doppler ultrasound diagnosis of a pseudoaneurysm of the hepatic artery following liver transplantation. J Clin Ultrasound. 1994;22(7):461–5.
51. Jeng KS, Huang CC, Lin CK, Lin CC, Liang CC, Chung CS, et al. Early detection of a hepatic artery pseudoaneurysm after liver transplantation is the determinant of survival. Transplant Proc. 2016;48(4):1149–55.
52. Mullan CP, Siewert B, Kane RA, Sheiman RG. Can Doppler sonography discern between hemodynamically significant and insignificant portal vein stenosis after adult liver transplantation? AJR Am J Roentgenol. 2010;195(6):1438–43.
53. Farid WR, de Jonge J, Slieker JC, Zondervan PE, Thomeer MG, Metselaar HJ, et al. The importance of portal venous blood flow in ischemic-type biliary lesions after liver transplantation. Am J Transplant. 2011;11(4):857–62.
54. Hamady M, Rela M, Sidhu PS. Spontaneous resolution of a portal vein stenosis over a 21-month period in a "split-liver" transplant: demonstration by colour Doppler ultrasound, catheter angiography and splenic pulp pressures. Eur Radiol. 2002;12(9):2280–3.
55. Ko EY, Kim TK, Kim PN, Kim AY, Ha HK, Lee MG. Hepatic vein stenosis after living donor liver transplantation: evaluation with Doppler US. Radiology. 2003;229(3):806–10.
56. Darcy MD. Management of venous outflow complications after liver transplantation. Tech Vasc Interv Radiol. 2007;10(3):240–5.
57. Rossi AR, Pozniak MA, Zarvan NP. Upper inferior vena caval anastomotic stenosis in liver transplant recipients: doppler US diagnosis. Radiology. 1993;187(2):387–9.
58. Brouwers MA, de Jong KP, Peeters PM, Bijleveld CM, Klompmaker IJ, Slooff MJ. Inferior vena cava obstruction after orthotopic liver transplantation. Clin Transpl. 1994;8(1):19–22.
59. Navarro F, Le Moine MC, Fabre JM, Belghiti J, Cherqui D, Adam R, et al. Specific vascular complications of orthotopic liver transplantation with preservation of the retrohepatic vena cava: review of 1361 cases. Transplantation. 1999;68(5):646–50.
60. Akun E, Yaprak O, Killi R, Balci NC, Tokat Y, Yuzer Y. Vascular complications in hepatic transplantation: single-center experience in 14 years. Transplant Proc. 2012;44(5):1368–72.
61. Ferro C, Andorno E, Guastavino A, Rossi UG, Seitun S, Bovio G, et al. Endovascular treatment with primary stenting of inferior cava vein torsion following orthotopic liver transplantation with modified piggyback technique. Radiol Med. 2014;119(3):183–8.
62. Viteri-Ramirez G, Alonso-Burgos A, Simon-Yarza I, Rotellar F, Herrero JI, Bilbao JI. Hepatic venous outflow obstruction after transplantation: outcomes for treatment with self-expanding stents. Radiologia. 2015;57(1):56–65.
63. Chu HH, Yi NJ, Kim HC, Lee KW, Suh KS, Jae HJ, et al. Longterm outcomes of stent placement for hepatic venous outflow obstruction in adult liver transplantation recipients. Liver Transpl. 2016;22(11):1554–61.
64. Lee JM, Ko GY, Sung KB, Gwon DI, Yoon HK, Lee SG. Long-term efficacy of stent placement for treating inferior vena cava stenosis following liver transplantation. Liver Transpl. 2010;16(4):513–9.

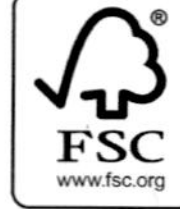